# THE MESOCORTICOLIMBIC DOPAMINE SYSTEM

ANNALS OF THE NEW YORK ACADEMY OF SCIENCES
Volume 537

# THE MESOCORTICOLIMBIC DOPAMINE SYSTEM

Edited by Peter W. Kalivas and Charles B. Nemeroff

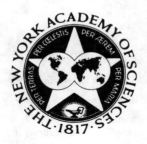

The New York Academy of Sciences
New York, New York
1988

*The illustration on the cover of the soft-bound edition of this volume is an artist's rendering of a three-dimensional reconstruction from serial sections of the ventral tegmental area (green) lying medial to the substantia nigra pars compacta (white), which is above the substantia nigra pars reticulata (orange). (Reconstruction by Valerie Domesick.)*

**Library of Congress Cataloging-in-Publication Data**

The Mesocorticolimbic dopamine system.

(Annals of the New York Academy of Sciences, ISSN 0077-8923; v. 537)

Based on a conference held by the New York Academy of Sciences in Miami, Florida on May 4–6, 1987.

Includes bibliographies and index.

1. Limbic system — Congresses. 2. Dopaminergic mechanisms — Congresses. 3. Neuropsychiatry — Congresses. 4. Schizophrenia — Pathophysiology — Congresses. I. Kalivas, Peter W., 1952– . II. Nemeroff, Charles B. III. New York Academy of Sciences. IV. Series. [DNLM: 1. Behavior — drug effects — Congresses. 2. Dopamine — physiology — Congresses. 3. Limbic System — physiology — Congresses. 4. Mental Disorders — physiopathology — Congresses. 5. Mesencephalon — physiology — Congresses. W1 AN626YL v.537 / WK 725 M582 1987]

Q11.N5 vol. 537          500 s          88-25476
[QP383.2]          [599'.0188]
ISBN 0-89766-470-1
ISBN 0-89766-471-X (pbk.)

CCP
*Printed in the United States of America*
**ISBN 0-89766-470-1 (Cloth)**
**ISBN 0-89766-471-X (Paper)**
**ISSN 0077-8923**

ANNALS OF THE NEW YORK ACADEMY OF SCIENCES

*Volume 537*
*October 15, 1988*

# THE MESOCORTICOLIMBIC
# DOPAMINE SYSTEM[a]

*Editors and Conference Organizers*
PETER W. KALIVAS and CHARLES B. NEMEROFF

## CONTENTS

[a] This volume is the result of a conference entitled The Mesocorticolimbic Dopamine System
held by the New York Academy of Sciences in Miami, Florida on May 4–6, 1987.

### Part III. Behavioral Properties

### Part IV. Clinical Medicine (I)

**Major funding was provided by:**

- NATIONAL INSTITUTE OF MENTAL HEALTH/NIH
- NATIONAL INSTITUTE OF DRUG ABUSE/NIH

**Additional financial assistance was received from:**

- ABBOTT LABORATORIES
- ASTRA ALAB AB
- AYERST LABORATORIES
- BERLEX LABORATORIES INC.
- BRISTOL-MEYERS COMPANY
- ELI LILLY AND COMPANY
- HOECHST-ROUSSEL
- HOFFMANN-LAROCHE INC.
- LOREX INC.
- McNEIL PHARMACEUTICAL
- MERCK SHARP AND DOHME RESEARCH LABORATORIES
- MILES LABORATORIES, INC./BAYER AG
- NATIONAL SCIENCE FOUNDATION
- OFFICE OF NAVAL RESEARCH, DEPARTMENT OF THE NAVY
- PFIZER CENTRAL RESEARCH
- SEARLE RESEARCH AND DEVELOPMENT
- SCHERING CORPORATION
- THE COCA-COLA COMPANY
- THE UPJOHN COMPANY

# Preface

PETER W. KALIVAS

*Department of Veterinary and Comparative
Anatomy, Pharmacology, and Physiology
College of Veterinary Medicine
Washington State University
Pullman, Washington 99164-6520*


CHARLES B. NEMEROFF

*Departments of Psychiatry and Pharmacology
Duke University Medical Center
Durham, North Carolina 27706*

The mesocorticolimbic dopamine system arises from perikarya in the ventromedial mesencephalon and innervates a number of cortical and limbic regions. It has become clear that this system is in many ways qualitatively distinct from the better-characterized nigrostriatal dopamine system. This is especially true of its postulated physiological functions and role in the pathophysiology of certain neuropsychiatric disorders. The proceedings contained in this volume address the role of the mesocorticolimbic dopamine system in mammalian behavior and neuropsychiatric disorders. To this end, the conference from which this volume is derived was organized into preclinical and clinical sections, with the express goal of promoting communication between these two groups of investigators.

We were fortunate in assembling many leading clinical and preclinical investigators to address the anatomical, cellular and functional properties of the mesocorticolimbic dopamine system. We wish to especially acknowledge the participation of Jacques Glowinski, Michel Le Moal, and Robert Roth, whose work was seminal in the evolution of our appreciation of the mesocorticolimbic dopamine system as a functionally distinct entity from the nigrostriatal system. The first two parts of this book are concerned with forming a framework of basic information regarding anatomy, electrophysiology, and neurochemistry. Thus, issues of co-localization of dopamine with other putative neurotransmitters are discussed, as is a role of the A8 dopamine cell group in innervating limbic and cortical regions of the brain. Intracellular and extracellular electrophysiological properties of dopamine neurons and their target cells are described. The neurochemical properties of the dopamine neurons are discussed in terms of anatomical heterogeneity and in response to environmental and pharmacological perturbation. The next preclinical part discusses some of the behavioral properties of the system and places a special emphasis on relationships to postulated clinically relevant functions. Thus, papers are included that describe a putative role in reward processes and drug addiction, and in sensitization to psychostimulant drugs. The final preclinical part of the volume is devoted to interactions between mesocorticolimbic dopamine and other neurotransmitters. Particular attention is given to those transmitters that are co-localized with dopamine, including cholecystokinin and neurotensin. Electrophysiological, neurochemical and behavioral evidence are presented to support an interaction between dopamine and these neuropeptides.

The first clinical part of this volume focuses on the "dopamine hypothesis of schizophrenia." This includes evaluation of the psychostimulant model of schizophrenia and discussion of a role for sensitization processes in the nervous system. In addition cerebrospinal fluid and plasma measures of dopamine metabolites and neuropeptides are suggested as potential indices of psychosis. Data are also presented supporting the novel possibility that schizophrenia may result from a deficit of dopaminergic transmission in the prefrontal cortex. The second clinical part focuses on the use of dopamine receptor antagonists in the treatment of neuropsychiatric disorders, and there is a discussion of the susceptibility of dopamine neurons to destruction by MPTP and a role for the mesocorticolimbic system in nonpsychotic disorders.

We gratefully acknowledge the invaluable assistance and organizational efforts provided by the New York Academy of Sciences. Special thanks are extended to the Conference Department in the persons of Ellen Marks and Cindy Wishengrad, whose continuous efforts and efficiency were invaluable. We acknowledge the punctilious editorial work done by Trumbull Rogers and his colleagues in the Editorial Department. And we would like to thank the session chairs, who often sparked lively discussion and were remarkably efficient at maintaining a smooth and stimulating exchange of ideas. Finally, we extend our appreciation to the financial sponsors of this conference, especially the National Institute of Drug Abuse and the National Institute of Mental Health.

# Topographic Organization of Ascending Dopaminergic Projections[a]

JAMES H. FALLON

*Department of Anatomy and Neurobiology*
*College of Medicine*
*University of California at Irvine*
*Irvine, California 92717*

## DEVELOPMENT OF CONCEPTS

Our understanding of the topographic organization of ascending dopaminergic projections from the midbrain has changed during the past quarter century. The years from 1964 to 1978[1-5] were dominated by the concept that dopamine (DA) neurons of the substantia nigra pars compacta (SN), also known as the A9 group, project to the striatum, forming the nigrostriatal pathway. The DA neurons of the ventral tegmental area (VTA) were thought to give rise to the mesolimbic and mesocortical pathways. Thus, the nigrostriatal and mesocorticolimbic systems could be separated on the basis of the lateral–medial (A9–A10) position of the parent DA neurons in the midbrain.

In 1978, it was shown that there is another level of complexity in the topography of ascending DA projections.[6,7] Using combined histochemical, biochemical, anterograde autoradiographic tracing, and HRP retrograde tracing techniques, we observed that the A9 and A10 neurons formed a continuum, with both groups contributing to the nigrostriatal and mesocorticolimbic systems. The topography of the projections were organized in three planes, including a medial–lateral organization, a crude anterior–posterior organization, and a reversed dorsal–ventral organization. It appeared that it was the dorsal–ventral plane that segregated the nigrostriatal and mesocorticolimbic projections. The ventral sheet of A9 and A10 neurons project to the striatum and the dorsal A9 and A10 neurons give rise to the mesocorticolimbic and, to a lesser extent, the nigrostriatal pathways[6,7] (the A8 projections are dealt with by A. Deutch in this volume). Because of the dual contribution of the A9 and A10 neurons to both the nigrostriatal and mesocorticolimbic projections, the ascending midbrain DA projections to the forebrain were renamed the mesotelencephalic system, with the subsystems named the mesostriatal and mesocorticolimbic (or mesolimbocortical) systems (for a review, see reference 8).

New levels of complexity in these DA systems have recently been presented. It is becoming apparent that "limbic" structures such as the nucleus accumbens, amygdala, and olfactory tubercle have "striatal" components and that "striatal" structures such as the caudate–putamen have limbic components (for a review, see reference 9). For example, the caudate–putamen can be subdivided into "patch" and "matrix" compartments, with the patch compartment receiving a prelimbic cortical input and the matrix compartment receiving a neocortical input. The DA input to the patch compart-

[a] This work was supported in part by NIH Grant NS 15321 and in part by a grant from the United Parkinson Foundation.

ment may arise from ventral A9 neurons, and the DA input to the matrix compartment may arise from intermediate (in a dorsal–ventral sense) A9 neurons.[10] Thus, when talking about the mesostriatal and mesocorticolimbic systems, we should consider the dual nature of both the DA cells of origin and the heterogeneity of forebrain targets as well. With this brief history in mind, we may now turn to some of the details of the topography of ascending DA systems.

## TOPOGRAPHY OF ASCENDING DOPAMINERGIC PROJECTIONS

The DA projections are predominantly ipsilateral, with a small contralateral (but not bilateral) component ranging from 1% to 5% of the ipsilateral component.[11] The overall projections to each forebrain structure arise from a circumscribed region of the SN-VTA (FIG. 1). The projections to the caudate–putamen (CPu) arise predominantly from the ventral and intermediate sheets of DA neurons in the SN and VTA (FIG. 1). The projections to the lateral septum (LS) arise from the ventral (paranigralis subnucleus) VTA. The nucleus accumbens (Acb) receives input from the dorsal (parabrachialis pigmentosus subnucleus) VTA and medial SN. The olfactory tubercle (Tu) receives input from the dorsal VTA and dorsal sheet of the medial SN. The amygdala (Amyg) and bed nucleus of the stria terminalis input arises from a broad area of the dorsal sheet of the SN-VTA, and most notably from the SN pars lateralis and dorsal VTA. The cor-

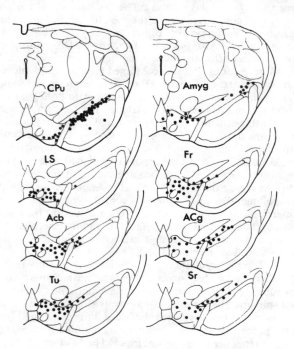

**FIGURE 1.** Location of DA neurons at a midrostral level of the SN-VTA projecting to caudate–putamen (CPu), lateral septum (LS), nucleus accumbens (Acb), olfactory tubercle (Tu), amygdala (Amyg), prefrontal cortex (Fr), anterior cingulate cortex (ACg), and suprahinal cortex (Sr).

tical regions receive input from the dorsal sheet of the SN–VTA, with the prefrontal (Fr) input arising from the VTA and medial-most SN, the anterior cingulate (ACg) input arising from the VTA and a broad region of the dorsal SN, and the suprarhinal (Sr) input arising from the entire width of the dorsal SN–VTA complex. Not shown in FIGURE 1 are the dorsal SN–VTA and A8 projections to the piriform cortex; entorhinal cortex and the minor VTA projections to the hippocampal formation and neocortices.

As introduced in the first section, DA neurons project to the forebrain in a topographical manner.[6] This topography is not as strict as found in the ascending sensory systems, but certain patterns are obvious. In general, medially situated DA neurons in the SN–VTA project to the medial (and somewhat anterior) sectors of forebrain structures, and laterally situated DA neurons project to the lateral (and somewhat posterior) sectors of the same forebrain structures. There is some overlap but little collateralization, of the DA projections to the medial and lateral sectors of a forebrain region such as the caudate–putamen.[12]

There is a slight anterior–posterior topography in the DA projections with anteriorally placed DA neurons projecting to anterior sectors of the forebrain region and posteriorally placed DA neurons projecting to posterior sectors. This crude topography may parallel and reflect the broad anterior–posterior trajectory of other forebrain inputs; for example, the corticostriatal projections are known to extend throughout extensive anterior–posterior domains of the caudate–putamen.

The dorsal–ventral topography of the DA projections provide an interesting separation of the mesostriatal and mesocorticolimbic projection systems. Ventrally situated SN–VTA neurons project to more dorsal subcortical areas such as the caudate–putamen and septum (FIG. 2). When a retrograde tracer such as HRP is injected into the caudate–putamen, the ventral sheet of DA neurons in the SN (which send their dendrites into the substantia nigra pars reticulata in dendritic bundles – see b in lower photograph of FIG. 3) are retrogradely labeled. Several more dorsally situated neurons are also retrogradely labeled. When a retrograde tracer is injected into cortical or ventral subcortical structures such as the amygdala, the dorsal sheet neurons are preferentially labeled. Many of these dorsal DA neurons have a fusiform shape with dendrites extending mediolaterally into the pars compacta of the SN (upper photograph in FIG. 3).

This dorsal–ventral "switch" has important implications for the circuitry of mesotelencephalic and telomesencephalic loops and the integration of topographical and nontopographical motor and limbic systems.[9,10]

## AXON COLLATERALIZATION PATTERNS

Although a given zone of the SN–VTA projects topographically to a particular forebrain site, it is apparant (FIG. 1) that there is overlap of the origins of these projections to multiple forebrain regions. The area of overlap is greatest in the intermediate sheet of the medial SN and lateral VTA. The locations of the dorsal (d), intermediate (I), and ventral (V) sheets are illustrated in FIGURE 4. In order to determine whether individual SN–VTA neurons project to multiple forebrain sites, different retrograde tracers (Fluoro-Gold, Fast Blue, True Blue, Propidium Iodide, Nuclear Yellow) were injected into various forebrain sites[13,14] (FIG. 5). Following these injections, numerous double- and a few triple-labeled neurons could be found in the intermediate sheet of medial SN and extreme lateral VTA (dense stippling in FIG. 6), especially in the regions bordering the medial terminal nucleus (mtn) of the accessory optic tract. Adjacent regions

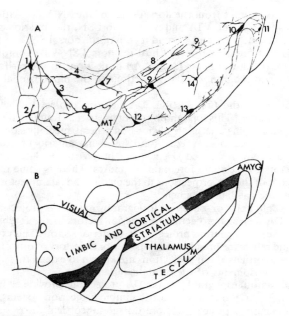

**FIGURE 2.** (A) Representation of the shapes of neurons (from Golgi reconstructions) found in different regions of the SN–VTA. Their shape, position, and neurotransmitter content and projections are described in detail elsewhere (see reference 9). (B) Drawing of the same level of SN–VTA shown in part A and depicting the forebrain and brainstem targets of SN–VTA neurons. Note the layered projection scheme, with SN pars reticulata projections to thalamus and tectum, the SN pars compacta projections from the ventral sheet to striatum, and the dorsal sheet projections to limbic and cortical structures.

of the medial SN contained fewer double-labeled neurons (moderate-density stippling in FIG. 6). Other regions of the SN–VTA rarely contained double-labeled neurons. Therefore, some medial SN and lateral VTA neurons have highly collateralized axons that could influence the function of widely separated forebrain regions (medial caudate–putamen, nucleus accumbens, septum, olfactory tubercle, prefrontal cortex, anterior cingulate cortex) simultaneously.

## NEUROCHEMICAL CORRELATES

Traditionally, the SN–VTA are considered to provide DA input to diverse forebrain structures. Recent evidence has pointed out the neurochemical heterogeneity of SN–VTA neurons in that subpopulations of DA neurons are known to contain cholecystokinin (CCK)[15,17] and/or neurotensin (NT).[18] We have recently examined some of the forebrain projections of SN–VTA neurons that co-localize DA and CCK[16,17] and CCK and NT.[19] These results can be summarized as follows: CCK is extensively co-localized with DA in the SN–VTA. There is a greater percentage of CCK-containing neurons in the

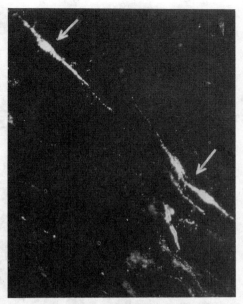

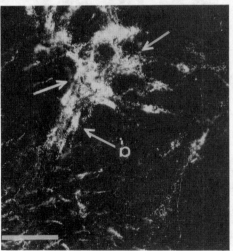

**FIGURE 3.** Photomicrographs of retrograde labeling of SN neurons with HRP (DAB technique) following injections of HRP into the amygdala (*top*) or caudate–putamen (*bottom*).[6] Note that the mesolimbic projections arise primarily from dorsal sheet neurons with a fusiform shape (*arrows at top*), whereas the mesostriatal projection arises from ventral sheet neurons (*arrows*) with dendritic bundles (b) extending ventrolaterally into the SN pars reticulata (*bottom*).

rostal half of the SN–VTA complex. The VTA, dorsal, and intermediate sheets of the SN and lateral SN contain the greatest percentage of co-localized CCK and DA. Ninety-six percent of the NT-containing neurons throughout the SN–VTA also contain CCK, although only 10–15% of CCK-containing neurons contain NT. Thus, CCK-containing neurons far outnumber NT-containing neurons. The NT/CCK neurons are localized

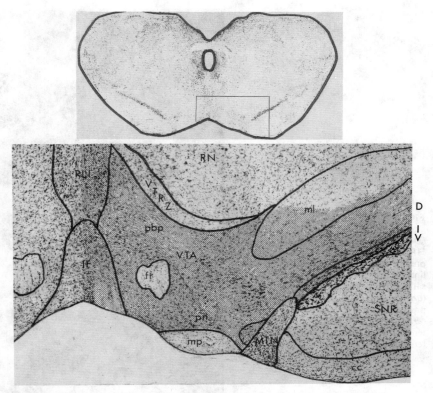

**FIGURE 4.** Photomicrograph of the SN–VTA at a midrostral level (*top*) and a higher magnification of the boxed-in area at top shown at the *bottom*. Note in particular the dorsal (D), intermediate (I), and ventral (V) sheets of SN neurons.

primarily in the dorsal and lateral VTA rostrally, and interspersed among the nerve III rootlets and paranigralis subnucleus of the VTA more caudally. The NT/CCK neurons are also present in the medial SN, with fewer present in the middle and lateral SN. The NT neurons that do not also contain CCK are located above the SN pars lateralis. In summary, NT-containing neurons form a small subset of CCK-containing neurons in the SN–VTA. Since they are extensively co-localized and since the majority of CCK-containing neurons also contain DA, it can be proposed that a heterogeneous population of DA, DA/CCK, and DA/CCK/NT neurons are present in the SN–VTA.

We have used combined immunofluorescence and fluorescent retrograde tracing techniques to demonstrate the connections of DA/CCK-[16,17] and CCK/NT-containing[19] neurons in the SN–VTA. It was found that the projections of the DA/CCK neurons to prefrontal cortex, nucleus accumbens, or amygdala were very similar, and virtually indistinguishable, from the DA projections previously discussed. Thus, the topography of their projections can be predicted on the basis of their position in the SN–VTA. An unresolved issue still exists for the DA/CCK projections to caudate–putamen. Fol-

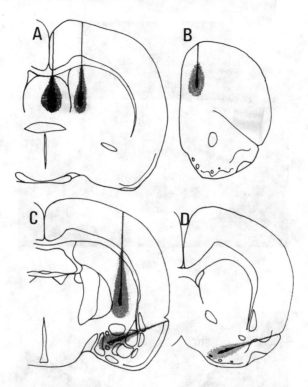

**FIGURE 5.** Location of injection sites of three different retrograde tracers in two rats (**A,B**—one animal; **C,D**—second animal) to determine the axon collateralization patterns of SN–VTA neurons (see FIG. 6).

lowing the retrograde fluorescence injections into the caudate–putamen combined with CCK immunofluorescence processing, it has been shown that CCK-containing neurons project to the caudate–putamen, especially to the rostral, medial, and ventral sectors.[16,17] In view of the predominance of CCK in neurons of the dorsal and intermediate sheets of SN neurons (especially rostrally), it could be predicted that the CCK innervation from the SN is primarily to the matrix compartment of the caudate–putamen. This issue is still unresolved.

The NT/CCK-containing neurons have a more restricted projection to the forebrain. These neurons have been shown to topographically innervate nucleus accumbens, prefrontal cortex, and amygdala, but not the caudate–putamen.

## CONCLUSIONS

It can be concluded that the SN–VTA projects topographically to the forebrain in three planes. Some neurons in the medial SN and lateral VTA provide highly collateralized

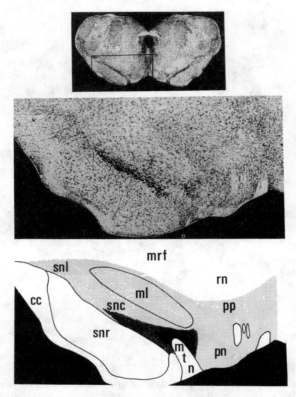

**FIGURE 6.** Representation of the locations of highly collateralized (*dense stippling at bottom*), moderately collateralized (*medium stippling*), and poorly collateralized (*light stippling*) neurons in the SN–VTA.

projections to cortical, limbic, and striatal targets. The SN–VTA is further composed of unique subpopulations of DA, DA/CCK, NT/CCK, and DA/CCK/NT neurons whose neurochemical characteristics are unique, but whose projections follow the basic topographical patterns of projections.

## REFERENCES

1. DAHLSTROM, A. & K. FUXE. 1964. Acta Physiol. Scand. **62** (Suppl. 232): 1–55.
2. UNGERSTEDT, U. Acta Physiol. Scand. Suppl. **367**: 1–49.
3. BERGER, B., J. P. TASSIN, G. BLANC, M. MOYNE & A. M. THIERRY. 1974. Brain Res. **81**: 332–337.
4. HÖKFELT, T., K. FUXE, O. JOHANSSON & A. LJUNGDAHL. 1974. Am. J. Pharmacol. **25**: 108–112.
5. LINDVALL, O., A. BJÖRKLUND, R.Y. MOORE & U. STENEVI. 1974. Brain Res. **81**: 325–331.
6. FALLON, J. H. & R. Y. MOORE. 1978. J. Comp. Neurol. **180**: 545–580.
7. FALLON, J. H., J. RILEY & R.Y. MOORE. 1978. Neurosci. Lett. **7**: 157–162.

8. LINDVALL, O. & A. BJÖRKLUND. 1984. Monoamine Innervation of Cerebral Cortex. 9–40. Alan Liss. New York.
9. FALLON, J. H. & S. E. LOUGHLIN. 1987. Cerebral Cortex, Vol. 6. Plenum. New York. In press.
10. GERFEN, C .R., M. HERKENHAM & J. THIBAULT. 1987. J. Neurosci. In press.
11. LOUGHLIN, S. E. & J. H. FALLON. 1982. Neurosci. Lett. **32:** 11–16.
12. VAN DER KOOY, D. 1979. Brain Res. **169:** 381–387.
13. FALLON, J. H. 1981. J. Neurosci. **1:** 1361–1368.
14. FALLON, J. H. & S. E. LOUGHLIN. 1982. Brain Res. Bull. **9:** 295–307.
15. HÖKFELT, T., C. SKIRBOLL, J. REHFELD, M. GOLDSTEIN, K. MARKEY & O. DANN. 1980. Neurosci. **5:** 2093–2124.
16. FALLON, J. H., R. HICKS & S. E. LOUGHLIN. 1983. Neurosci. Lett. **37:** 29–35.
17. FALLON, J. H. & K. B. SEROOGY. 1985. Ann. N.Y. Acad. Sci. **448:** 596–597.
18. KALIVAS, P. W. 1984. J. Comp. Neurol. **226:** 495–507.
19. SEROOGY, K. B., A. MEHTA & J. H. FALLON. 1987. Exp. Brain Res. **68:** 277–289.

# Neuroanatomical Organization of Dopamine Neurons in the Ventral Tegmental Area[a]

VALERIE B. DOMESICK

*Mailman Research Center*
*McLean Hospital*
*Belmont, Massachusetts 02178*

*Harvard Medical School*
*Boston, Massachusetts 02115*

## INTRODUCTION

This review will summarize work from our laboratory on several aspects of the neuroanatomical organization of the ventral tegmental area (VTA), namely, shape and volume, the cytology of dopaminergic and nondopaminergic cells,[1] afferent,[2-4] and efferent connections,[5] and conduction lines through the ventral pallidum, thalamus and cortex.[6,7] It is based on evidence from experiments using a variety of techniques such as computer-aided three-dimensional reconstruction, histology, electron microscopy, and anterograde and retrograde neuronal tracing. Three main points will be emphasized: (1) The dopamine cells of the ventral tegmental area lie in a continuum with those of the pars compacta of the substantia nigra. (2) The VTA projects to the nucleus accumbens, and also projects to a region of the striatum considerably larger than usually recognized, namely to a ventromedial sector of the striatum which extends dorsalward from the nucleus accumbens. This region of the striatum is closely associated with the "limbic" system by the number of afferent projections it receives from the amygdala, medial frontal and cingulate cortex, the thalamus, the VTA, and the raphe nuclei. This "limbic" striatum projects to the ventral pallidum, which in turn projects to these same areas, namely the amygdala, medial frontal and cingulate cortex, the mediodorsal thalamic nucleus, the VTA, and the raphe nuclei. (3) The VTA has multiple projections to these structures of the limbic system by direct projections and by conduction lines through the ventral pallidum and the thalamus.

[a] Support for the research reported in this paper was received from NIMH Grants MH31154 and MH43018.

ABBREVIATIONS: a, nucleus accumbens; aa, nucleus anterior amygdalae; ac, nucleus centralis amygdalae; aco, nucleus corticalis amygdalae; alp, nucleus lateralis posterior amygdalae; am, nucleus medialis amygdalae; avt, ventral tegmental area; bs, bed nucleus of stria terminalis; cg, substantia grisea centralis; cl, nucleus centralis lateralis; cm, nucleus centralis medius; cp, caudatoputamen; db, nucleus of the diagonal band; dt, dorsal tegmental nucleus; ea, entorhinal area; FR, fasciculus retroflexus; gp, globus pallidus; hl, lateral hypothalamic region; hm, medial hypothalamic region; ip or IP, interpeduncular nucleus; lc, locus coeruleus; ld, laterodorsal nucleus; lh, lateral habenular nucleus; mc, mammillary body; md, mediodorsal nucleus; ML, medial lemniscus; MP, mammillary peduncle; mr, medial raphe nucleus; ntdl, nucleus tegmenti dorsalis lateralis.

## MATERIALS AND METHODS

The subjects in all our studies were adult albino rats (Charles River Laboratories). The animals were anesthetized with Chloropent (1.0 ml/300 g body weight) for all surgical and intracardial perfusion techniques.

The computer-aided three-dimensional constructions were prepared from a set of serial sections stained with cresylecht violet. Outlines of the entire section with interior outlines of the striatum, ventral tegmental area and substantia nigra were entered into the computer and converted electronically to digital form for management by programs that permit acquisition and storage of manually traced and aligned outlines as a series of three-dimensional coordinates. In order to facilitate the visualization of a three-dimensional reconstruction in color, we are using software for three-dimensional data entry and reconstruction provided by Dr. John Kinnamon (University of Colorado), running on a PC Limited (IBM PC-AT-compatible) with a Vega EGA, interfaced to a Summagraphics Summasketch digitizing tablet and a NEC Multisync high-resolution monitor.

Using this system, areas of interest can be digitized one plane at a time, then graphically reconstructed as a three-dimensional object, and rotated to an optimum viewing angle. This creates a database to be used for quantitative analysis of size and volumes as well as three-dimensional views of the structures of interest.

Semi-thin sections and ultrathin sections of the VTA were prepared from tissues fixed by a two-stage perfusion technique (1% formaldehyde, 1.25% glutaraldehyde in 0.1M cacodylate buffer, pH 7.4, followed by concentrated solution containing four times the amounts of aldehydes). The tissue was embedded in Spurr's epoxy resin and cut on a Sorvall Porter Blume MT-2 ultramicrotome. Semi-thin (1 micron) sections were stained with Toluidine blue for examination in a Zeiss Universal microscope. Ultrathin sections were contrasted with lead citrate and examined in a Siemens Elmiskop 1 electron microscope.

The projections of the ventral tegmental area were traced anterogradely by autoradiography or retrogradely by horseradish peroxidase (HRP) histochemistry (see refs. 3, 5 for details).

Rats received a single small injection of [³H] proline and [³H] leucine (New England Nuclear) or HRP in the ventral tegmental area, delivered by microelectrophoresis from a stereotaxically inserted glass micropipette; the driving force was supplied by passing a cathodal, direct current of 0.5–1.5 micro-amps in 7.5-Hz square-wave pulses, between the pipette solution and a ground wire attached to exposed periosteum.

After survival times ranging from 5 to 10 days, the rats were perfused with 10% formol-saline. The brains were immediately dissected out and prepared for autoradiography or HRP histochemistry.

## RESULTS

### *Computer-Aided Three-Dimensional Reconstruction*

As first demonstrated by the now classic histofluorescent methods,[8,9] the majority of mesencephalic dopaminergic cells are located in the pars compacta of the substantia nigra (SNc), cell group A9 of Dahlstrom and Fuxe;[8] in the medially adjacent ventral tegmental area of Tsai,[10,11] cell group A10; and most caudolaterally in cell group A8. Visualized by histofluorescence[8,9,12] and more recently by immunocytochemistry,[13,14] the dopamine cells of these three groups can be seen to form a continuum. As shown

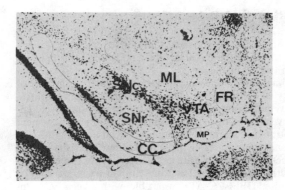

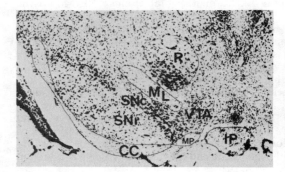

**FIGURE 1.** A Nissl-stained (cresylecht violet) series of coronal sections through the anterior, middle, and posterior VTA of the rat midbrain. Note the relationships between the ventral tegmental areas (VTA) and the substantia nigra pars compacta (SNc) and substantia nigra pars reticulata (SNr).

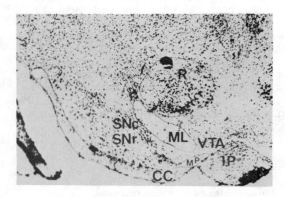

by Hanaway,[15] this continuum is clearly seen in the cytoarchitectonics of the VTA as illustrated by a set of coronal sections stained for in Nissl (FIG. 1). Anteriorly, cells of the VTA form a wedge-shaped group which appears as a dorsomedial extrusion from the medial pars compacta of the substantia nigra (SNc), which is a narrow dorsal stratum of densely packed cells overlying the larger ventral sector of the substantia nigra, the pars reticulata (SNr), lying in the curve formed by the crus cerebri (CC).

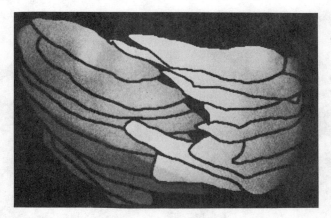

**FIGURE 2.** A three-dimensional reconstruction from outlines of the ventral tegmental area (*right*) lying dorsal to the substantia nigra pars compacta and pars reticulata (*left*) taken from serial coronal sections.

Further caudally the medial lemniscus lies between the VTA and SNc. At posterior levels (not shown) the cells of the VTA merge with those of the retrorubral nucleus, which in turn merge with cell group A8.

The boundaries of the VTA and substantia nigra (SNc and SNr) were outlined on another set of serial, coronal Nissl pictures. Using these outlines, a computer-aided three-dimensional reconstruction of the VTA and substantia nigra were made (FIG. 2). The volumes of the VTA, SNc, and SNr are given in TABLE 1. These agree with those reported by Halliday.[16]

## Cytology

Although electrophysiological experiments[17,18] demonstrated a difference in the electrophysiological properties of dopaminergic and nondopaminergic cells, there was considerable disagreement as to the existence of corresponding cytological differences.[1]

Inspection at higher magnification, in Nissl preparations, of the cells in the ventral tegmental area and substantia nigra reveals two classes of cells. In a series of experiments,[1] we showed that: (1) a dark-staining, basophilic cell corresponded to the dopaminergic cell, while (2) a light-staining cell corresponded to the nondopaminergic cell. Both types are found in the VTA, where they are intermingled rather than grouped in separate strata as they are in the substantia nigra. The morphological distinction between these two cell types is shown in photomicrographs (FIG. 3) of cells from a semi-thin (1μ) plastic section taken from a long series of 25 serial sections stained with

**TABLE 1.** Volumes of the Nigral Complex

| Area | Volume (mm³) |
|------|--------------|
| Ventral tegmental area (A10) | 1.2748 |
| Substantia nigra, pars compacta (A9) | 0.4024 |
| Substantia nigra, pars reticulata | 2.126 |
| Total Region | 3.8032 |

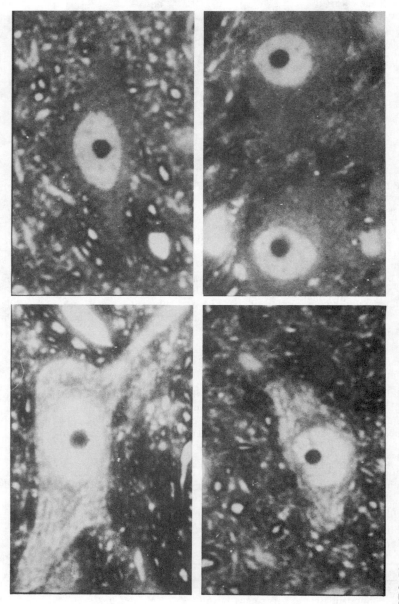

**FIGURE 3.** Photomicrographs contrast the darker-staining, basophilic dopaminergic cells (*right*) with the lighter-staining nondopaminergic cells (*left*). Toluidine blue stain, 1-µm section.

a basic stain, toluidine blue. The characteristically basophilic appearance of the dark-staining cells is due to massive aggregations of Nissl substance, which almost completely fill the cytoplasm.

In contrast, the cytoplasm of the lighter-staining cell appears translucent because the Nissl substance is loosely arranged in a diffuse pattern, leaving large spaces apparently not filled with ribosomes. This is illustrated by electron micrographs (see ref. 1) which show that the massive blocks of Nissl substance of the basophilic dopaminergic cells are composed of a large number of well-organized stacks of RER cisternae, densely interspersed by free ribosomes or other organelles. In contrast, the single or loosely organized short stacks of RER are interspersed with electronlucent perikaryal spaces in the nondopaminergic cells. Both Nissl patterns appear in cells of various shape: ovoid, spheroidal, multipolar or fusiform; and size: small, medium or large; so that neither shape nor size can be used to distinguish the two cell classes. A similar heterogenity of neuronal shapes, size and dendritic processes were also described by Phillipson[19] in observations taken from Golgi preparations. It is possible that subgroups will eventually correlate with differences reported for dopamine cells in amine turnover,[20] neuronal discharge rates,[21] or subpopulations of neurons in which cholecystokinin (CCK)[22] or acetylcholinesterase[23] colocalize with dopamine.

## Afferents

The majority of afferents to the ventral tegmental area originate from structures associated with the limbic system. The telencephalic structures of the limbic system are Broca's limbic lobe (the cingulate and parahippocampal gyri and hippocampal formation), the amygdala and the septum (see ref. 4). These limbic areas are connected with an uninterrupted continuum of subcortical grey matter that stretches in a paramedian zone, caudalward from the septum, over the preoptic region and hypothalamus to the "limbic midbrain area,"[24,25] which includes the ventral tegmental area, the ventral half of the central gray substance, the dorsal and median raphe nuclei, the interpeduncular nucleus, and the dorsal and ventral tegmental nuclei of Gudden. Reciprocal ascending and descending connections ("limbic forebrain–midbrain circuit") between the components of the continuum largely follow the longitudinal fiber system of the medial forebrain bundle, which is interspersed throughout its extent. The gray matter of the nucleus of the diagonal band, the lateral preoptic nucleus, lateral hypothalamic nucleus, and ventral tegmental area, receive and add fibers to the bundle in either the caudal or rostral direction, or both. Afferents to the ventral tegmental area in this system have specifically been identified from the raphe nuclei,[26] the lateral hypothalamus,[27] the lateral preoptic area,[28] the nucleus of the diagonal band,[29,30] the septum,[30] the ventral pallium,[7] the amygdala[31] and the orbitofrontal cortex.[32] These afferents have also been described by Phillipson[33] in a study using retrograde tracing.

In addition, afferents from the nucleus accumbens[3] to the ventral tegmental area and substantia nigra have been reported to follow a similar course in the medial forebrain bundle and to be distributed much like the larger number of fibers descending from the hypothalamus (FIG. 4).

## Efferent Projections of the Ventral Tegmental Area (VTA)

From the results of histofluorescence studies, Ungerstedt[34] introduced the term mesolimbic system when he noted that the ascending dopaminergic projections originating from the VTA (dopamine cell group A10) innervated structures associated

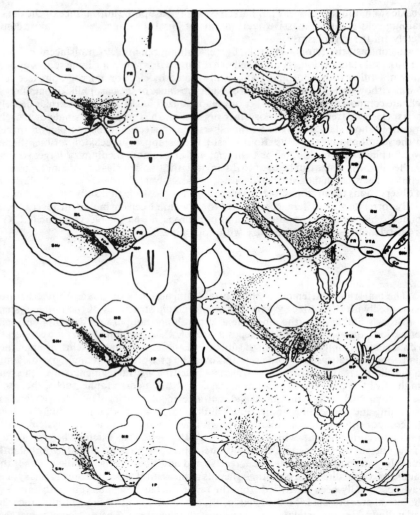

**FIGURE 4.** Chartings of the fiber distribution to the nigral complex after isotope injections in the nucleus accumbens (*left column*) and hypothalamus (*right column*).

with the limbic system including the central nucleus of the amygdala, the bed nucleus of the stria terminalis, the septum, the olfactory tubercle, and the nucleus accumbens. Subsequent studies[35-37] confirmed the existence of these A10 projections to the limbic system and showed additional evidence of dopaminergic A10 projections to the limbic cortex, including the medial frontal, cingulate, anterior suprarhinal, and entorhinal cortex.[38-42]

Studies by anterograde and retrograde labeling methods[5,43-46] have demonstrated that there is a wider distribution of VTA efferents, to the thalamus (the mediodorsal nucleus, the ventromedial nucleus, the nucleus reunions, and the lateral habenular nucleus), the midbrain reticular formation, the central gray, the median and dorsal raphe nuclei, and the locus coeruleus; the results of these tracing methods allow no conclusions regarding the dopaminergic nature of the projections.

The fibers traced autoradiographically from an injection in the ventral tegmental area (VTA) are charted in frontal sections in FIGURES 5 and 6.

The injection site (FIG. 5D) in this case was centered in an anterior VTA region rostral to the interpeduncular nucleus and separated from the pars compacta by the medial terminal nucleus of the accessory optic tract (AOT).

From the injection site numerous labeled axons spread lateralwards over the ipsilateral substantia nigra in which they are distributed over the entire rostrocaudal extent of the pars compacta, and in lesser number to the most dorsal zone of the pars reticulata (FIGS. 5C, 5D, and 6E). Other fibers passed dorsocaudally into median and paramedian parts of the midbrain tegmentum, while a large contingent ascended in the medial forebrain bundle.

## Descending Projections of VTA

Labeled fibers descending from VTA spread caudally and dorsally over a wide medial zone of the midbrain tegmentum, including the median raphe nucleus, and continued dorsally into the ventral region of the central gray substance, including the dorsal raphe nucleus (FIGS. 5B, 5C). At more caudal levels, the dorsal and ventral peribrachial areas showed sparse labeling that continued medially and caudally over the locus coeruleus and an adjacent lateral part of the nucleus tegmenti dorsalis lateralis (FIG. 5A). The dorsal and ventral tegmental nuclei of Gudden were free from label, and neither did label above background appear in the brain stem caudal to the locus coeruleus. A small group of labeled fibers was seen to cross the midline to descend in a pattern similar to that of the ipsilateral descending fibers.

## Ascending Projections of the VTA

*Diencephalon.* Labeled axons ascended from the injection site through the ipsilateral medial forebrain bundle. At the level where the fasciculus retroflexus passes medial to the forebrain bundle a few labeled fibers deviated dorsally from the medial forebrain bundle to be traced alongside the fasciculus retroflexus to the lateral half of the lateral habenular nucleus (FIGS. 6E, 6F).

Because of the diffuse distribution of label throughout the length of the medial forebrain bundle, it is uncertain whether any VTA fibers actually terminate in the lateral hypothalamic region. Farther rostrally, offsets from the main ascending path passed dorsalwards through the subthalamic region to the extreme ventromedial part of the ventromedial thalamic nucleus, the nucleus reuniens, the nucleus centralis medius, and the marginal zone of the mediodorsal nucleus, where labeling was densest in the medial region bordering the periventricular nucleus (FIG. 6G).

*Basal Forebrain.* Near the level of the rostral pole of the thalamus, dorsal offsets from the main group of labeled fibers spread into the preoptic part of the bed nucleus of the stria terminalis (FIG. 6H); more anterior parts of the bed nucleus were free of label. Finally, at levels rostral to the transverse limb of the anterior commissure, diffusely arranged labeled fibers from the medial forebrain bundle entered the nucleus of the diagonal band of Broca, the ventral pallidum, and the medial half of the lateral septal nucleus (FIGS. 6I, 6J).

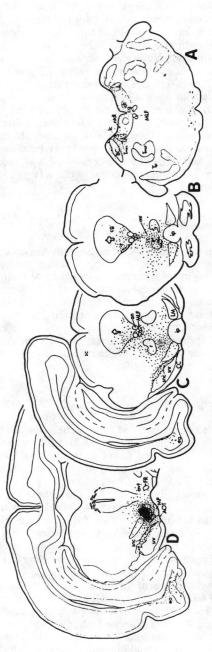

**FIGURE 5.** Charting of labeled, descending fiber projections from the ventral tegmental area, resulting from an isotope injection shown in FIGURE D.

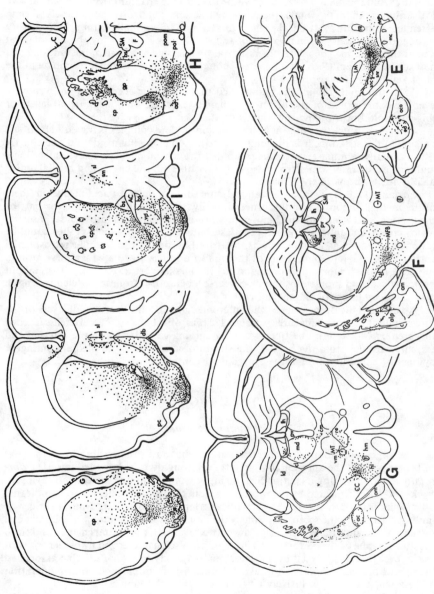

**FIGURE 6.** Charting of labeled, ascending fiber projections from the ventral tegmental area, resulting from an isotope injection shown in FIGURE 5.

*Striatum*. Within the striatum labeled VTA fibers are more widely distributed than previously described. At middle hypothalamic levels labeled fibers began to spread laterally from the medial forebrain bundle to enter the striatum from the ventral side to distribute to the entire fundus region of the striatum. At all rostrocaudal levels labeling extended from this most basal region dorsalwards in gradually diminishing density throughout the ventromedial extent of the striatum, avoiding only the dorsolateral half of the striatum. Thus, VTA fibers appear to innervate nearly all of the ventromedial half of the striatum (FIGS. 6H–K), even though their largest number terminate in the most ventral striatal region.

At rostral levels the labeling continued to the nucleus accumbens and ventrally over the entire extent of the olfactory tubercle (FIGS. 6J, 6K), marking all layers of this structure but avoiding the islands of Calleja.

*Amygdala*. Since the anterior half of the amygdaloid complex is traversed by fibers passing to the striatum, it is difficult to determine in which amygdaloid nuclei VTA fibers actually terminate. It seems certain that the central nucleus receives such fibers and farther rostrally some termination of VTA fibers in the lateral and medial amygdaloid nuclei seems likely (FIGS. 6F, 6G).

*Cortex*. At levels rostral to the callosal genu some of the most medial labeled fibers in the medial forebrain bundle turned dorsally, traversed the most anterior part of the septum, and deep into the hippocampal rudiment gathered into slender fascicles which curved caudalwards, joining the fasciculus cinguli (C), in which they could be followed to a level as far caudally as the rostral border of the granular retrosplenial cortex (FIGS. 6G–K). Some fibers of the same group described a wider curve around the genu through more anterior regions of the medial cortex (FIG. 6K). Throughout its precallosal and supracallosal course, sparse label spread from the fasciculus cinguli over the deep layers of the medial cortex.

Apart from the deep strata of the anteromedial and sulcal cortex, all layers of the rostral half of the entorhinal area were labeled (FIG. 6E). Labeled VTA efferents reached this area by two routes: one fiber group by curving caudalwards in the external and extreme capsules from the base of the striatum; a second, more medial contingent by passing caudally through the amygdaloid complex.

## DISCUSSION

### The Limbic Striatum

The larger, anterior part of the striatum (i.e., that part situated anterior to the level of the crossing of the anterior commissure) can roughly be subdivided into (1) a *dorsolateral half*, receiving its major cortical input from the motor cortex, and (2) a *ventromedial half* delineated by the projection from the vental tegmental area (indicated by stipple in FIG. 7). It receives partially overlapping projections from a variety of limbic structures in the forebrain; namely the hippocampal formation,[47] the basolateral nucleus of the amygdala,[48] the cingulate cortex,[49] and the prefrontal cortex[50] and from the dorsal raphe of the midbrain.[51] This region is also characterized by higher somatostatin levels[52] and is labeled by a monoclonal antibody to LAMP (limbic-associated membrane protein) developed by Levitt[53] from a hippocampal membrane preparation and shown to almost exclusively label structures of the limbic system.

As defined by its afferents, the "limbic striatum" corresponds to the entire anteroventromedial sector of the striatum, and continues anteriorly to the nucleus accumbens and olfactory tubercle. Outlines of the striatum from a series of coronal sections through

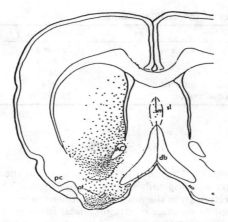

**FIGURE 7.** Ventromedial and dorsolateral halves of the anterior part of the striatum.

its anteroposterior extent were used to three-dimensionally reconstruct the striatum (FIG. 8). Three regions of the striatum were delineated; namely, the dorsolateral, ventromedial and nucleus accumbens. The volumes (TABLE 2) show that the limbic striatum (ventromedial sector plus the nucleus accumbens) comprises nearly 40% of the striatum.

The dualism of the limbic and the nonlimbic striatal sectors are reflected in the descending striatofugal conduction lines through the pallidum.[7,54]

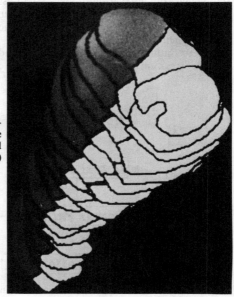

**FIGURE 8.** Three-dimensional reconstruction from outlines of the three sectors of the striatum: dorsolateral (*top*), ventromedial (*middle*), and nucleus accumbens (*bottom*) sector of the striatum.

**TABLE 2.** Volumes of the Striatal Complex

| Area | Volume (mm³) |
|---|---|
| Caudatoputamen | 22.4369 |
| Limbic | 6.8718 |
| Nonlimbic | 15.5651 |
| Nucleus accumbens | 2.9543 |
| Total region | 25.39119 |

### The Ventral Pallidum

A ventral extension of the globus pallidus, lying below the anterior commissure in the basal forebrain was originally recognized by Heimer.[55,56] He noted that it received a dense projection from the nucleus accumbens, whose mode of termination resembled the sleeve-like plexuses of striatopallidal fibers surrounding dendrites in the dorsal pallidum. The ventral pallidum, like the overlying dorsal pallidum, receives afferent input from the subthalamic nucleus,[57] has a high iron content[58] and strong enkephalin-like[59-61] and glutamic-acid-decarboxylase-like immunoreactivity.[62] The ventral pallidum can be distinguished from the dorsal pallidum by its innervation of a dense substance-P-positive fiber plexus.[59,60] The striatopallidal projection from the "nonlimbic," dorsolateral striatal sector projects to the dorsal pallidum and entopeduncular nucleus; the "limbic," ventromedial striatal region and nucleus accumbens project topographically to the entire extent of the ventral pallidum as defined by its dense substance-P-positive fiber plexus.[54]

While the main outflow from the dorsal pallidum and entopeduncular nucleus is to the subthalamic nucleus, substantia nigra and ventral thalamic nuclei, the efferent projections of the ventral pallidum[7] involve not only the subthalamic nucleus and substantia nigra but also various limbic-system-associated structures: the amygdala, medial frontal and cingulate cortex, lateral habenular nucleus, mediodorsal thalamic nucleus, hypothalamus, ventral tegmental area, and more caudal and dorsal regions of the midbrain tegmentum.

These findings indicate the ventral pallidum can convey striatal input from the "limbic" striatum into both extrapyramidal and limbic circuits.

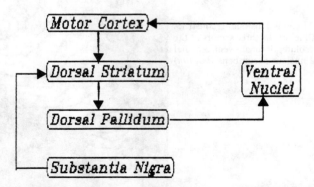

**FIGURE 9.** Circuit diagram of transthalamic circuitry of the "nonlimbic," dorsolateral striatum.

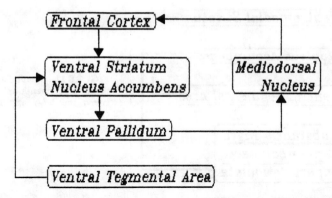

**FIGURE 10.** Circuit diagram of transthalamic circuitry of the "limbic" striatum.

### Conduction Lines to the Cortex

The limbic–nonlimbic dichotomy in the innervation of the striatum is also reflected in the existence of two distinct transthalamic striatal output loops. FIGURE 9 illustrates the "extrapyramidal motor circuit," which leads from motor cortex → striatum → pallidum → ventral thalamus (ventroanterior and ventrolateral [VA-VL] complex) → motor cortex. A second parallel circuit (FIG. 10) involves limbic counterparts: frontal cortex → ventral striatum and nucleus accumbens → ventral pallidum → mediodorsal thalamic nucleus → frontal cortex.

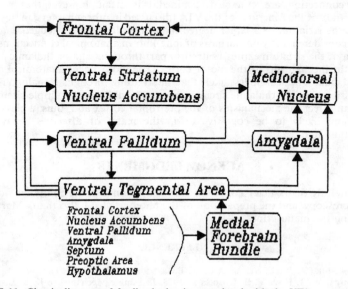

**FIGURE 11.** Circuit diagram of feedback circuits associated with the VTA.

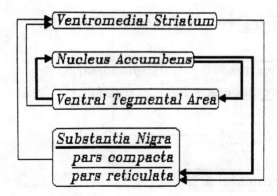

**FIGURE 12.** Circuit diagram of the "loop" and "open-loop" circuits between the VTA and the striatal complex.

Thus, by virtue of its projection to the ventromedial striatum, the ventral tegmental area is involved in complex circuitry (FIG. 11), composed of several feedback loops. The circuitry includes projections from the ventral tegmental area to the ventral pallidum, amygdala, mediodorsal nucleus, and frontal cortex. Not diagrammed are the projections from the ventral pallidum to all the "limbic" structures (frontal cortex, nucleus accumbens, amygdala, hypothalamus) which are shown to project to the ventral tegmental area via the medial forebrain bundle.

Also to be noted (FIG. 12) is the absence of a return projection from the ventromedial striatum to the ventral tegmental area which suggests an "open" or "nonloop" connection where the projection from the VTA to the striatum has no reciprocating striatal feedback.[63] The nucleus accumbens, which is considered part of the striatal complex, does project back to the VTA (see FIG. 12 and FIG. 4). The functional counterparts of these connections are yet to be determined. It is certain, however, that the anatomical substrate of the functions of the VTA (discussed in other chapters, in this volume) involves the striatum to a larger degree than heretofore acknowledged.

It is considered likely on the basis of long-known anatomical connections that the function of the striatum expresses itself in part through a major thalamic circuit affecting the mechanisms of the motor cortex. The more recent anatomical data here reviewed make it appear no less likely that the striatum, through an analogous, though less massive, "limbic" thalamic circuit, mediated by direct and multiple circuits of the VTA, can affect the mechanisms of the prefrontal cortex and, thus, a class of functions more likely to be cognitive or in the realm of affective behavior than skeletomuscular.

## ACKNOWLEDGMENTS

I gratefully thank Peter Paskevich for his assistance in the computer work, electron microscopy, and the preparation of the photographs. I also thank Martha Shea for typing the manuscript.

## REFERENCES

1.  DOMESICK, V. B., L. STINUS & P. A. PASKEVICH. 1982. Neuroscience **8:** 743–765.
2.  NAUTA, W. J. H. & V. B. DOMESICK. 1978. *In* Limbic Mechanisms. K. E. Livingston & O. Hornykiewicz, Eds.: 75–93. Plenum Press. New York.

3. NAUTA, W. J. H., G. P. SMITH, R. L. M. FAULL & V. B. DOMESICK. 1978. Neuroscience 3: 385-401.
4. NAUTA, W. J. H. & V. B. DOMESICK. 1982. In Neural Substrates of Behavior. A. Beckman, Ed.: 175-206. Spectrum Publications. New York.
5. BECKSTEAD, R. M., V. B. DOMESICK & W. J. H. NAUTA. 1979. Brain Res. 175: 191-217.
6. NAUTA, W. J. H. & V. B. DOMESICK. 1984. Afferent and efferent relationships of the basal ganglia. Ciba Foundation Symposium 107: 3-23. Pittman Press. London.
7. HABER, S. N., H. J. GROENEWEGEN, E. A. GROVE & W. J. H. NAUTA. 1985. J. Comp. Neurol. 235: 322-335.
8. DAHLSTROM, A. & K. FUXE. 1964. Acta Physiol. Scand. 62 (Suppl. 232): 1-55.
9. LINDVALL, O. & A. BJORKLUND. 1974. Acta Physiol. Scand. (Suppl. 412): 1-48.
10. TSAI, C. 1925. J. Comp. Neurol. 39: 173-216.
11. PHILLIPSON, O. T. 1979. J. Comp. Neurol. 187: 85-98.
12. MOORE, R. Y. & F. E. BLOOM. 1978. Am. Rev. Neurosci. 1: 129-169.
13. PICKEL, V. M., T. H. JOH & D. J. REIS. 1977. In Nonstriatal Dopaminergic Neurons. E. C. Costa & G. L. Gessa, Eds.: 321-329. Adv. Biochem. Psychopharmacol. Raven Press. New York.
14. SWANSON, L. W. 1982. Brain Res. Bull. 9: 321-353.
15. HANAWAY, J., M. A. McCONNELL & M. G. DETSKY. 1970. Am. J. Anat. 129: 417-438.
16. HALLIDAY, G. M. & I. TORK. 1986. J. Comp. Neurol. 252: 423-445.
17. THIERRY, A. M., J. M. DENIAU, D. HERVE & G. CHEVALIER. 1980. Brain Res. 201: 210-214.
18. YIM, C. Y. & G. J. MOGENSON. Brain Res. 181: 301-313.
19. PHILLIPSON, O. T. 1979. J. Comp. Neurol. 187: 99-115.
20. AGNATI, L. F., K. FUXE, K. ANDERSSON, F. BENFENATI, P. CORTELLI & R. D'ALESSANDRO. 1980. Neurosci. Lett. 18: 45-51.
21. CHIODO, L. A., S. M. ANTELMAN, A. R. CAGGIULA & C. G. LINEBERRY. Brain Res. 189: 544-549.
22. HOKFELT, T., L. SKIRBOLL, J. F. REHFELD, M. GOLDSTEIN, K. MARKEY & O. DANN. 1980. Neuroscience 5: 2093-2124.
23. PALKOVITS, M. & D. M. JACOBOWITZ. 1974. J. Comp. Neurol. 157: 29-42.
24. NAUTA, W. J. H. 1958. Brain 81: 319-340.
25. NAUTA, W. J. H. & W. HAYMAKER. 1969. In The Hypothalamus. W. Haymaker et al., Eds.: 136-209. Charles C Thomas. Springfield, Ill.
26. BOBILLIER, P., S. SEQUIN, A. DEGUEURCE, B. D. LEWIS & J. F. PUJOL. 1979. Brain Res. 166: 1-8.
27. SAPER, C. B., L. W. SWANSON & W. M. COWAN. 1978. J. Comp. Neurol. 183: 689-706.
28. SWANSON, L. W. 1976. J. Comp. Neurol. 167: 227-256.
29. DOMESICK, V. B. 1976. Anat. Rec. 184: 319-320.
30. SWANSON, L. W. & W. M. COWAN. 1979. J. Comp. Neurol. 186: 621-656.
31. KRETTEK, J. E. & J. L. PRICE. 1978. J. Comp. Neurol. 178: 225-254.
32. BECKSTEAD, R. M. 1979. J. Comp. Neurol. 184: 43-62.
33. PHILLIPSON, O. T. 1979. J. Comp. Neurol. 187: 117-144.
34. UNGERSTEDT, U. 1971. Acta Physiol. Scand. (Suppl. 367): 1-48.
35. FALLON, J. H., D. A. KOZIELL & R. Y. MOORE. 1978. J. Comp. Neurol. 180: 509-532.
36. FALLON, J. H. & R. Y. MOORE. 1978. J. Comp. Neurol. 180: 545-580.
37. MOORE, R. Y. 1978. J. Comp. Neurol. 177: 665-684.
38. THIERRY, A. M., G. BLANC, A. SOBEL, L. STINUS & J. GLOWINSKI. 1973. Science 182: 499-501.
39. BERGER, B., J. P. TASSIN, G. BLANC, J. A. MOYNE & A. M. THIERRY. 1974. Brain Res. 81: 332-337.
40. FUXE, K., T. HOKFELT, O. JOHANSSON, G. JONSSON, P. LIDBRINK & A. LJUNGDAHL. 1974. Brain Res. 82: 349-355.
41. LINDVALL, O., A. BJORKLUND, R. Y. MOORE & U. STENEVI. 1974. Brain Res. 81: 325-331.
42. LINDVALL, O., A. BJORKLUND & I. DIVAC. 1978. Brain Res. 142: 1-24.
43. SIMON, H., M. LE MOAL, D. GALEY & B. CARDO. 1976. Brain Res. 115: 215-231.
44. CARTER, D. A. & H. C. FIBIGER. 1977. Neuroscience 2: 569-576.
45. SIMON, H., M. LE MOAL & A. CALAS. 1979. Brain Res. 178: 17-40.
46. PHILLIPSON, O. T. & A. C. GRIFFITH. 1980. Brain Res. 197: 213-218.
47. KELLEY, A. E. & V. B. DOMESICK. 1982. Neuroscience 7: 2321-2336.

48. KELLEY, A. E., V. B. DOMESICK & W. J. H. NAUTA. 1982. Neuroscience 7: 615–630.
49. DOMESICK, V. B. 1969. Brain Res. 12: 296–320.
50. LEONARD, C. M. 1969. Brain Res. 12: 321–343.
51. STEINBUSCH, H. W. M. 1981. Neuroscience 6: 557–618.
52. BEAL, M. F., V. B. DOMESICK & J. B. MARTIN. 1983. Brain Res. 278: 103–108.
53. LEVITT, P. 1984. Science: 299–301.
54. DOMESICK, V. B., P. PASKEVICH & S. W. MATTHYSSE. 1986. Neurosci. Abst.
55. HEIMER, L. & R. D. WILSON. 1975. In Golgi Centennial Symposium. M. Santini, Ed.: 177–193. Raven Press. New York.
56. HEIMER, L. 1978. In Limbic Mechanisms. K. E. Livingston & O. Hornykiewicz, Eds.: 95–187. Plenum Press. New York.
57. RICARDO, J. 1980. Brain Res. 202: 257–271.
58. HILL, J. M. & R. C. SWITZER. 1984. Neuroscience 11: 595–603.
59. SWITZER, R. C., J. HILL & L. HEIMER. 1982. Neuroscience 7: 1891–1904.
60. HABER, S. N. & R. ELDE. 1981. Neuroscience 6: 1291–1298.
61. HABER, S. N. & W. J. H. NAUTA. 1983. Neuroscience 9: 245–260.
62. FALLON, J. H. & C. E. RIBAK. 1980. Soc. Neurosci. Abstr. 6: 114.
63. DOMESICK, V. B. 1981. In Apomorphine and Other Dopaminomimetics. Basic Pharmacology, Vol. 1. G. L. Gessa & G. U. Corsini, Eds.: 27–39. Raven Press. New York.

# Telencephalic Projections of the A8 Dopamine Cell Group

ARIEL Y. DEUTCH,[a,b] MENEK GOLDSTEIN,[c]
FRANK BALDINO, JR.,[d] AND ROBERT H. ROTH[a]

[a] *Departments of Pharmacology and Psychiatry*
*Yale University School of Medicine*
*New Haven, Connecticut 06510*

[c] *Department of Psychiatry*
*New York University School of Medicine*
*New York, New York 10016*

[d] *Biomedical Products Division*
*E. I. DuPont and Co.*
*Wilmington, Delaware 19801*

## INTRODUCTION

The mesencephalic dopamine cell groups form a continuous band of neurons located along the ventral aspects of the mesencephalon, extending caudally to occupy a more dorsal position at the pontomesencephalic juncture. These dopamine (DA) neurons do not exhibit significant ontogenetic differences,[1,2] nor are there clear boundaries demarcating the mesencephalic cell groups.[3] Accordingly, it has been suggested that these DA neurons be collectively designated the mesotelencephalic dopamine system.[4]

Although the midbrain DA neurons exhibit a broad topographic organization in their projections onto the telencephalon,[5] there is a considerable degree of overlap of these dopaminergic projections. Thus, while the medially situated DA neurons of the A10 cell group (centered in the ventral tegmental area) project to the medially situated septum and nucleus accumbens septi (NAS), the A10 DA neurons also project to the more lateral striatum (CP). Conversely, the A9 DA neurons of the substantia-nigra, pars compacta (SNpc) project not only to the striatum, but also to mesolimbic areas such as the NAS.

The A8 DA cell group has generally been considered to represent a caudal extension of the A9 DA neurons of the SN. The A8 neurons are located dorsal and caudal to the SN. The location of these neurons roughly corresponds to the region designated the retrorubral nucleus in the cat by Berman;[6] the nuclear groupings in this region of the rat [the retrorubral field (RRF)] are not as clearly defined. The dopaminergic neurons of the rostral and ventral aspects of the A8 cell group cannot be clearly differentiated from the contiguous A9 DA neurons of the caudal and lateral SN, nor is there a clear demarcation between the most medial A8 DA cells and the dopaminergic neurons of the caudal and lateral aspects of the A10 cell group in the nucleus parabrachialis pigmentosus.[3,4,7]

[b] To whom correspondence should be addressed.

27

Anatomical studies in a number of species have demonstrated that neurons situated within the RRF project to the striatum;[5,8-16] however, most of these investigations did not determine if the RRF neurons that project to the CP are dopaminergic. Nauta and colleagues[17] noted that neurons situated within the A8 cell group region project to the nucleus accumbens as well as the striatum, and thus innervate both mesolimbic and striatal areas; these conclusions were subsequently confirmed by a number of groups.[18-21] Lenard and Nauta,[22] using autoradiographic methods, demonstrated that neurons of the RRF contribute widely to mesolimbic regions, and suggested that the A9 DA neurons of the SN are embedded in a matrix of mesolimbic DA neurons, those of the A10 cell group medially and those of the A8 cell group on the dorsal and lateral borders. Subsequently, Swanson[23] demonstrated that DA neurons within the RRF contributed to the mesolimbic innervation.

In light of these studies suggesting that the DA neurons of the A8 cell group contribute to the striatal and mesolimbic innervations originating from the RRF, we decided to systematically examine the telencephalic projections of the A8 DA neurons. This was accomplished by initially determining the efferent projections of the RRF using an anterograde tract tracing method. The anterograde data were then used to guide the systematic examination of the contribution of A8 DA cells to telencephalic sites, using a combined retrograde tracer–immunohistochemical method.

## DELINEATION OF THE A8 CELL GROUP

General mapping of the extent of the A8 DA cell group was accomplished using immunohistochemical examination of tyrosine hydroxylase-like immunoreactive neurons. Both tyrosine hydroxylase (TH) and dopamine-beta-hydroxylase (DBH) immunoreactive elements in the region were examined.

The location of the A8 DA cells in the rat was consistent with previous observations.[3,7,24,25] The A8 cells appear rostrally as a small group of neurons forming a cell bridge joining the dopaminergic neurons of the nuc. parabrachialis pigmentosus of the A10 cell group and the A9 neurons of the SN; some of these rostral A8 DA neurons are embedded in the medial lemniscus (see FIG. 1). More caudally, two prominent aggregates of A8 DA neurons become apparent. At this level a dorsally situated cell-dense portion can be seen, and ventrally a rather diffuse population of neurons exhibiting TH-like immunoreactivity is present. Still more caudally, the ventral diffuse population disappears, and the compact portion of the A8 cell group moves dorsally, initially to the region ventral to the deep mesencephalic nucleus, and still more caudally to a position dorsal and medial to the nucleus pedunculopontinus tegmentalis, partially overlapping the rostral aspect of the cuneiform nucleus. Sections adjacent to those processed for TH immunohistochemistry were examined for the presence of DBH-positive perikarya, in order to determine if any of the TH-positive neurons in the A8 cell group region were noradrenergic. Although DBH-like immunoreactivity was clearly present in fibers coursing through the A8 region (the ventral noradrenergic bundle), no DBH-positive neurons were observed within the A8 cell group region.

A similar organization of the A8 neurons was observed in the brains of two non-human primate species examined, the African green monkey (Circopithecus aethiops) and the stump-tailed macaque (Macaca arctoides). Although slight differences in the number of neurons comprising the A8 cell group and the positioning of these neurons within the mesencephalon were present, as has been previously reported,[26] the basic organization in the two species was very similar. In the primate, as in the rat, A8 DA neurons are continuous with the lateral aspects of the SN, and form cell bridges con-

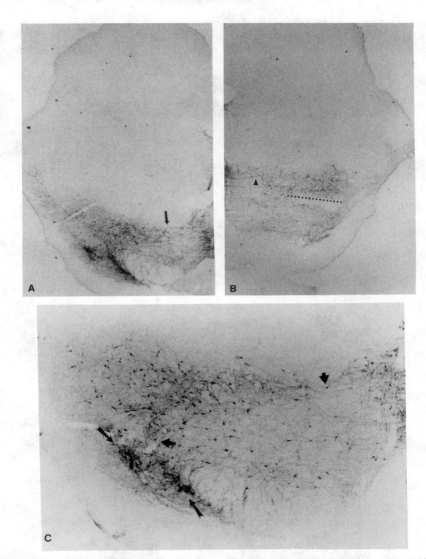

**FIGURE 1.** A8 DA neurons of the rat, as revealed by TH immunohistochemistry. The bridge of A8 neurons crossing from the dorsal and lateral SN to the lateral VTA is illustrated in panels **A** and **C** (*enlargement of* **A**). The caudal-most A9 neurons of the SN (*large arrows in* **C**) and the lateral A10 neurons merge without clear boundaries (*arrowheads in* **A** and **C**) with the A8 neurons of the RRF. More caudally (**B**) the dorsal (cell-dense) portion of the A8 cell group can be differentiated from the ventral-sparse region, as shown by the dotted line. The transition zone between the A8 neurons and the dorsal and medial A10 neurons at this level is marked by an arrowhead.

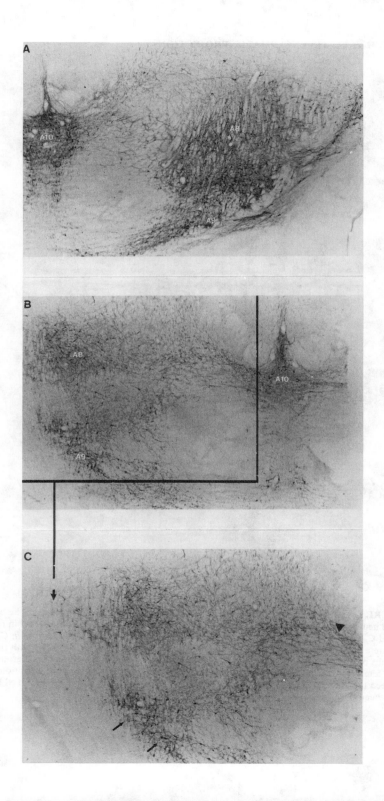

necting the A9 neurons of the SN and the A10 neurons of the ventral tegmental area (VTA) (FIG. 2); again, some of the TH-positive A8 neurons are embedded in the medial lemniscus. More caudally, A8 neurons are situated medial to the lemniscus, and formed a dorsal cell-dense region and a more diffusely organized ventral region. Still more caudally, the A8 DA neurons gradually shift to a more dorsal position, dorsomedial to and overlapping with the nucleus pedunculopontinus tementalis and partially within the nucleus subcuneiformis and ventral aspects of the nucleus cuneiformis.

Examination of the distribution of TH-positive neurons within the midbrain of the human revealed A8 DA neurons situated dorsal and medial to the medial lemniscus (FIG. 3), and extending caudally for a considerable distance. It shoud be noted that several types of TH-positive neurons appear within the area we and others[27,28] consider to represent the A8 cell group. The A8 region in the human appears to correspond to the perirubral area of Foix and Nicolescu.[29] The parallel organization of the midbrain DA cell groups in the human and nonhuman primate can be best appreciated if the plane of section in the human brain is maintained perpendicular to the ventral surface of the hypothalamus, rather than the plane of section used in traditional pathological examination of the brain.

It should be noted that while the position of the A8 DA neurons within the midbrain remains roughly comparable across mammalian species, other features of the mesencephalic DA neurons may differ. For example, certain mesencephalic DA neurons of the rat also contain the peptide neurotensin.[30] However, in preliminary studies of the primate midbrain, we have been unable to visualize the neurotensin perikarya. If confirmed, these studies suggest that the multiple levels of organization present in the midbrain DA neurons differ significantly across species, and that theoretical extrapolations from rodent to man will have to be reevaluated.

The distribution of the dopamine neurons of the mesencephalon have recently been examined by establishing the location of mRNA encoding for TH in midbrain neurons, as detected by *in situ* hybridization histochemistry (see Baldino *et al.*, this volume). There is a virtual complete correspondence of TH-positive perikarya and neurons which express the TH gene.

## ANTEROGRADE STUDIES

Anterograde tracer studies in the rat were accomplished using *Phaseolus vulgaris* leucoagglutinin (PHA-L) histochemistry.[31] Following iontophoretic injection, PHA-L is taken up by local neurons and anterogradely transported; the lectin is not accumulated by fibers of passage. In the present study, discrete iontophoretic injections of the lectin were placed in various aspects of the retrorubral field, or into the substantianigra, the SN pars lateralis, or the VTA.

A charting of a case in which the PHA-L deposit was centered in the retrorubral field is shown in FIGURE 4. Following this PHA-L injection, labeled fibers were seen in a variety of mesolimbic, mesocortical, and striatal areas. Axons ascending to the

---

◄ **FIGURE 2.** The primate A8 cell group, shown with TH immunohistochemistry. At the rostral pole of the A8 cell group (**A**), the A8 neurons arise as a dorsal extension of the SN A9 neurons, and form a bridge to the A10 neurons. More caudally (**B** and **C**) the A8 neurons can be seen to be more dorsal, but still occupying a position between the caudal-most A9 neurons (*small arrows*) and the lateral wings of the caudal A10 cell group (*arrowhead*). The similarities in organization between the primate A8 cell group and the rodent A8 cell group (FIG. 1) are readily apparent.

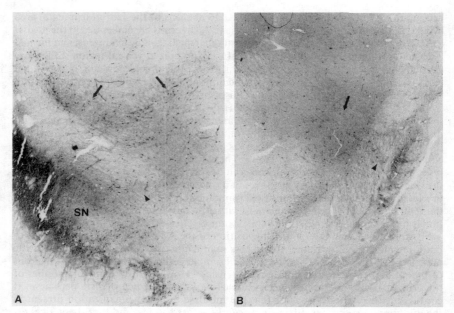

**FIGURE 3.** TH-immunoreactive neurons of the A8 cell group in the human brain stem. The lateral A9 neurons of the SN (*panel* **A**, and more caudally in *panel* **B**) are separated from the A8 neurons by the medial lemniscus. Some neurons can be seen to bridge the across the medial lemniscus (*arrowheads*).

telencephalon were observed to take two routes. A large axonal bundle could be seen traversing the pars compacta of the SN and the region dorsal to the pars compacta before turning rostrally in the VTA to ascend as part of the median forebrain bundle (MFB). Also observed was a very small projection that initially coursed rostrally running dorsal to the medial lemniscus before turning ventromedially to join the MFB in the hypothalamus; this bundle has been previously described.[32]

Diencephalic projections of the RRF were derived from both this latter dorsal projection and from the main axonal bundle. In particular, the RRF was noted to innervate the dorsomedial and lateral hypothalamus; a small cluster of fibers was also observed immediately dorsal to the mammillothalamic tract. Terminal labeling was observed in the subthalamic nucleus and the zona incerta. Thalamic labeling was present in the ventral aspects of the thalamus as well as in the mediodorsal nucleus.

Telencephalic projections of the RRF included a number of mesolimbic, striatal, and allocortical regions. Following PHA-L injections into the RRF, a broad band of fibers was observed to emerge from the MFB and turn dorsal and laterally to innervate the bed nucleus of the stria terminalis, the ventral pallidal region, and the amygdala.

The dorsal and ventral divisions of the bed nucleus of the stria terminals received RRF projections; the ventral (including subcommissural) aspects of the nucleus were more densely labeled. The ventral pallidal region was heavily labeled following PHA-L injections of the RRF. Ventral pallidal labeling was heterogeneous, such that clusters or bands of fibers were interspersed with areas relatively devoid of terminal labeling.

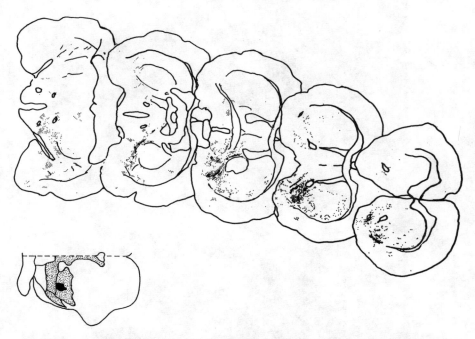

**FIGURE 4.** Charting of the distribution of PHA-L-labeled fibers following iontophoretic deposit of the anterograde tracer into the RRF (*inset*). The broad band of fibers running across the ventral pallidum with the ansa peduncularis/vantral amygdalofugal pathway fibers can be seen to be heterogeneously distributed across this region. Striatal labeling is particularly prominent in the "ventral pocket" region, and RRF efferents can be seen to innervate both "limbic" (e.g., nuc. accumbens) and "motor" striatal (lateral caudatoputamen) sectors. A small contralateral projection to the ventral pallidal and ventral striatal regions can also be seen. Although allocortical regions (pyriform and entorhinal cortices) are labeled, no RRF-derived fibers are present in the neocortex.

Some very fine fibers were observed in the globus pallidus. The broad band of fibers running across and innervating the ventral pallidum continued laterally to innervate the striatum and amygdala. The amygdaloid innervation was relatively restricted; the RRF appeared to project to the central nucleus and the transition zone between the central and basolateral nuclei (FIG. 5). Labeling of the anterior intercalated nuclei was also observed. Immediately dorsal to the amygdala the transition zone between the amygdala and the striatum, was densely labeled, as was the ventral tail of the CP. The ventral pallidal/subcommissural band of fibers appeared to contribute fibers to both the pyriform cortex rostrally, and the entorhinal cortex caudally.

The most massive projection of the RRF was onto the ventral striatum, including the nucleus accumbens (FIG. 5). Both the striatal and NAS innervations were distinctly patchy. Terminal labeling was observed throughout the NAS, but was sparse in the dorsomedial aspects of the structure. PHA-L labeling was also observed in the lateral olfactory tubercle. The most dense terminal labeling was observed in the lateral NAS

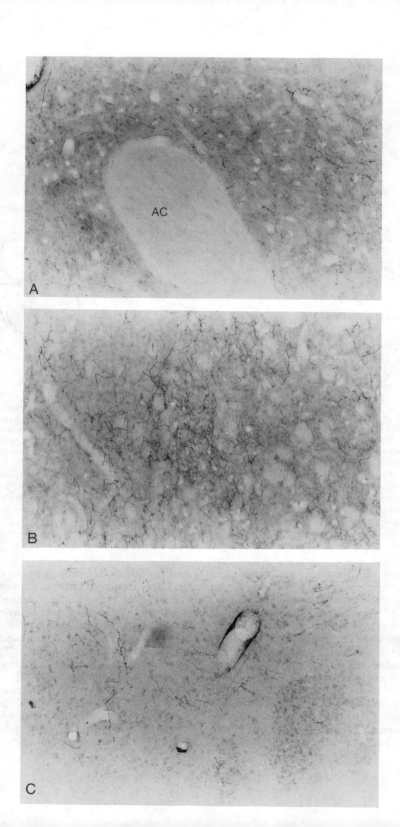

and the ventral striatum lateral to the NAS, the so-called "ventral pocket."[17] Striatal labeling was also observed along the entire lateral aspects of the structure, extending dorsally to curve under the corpus callosum.

While the RRF projection to the striatum and mesolimbic sites are widespread, injections of PHA-L into the very lateral aspects of the DA neurons of the SN (the dopaminergic portions of the pars lateralis) resulted in much more restricted telencephalic labeling (see FIG. 6). Thus, injections of PHA-L involving only the pars lateralis yielded anterograde labeling of the most ventral and lateral aspects of the striatum, and the ventrally contiguous amygdala; the amygdalostriatal transition zone was densely innervated. The pars lateralis projection fields therefore resemble a subset of RRF projections.

In summary, the RRF was observed to project to most mesolimbic areas (including the bed nucleus of the stria terminalis, olfactory tubercle, nucleus accumbens, and amygdala), the striatum (especially the ventral and lateral aspects of the CP), and some allocortical sites (the pyriform and entorhinal cortices). No consistent RRF projection to neocortical regions such as the anteromedial prefrontal cortex was observed, although an occasional labeled fiber was seen in the supragenual (cingulate) cortex. The anterograde tracer studies also revealed a crude topographical organization of RRF projections onto the telencephalon, such that more medial injections resulted in a greater degree of more medial (for example, nucleus accumbens) labeling, whereas more lateral injections resulted in heavier labeling in the striatum and amygdala. These results confirm previous reports using retrograde tracing methods that indicated a mediolateral topography of RRF projections onto the striatum[5,11,14] as well as the nucleus accumbens.[21] Although it was not possible to discern a consistent rostrocaudal topography, when placed in context of other projections originating from the mesencephalic DA cell body areas the RRF appeared to label more heavily the more caudal aspects of the nucleus accumbens, and to a lesser degree of the striatum; injections into the more rostral SN or VTA resulted in a greater degree of labeling in the more rostral aspects of the NAS and CP. However, since we did not have sufficient cases in which the PHA-L injections were restricted to the caudal (dorsal) aspects of the RRF, it is conceivable that a more consistent rostrocaudal topography of the A8 cell group projections is present.

## COMBINED RETROGRADE TRACER–IMMUNOHISTOCHEMICAL STUDIES

A combined retrograde tracer–immunohistochemical method was used to determine the contribution of the DA neurons of the A8 cell group to the RRF-derived innervation of the telencephalon. Discrete iontophoretic deposits of horseradish peroxidase–conjugated wheat germ agglutinin (WGA–HRP) were placed in various mesocortical, mesolimbic, or striatal sites. Animals were subsequently sacrificed and the brains processed to reveal retrogradely labeled neurons that exhibited tyrosine hydroxylase-

---

◀ **FIGURE 5.** PHA-L-labeled fibers in striatal and mesolimbic terminal fields following tracer injection into the RRF. In all panels dorsal is up and medial is to the left. (**A**) Labeled fibers in the nucleus accumbens. Fibers are more dense in the lateral aspects of the accumbens, but can also be seen in the ventromedial and dorsomedial sectors. AC = anterior commissure. (**B**) A cluster of PHA-L-labeled fibers in the "ventral pocket" region of the striatum. Note the patch organization, labeled fibers surrounded by an area relatively devoid of RRF afferents. (**C**) PHA-L-labeled fibers in the amygdala.

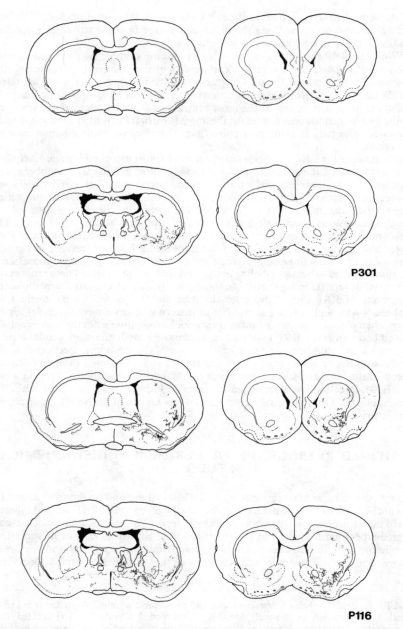

**FIGURE 6.** Chart comparing the efferent projections of the RRF (case P116) and SN pars lateralis (SNpl; case P301) onto the telencephalon. The SNpl projections, seen in the top panel, appear to define a subset of the RRF projections (*bottom panel*) seen following PHA-L deposit into the rostral and lateral RRF.

like immunoreactivity. Iontophoretic deposits of the peroxidase-conjugated lectin were used in order to minimize any contribution of uptake of the label by fibers of passage.

Injections of WGA–HRP into all fields of the striatum resulted in retrograde labeling of the dopaminergic neurons of the A8 cell group. In addition, nondopaminergic neurons were also retrogradely labeled (FIG. 7). Significantly greater numbers of retrogradely labeled A8 neurons were seen following tracer injections into the lateral and ventral aspects of the striatum that were observed following dorsomedial striatal injections.

A8 DA neurons were also retrogradely labeled after WGA–HRP injections into the nucleus accumbens (FIG. 8). Although labeled A8 neurons could be observed following tracer deposits into any portion of the NAS, iontophoretic injections centered in the ventrolateral NAS resulted in a greater number of retrogradely labeled A8 neurons.

Other mesolimbic areas also received both dopaminergic and non-dopaminergic projections originating in the A8 cell group. Thus, WGA–HRP injections restricted to the olfactory tubercle resulted in A8 labeling, as did injections into the bed nucleus of the stria terminalis; tracer injections of the lateral septal nucleus did not label any DA neurons in the RRF.

A8 neurons were retrogradely labeled following WGA–HRP injections into the amygdala (FIG. 7). Injections centered in the central nucleus, but which also involved the aspects of the lateral and basolateral nuclei, resulted in A8 labeling. It was not possible to determine unambiguously whether injections centered in the central amygdaloid nucleus extended dorsally to involve the striatum, although they almost certainly involved the amygdalostriatal transition zone. However, a clear pattern of retrograde labeling of the midbrain DA neurons emerged by assessing the distribution of labeled neurons following tracer deposits into successively more ventral injections of the striatum, culminating in tracer deposits involving the ventral aspects of the central nucleus and the intercalated nuclei of the amygdala. Thus, injections of WGA–HRP into the dorsal striatum overlying the amygdala resulted in retrogradely labeled DA neurons forming a broad band across the entire SNpc, and extending to include the A8 DA neurons. Tracer injections of the ventral aspects of the posterior striatum also resulted in A8 labeling, but the labeling of the SNpc was restricted to the medial and lateral thirds of the SN, that is, a conspicuous central sector of the DA neurons of the SNpc was not retrogradely labeled. Finally, injections into the amygdala, which involved the ventral half of the central nucleus but did not encroach upon the overlying striatum, resulted in retrograde labeling of the A8 neurons, the lateral DA neurons of the A10 cell group merging with the most medial A9 neurons, and the DA neurons situated in the pars lateralis of the SN. These results are schematically depicted in FIGURE 9.

WGA–HRP injections were placed in the ventral pallidum in order to determine if A8 DA neurons project to the region. Both iontophoretic deposits and a limited number of pressure injections of the retrograde tracer were placed in the ventral pallidum. Iontophoretic deposits revealed that DA neurons of the A8 cell group as well as A10 neurons contribute to the dopaminergic innervation of the ventral pallidum (FIG. 8). Pressure injections resulted in a significantly greater number of retrogradely labeled neurons in the ventral mesencephalon, including both DA and non-DA neurons of the SNpc as well as VTA and RRF neurons. The majority of retrogradely labeled neurons following either pressure or iontophoretic injections of the VP were non-dopaminergic.

Tracer deposits into two allocortical sites, the pyriform and entorhinal cortices, resulted in retrogradely labeled A8 neurons. A greater number of labeled A8 neurons were observed following tracer injections of the pyriform cortex than were seen after entorhinal cortex injections. Entorhinal cortical injections resulted in labeling of more medial A8 DA neurons, whereas injections of the pyriform cortex resulted in lateral A8 neurons being more frequently labeled.

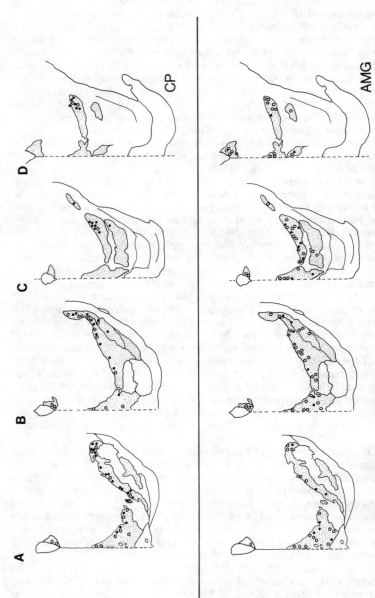

**FIGURE 7.** Distribution of retrogradely labeled TH-positive neurons (*filled circles*) and retrogradely labeled nondopaminergic neurons (*open circles*) following WGA–HRP deposits into the caudal striatum (CP) and the central amygdaloid region (AMG). The DA cell body regions of the midbrain are the lightly stippled regions. The caudal striatal projection originates from all three midbrain DA cell groups: neurons of the lateral A10 and lateral A8 areas innervate this striatal region, whereas the A9 neurons of the medial and lateral SN contribute heavily to the innervation of the tail of the caudate. Some non-dopaminergic neurons are also seen labeled, particularly in the VTA, lateral SN, and rostral RRF regions. Injections of WGA–HRP into the amygdala labeled significantly fewer DA neurons, and a substantial number of non-dopaminergic neurons were retrogradely filled. In addition, amygdala deposits of the retrograde-tracer-labeled neurons in the lateral A10 and medial and lateral A9 regions.

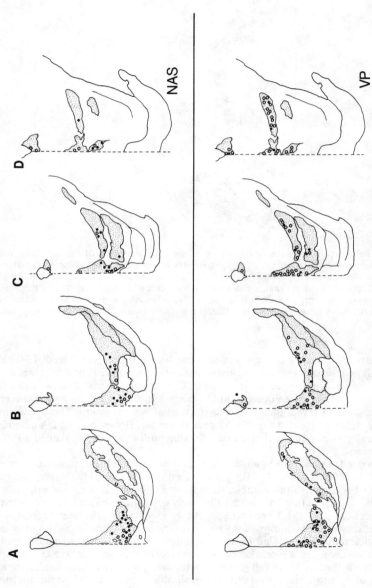

**FIGURE 8.** Charting of retrogradely labeled TH-positive neurons (*filled circles*) and retrogradely labeled non-dopaminergic neurons (*open circles*) in the DA cell group regions of the mesencephalon (*stippled areas*). WGA–HRP-labeled DA neurons are present in the lateral VTA and medial A8 cell group following tracer deposit restricted to the ventromedial area of the nucleus accumbens (NAS). Although large numbers of nondopaminergic neurons were retrogradely labeled following iontophoretic deposits of WGA–HRP into the ventral pallidum (VP), relatively few dopaminergic neurons were retrogradely filled. These are scattered across the A8 cell group and the A10 region.

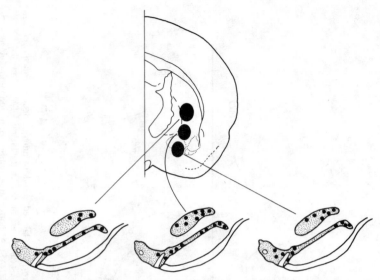

**FIGURE 9.** Schematic illustration of the source of the DA innervation of the amygdala and caudal striatum. WGA–HRP injections of progressively more ventral sites within the striatum (*dorsally*) and the central amygdaloid region (*ventrally*) result in the progressive appearance of a large central region in the SN that is characterized by a lack of retrogradely labeled neurons. The A8 neurons (*dorsally situated oval*) are labeled following these injections, but are most heavily labeled when the tracer deposit involves the transition region between the striatum and amygdala (*bottom center*).

Injections of WGA–HRP into neocortical areas, such as the pregenual medial frontal cortex (PFC) and the supragenual cingulate cortex, did not result in consistent labeling of A8 DA neurons. Tracer injections into the PFC or cingulate cortical tracer deposits resulted in the labeling of an occasional DA neuron in the transition zone between the lateral aspects of the caudal VTA and the medial A8 cell group. These neurons could not be clearly designated as either A8 or A10 neurons. However, other DA neurons of the A10 cell group were clearly labeled following both anterior cingulate and PFC tracer injections.

The retrograde tracer–immunohistochemical data confirm the anterograde tracer data, and indicate that neurons of the A8 cell group contribute to the dopaminergic innervation of widespread mesolimbic, striatal, and allocortical sites. Indeed, virtually all of the structures that have been collectively designated the mesolimbic system receive projections from the A8 cell group, with the exception of the lateral septal nucleus. A mediolateral topography of A8 projections onto the mesolimbic system was observed, such that more medial A8 neurons innervate more medial structures such as the nucleus accumbens, whereas lateral structures such as the amygdala receive inputs from neurons of the lateral A8 cell group. In addition, a more restricted mediolateral topography of A8 projections onto certain mesolimbic structures, such as the nucleus accumbens, was present. A dorsoventral topography of the A8 DA neurons was not apparent. However, there was a suggestion of a topography of A8 efferents to the telencephalon along the anterior–posterior dimension, such that more rostral A8 neurons tended to be labeled following more anterior tracer deposits, while injections into more caudal structures resulted in a somewhat greater number of more posterior A8 neurons being labeled. It should be noted, however, that neurons in the most posterior aspects of the A8 cell group were infrequently labeled; the possibility that the most caudal A8 neurons project to non-telencephalic sites must be entertained.

The greatest number of retrogradely labeled A8 DA neurons was observed after striatal injections of WGA–HRP. All striatal areas appear to receive A8 inputs, although ventrolateral regions including the "ventral pocket" appear to receive particularly dense dopaminergic innervations from the A8 cell group. Few retrogradely labeled A8 neurons were observed following WGA–HRP deposits into the most anterior striatal regions. Similarly, injections into the dorsomedial sector of the striatum at all anteroposterior levels labeled very few A8 neurons.

WGA–HRP injections into allocortical regions retrogradely labeled A8 neurons. In contrast, tracer deposits into neocortical sites, such as the PFC and anterior cingulate cortex, did not result in unambiguous A8 labeling. The mediolateral topography that appears to characterize A8 efferents to mesolimbic and striatal areas does not appear to be present in A8 projections to cortical regions, although it should be noted that only a few cortical regions have been systematically investigated.

## INTERCONNECTIONS OF THE MIDBRAIN DOPAMINE NEURONS

The axons of A8 DA neurons ascend to telencephalic sites by projecting through the SNpc and the region immediately dorsal to coalesce with the nigrostriatal DA axons before turning rostrally in the VTA. PHA-L labeling of A8 DA neurons revealed axons of passage coursing through the SN and VTA, but in addition showed axonal varicosities and specializations consistent with areas of synaptic contact[33] (see FIG. 10). In light of these observations we examined the possibility of interconnections between the neurons of the different DA cell groups, such as A8 projections to the VTA. This was accomplished using both combined anterograde tracer–immunohistochemical and combined retrograde tracer–immunohistochemical methods.

PHA-L labeled fibers originating in the RRF were observed in the SN and VTA. While the majority of these fibers appear to be axons of passage, varicose fibers that branched and exhibited disc-like swellings suggestive of terminal specializations could be observed in the VTA (FIG. 11); these were especially prominent in the nucleus paranigralis. Furthermore, labeled fibers could be observed to traverse the midline aspects of the A10 cell group (nuc. interfascicularis, and rostral and central linear nuclei; see Phillipson[34]), to innervate the contralateral VTA, and to course along the contralateral SNpc to terminate in the RRF. Combined PHA-L-TH immunohistochemical studies revealed occasional pericellular axonal arrays surrounding TH-positive neurons of the A10 cell group.

Combined retrograde tracer–immunohistochemical studies were undertaken in order to confirm the impression suggested by the anterograde data. WGA–HRP was iontophoretically deposited into the VTA using relatively low (1.0–1.5 μA) ejection currents; when used under these conditions WGA–HRP appears to result in minimal retrograde labeling on neurons secondary to uptake by fibers of passage. Furthermore, in a limited number of cases we iontophoretically deposited the fluorescent retrograde tracer fluorogold that has recently been reported not to be taken up by fibers of passage.[35] Both methodologies led to the same conclusions, although a greater number of retrogradely labeled neurons was observed using FG injections. Thus, neurons within the RRF were retrogradely labeled following tracer injections into the VTA; approxi-

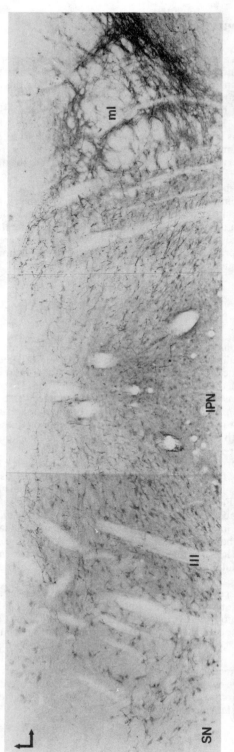

**FIGURE 10.** Photomicrograph illustrating PHA-L-labeled fibers in the ventral mesencephalon following tracer deposit into the RRF. Arrow pointing up indicates dorsal; arrow pointing right indicates medial. PHA-L-labeled fibers can be seen to traverse the pars compacta of the SN and the region dorsal to the SN, as well as the region dorsal to the medial lemniscus (ml) before entering the VTA, where most of the fibers run in a dorsolateral position before ascending to the forebrain. Some fibers can be seen to cross the VTA overlying the interpeduncular nucleus (IPN), cross the contralateral VTA and through the oculomotor roots (III) before entering the contralateral SN to run along the pars compacta before turning to innervate the contralateral RRF.

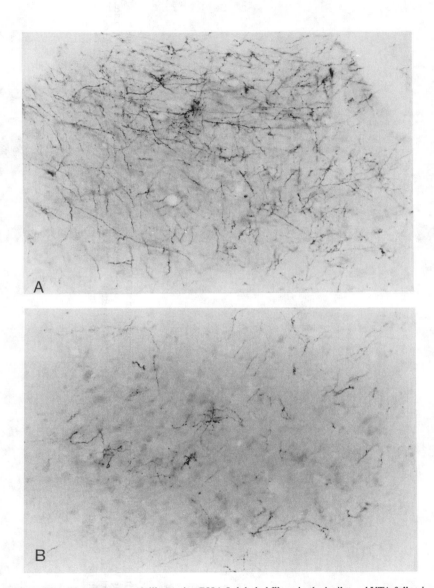

**FIGURE 11.** Photomicrograph illustrating PHA-L-labeled fibers in the ipsilateral VTA following injection of the tracer into the RRF. While a large number of these fibers appear to represent fibers of passage (*upper portion of panel A*), there are areas in which terminal swellings and varicosities suggestive of areas of terminal specialization are present, here shown in the nuc. paranigralis (*panel B*).

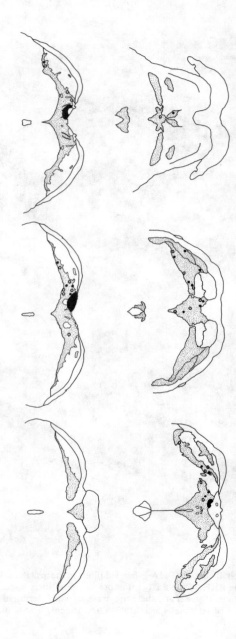

**FIGURE 12.** Charting of the distribution of retrogradely labeled TH-positive neurons (*filled circles*) in the ventral mesencephalic DA cell group areas (*stippled*) following WGA–HRP iontophoretic deposit into the VTA (*dense black zone*). Nondopaminergic neurons that were retrogradely labeled are shown as open circles. Both retrogradely labeled DA and non-DA neurons are present in the A8 cell group; in contrast, very few retrogradely labeled neurons are seen in the SN. Neurons in the regions immediately adjacent to the injection site were not charted.

mately half of these neurons were dopaminergic (FIG. 12). A very small number of A9 neurons were also labeled. Retrograde tracer injections into the most rostral portions of the VTA (in the supramammillary region), a DA cell-sparse region where the ascending dopaminergic bundle is well defined, did not result in significant retrograde labeling of either the A8 or A9 cell groups, suggesting that uptake of the tracer by fibers of passage did not occur to a significant degree.

Thus, A8 neurons appear to provide a dopaminergic innervation of other midbrain DA neurons, particularly those of the A10 cell group. Reciprocal projections from the VTA to the RRF, both dopaminergic and nondopaminergic, are also present. Very few retrogradely labeled A8 (or A10) neurons were observed following tracer injections into the SN, suggesting that the accumulation of the retrograde tracer by fibers of passage did not contribute to the observed results.

## FUNCTIONAL IMPLICATIONS OF THE ORGANIZATION OF THE A8 CELL GROUP

The distribution of A8 DA neurons to widespread mesolimbic, striatal, and allocortical dopamine terminal fields suggests that the A8 neurons may be uniquely organized such that they may be able to influence the activity of multiple forebrain sites. The present data confirm and extend previous observations indicating that RRF neurons innervate the striatum and also innervate mesolimbic areas.[5,7,17,19–23,36,37] Furthermore, these data specifically indicate that the A8 DA neurons as well as non-dopaminergic neurons of the RRF contribute to these telencephalic sites, in accord with the observations of Swanson.[23] Moreover, an A8 projection to the ventral pallidum was observed. Previous studies have indicated a discrete dopaminergic innervation of this region in addition to the DA fibers traversing the area,[38,39] and a recent study has reported that the ventral pallidum receives projections from the RRF.[37] The A8 projections to the entorhinal and pyriform cortex are consistent with previous observations.[23] However, we did not observe neocortical projections of the A8 DA neurons, in contrast to the findings of Swanson;[23] this discrepancy may reflect our uncertainty concerning the assignment of the retrogradely labeled neurons to the A8 cell group.

RRF neurons were also noted to innervate a number of diencephalic sites, including the zona incerta, subthalamic nucleus, ventral thalamus, and lateral and dorsomedial hypothalamus. At present, we have no retrograde data on these projections. However, previous retrograde tracer studies indicate projections from the region of the RRF in the ventrolateral mesencephalic reticular formation to these diencephalic sites.[40,41]

It appears that the major telencephalic target of the A8 DA neurons is the striatum, including the ventral striatum (nucleus accumbens). A8 neurons project onto the nucleus accumbens and striatum in a topographically organized fashion; previous reports have also suggested that the striatal innervation derived from RRF neurons was topographically organized.[11,14] The RRF projections onto the striatum are heterogeneous and are characterized by distinct clusters of fibers surrounded by areas with relatively sparse RRF-derived input. Olson *et al.*[42] noted that the striatal DA innervation of the neonatal rat is heterogeneous, being comprised of highly fluorescent DA islands (the islandic or patch innervation) and a less-intensely fluorescent matrix compartment. In the adult rat the compartmental organization of the striatum is difficult to visualize in the adult rat using monoamine fluorescent histochemical methods or tyrosine hydroxylase immunohistochemistry; however, the patchy nature of the dopaminergic innervation of the rat striatum is clearly visible when examined with DA immunohistochemistry,[38] or after pharmacological manipulation.[43,44] The patchy nature of the striatal dopaminergic innervation is prominent in adult primates and felines. Graybiel and associates[37,45-49] and Gerfen and co-workers[36,50-53] have characterized the histochemical compartmentalization of the striatum. Both groups have recently reported that the A8 DA neurons project predominantly to the matrix compartment of the striatum.[36,37]

These recent studies suggest that the compartmental organization of the striatum is paralleled by a spatial and biochemical heterogeneity of midbrain DA neurons. Thus, Jimenez-Castellanos and Graybiel[37] have reported that whereas the A8 neurons contribute to the striatal matrix, a distinct (caudal and medial) group of A9 neurons appears to project predominantly to the striosomal (patch) striatal compartment of the cat. Furthermore, the midbrain correspondents of striatal histochemical compartments can be defined on biochemical grounds, for example, those midbrain DA neurons that innervate the striatal matrix contain a 28 kDa calcium binding protein.[36] Recent data suggest that the A8 DA neurons may be preferentially vulnerable to the neurotoxic actions of 1-methyl-4-phenyl-1,2,3,6-tetrahydropyridine[54] (MPTP). Since the A8 neurons appear to contribute to the matrix compartment of the striatum, the finding that A8 neurons differ from most other midbrain neurons in their susceptibility to an environmental insult may indicate that the patch and matrix compartments of the striatum may be functionally dissociated. The definition of distinct aggregates of midbrain DA neurons on the basis of efferent projections and on the basis of such features as transmitter colocalization, occurrence of non-transmitter proteins, presence of transmitter receptors, and other biochemical markers will clearly be a hallmark of future attempts to classify the midbrain DA neurons. The definition of distinct subsets of midbrain DA neurons on the basis of biochemical characteristics suggests that functional domains of neuronal systems will not be defined on gross hodological grounds, but will require the placement of these neurons into a hierarchical classification system recognizing biochemical and molecular characteristics.[55] For example, we have previously suggested that the DA neurons of the SN pars lateralis may constitute a functional subset of the A8, rather than A9, cell group; this suggestion was based on similarities in the biochemical responsiveness of these neurons to neuroleptics and the efferent projections of these neurons.[56] However, Jimenez-Castellanos and Graybiel[37] noted that the pars lateralis DA neurons contribute to both the matrix and striosomal striatal compartments, and can thus be differentiated from the A8 DA neurons. These data, in conjunction with assessment of such features as incorporation of precursor into these neurons,[57] the responses of these neurons to environmental and pharmacological challenges,[54,56] and the behavior subserved by these neurons [for example, what are the midbrain correspondents of the striatal sector in which local injections of amphetamine can elicit stereotypy? (see Kelley et al.[58])] will be required to unravel the rationale underlying the organization of midbrain DA neurons.

The classical organization scheme for the functional compartmentalization of the striatum is based on the observation that there are topographically organized projections from the entire cortical mantle onto the striatum. Thus, the motor cortex of the rat projects to the dorsolateral striatum, whereas the prelimbic cortex innervates the medial striatum.[59] A broad functional organization along similar lines has been proposed for the DA innervations of the striatum: a lateral striatal DA innervation derived from the SN, subserving motoric acts and sensorimotor integration, and the ventromedial striatal (including the nucleus accumbens) DA input, derived from the VTA, involved in motivation and affect.[60] The A8 DA projections appear to be unique in that they clearly contribute to both the "motor" and "limbic" striatum. As such, the A8 DA neurons may be situated in a key position to regulate activity within both striatal domains. It is not known if the A8 DA neurons collateralize to innervate both ventromedial and dorsolateral striatal sites, or alternatively if A8 DA neurons are electrotonically coupled as are certain nigral DA neurons;[61] both mechanisms could subserve simultaneous regulation of different striatal sectors.

The regulation of both limbic and motor striatal sectors by the A8 DA neurons may be mirrored by a larger degree of interrelationships between the mesocorticolimbic and nigrostriatal DA systems. The interconnections of the midbrain DA neurons provides a mechanism whereby the functional activity within one DA system either influences or is influenced by the activity of another DA system. For example, the impetus ("motivation") to execute a motor act may occur at the level of the terminal fields, or alternatively via regulation of the firing rate or pattern of neuronal activity of nigral (dorsolateral striatal–motor) neurons by RRF or VTA (ventromedial striatal–motivational) DA neurons. It is not clear to what degree the interconnections of the midbrain DA neurons represent collateralized projections, such that an axon ascending to a forebrain site collateralizes to innervate certain mesencephalic DA neurons; local circuit interactions via the long dendritic trees of many DA neurons[62-64] may provide another avenue for interdependence in the functional activity of midbrain DA cells. Whatever varieties of anatomical arrangements subserve the interrelationships of the midbrain

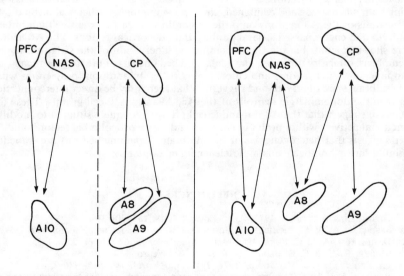

**FIGURE 13.** Schematic depiction of the interrelationships of the A8, A9, and A10 DA cell groups of the ventral mesencephalon. The original conception of the organization of the midbrain DA neurons and their efferent targets is shown in the left; the A8 cell group was thought to represent a dorsal extension of the A9 neurons of the SN and project solely to the striatum (CP). Current data suggest that there is a substantial degree of overlap of the midbrain DA cell body regions onto the telencephalic terminal fields, such that the A10 neurons provide a large part of the DA innervation of the meso(neo)cortical system (such as the prefrontal cortex, PFC) and the mesolimbic system (such as the nucleus accumbens, NAS); there is also a substantial (not shown) projection from the A10 cell group to the striatum. The A9 neurons of the SN innervate both the striatal and mesolimbic areas, the latter to a lesser degree; there is also a small nigral projection to the neocortex (e.g., anterior cingulate cortex). The A8 DA neurons provide part of the mesolimbic and striatal dopaminergic innervations. Reciprocal projections from the terminal field areas also integrate the midbrain DA system, as do direct interconnections between the DA cell body areas. These data suggest the function of an integrated mesotelencephalic DA system.

DA neurons, it is becoming increasingly clear that a view encompassing independent mesolimbic, mesocortical, and nigrostriatal DA systems no longer is appropriate. Rather, heterogeneities of the midbrain DA neurons appear to be embedded within a larger homogeneous mesotelencephalic system with integrative properties.

The A8 DA neurons may represent loci of integration of limbic and striatal information within the larger mesotelencephalic DA system. Originally conceptualized as an extension of the substantia nigra, the A8 DA cell group appears to share projections and perhaps functional attributes with both the SN and the VTA, mirroring the interrelationships that occur at the terminal field level (see FIG. 13). The elucidation of the organizing principles that govern the functional array designated the mesotelencephalic DA system will require the understanding of the hierarchy of features, including intrinsic regulatory controls, common to all DA neurons, as well as the features defining distinct subsets of midbrain DA neurons.

# SUMMARY

The telencephalic projections of the A8 dopamine cell group of the rat were assessed using both anterograde and combined retrograde–immunohistochemical methods. The projections of the A8 neurons onto the forebrain were more extensive than hitherto realized, and encompassed striatal, limbic, and allocortical regions. The A8 neurons were shown to contribute to the dopaminergic innervation of the striatum, nucleus accumbens, olfactory tubercles, amygdala, and bed nucleus of the stria terminalis, and also innervate the pyriform and entorhinal cortices. In addition, projections within the midbrain were observed, and suggested that there may be direct interconnections between the dopaminergic neurons of the A8, A9, and A10 cell groups. These data therefore suggest that the A8 dopamine cell group is uniquely situated to modulate functional activity within both nigrostriatal and mesocorticolimbic regions, and further suggests that heterogeneities of the midbrain dopamine neurons are embedded within a larger homogeneous mesotelencephalic dopamine system.

## REFERENCES

1. OLSON, L. & A. SEIGER. 1972. Anat. Entwick.-Ges. **137**: 301–316.
2. SPECHT, L. A., V. M. PICKEL, T. H. JOH & D. J. REIS. 1981. J. Comp. Neurol. **199**: 255–276.
3. DAHLSTROM, A. & K. FUXE. 1964. Acta Physiol. Scand. **62** (Suppl. 232): 1–55.
4. MOORE, R. Y. & F. E. BLOOM. 1978. Ann. Rev. Neurosci. **1**: 129–169.
5. FALLON, J. H. & R. Y. MOORE. 1978. J. Comp. Neurol. **180**: 545–580.
6. BERMAN, A. L. 1968. The Brainstem of the Cat. A Cytoarchitectonic Atlas with Stereotaxic Coordinates. Univ. of Wisconsin Press. Madison.
7. LINDVALL, O. & A. BJORKLUND. 1984. Dopamine-containing systems in the CNS. *In* Handbook of Chemical Neuroanatomy, vol. 2: Classical Transmitters in the CNS, Part I. A. Bjorklund & T. Hokfelt, Eds.: 55–122. Elsevier, Amsterdam.
8. ROYCE, G. J. 1978. Brain Res. **153**: 465–475.
9. VANDERMAELEN, C. P., J. D. KOCSIS & S. T. KITAI. 1978. Brain Res. Bull. **3**: 639–644.
10. BENTIVOGLIO, M., D. VAN DER KOOY & H. G. J. M. KUYPERS. 1979. Brain Res. **174**: 1–17.
11. VAN DER KOOY, D. 1979. Brain Res. **169**: 381–387.
12. SZABO, J. 1980. Brain Res. **188**: 3–21.
13. SZABO, J. 1980. J. Comp. Neurol. **189**: 307–321.
14. VEENING, J. G., F. M. CORNELISSEN & P. A. J. M. LIEVEN. 1980. Neuroscience **5**: 1253–1268.
15. PARENT, A., A. MACKEY & L. DE BELLEFEUILLE. 1983. Neuroscience **10**: 1137–1150.
16. MORGAN, S., H. STEINER, C. ROSENKRANZ & J. P. JUSTON. 1986. Neuroscience **17**: 609–614.

17. NAUTA, W. J. H., G. P. SMITH, R. L. M. FAULL & V. B. DOMESICK. 1978. Neuroscience **3:** 385–401.
18. GROENEWEGEN, H. J., N. E. H. M. BECKER & A. H. M. LOHMAN. 1980. Neuroscience **5:** 1903–1916.
19. JAEGER, C. B., T. H. JOH & D. J. REIS. 1983. J. Comp. Neurol. **218:** 74–90.
20. DEUTCH, A. Y., M. GOLDSTEIN, B. S. BUNNEY & R. H. ROTH. 1984. Soc. Neurosci. Abst. **10:** 9.
21. PHILLIPSON, O. T. & A. C. GRIFFITH. 1985. Neuroscience **16:** 275–296.
22. LENARD, L. & W. J. H. NAUTA. 1979. Neurosci. Lett. Suppl. 3: S52.
23. SWANSON, L. W. 1982. Brain Res. Bull. **9:** 321–353.
24. KOHLER, C. & M. GOLDSTEIN. 1984. J. Comp. Neurol. **223:** 302–311.
25. HOKFELT, T., O. JOHANSSON, K. FUXE, M. GOLDSTEIN & D. PARK. 1977. Med. Biol. **55:** 21–40.
26. FELTEN, D. L. & J. R. SLADEK, JR. 1983. Brain Res. **10:** 171–284.
27. PEARSON, J., M. GOLDSTEIN, K. MARKEY & L. BRANDEIS. 1983. Neuroscience **8:** 3–32.
28. GASPAR, P., B. BERGER, M. GAY, M. HAMON, F. CESSELIN, A. VIGNY, F. JAVOY-AGID & Y. AGID. 1983. J. Neurol. Sci. **58:** 247–267.
29. NICOLESCO, J. & C. FOIX. 1925. Anatomie Cerebrale — Les Noyaux Gris Centraux et la Region Mesencephalo-sous-optique. Masson, Paris.
30. HOKFELT, T., B. J. EVERITT, E. THEDORSSON-NORHEIM & M. GOLDSTEIN. 1984. J. Comp. Neurol. **222:** 543–559.
31. GERFEN, C. R. & P. E. SAWCHENKO. 1985. Brain Res. **343:** 144–150.
32. LINDVALL, O. & A. BJORKLUND. 1974. Acta Physiol. Scand. (Supp. 412): 1–48.
33. WOUTERLOOD, F. G. & H. J. GROENEWEGEN. 1985. Brain Res. **326:** 188–191.
34. PHILLIPSON, O. T. 1979. J. Comp. Neurol. **187:** 85–98.
35. SCHMUED, L. & J. H. FALLON. 1986. Brain Res. **337:** 147–154.
36. GERFEN, C. R., M. HERKENHAM & J. THIBAULT. 1987. J. Neurosci. **7:** 3915–3934.
37. JIMENEZ-CASTELLANOS, J. & A. GRAYBIEL. 1987. Neuroscience **23:** 223–242.
38. VOORN, P., B. JORRITSMA-BYHAM, C. VAN DIJK & R. M. BUIJS. 1986. J. Comp. Neurol. **251:** 84–99.
39. LINDVALL, O. & U. STENEVI. 1978. Cell. Tis. Res. **190:** 383–407.
40. SHAMMAH-LAGNADO, S. J., N. NEGRAO & J. A. RICARDO. 1985. Neuroscience **15:** 109–134.
41. ROGER, M. & J. CADUSSEAU. 1985. J. Comp. Neurol. **241:** 480–492.
42. OLSON, L., A. SEIGER & K. FUXE. 1972. Brain Res. **44:** 283–288.
43. FUXE, K., B. B. FEDHOLM, L. F. AGNATI & H. CORRODI. 1978. Brain Res. **146:** 295–311.
44. FUKUI, K., H. KARIYAMA, A. KASHIBA, N. KATO & H. KIMURA. 1986. Brain Res. **382:** 81–86.
45. GRAYBIEL, A. M. 1984. Neuroscience **13:** 1157–1187.
46. GRAYBIEL, A. M. & C. W. RAGSDALE, JR. 1978. Proc. Natl. Acad. Sci. U.S.A. **75:** 5723–5726.
47. GRAYBIEL, A. M. 1984. Neurochemically specified subsystems in the basal ganglia. *In* Functions of the Basal Ganglia. D. Evered and M. O'Connor, Eds.: 114–149. Ciba Foundation Symposium 107. Pitman. London.
48. GRAYBIEL, A. M. 1986. DA-containing innervation of the striatum: Subsystems and their striatal correspondents. *In* Recent Developments in PD. S. Fahn, C. D. Marsden, and P. Jenner, Eds.: 1–16. Raven Press. New York.
49. GRAYBIEL, A., E. C. HIRSCH & Y. A. AGID. 1987. Proc. Natl. Acad. Sci. U.S.A. **84:** 303–307.
50. GERFEN, C. R. 1984. Nature **311:** 461–464.
51. GERFEN, C. R. 1985. J. Comp. Neurol. **236:** 454–476.
52. GERFEN, C. R., K. G. BAIMBRIDGE & J. J. MILLER. 1985. Proc. Natl. Acad. Sci. U.S.A. **82:** 8780–8784.
53. GERFEN, C. R., K. G. BAIMBRIDGE & J. THIBAULT. 1987. J. Neurosci. **7:** 3935–3944.
54. DEUTCH, A. Y., J. D. ELSWORTH, M. GOLDSTEIN, K. FUXE, D. E. REDMOND, JR., J. R. SLADEK, JR., & R. H. ROTH. 1986. Neurosci. Lett. **68:** 51–56.
55. ROTH, R. H., M. E. WOLF & A. Y. DEUTCH. 1987. Neurochemistry of midbrain dopamine neurons. *In* Psychopharmacology. The Third Generation of Progress. H. Y. Meltzer, Ed.: 81–94. Raven Press. New York.
56. DEUTCH, A. Y., M. GOLDSTEIN & R. H. ROTH. 1985. Soc. Neurosci. Abstr. **11:** 208.
57. BUTCHER, L., J. ENGEL & K. FUXE. 1970. J. Pharm. Pharmacol. **22:** 313–317.
58. KELLEY, A. E., C. G. LANG & A. M. GAUTHIER. 1988. Psychopharmacology. In press.
59. DONOGHUE, J. P. & M. HERKENHAM. 1986. Brain Res. **365:** 397–403.

60. IVERSEN, S. D. 1984. Behavioral effects of manipulation of basal ganglia neurotransmitters. *In* Functions of the Basal Ganglia. D. Evered and M. O'Connor, Eds.: 183–195. Ciba Foundation Symposium 107. Pitman. London.
61. GRACE, A. A. & B. S. BUNNEY. 1983. Neuroscience **10:** 333–348.
62. JURASKA, J. M., C. J. WILSON & P. M. GROVES. 1977. J. Comp. Neurol. **172:** 585–600.
63. PRESTON, R. J., R. A. MCCREA, H. T. CHANG & S. T. KITAI. 1981. Neuroscience **6:** 331–344.
64. PHILLIPSON, O. T. 1979. Comp. Neurol. **187:** 99–116.

# In Vivo and in Vitro Intracellular Recordings from Rat Midbrain Dopamine Neurons[a]

ANTHONY A. GRACE[b]

*Departments of Behavioral Neuroscience and Psychiatry*
*University of Pittsburgh*
*Pittsburgh, Pennsylvania 15260*

## INTRODUCTION

The study of dopamine (DA) neuron activity using electrophysiological recording techniques has engendered significant contributions in advancing our understanding of the physiology of the nigrostriatal and mesolimbic dopaminergic systems. This has been particularly evident in studies related to the neuronal effects of therapeutic drug actions. Most of these studies have used extracellular recording techniques to ascertain the involvement of DA neurons in a variety of central drug effects, such as the amphetamine-induced inhibition of DA neuron firing via activation of striatonigral feedback loops,[1] the differential effects of acute and chronic neuroleptic administration on DA cell activity,[2] and the involvement of autoreceptors in the complementary behavioral effects produced by low versus high doses of the DA agonist apomorphine.[3] However, although extracellular recording proved useful in assessing how neuronal firing rates are affected by drugs and stimuli, this technique is nevertheless comparatively limited in its ability to address the actual mechanisms underlying these phenomena. In contrast, the application of intracellular recording techniques to the *in vivo* preparation enabled the investigation of DA system activity at this more basic level of analysis. Thus, the DA cell responses previously characterized during extracellular recording could be reexamined at the level of membrane voltage and conductance changes. *In vivo* intracellular recordings also allowed a direct correlation to be made between specific neuronal electrophysiological characteristics and neurochemically identified DA cells. This electrophysiological identification thus enabled DA cell identification in subsequent experiments to be based on this defined set of unique electrophysiological criteria. Moreover, initial studies on DA neuron action potential generation using intracellular recording techniques provided basic information on DA cell regulation that would have been difficult if not impossible to infer based solely on the information provided by extracellular recordings. This included the driving of spontaneous spike generation by an endogenous pacemakerlike slow depolarizing current, and the calcium-mediated transition of firing patterns from single spiking to burst firing.[4,5]

Despite the higher information content of data afforded by intracellular recordings in the intact preparation, the *in vivo* preparation nonetheless is constrained by the inability to conclusively determine the ionic mechanisms underlying these observa-

[a] This work was supported by U.S. Public Health Service Grants MH42217 and MH30915.
[b] The author is a Sloan Fellow.

51

tions. Thus, the limited access of the extracellular environment to experimental manipulations complicates the use of most ion channel blockers and prohibits alterations of extracellular ionic concentrations, thereby impeding precise determinations of the ionic currents of spike-generating regions underlying the cellular responses studied. Furthermore, it is often difficult to distinguish which responses are due to the direct actions of drugs on neurons versus those arising from the indirect actions induced by the drug on afferent neurotransmitter systems that may ultimately influence DA cell firing. These shortcomings were circumvented by the development of the *in vitro* brain slice technique, where neuronal physiology could be examined in an easily accessible, semi-isolated preparation. This methodology enabled the investigation of neuronal activity in a mechanically stable and accessible environment, while still preserving the morphological structure of the neuron and local synaptic and dendritic interactions with neighboring neurons. As applied to DA neurons, this preparation enabled more comprehensive and precise determination of the ionic conductance changes that occur in response to various neurotransmitters or drug administration. Furthermore, the direct effects of DA agonists, neuroleptics, and other drugs on DA cell responses could be determined without confounding influences from their indirect effects on striatonigral feedback loops or other afferent neurotransmitter systems.[6] However, this should not be taken to suggest that the *in vitro* technique alone is the single best approach to studying DA system electrophysiology. Indeed, with respect to the ultimate goals of this research — that is, an understanding of DA cell regulation in the behaving animal or its dysfunction in the psychiatric patient — the combination of information gained by these distinct techniques provides a more comprehensive model of DA cell function than could be obtained by the use of any single technique alone. This is a consequence of the unique perspective afforded by each preparation in examining *different* but *related* areas of DA cell function. Thus, extracellular recording *in vivo* has the advantage of sampling the responses of a large number of neurons to particular experimental manipulations without introducing artifacts due to neuron population bias, as can occur with intracellular recording, and without possible artifacts associated with electrode impalement. In contrast, *in vivo* intracellular recording permits analysis of the changes in membrane potentials that underlie DA cell responses while the neurons are in their normal cellular microenvironment, with intact afferent processes and hormonal influences. This would be of particular significance in the determination of changes in overall membrane conductance in response to systemic drug administration, chronic drug treatments, or stimulation of long-loop afferent processes, factors that are particularly important in assessing the neuropharmacological actions of drugs on brain systems. Finally, *in vitro* recording facilitates the examination of direct drug actions on single neurons at the level of ion conductance changes, and without the potential artifacts arising from drug-induced changes in other associated brain regions. Thus, taken together, these preparations afford multiple levels of analyses for investigating DA and other neuronal systems that are unavailable when using any single technique alone, thereby yielding a more comprehensive picture of DA cell regulation.

The following review concentrates on results obtained using intracellular recording techniques. The interested reader is directed to other reviews for information dealing with extracellular recordings of DA cell physiology.[7,8] Information gained from each of the intracellular recording preparations are presented in the following sections on DA cell regulation. The *in vivo* intracellular recording data are drawn from the cited publications, and the *in vitro* electrophysiology is derived from more recent work presented at symposiums[6,9,10] or that are currently in preparation for publication. With regard to the location of the neurons recorded, both nigral and ventral tegmental DA neurons were used in this analysis, since no obvious differences in their properties with respect to the characteristics examined here were noted. Thus, any differences between these classes of DA cells with regard to basic DA cell physiology or firing characteristics may arise more from their interconnections than from differences in the basic neuronal properties reviewed here.

## GENERAL CONSIDERATIONS

Dopamine neurons recorded intracellularly in the substantia nigra (SN) and in the ventral tegmental area (VTA) of albino male rats displayed significantly different properties when recorded in the *in vivo* preparation versus those observed *in vitro*. In both preparations, only cells with stable membrane potentials and firing patterns were used in the data analysis. Due to the inherent difficulties with the physical stability of the *in vivo* preparation, the frequency of obtaining stable intracellular impalements was comparatively low. Nonetheless, when stable penetrations were achieved, they could be maintained for an extended period of time (up to 2.5 hours), during which the DA neurons were firing spontaneously with firing rates, patterns, and action potential durations equivalent to those recorded extracellularly from identified DA neurons.[11,12] Furthermore, computer differentiation of the intracellular action potentials produced waveforms that were identical to those observed during extracellular recordings from DA neurons.[11,12] Since the extracellularly recorded current transients should be equivalent to the first derivative, or rate of change, of intracellularly recorded membrane voltages,[13,14,15] DA neurons injured by electrode penetration should have alterations in their differentiated spike waveforms and waveform durations resembling those seen in injured neurons recorded extracellularly — that is, increasingly longer duration action potentials with rapidly decreasing amplitudes. Injured neurons would also show marked alterations in firing rates and patterns from those typically observed *in vivo* during extracellular recording, such as an acceleration of firing rates and atypically short (i.e., <50 msec) interspike intervals, progressing to a cessation of spontaneous activity. In addition, cell injury during intracellular recording would yield unstable, decaying membrane potentials and declining input resistances. Since none of these artifacts were observed in the DA neuron penetrations meeting our stability criteria,[11] indications are that the DA neurons recorded intracellularly *in vivo* had penetrations of sufficient stability to ensure the collection of highly reproducible data. The reported higher input resistances, larger amplitude/shorter duration action potentials, and absence of spike pattern variations in DA cells recorded *in vitro* is most likely due to the altered cellular environment or absence of afferent neurotransmitters.

## DOPAMINE CELL IDENTIFICATION

In attempting to correlate electrophysiological recordings of neuronal activity with drug-induced changes in postsynaptic neurotransmitter release measured biochemically, it is necessary to first verify that the class of cells being recorded are indeed the neurons that contain and release the particular neurotransmitter under investigation. Using *in vivo* intracellular recordings, the dopaminergic identity of a subset of midbrain neurons was directly confirmed by neurochemically identifying single neurons injected intracellularly with neurotransmitter-specific marker compounds. This was done by taking advantage of a histochemical technique whereby the catecholamines within neurons are caused to fluoresce after treatment with glyoxylic acid,[16] the resultant fluorescent intensity of the neurons being proportional to the amount of catecholamine the neurons contain. Thus, after injecting putative DA neurons intracellularly with the DA precursor L-DOPA, it was possible to directly verify the dopaminergic identity of these single electrophysiologically defined cells based on their increased

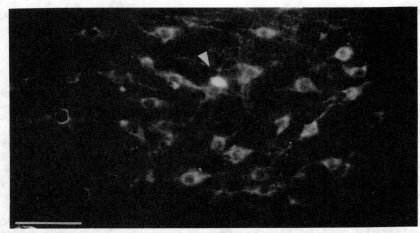

**FIGURE 1.** Identification of DA neurons by *in vivo* intracellular labeling and catecholamine histofluorescence. Treatment of slices of rat midbrain with glyoxylic acid causes the DA contained in midbrain DA neurons to fluoresce when examined under a fluorescence microscope. Intracellular injection of the DA precursor L-DOPA into substantia nigra neurons induces increased levels of DA only when injected into the DA-containing neurons of this region. This results in a dramatically increased level of fluorescent intensity within the DA neuron injected with the L-DOPA (*arrow*) as compared to the noninjected neighboring DA neurons fluorescing at their more typical levels of intensity. The fact that only neurons in the substantia nigra showing a distinctive electrophysiological pattern demonstrated enhanced fluorescence levels after L-DOPA injection confirmed the validity of DA cell identification based on a defined set of electrophysiological criteria. (Calibration bar = 50 µm)

fluorescent intensity as compared to that of the noninjected neighboring DA neurons[17] (FIG. 1). This was further substantiated by intracellular injection of one of two other compounds that also selectively increase the fluorescent intensity of the injected DA neurons by increasing intraneuronal DA levels. These compounds were (1) tetrahydrobiopterin, the cofactor for the rate-limiting catecholamine synthetic enzyme tyrosine hydroxylase, and (2) colchicine, to interfere with cellular transport mechanisms and thus cause a buildup of DA and tyrosine hydroxylase in the soma of the impaled cell. As predicted, in each experiment where one of these compounds was injected intracellularly into a neuron within the SN exhibiting the characteristic electrophysiological criteria associated with DA neurons, a single DA neuron displaying markedly enhanced levels of fluorescence was observed within a field of normally fluorescing DA neurons.[18]

Further evidence of the dopaminergic identity of these neurons was gathered based on additional criteria, such as verification of the anatomical location and morphology of DA neurons after intracellular staining, antidromic activation from postsynaptic targets in the striatum[11,12] or prefrontal cortex[18] at their characteristically slow axonal conduction velocity,[19] and their sensitivity to dopamine agonists.[20] Together, these studies directly demonstrated that recordings were made from a single neurochemical class of midbrain neurons containing DA. Futhermore, differentiation of the intracellular action potential in order to obtain a representation of the equivalent extracellularly recorded spike, as previously described, revealed the classically described DA neuron extracellular action potential waveform: a notch in the positive phase of the spike that corresponded to a delay between firing of the initial segment (IS) and somatodendritic (SD) components of the action potential, and the prominent negative component of the extracellular spike that arose from the slow repolarization phase of the action potential,[12] as reviewed in the CONCLUSIONS section of this paper. This finding substantiated earlier correlations of spike waveforms and DA neuron activity based on extracellular recordings in this brain region.[21]

## MORPHOLOGY OF DOPAMINE NEURONS

Intracellular injections of highly fluorescent dyes, such as Lucifer yellow,[22] have facilitated the analysis of single neuron morphology in brain tissues. Lucifer yellow injections have been used to investigate the morphology of DA cells in both the *in vivo*[12] and *in vitro*[6,10,27] preparations. Using the *in vitro* brain slice for morphological studies of this type has the advantages of being able to visually identify the locations of neurons before intracellular staining, and allowing examination of the morphology of intact cells within the brain slice without serial sectioning or reconstruction. In this study, DA neurons could be subdivided based on their morphology and the brain regions in which the neurons were located. The more dorsal, limbic-related[23] SN DA neurons typically exhibited smaller, fusiform somata about 15–30 μm in length, with beaded dendrites radiating from the neuronal poles and extending along the dorsal/ventral confines of the zona compacta (FIG. 2A). The more ventral nigrostriatal neurons, in contrast, had multipolar somata 20–35 μm in diameter with 3 to 5 major dendrites arising from the soma and, unlike the more dorsal fusiform neurons, had at least one major dendritic branch that extended deep into the zona reticulata (FIG. 2B). In the VTA, both fusiform and multipolar neurons were observed, with 2 to 5 fascicles of dendrites emanating in a more or less radial array from the soma (FIG. 2C). In all of the stained DA cells observed, the axons arose from major dendrites rather than directly from the soma. This morphology probably underlies the low conduction safety factor between the IS and SD spike components. Thus, only the IS spike is typically driven by antidromic activation, due to the inability of the IS spike to trigger the SD spike without concurrent depolarization of the soma by the slow depolarization.[12]

## BASIC PROPERTIES

Although DA neurons recorded intracellularly in both preparations exhibited the distinctive slow depolarization preceding spontaneous action potentials, other electrophysiological characteristics showed markedly different attributes when recorded *in vitro*. The input resistance of dopamine neurons recorded *in vivo* averaged 31 ± 7 megohms[11] (FIG. 3A) with action potential amplitudes in spontaneously firing cells reaching amplitudes of 60–65 mV. The input resistance of DA cells *in vitro*, on the other hand, ranged from 100 to 350 megohms (MΩ)[9,10] (FIG. 3B), which is 5 to 10 times higher than that observed in intact animals, but similar to other reports of input resistances of SN zona compacta neurons recorded *in vitro*.[24–27] Furthermore, the action potentials were generally 70–90 mV in amplitude in the slice. Although one may infer that a comparatively less stable penetration of the DA neurons in the *in vivo* preparation could account for these differences, the evidence indicates that poor penetration could not adequately account for the marked discrepancies observed, given the evidence just presented. Interestingly, intracellular injection of the calcium chelator EGTA into DA cells *in vivo* altered their electrophysiological characteristics in such a way as to make the firing pattern and action potential amplitudes resemble those observed *in vitro* — that is, an invariant pacemaker firing pattern with action potentials more than 80 mV in amplitude.[4] The common attributes underlying the similari-

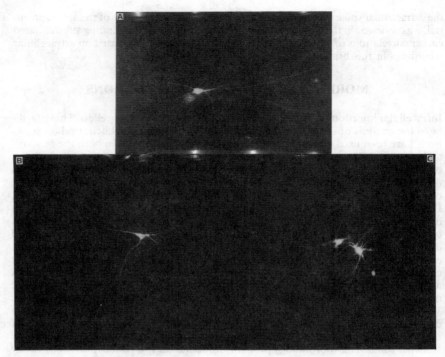

**FIGURE 2.** The morphology of physiologically identified DA neurons can be examined after intracellular injection of highly fluorescent dyes, such as Lucifer yellow. DA neurons in the substantia nigra can be subdivided into two classes based on their morphology: (**A**) the more dorsal DA neurons that project primarily to limbic regions of the brain are fusiform in shape, with their dendrites oriented mediolaterally, running parallel to and contained within the confines of the zona compacta region; and (**B**) the more ventral nigrostriatal DA neurons that are multipolar in shape and that, in addition to having dendrites oriented along the zona compacta, also have one or more dendritic fascicles extending ventrally into the zona reticulata. (**C**) In contrast, the somata of ventral tegmented DA neurons are either fusiform or multipolar in shape, with dendrites emanating from the somata in a more radial pattern. Two neurons were recovered from injections in the ventral tegmentum, although it could not be confirmed that this resulted from injection of a single neuron. Within each brain region studied, DA cell axons were found to arise from a major dendrite or somatic appendage rather than directly from the soma.

ties in firing regulation between these two dissimilar preparations has not as yet been fully analyzed.

The apparent spike threshold for DA neuron action potentials measured at the soma occurs at significantly more depolarized levels than those reported for other mammalian neurons. DA cell thresholds average $-41 \pm 4$ mV (mean $\pm$ SD) *in vivo*, although somewhat more variation in threshold levels were noted *in vitro*, with some spontaneously firing cells having thresholds above $-35$ mV. Hyperpolarizing pulses revealed the presence of two voltage-sensitive outward currents in both preparations, although they were somewhat more pronounced in the *in vitro* case owing to the higher membrane resistance. These currents were: a rapidly developing anomalous rectification, revealed by the sag in the membrane potential response to injection of a hyper-

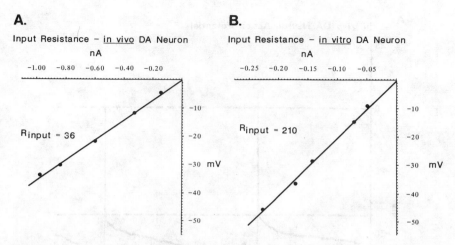

**FIGURE 3.** The membrane resistance of DA neurons can be estimated by calculating the overall input resistance of the cell. The input resistance is derived from the slope of the line relating the amplitude of intracellularly injected hyperpolarizing current pulses to the membrane voltage deflections produced. (**A**) DA neurons *in vivo* typically exhibit input resistances between 20 and 50 MΩ. In this case, the peak input resistance of the DA neuron was 36 MΩ. (**B**) In contrast, DA neurons penetrated in the *in vitro* brain slice have input resistances ranging from 100 to 300 MΩ, or about 3 to 5 times higher than those recorded *in vivo*. The DA neuron examined here exhibited an input resistance of 210 MΩ, necessitating the use of much lower amplitude current injection pulses than in part (**A**).

polarizing current pulse; and a time- and voltage-dependent putative $A$ current ($I_A$), which delayed repolarization to resting potentials after the offset of a hyperpolarizing pulse. The identity of this $I_A$ in DA cells is considered tentative at present, given the inability to block this conductance pharmacologically using 4-aminopyridine.[28-30] The significance of these currents as they relate to DA cell activity are reviewed below.

## PACEMAKER POTENTIALS AND AFTERHYPERPOLARIZATIONS

The spontaneous activity of DA neurons appears to be regulated by the interaction of two transmembrane currents: an inward voltage-sensitive pacemaker current (slow depolarization) that depolarizes the membrane to spike threshold, and an outward calcium-activated potassium current responsible for postspike afterhyperpolarization (AHP). However, these currents appear to affect DA cell firing differently in the two preparations.

### In Vivo *Recordings*

Most of the DA neurons recorded intracellularly and extracellularly *in vivo* were spontaneously active, with the extended repolarization phase of intracellularly recorded action potentials giving rise to the prominent negative component of extracellularly recorded spikes. Furthermore, DA cells *in vivo* exhibited a diversity of firing patterns,

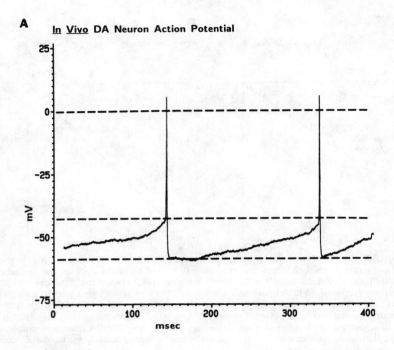

**A** In _Vivo_ DA Neuron Action Potential

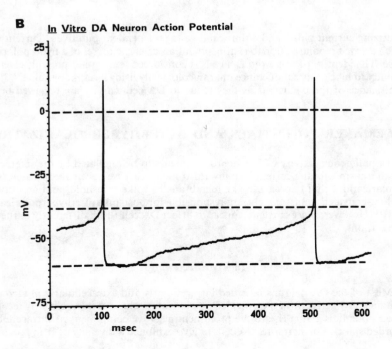

**B** In _Vitro_ DA Neuron Action Potential

ranging from irregular single spiking to burst firing.[4,5] Spontaneous activity was driven by a self-generated slow depolarization, which is the most distinctive feature of DA neuron action potentials recorded intracellularly in spontaneously firing DA neurons. This slow depolarization has many characteristics in common with the pacemaker potentials described in various invertebrate neurons.[31] It is a long-duration pacemakerlike depolarization, which depolarizes the DA neuron membrane potential from a resting potential of about $-55 \pm 3$ mV (mean $\pm$ SD) to a spike threshold of $-41 \pm 4$ mV[4] (FIG. 4A), that is comparatively high with respect to mammalian neurons investigated to date. *In vivo*, this slow depolarization typically began $80 \pm 40$ msec prior to the action potential, and attained amplitudes averaging $14 \pm 3$ mV. The slow depolarizations are endogenously generated by the DA cell rather than by synaptic input, since their expression is regulated by the membrane potential — that is, the rate of activation of the slow depolarization is proportional to the membrane potential, they can be triggered by depolarizing pulses, and hyperpolarizing pulses reset the ongoing depolarizations back to the resting membrane potential.[4]

Due to the comparatively depolarized spike threshold (at least as measured at the soma) and consequently the amount of current required to depolarize the DA cell membrane from resting potentials to this threshold (i.e., 10–15 mV of depolarization), it is apparent that this slow depolarization actually *drives* the firing of the DA neuron. Indeed, this self-generated rhythmicity may be a major factor enabling transplanted DA neurons to supply DA to denervated striata in the absence of an afferent excitatory drive. This may also account for the conspicuous absence of spontaneous excitatory postsynaptic potentials (EPSPs) during intracellular recordings from DA neurons, although in the *in vivo* preparation there is a notable presence of a continuous bombardment of chloride-mediated inhibitory postsynaptic potentials (IPSPs).[32] Thus, the evidence collected to date suggests that DA neuron activity is self-driven, with its firing rate modulated primarily in an inhibitory manner by afferent inputs,[32] although a slower peptide-mediated excitation has not been ruled out. The importance of this slow depolarization in driving DA cell firing could make its site of generation an important region for afferent regulation of DA cell activity.

The action potentials triggered by these slow depolarizations are followed by a prominent AHP, which is at least partially mediated by a calcium-activated potassium current ($I_{K(Ca)}$).[33] In the *in vivo* preparation, it is this current that appears to break the pacemaker pattern into an irregular, single-spike firing pattern.[4] Thus, during *in vivo* recordings from DA neurons, intracellular injection of sufficient amounts of the calcium chelator EGTA to prevent spike AHPs led to a transformation from the irregular firing pattern into a pacemaker pattern, as well as increasing the action potential amplitude by 20 mV or more[4] (FIG. 5A).

A second firing pattern observed *in vivo* was one of burst firing, in which DA neurons

---

◄FIGURE 4. The generation of spontaneous action potentials appears to be regulated by similar processes in both the *in vivo* and the *in vitro* preparations. (A) *In vivo* intracellular recordings revealed that DA neuron action potentials are driven by a slow depolarization preceding spontaneous spikes, which brings the membrane potential from its resting level ($-55$ to $-60$ mV) to the comparatively high spike threshold characteristically observed in these cells (i.e., $-40$ to $-45$ mV). The spikes are followed by an AHP, which resets the membrane potential to resting levels prior to the initiation of the next slow depolarization. (B) In a similar manner, DA neurons recorded *in vitro* are also driven by the slow depolarization. The slow depolarization has a more uniform rate of rise with a duration close to that of the interspike interval, and is larger in amplitude due to the more negative membrane potentials typically recorded in DA neurons *in vitro*. The action potentials and the spike AHPs are also larger in amplitude in the *in vitro* preparation.

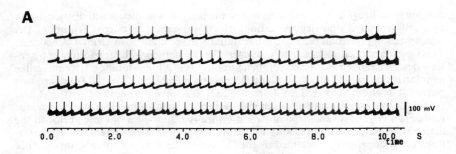

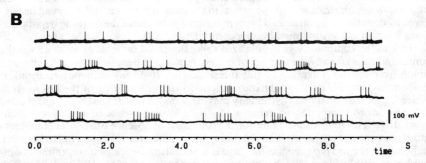

**FIGURE 5.** The firing pattern of DA neurons recorded *in vivo* is regulated by intracellular calcium. DA neurons recorded *in vivo* typically fire in two different spike patterns: an irregular single spiking pattern and burst firing. The irregular firing pattern arises from an interaction of the slow depolarizing pacemaker current and the calcium-mediated AHP. Blockade of the AHP by intracellular injection of increasing amounts of the calcium chelator EGTA (electrodes contained 0.1 M EGTA in 3 M potassium acetate) transforms the irregular firing pattern (**A:** *first trace*) into a regular, pacemakerlike pattern (**A:** *last trace*). In contrast, intracellular injection of calcium by diffusion from a calcium-containing electrode (20 mM calcium chloride in 3 M potassium acetate) causes a transition from the irregular spike pattern of discharge (**B:** *first trace*) to one of burst firing (**B**). Tracings are representative 9–10 sec segments of *in vivo* intracellular recordings taken over a 15–20 min period show the progressive change in firing patterns induced.

fire spikes in groups of 3 to 8 action potentials of decreasing amplitude and increasing duration (FIG. 5B). This firing pattern showed little dependency on the baseline firing rate, although increases in activity typically caused a transition into the burst firing mode.[5] This alteration of firing pattern was probably triggered by increasing levels of calcium entry into the DA neurons as a consequence of increased spike firing. Thus, burst firing was initiated in DA cells *in vivo* by intracellular injections of calcium (FIG. 5B), whereas intracellular injections of EGTA prevented cell depolarization from eliciting the burst firing patterns.

### In Vitro *Recordings*

As observed *in vivo*, most DA neurons recorded *in vitro* exhibited spontaneous activity. The DA neurons *in vitro* were also driven by a pacemaker current with similar voltage-dependent properties (FIG. 4B). However, despite the presence of a prominent

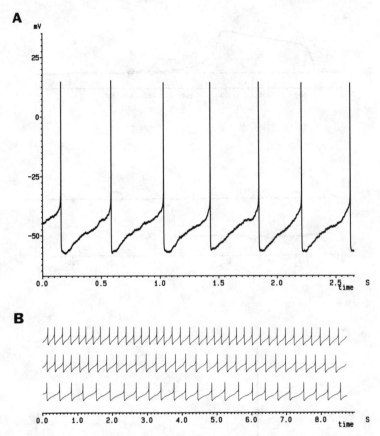

**FIGURE 6.** DA neuron firing pattern recorded *in vitro*. (**A**) In contrast to the varied firing patterns recorded *in vivo*, DA neurons recorded in the *in vitro* preparation fire exclusively in a very regular pacemaker pattern. (**B**) This pacemaker pattern is not affected by alterations in membrane potential, since depolarization (*upper trace*) or hyperpolarization (*lower trace*) of the membrane by current injection only alters the firing rate of the DA neuron without altering the highly uniform pacemaker pattern of discharge observed in the resting state (*center trace*; spike peaks are truncated by chart recorder).

$I_{K(Ca)}$ in DA neurons in this preparation neither the irregular firing pattern nor burst firing was observed. Instead, only a markedly uniform pacemaker pattern of spike discharge was encountered[6,10,25-27] (FIG. 6A). This pacemaker pattern is quite similar to the very regular firing pattern observed *in vivo* following intracellular injection of EGTA, as previously reviewed. Also, whereas depolarization did increase the spontaneous firing rate of DA neurons recorded *in vitro*, it did not alter the firing pattern, as shown for depolarization of DA neurons *in vivo*.[5] Instead, depolarization only produced a faster pacemaker pattern (FIG. 6B). The slow depolarization, in agreement with the *in vivo* data, is also voltage-dependent, since (1) it can be triggered by depolarizing pulses (FIG. 7A) or by the rebound of hyperpolarizing pulses (FIG. 7B),

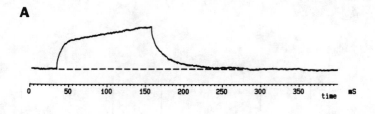

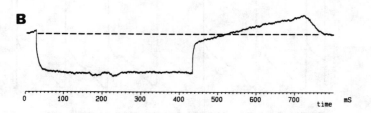

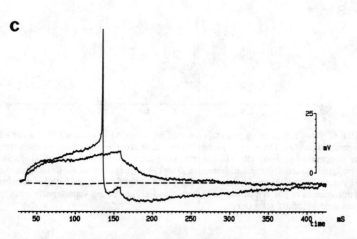

**FIGURE 7.** Voltage and ionic dependency of the slow depolarization recorded *in vitro*. The slow depolarization can be triggered in a quiescent DA neuron by intracellular injection of a depolarizing pulse (**A**). In this example, the slow depolarization does not return to baseline until 100 msec following the termination of the depolarizing pulse. The slow depolarization can also be triggered by the rebound from the offset of a hyperpolarizing current pulse (**B**). This pacemakerlike current can be reset to baseline levels by injecting hyperpolarizing current pulses (not shown) or by the AHP following an action potential (**C**). The slow depolarization is mediated by an inward sodium current, since it can be blocked by administration of the sodium channel blocker tetrodotoxin (TTX) to the Ringer's solution ($D_1$, $D_2$). After TTX application, a small-amplitude, low-threshold calcium current also triggered by the depolarizing pulse is revealed ($D_2$, *dashed line*).

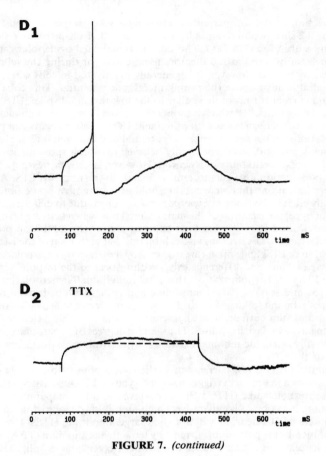

**FIGURE 7.** *(continued)*

and (2) it can be reset to resting membrane potentials by a hyperpolarizing pulse or the AHP from an action potential (FIG. 7C).

The *in vitro* preparation permitted a rigorous examination of the membrane conductance changes underlying this slow depolarization. Thus, administration of the sodium channel blocker tetrodotoxin (TTX) into the superfusion medium resulted in blockade of spontaneously occurring slow depolarizations (FIG. 7D$_1$ and D$_2$), providing strong evidence that the slow depolarization is mediated by an inward sodium current. Blockade of the slow depolarization also revealed a second voltage-dependent inward current, which is discussed below.

## LOW- AND HIGH-THRESHOLD CALCIUM CURRENTS

The greater accessibility of the *in vitro* preparation allows one to examine the ionic components of membrane currents after selective ion channel blockade, thereby enabling dissection of the ion currents underlying a given response. Thus, following blockade of the slow depolarization by TTX, a second, TTX-insensitive slow inward current can be observed (FIG.7D$_2$). This current is activated by depolarization of the DA neuron from hyperpolarized membrane potentials or during the rebound from hyperpolarizing pulses. However, it is generally inactivated in cells where the membrane potential is at or above the resting membrane potential. This cobalt-sensitive slow calcium current is thus quite similar to the low-threshold spike (LTS) described by Llinás and colleagues,[34–38] which is thought to be found only in mammalian neurons. As shown in other neuron types with prominent LTSs, these currents can profoundly alter the relationship between membrane potential and cell excitability. Hyperpolarization in many preparations is commonly believed to inhibit spontaneous firing and decrease the state of excitability of a neuron. However, in cells expressing a prominent LTS, hyperpolarization also acts to remove inactivation from this LTS. As a consequence, depolarizations that were subthreshold at resting membrane potentials will preferentially elicit spike firing in *hyperpolarized* neurons due to deinactivation of the LTS by prior hyperpolarization of the membrane. Thus, when activated from a hyperpolarized level, the LTS will more than compensate for the inhibition produced by the hyperpolarization. DA neurons also exhibit this deinactivation of the LTS by hyperpolarization, since LTSs and spiking are triggered by the offset of hyperpolarizing pulses. Nonetheless, a significant difference exists with respect to the responsiveness of the DA neuron LTS to hyperpolarization; that is, although small hyperpolarizations elicit rebound LTSs and spiking, larger amplitude hyperpolarizations instead result in an *attenuation* of rebound spiking (FIG. 8). This is apparently due to activation of a voltage-dependent potassium current, with characteristics similar to the $A$ current ($I_A$), following strong hyperpolarizing pulses. Thus, larger degrees of hyperpolarization in DA neurons actually attenuate rebound excitation by activating conductances that block activation of the LTS.[9,10]

Intracellular injection of currents of sufficient amplitude to strongly depolarize the membrane of a neuron can trigger a second type of TTX-insensitive spike, known as the high-threshold spike (HTS[38–42]). As observed in other preparations after TTX administration, injection of comparatively high-amplitude depolarizing current pulses into the somata of DA neurons will not elicit large-amplitude HTSs. However, after blockade of membrane potassium currents by tetraethylammonium (TEA), even lower amplitude depolarizing current pulses can readily trigger large-amplitude (>50 mV), cobalt-sensitive, all-or-none spikes (FIG. 9). This ability of TEA to decrease spike thresholds is dependent on the relative locations of the spike-generating sites of the neuron.[24] Analysis of DA neuron spike-generating regions using TEA is described in detail in the CONCLUSIONS section of this paper.

## PHARMACOLOGY OF THE DOPAMINE NEURON AUTORECEPTOR

Dopamine neurons are very sensitive to the inhibitory actions of DA and DA agonists, such as apomorphine, when they are applied to the DA cell body autoreceptor.[21] Indeed, systemically administered apomorphine acts preferentially on the DA cell body autoreceptor to inhibit DA cell firing at doses too low to exert an influence on postsynaptic target neurons, at least with respect to the nigrostriatal system.[3] As a consequence, the administration of low doses of apomorphine causes a net *decrease* in postsynaptic DA receptor stimulation, since the direct inhibition of DA cell firing removes

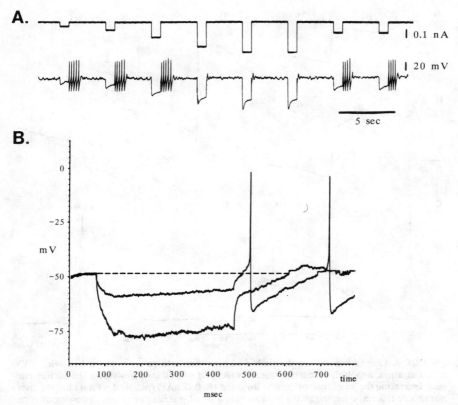

**FIGURE 8.** The low-threshold calcium current and the ensuing rebound spiking can be activated by the offset of small-amplitude hyperpolarizing current pulses (**A**, current pulses 1–3; current injection amplitude indicated in *top trace*, membrane potential on *bottom trace*). However, if larger amplitude hyperpolarizing current pulses are injected, the rebound spike activity is blocked (**A**, current pulses 4–6). Examination of this phenomenon at a faster time base (**B**) shows that larger hyperpolarizations trigger another current, a putative $A$ current ($I_A$). This potassium current attenuates the repolarization of the membrane to resting potentials, thereby blocking the rebound low-threshold spikes and action potentials. In contrast, injection of a hyperpolarizing current pulse at an amplitude that is subthreshold with respect to activation of the $I_A$ elicits a rebound low-threshold current and two action potentials.

more DA input from postsynaptic receptor sites than is gained by the direct action of apomorphine at these sites.

## In Vivo *Studies*

Administration of systemic apomorphine in low, primarily presynaptic doses (maximum 20 µg/kg, iv) resulted in a dose-dependent inhibition of DA cell firing in the SN and VTA (with the exception of a class of mesocortical neurons lacking sensitivity

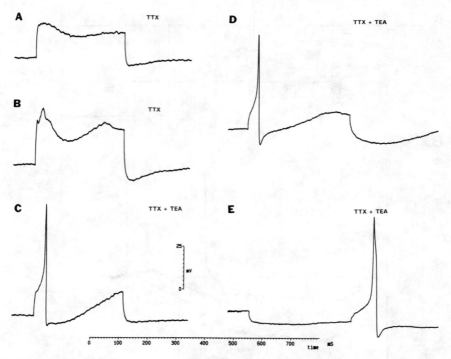

**FIGURE 9.** Comparison of low-threshold and high-threshold calcium spikes. Following TTX administration, depolarizing current injection (**A**: 0.08 nA) elicits a low-threshold calcium current. Increasing the amplitude of current injection (**B**: 0.18 nA) typically does not alter the components of this response, triggering at most only a small spikelike response. Following application of the potassium blocker tetraethylammonium (TEA), intracellular injection of previously subthreshold levels of current (0.08 nA) triggers a large-amplitude, high-threshold dendritic calcium spike (**C**). In the presence of TEA, this spike can be triggered by comparatively low amplitudes of depolarizing current injection (**D**: 0.05 nA) or by the rebound from a hyperpolarizing current pulse (**E**: −0.03 nA).

to DA agonists[18,43]). In extracellular recordings of DA neurons, apomorphine caused a progressive slowing of DA cell firing, accompanied by an increase in spike amplitude, a decrease in spike duration, and an alteration of the firing pattern to a pacemaker-like sequence, until complete inhibition of cell firing was produced. During *in vivo* intracellular recordings, systemic apomorphine also inhibited DA cell firing in a dose-dependent manner. Intravenous administration of apomorphine in doses between 10 and 20 µg/kg elicited two responses in DA neurons: (1) an inhibition of firing accompanied by a hyperpolarization of the membrane potential, and (2) an increase in the input resistance (decreased membrane conductance).[20] In order to ascertain which membrane currents mediated these actions of apomorphine, the reversal potential of these effects was calculated. This was done by measuring the membrane potentials reached in response to a series of hyperpolarizing current pulses administered before and after drug administration, and plotting the resultant regression lines for the current/voltage relationships for each condition. The intersection of the two regression lines representing data acquired before and after drug administration occurs at the membrane potential at which apomorphine administration would cause no net change in membrane potential. This membrane potential, by definition, would thus be the reversal potential for the apomorphine-induced changes in membrane ion conductance(s). *In vivo*, small doses of apomorphine produced a hyperpolarization with a reversal potential near $-40$ mV. This value is not a reversal potential commonly associated with a single characterized ionic conductance; therefore, this result was probably due to an activation of two or more conductances. In order to separate these putative response classes, the main afferent system to the SN, which arises from the striatum, was transected. This operation resulted in an attenuation of most of the increased input resistance induced by apomorphine without affecting the hyperpolarization and cessation of firing produced.[20] The reversal potential for this more circumscribed response was difficult to determine precisely, due to the small change in membrane conductance induced, but appeared to be positive to 0 mV. This is consistent with an effect mediated by decreased conductance of an inward current. Since the hyperpolarization of 4–8 mV was accompanied by a cessation of the slow depolarization and spiking, and given that the slow depolarization cannot be blocked by directly hyperpolarizing the soma by this magnitude, it was concluded that apomorphine inhibited DA neuron activity by attenuating the slow depolarizing pacemaker current.[11,20] This was the most likely explanation for the data, given: (1) the inability of larger (e.g., 10–15 mV) hyperpolarizations to block the slow depolarization, (2) the triggering of a small increase in input resistance and a hyperpolarization by apomorphine, which is consistent with a decreased inward current flow, and (3) the relative significance of the slow depolarization in driving the spontaneous activity of DA neurons, thereby allowing inhibitory stimuli applied at this site to have greater efficacy in inhibiting DA neuron spontaneous activity. The increased input resistance, arising from the striatonigral feedback loops, probably arises from disinhibition of striatonigral neurons secondary to the apomorphine-induced inhibition of striatal DA release.[20,32]

## In Vitro *Studies*

The primary difficulty in establishing the actions of apomorphine on DA cell electrophysiology *in vivo* was in separating the direct effects of the agonist from those mediated by effects on neighboring neurons or afferent projections. Indeed, the striatonigral transections in the preceding investigation ruled out only a single, albeit major, possible source of artifact arising from indirect effects of apomorphine. It is possible that some indirect effects of apomorphine could be due to its actions on DA-sensitive neurons in the zona reticulata[44,45] or on the DA receptors located on striatonigral afferents[46] that may retain their DA reactivity after the transection. The *in vitro* preparation could circumvent some of these difficulties but, of course, introduces other confounding variables, such as penetration of DA into the slice, stability of added DA in oxygenated and carbonate buffered Ringer's solutions, and inactivation of exogenous DA by reuptake or metabolizing enzyme activity. Thus, despite the accessibility of this preparation for testing the effects of direct administration of neurotransmitters, the DA agonist apomorphine was chosen instead of the neurotransmitter DA for this study based on (1) its greater stability in the Ringer's solution, (2) its faster penetration into tissues, (3) its higher specificity, especially with regard to the absence of an interaction with noradrenergic *alpha* receptors, (4) the lack of uptake into dendritic processes or glial cells, and (5) its resistance to degradation by metabolic enzymes. The effects of this drug were examined on neurons in the SN and lateral VTA. Since a population of neurons within the medial VTA has been shown to be insensitive to DA,[18,43] and since they cannot be identified by antidromic activation in the *in vitro* preparation, a negative response to apomorphine in VTA DA cells would be difficult to interpret.

Thus, in order to maximize the probability of recording from DA neurons containing active autoreceptors, the SN and more lateral VTA DA neurons were studied. The general applicability of these findings to other DA neuronal subtypes will be examined in subsequent studies.

One problem arises when attempting to measure the input resistance and membrane potential responses to drugs in a neuron that is generating continuous pacemaker potentials and action potentials — that is, where does one draw the baseline membrane potential? This was not as troublesome in the *in vivo* example previously outlined, since both the irregular firing pattern as well as the bursting pattern exhibited periods where no spiking or slow depolarizations were present, thus facilitating the determination of membrane potential and input resistance changes using hyperpolarizing current pulses. One may choose to circumvent this difficulty by examining a DA neuron that is nonfiring, or to suppress spontaneously active DA cells by injecting sufficient levels of hyperpolarizing current to attenuate the pacemaker current. Of course, if DA agonists do exert their inhibitory action on DA neurons through an action on this pacemaker current, inactivation of this current by blocking cell firing would yield misleading information concerning the action of DA agonists on autoreceptors and how they regulate DA neuron activity.

In this series of studies, attempts at obtaining accurate information about apomorphine effects during spontaneous spike generation were made by comparing the membrane voltage changes produced by constant amplitude current pulses administered repeatedly. Since a current pulse can reset the slow depolarization to baseline (thereby giving an exaggerated measure of input resistance) and will be attenuated if it occurs during the spike AHP, values for average deflections were obtained from a series of pulses occurring at the same point in the course of the slow depolarization. Furthermore, long-duration (>500 msec) current pulses were used to allow the membrane potential to achieve equilibrium. In this way, it was hoped that the confounding nature of the AHP and slow depolarization on input resistance measurements could be circumvented, or at least minimized. Administration of apomorphine to the bath caused a dose-dependent hyperpolarization and inhibition of DA cell firing. Initial slowing of DA cell firing occurred at threshold doses of about 2–5 µM apomorphine, although apomorphine doses greater than 80 µM were usually required for complete inhibition of firing. This inhibition was accompanied by a hyperpolarization of 6–8 mV from resting potentials. Again, although difficult to establish accurately, the input resistance of the DA cell was found to increase by about 25%; in the case in FIGURE 10, the DA cell input resistance changed from approximately 110 to 145 MΩ. The slowing of DA cell firing was associated with a delayed activation of the slow depolarization. The slow depolarization can also be attenuated by hyperpolarizing the membrane by intracellular current injection, since the rate of rise of this current is strongly dependent on membrane potential.[4] However, in order to match the slowing of the slow depolarization and decreased firing rate produced by a moderate dose of apomorphine (5–10 µM), it was necessary to hyperpolarize the DA neuron membrane potential to a level 5 mV *more* hyperpolarized than the hyperpolarization produced by the apomorphine. At this more hyperpolarized membrane potential, the slow depolarizations are attenuated to a similar extent, as occurs after apomorphine administration in the absence of hyperpolarizing current injection (FIG. 10A). Finally, if sufficient negative current is injected to adjust the membrane potential to the hyperpolarized level produced by apomorphine, it is clear that the hyperpolarizing current caused less slowing of the DA cell firing rate and slow depolarization time course than the hyperpolarization produced by the apomorphine alone (FIG. 10B). Note that this difference was not a consequence of electrode imbalance, since the electrode bridge balance was confirmed continuously during the repeated injections of hyperpolarizing current pulses. The changes observed in the action potential amplitudes and spike thresholds at these different membrane potentials, as shown in FIGURE 10, are characteristic of DA neuron electrophysiology, and have been described previously.[11,12]

Thus, this evidence indicates that apomorphine inhibits spontaneous DA neuron slow depolarizations and spiking. Nonetheless, this activity can still be reinstated after apomorphine by depolarizing the membrane to voltages significantly above the pre-apomorphine resting membrane potential. Therefore, although apomorphine does not block activation of the slow depolarization completely, it apparently does alter its voltage dependency, thus necessitating significantly enhanced levels of depolarization after apomorphine in order to reactivate spiking. The mechanism underlying this change in the voltage dependency of the slow depolarization is unknown at present. One possibility is that it occurs through a direct action of apomorphine on the sodium channel responsible for the slow depolarization, or alternately by an action on another conductance (e.g., potassium channels) located in the immediate vicinity of the site of generation of the slow depolarization, thereby shunting the depolarizing current away from the spike-generating regions. Indeed, this latter model of autoreceptor action could account for the potassium dependency of the DA response in hyperpolarized nonfiring substantia nigra zona compacta neurons reported by others.[47]

# CONCLUSIONS

Dopamine neuron action potentials, by all indications, are driven primarily if not exclusively by self-generated inward currents. This baseline excitatory drive is subsequently modulated into the characteristic DA neuron activity patterns through the influence of endogenous calcium currents and potassium conductances, in addition to afferent neurotransmitter inputs. Indeed, this high degree of self-regulation of DA cell activity derived from the unique properties of the DA cell membrane could contribute to the ability of transplanted DA neurons to functionally reinnervate the DA-depleted striatum despite the absence of the normal complement of afferent processes. Nevertheless, these afferents undoubtedly have a significant role in the fine-tuning of nigral DA cell populations, such as in the activation of specific subgroups of DA cells or alternately in providing for a rapid or transient enhancement of DA release. One manner through which these afferents could effectively modulate DA neuron firing over a comparatively wide range of parameters would be through an action at the sites of the aforementioned endogenous regulatory currents. Hence, in order to infer the possible modulatory actions the afferent inputs can exert on DA cell activity patterns, in addition to analyzing the functional compartmentalization of the DA neuron, it would be useful to know the general cellular location of these active membrane regions.

The location and ionic nature of these currents can be inferred from studies of *in vivo* extracellular and intracellular recordings combined with the data presented here on *in vitro* DA neuron electrophysiology. The neuronal sites of current flow can be estimated, with respect to proximity to the soma, by comparing intracellular and extracellular action potential waveforms[12,37,48,49] and by observing changes in spike threshold after potassium channel blockade.[24] Thus, whereas intracellular recordings reflect the membrane voltage changes accompanying spiking, the extracellular records depict local current flow across the membrane, in the form of a voltage induced across the extracellular electrode. Thus, the extracellular electrode measures transmembrane current or, in essence, the rate of change of the membrane voltage.[13-15] Hence, the extracellularly recorded waveform pattern can be predicted from the absolute value of the differentiated intracellular voltage change that occurs with spike activity. The polarity

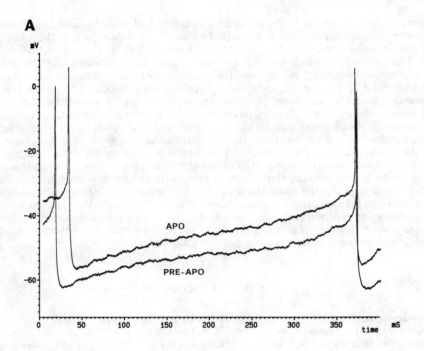

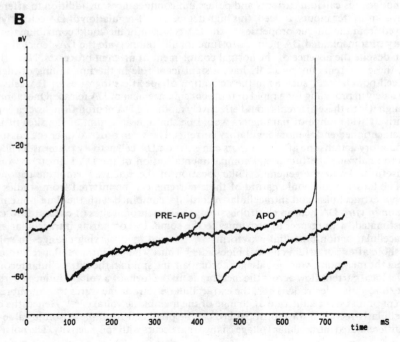

of these currents depends on the site of inward current flow across the membrane — if the site of inward current flow (i.e., the active spiking region) is at the location of the extracellular electrode (i.e., the soma), a negative extracellular voltage spike would be recorded secondary to the local depletion of positive ions. If, however, the site of inward current flow occurs distal to the recording site (e.g., the dendrites), then the return path of the distal inward current flow would occur via induction of a parallel outward current flow across the membrane at the soma, causing a positive deflection in the extracellular electrode located outside of the soma. Since DA neuron action potentials have positive-going IS and SD spike components, both of these spikes must be generated distal to the recording site at the soma. The low safety factor for antidromic invasion of DA neurons,[12] coupled with the observed dendritic origin of the axon,[9,12,50,51] supports this hypothesized distal origin of IS spike generation.

The data acquired from the *in vitro* experiments extends this information concerning the location of the active spiking regions of the cell. Spike thresholds measured *at the active membrane site* are usually rather constant in the absence of drugs or neurotransmitter influences. If the soma is located electrotonically near the source of the spike, both regions should be at or near the same membrane potential. Hence, the spike threshold recorded at the soma during injection of depolarizing current into the soma should be similar to the spike threshold that would be measured at this proximal active spiking zone. Furthermore, decreasing the membrane conductance with potassium channel blockers would have little effect on altering this threshold, since the membrane potential at the spike-generating region would still vary in concert with the membrane potential measured at the soma during current injection. However, if the site of spike generation is electrotonically distal to the soma, then there is a greater likelihood that the active spiking zone would *not* be isopotential with the soma, especially during current injection into the soma. Thus, during current injection, the soma would be depolarized to more positive potentials than the distal spike-generating region due to current loss across the membrane between sites of current injection and measurement (i.e., the soma) and the site where the spike is generated (i.e., the spike-generating regions on distal dendrites). As a consequence, the *apparent* dendritic spike threshold, as measured at the soma, would be much more depolarized than the *actual* spike threshold at the active site due to current loss occurring across the membrane between these regions. If, however, this current loss is limited by "plugging" dendritic "leakiness" (i.e., decreasing membrane conductance) with TEA, then the current injected into the soma would be conducted along the dendrites more efficiently to reach the distal dendritic regions without significant current loss. This would cause the active dendritic spike zone to be more isopotential with the soma. Therefore, TEA would

---

◄**FIGURE 10.** Comparison of apomorphine-induced inhibition of DA neuron firing *in vitro* with inhibition produced by hyperpolarizing current injection. Apomorphine exerts a stronger suppressive effect on DA cell firing than would be predicted by the amount of membrane hyperpolarization it produces. Thus, a larger amount of hyperpolarization (i.e., 5–10 mV more hyperpolarization than that produced by apomorphine) must be induced by current injection into untreated DA neurons (**A**: PRE-APO) to match the firing rate reduction produced by a low dose of apomorphine (**A**: APO; 50 mM). Furthermore, a DA neuron that is hyperpolarized by current injection to the same membrane potential reached in response to apomorphine administration (**B**: PRE-APO) exhibits a smaller inhibition of firing rate and less attenuation of the slow depolarization than occurs in response to apomorphine administration (**B**: APO). Thus, the apomorphine-induced inhibition of firing appears to be mediated by more than simple hyperpolarization of the membrane. One possibility would be a direct action of apomorphine on activation of the slow depolarization.

cause a drop in the *apparent* threshold of the dendritic spike. Thus, in general, if a spiking region exhibits lowered thresholds after TEA administration, it is probably located distal to the soma.[24] Since DA neuron high-threshold calcium spikes (HTSs) cannot be triggered by depolarizing current injected into the soma, but are easily triggered by depolarizing current pulses after TEA administration, the HTSs are probably located on distal dendrites, as found in some other neuronal types.[24,37,42] Indeed, given the comparatively high input resistance of DA neurons in the absence of TEA (i.e., 100 MΩ), this HTS must be generated at a considerable distance from the soma. In contrast, neither the slow depolarization nor the LTS appear to change in threshold after TEA administration, thus indicating that these regions are probably located at the soma or proximal dendritic regions.

Drawing from this information, the following model of DA neuron action potential generation was constructed: the sodium-dependent slow depolarization occurring near the soma depolarizes the soma and dendrites until the IS region reaches threshold. The IS spike then travels down the axon and across the already depolarized soma to invade the dendrites, where it elicits a calcium-mediated HTS. The calcium entering during the HTS would, in turn, activate a potassium current (i.e., the $I_{K(Ca)}$), resulting in a synchronous hyperpolarization of the entire DA neuron membrane after the spike. The rebound from this widespread hyperpolarization would activate the LTS, thereby triggering the next slow depolarization and spiking sequence.

By combining information about DA neuron physiology obtained in the *in vivo* and the *in vitro* preparations, a more complete picture of neuronal regulation may be garnered. Thus, DA neurons recorded *in vivo* display markedly different firing patterns, which appear to be regulated by the demands placed upon the neurons. At least one-third of the DA neurons in the substania nigra and ventral tegmental region are nonfiring in anesthetized rats,[2,52,53] immobilized nonanesthetized rats,[2] and in slices of rat midbrain. The process underlying this inactive, "reserve" state is currently not understood. One possible reason for this inactivity may be derived from the voltage-dependent currents associated with hyperpolarization and depolarization of the DA neuron membrane, as previously outlined. Thus, hyperpolarization in a number of other mammalian central neurons to voltages below the resting membrane potentials will deinactivate the LTS, causing it to trigger a burst of action potentials in response to subsequent depolarizing stimuli.[35,37,38] In fact, the rebound excitation triggered by repolarization from this hyperpolarized state may be more intense than that produced by a larger amplitude direct depolarization of the neuron. Based on these activation and inactivation characteristics, LTSs would thus serve to transpose neuronal hyperpolarization into a state of enhanced excitability by potentiating excitatory inputs. Indeed, DA neurons respond to small hyperpolarizing pulses by generating rebound LTSs. On the other hand, dopamine neurons can also respond to hyperpolarization in an *opposite* manner, depending on the membrane potential. Thus, spontaneously firing DA neurons appear to have factors that serve to maintain their ongoing activity, whereas prolonged hyperpolarization appears to trigger conductances that limit neurons to the inactive state. Accordingly, although a small hyperpolarizing pulse may lead to rebound spiking in DA neurons by deinactivation of the LTS, larger hyperpolarizations will activate the putative *A* current, thereby slowing membrane repolarization at the offset of the hyperpolarizing pulse and attenuating the rebound LTS. Therefore, strong hyperpolarizations will attenuate DA neuron activity by acting on at least two currents: (1) a hyperpolarization-mediated activation of the anomalous rectifying current, dampening the effects of excitation and attenuating the slow depolarization by enhancing membrane conductances and outward currents (i.e., essentially "shorting out" the depolarizing drive of the neuron), and (2) rebound activation of the *A* current upon depolarization from hyperpolarized membrane potentials, thereby limiting the ability of the DA neuron to repolarize. These processes would thus serve to augment the inhibition of hyperpolarized DA neurons, thereby preventing transition into a state of spontaneous activity. Indeed, initial results suggest that the nonfiring DA neurons recorded in the *in vitro* preparation may tend to have larger $A$ currents than spontaneously firing DA cells, to the extent that action potential AHPs in the nonfiring cells are of sufficient amplitude to activate the $A$ current.

Conversely, DA neurons that are spontaneously firing have forces acting upon them to maintain this active state. Thus, the slow depolarization, being voltage-dependent, has a faster activation rate at more depolarized membrane potentials.[4] Furthermore, depolarization would increase DA neuron input resistance,[5] making the slow depolarization more effective and enhancing the amplitude of the spike AHP. The enhanced spike AHP rebound would in turn activate the LTS, which would subsequently trigger another slow depolarization and begin the pacemaker cycle over again. Thus, spontaneously firing depolarized dopamine neurons would tend to maintain their state of activity and spontaneously inactive hyperpolarized DA cells would tend to remain in the silent ("on reserve") condition until sufficient levels of maintained depolarization, or possibly an as yet unidentified stimulus, could trigger this putative "switch" to allow the cell to enter into the active mode. Experimental evidence for this two-state model of DA neuron firing can be derived from studies of the relative levels of activity of populations of DA neurons in control and drug-treated rats. Thus, extracellular recordings in control, anesthetized rats showed that DA cell firing rates are normally distributed around an average frequency of 4.5 Hz ($\pm 1.7$ Hz SD, $n = 597$), with few cells firing below 1 Hz.[4] However, after systemic administration of the DA antagonist haloperidol, the number of spontaneously firing DA neurons found in 12 electrode passes increases by over 50% in both the SN[2] and the VTA,[52,54] indicating that a large proportion of previously inactive ("silent") DA neurons had been activated by the neuroleptic. Furthermore, inactive DA neurons will often begin firing after repeated iontophoretic applications of excitatory neurotransmitters.[2] Thus, DA neurons actually exist in two general states of activity, with one set of cells firing at 0.0 Hz (i.e., nonfiring) and the others firing spontaneously, with firing rates normally distributed around an average rate of 4.5 Hz.

The spontaneously active DA neurons recorded *in vivo* can be further subdivided into two groups on the basis of differential patterns of spike discharge: irregular single spiking and burst firing.[4,5] Thus, in the basal, nonstimulated states, DA neurons fire in a slow, irregular pattern with comparatively long interspike intervals. However, whenever the neurons are driven to faster firing rates, either by postsynaptic feedback, administration of excitatory neurotransmitters, or depolarization by intracellular current injection, the neurons transform their spontaneous discharge pattern into one of burst firing, characterized by groups of three to eight spikes of decreasing amplitude and increasing duration occurring at comparatively brief interspike intervals, and separated by prolonged interburst periods of quiescence. This pattern of activity appears to be triggered by increased calcium entry secondary to the accelerated spike activity, since intracellular injection of calcium will elicit burst firing in the absence of enhanced depolarization, and injection of the calcium chelator EGTA into DA neurons will prevent subsequent depolarizations from eliciting burst firing.[4,5]

What is the importance of the burst firing pattern in the regulation of DA systems? Although the answer to this question has not been determined conclusively, the potential relevance of burst firing to neuronal function may be drawn from studies of burst firing in other systems. Thus, the nerves innervating the cockroach salivary glands are known to release two to three times the amount of neurotransmitter when stimulated in a burst/pause pattern than when stimulated with an equivalent number of rhythmically occurring spikes.[55,56] In the mammalian hypothalamus, neurosecretory neurons were reported to be almost refractory to release of peptides in the absence of a burst firing pattern.[57-59] One study conducted on nigrostriatal pathway stimulation reported that stimulation of DA cell axons in a sequence patterned after DA neuron burst firing released more DA per impulse than stimuli delivered in a single spiking pattern.[60] Another functional model for burst-patterned activity can be derived from studies of mammalian sympathetic nerves. In this investigation, single spike patterns of stimulation lead to release of norepinephrine from the nerve terminal. However, if the pathway is stimulated in a bursting pattern, a preferential increase in the release of the peptide cotransmitter neuropeptide Y occurs.[61] Thus, upon demand, the DA system may actually be able to compensate for short-term increased DA requirements by altering neuronal firing patterns. This alteration could result in the enhancement of the amount of DA released per impulse, or alternately could lead to the preferential release of a cotransmitter that may function to enhance the postsynaptic efficacy of the released DA. This may be of particular significance in the mesolimbic system, where the DA neurons have been reported to fire a higher proportion of spikes in a bursting mode,[18] and subsets of DA neurons are known to contain and release the neuropeptide cholecystokinin (CCK) as a cotransmitter.[62]

In summary, the spontaneous electrophysiological activity of DA neurons recorded in both the *in vivo* and the *in vitro* preparation is self-driven by a voltage-dependent sodium-mediated slow depolarization, similar to the pacemaker currents detailed in invertebrate preparations. Unlike other neuronal types described to date, the activity of DA neuron populations can be subdivided into two general categories: (1) spontaneously active with few very slow firing cells, and (2) nonfiring and hypoexcitable, with the steady-state activity level of the DA neurons being maintained by their unique membrane properties. These firing and nonfiring activity states of DA neurons have been seen during extracellular and intracellular recordings in both preparations. The spontaneously active DA neurons recorded *in vivo* can be further subdivided based on their pattern of spike discharge — either an irregular single spiking pattern or, upon depolarization, burst firing. In contrast, spontaneously active DA neurons recorded in the *in vitro* preparation fire exclusively in a highly regular pacemaker pattern independent of the level of cell depolarization. These highly integrated, self-regulatory systems present in DA neuron membranes are also subject to further modification by afferent neurotransmitters through processes that are yet to be determined, to yield a multicompartmental functional neurotransmitter system unique in its ability to modulate central brain structures.

## ACKNOWLEDGMENTS

I would like to thank Dr. Benjamin S. Bunney and Dr. Rodolfo Llinás for their interest and time committed to my training, which made this research possible. I also thank Dr. Shao-Pii Onn for her advice and able assistance in carrying out the preliminary studies on DA neuron morphology and identification, and Jeff Hollerman for his valuable suggestions during the preparation of this manuscript.

## REFERENCES

1.  BUNNEY, B. S. & G. K. AGHAJANIAN. 1976. Science 192: 391–393.
2.  BUNNEY, B. S. & A. A. GRACE. 1978. Life Sci. 23: 1715–1728.
3.  SKIRBOLL, L. R., A. A. GRACE & B. S. BUNNEY. 1979. Science (N.Y.) 206: 80–82.
4.  GRACE, A. A. & B. S. BUNNEY. 1984. J. Neuroscience 4: 2866–2876.

5. GRACE, A. A. & B. S. BUNNEY. 1984. J. Neuroscience **4:** 2877-2890.
6. GRACE, A. A. 1987. *In* The Neurophysiology of Dopamine Systems. L. A. Chiodo and A. S. Freeman, Eds.: 1-67. Lake Shore. Detroit, Mich.
7. BUNNEY, B. S. 1979. *In* The Neurobiology of Dopamine. A. S. Horn, J. Korf, and B. H. C. Westerink, Eds.: 417-452. Academic Press, New York.
8. GRACE, A. A. 1983. Ph.D. Dissertation. Yale Univ., New Haven, Conn.
9. GRACE, A. A. 1987. Neuroscience **22** (Suppl.): S622.
10. GRACE, A. A. 1987. Soc. Neurosci. Abst. **13:** 537.
11. GRACE, A. A. & B. S. BUNNEY. 1983. Neuroscience **10:** 301-315.
12. GRACE, A. A. & B. S. BUNNEY. 1983. Neuroscience **10:** 317-331.
13. ARAKI, T. & T. OTANI. 1955. J. Neurophysiol. **18:** 472-485.
14. ARAKI, T. & C. A. TERZUOLO. 1962. J. Neurophysiol. **25:** 772-789.
15. TERZUOLO, C. A. & T. ARAKI. 1961. Ann. N.Y. Acad. Sci. **94:** 547-558.
16. DE LA TORRE, J. C. & J. W. SURGEON. 1980. Histochemistry **49:** 81-93.
17. GRACE, A. A. & B. S. BUNNEY. 1980. Science (N.Y.) **210:** 654-656.
18. CHIODO, L. A., M. J. BANNON, A. A. GRACE, R. H. ROTH & B. S. BUNNEY. 1984. Neuroscience **12:** 1-16.
19. GUYENET, P. G. & G. K. AGHAJANIAN. 1978. Brain Res. **150:** 69-84.
20. GRACE, A. A. & B. S. BUNNEY. 1985. Brain Res. **333:** 285-298.
21. BUNNEY, B. S., J. R. WALTERS, R. H. ROTH & G. K. AGHAJANIAN. 1973. J. Pharmacol. Exp. Ther. **185:** 560-571.
22. STEWART, W. W. 1978. Cell **14:** 741-759.
23. FALLON, J. H., J. N. RILEY & R. Y. MOORE. 1978. Neurosci. Lett. **7:** 157-162.
24. LLINÁS, R., S. A. GREENFIELD & H. JAHNSEN. 1984. Brain Res. **294:** 127-132.
25. SILVA, N. L. & B. S. BUNNEY. 1985. Soc. Neurosci. Abst. **12:** 1517.
26. PINNOCK, R. D. 1984. Brain Res. **332:** 337-340.
27. KITA, T., H. KITA & S. T. KITAI. 1986. Brain Res. **372:** 21-30.
28. CONNOR, J. A. & C. F. STEVENS. 1971. J. Physiol. (London) **213:** 1-19.
29. CONNOR, J. A. & C. F. STEVENS. 1971. J. Physiol. (London) **213:** 21-31.
30. CONNOR, J. A. & C. F. STEVENS. 1971. J. Physiol. (London) **213:** 31-53.
31. CARPENTER. D. O. 1982. Cellular Pacemakers. Vol. 1, Mechanisms of Pacemaker Generation. Wiley. New York.
32. GRACE, A. A. & B. S. BUNNEY. 1985. Brain Res. **333:** 271-284.
33. MEECH, R. W. 1978. Annu. Rev. Biophys. Bioeng. **7:** 1-18.
34. JAHNSEN, H. & R. LLINÁS. 1984. J. Physiol. (London) **349:** 205-226.
35. JAHNSEN, H. & R. LLINÁS. 1984. J. Physiol. (London) **349:** 227-247.
36. LLINÁS, R. & Y. YAROM. 1981. J. Physiol. (London) **315:** 549-567.
37. LLINÁS, R. & Y. YAROM. 1981. J. Physiol. (London) **315:** 569-584.
38. GRACE, A. A. & R. LLINÁS. 1985. Soc. Neurosci. Abst. **10:** 739.
39. LLINÁS, R. & M. SUGIMORI. 1980. J. Physiol. (London) **305:** 171-195.
40. LLINÁS, R. & M. SUGIMORI. 1980. J. Physiol. (London) **305:** 197-213.
41. SCHWARTZKROIN, P. A. & M. SLAWSKI. 1977. Brain Res. **135:** 157-161.
42. WONG, R. K. S., D. A. PRINCE & A. I. BUSBAUM. 1979. Proc. Nat. Acad. Sci. U.S. **76:** 986-990.
43. BANNON, M. J., R. L. MICHAUD & R. H. ROTH. 1981. Mol. Pharmacol. **19:** 270-275.
44. RUFFIEUX, A. & W. SCHULTZ. 1980. Nature (London) **285:** 240-241.
45. WASZCZAK, B. L. & J. R. WALTERS. 1983. Science (N.Y.) **220:** 218-221.
46. SPANO, P. F., M. TRABUCCI & G. DiCHIARA. 1977. Science (N.Y.) **196:** 1343-1345.
47. LACEY, M. G., N. B. MERCURI & R. A. NORTH. 1986. Soc. Neurosci. Abst. **12:** 1515.
48. FREYGANG, W. H. 1958. J. Gen. Physiol. **41:** 543-564.
49. HUBBARD, J. J., R. LLINÁS & D. M. J. QUASTEL. 1969. *In* Electrophysiological Analysis of Synaptic Transmission. 1-372. Williams & Wilkins, Baltimore.
50. JURASKA, J. M., C. J. WILSON & P. M. GROVES. 1977. J. Comp. Neurol. **172:** 585-600.
51. SCHWYN, R. C. & C. A. FOX. 1974. J. Hirnforschung. **16:** 95-126.
52. CHIODO, L. A. & B. S. BUNNEY. 1983. J. Neurosci. **3:** 1607-1619.
53. WHITE, F. J. & R. Y. WANG. 1983. Life Sci. **32:** 983-993.
54. WHITE, F. J. & R. Y. WANG. 1983. Science (N.Y.) **221:** 1054-1057.
55. GILLARY, H. L. & D. KENNEDY. 1969. J. Neurophysiol. **32:** 595-606.

56. GILLARY, H. L. & D. KENNEDY. 1969. J. Neurophysiol. **32:** 607–612.
57. DREIFUSS, J. J., B. H. GAHWILER & P. SANDOZ. 1978. *In* Abnormal Neuronal Discharges. N. Chalazonitis and M. Boisson, Eds.: 111–114. Raven Press. New York.
58. DREIFUSS, J. J., E. TRIBOLLET & M. MUHLETHALER. 1981. Biol. Reprod. **24:** 51–72.
59. LINCOLN, D. W. & J. B. WAKERLY. 1974. J. Physiol. (London) **242:** 533–554.
60. GONON, F. G. & M. J. BUDA. 1985. Neuroscience **14:** 765–774.
61. LUNDBERG, J. M., A. RUDEHILL, A. SOLLEVI, E. THEODORSSON-NORHEIM & B. HAMBERGER. 1986. Neurosci. Lett. **63:** 96–100.
62. HÖKFELT, T., L. SKIRBOLL, J. F. REHFELD, M. GOLDSTEIN, K. MARKEY & O. DANN. 1980. Neuroscience **5:** 2093–2124.

# Effects of Acute and Chronic Neuroleptic Treatment on the Activity of Midbrain Dopamine Neurons[a]

BENJAMIN S. BUNNEY

*Departments of Psychiatry and Pharmacology*
*Yale University School of Medicine*
*New Haven, Connecticut 06510*

## INTRODUCTION

Psychosis has probably afflicted humans for as long as they have been on the earth. For the great majority of this time nonbiological factors were believed to be the cause — for example, demonic possession, witchcraft, or ego-disintegration secondary to unresolved conflicts between the supergo and the id. However, in 1953, with the discovery of chlorpromazine and its remarkable ability to ameliorate some psychotic symptoms, these nonbiological etiologies began to seem less likely. On the other hand, discovery of a pharmacological treatment for psychosis forced us to face a new question: How can such a simple molecule produce such profound behavioral changes? Over thirty years later we are still asking the same question. In this chapter, we attempt to summarize the progress that has been made in addressing this issue using data collected primarily with the use of one technique, single unit recording. It should be acknowledged, however, that no single experimental approach can determine the "whole truth." Thus, discoveries made using biochemical techniques often point the way for electrophysiological experiments and vice versa. In addition, neither approach would be of much use without information gained from anatomical and behavioral studies.

## BACKGROUND

In order to understand the effects of antipsychotic drugs (ADs) on the functioning of central dopamine (DA) systems it is necessary to understand both their neuroanatomy and the way that they function under physiological, nondrug conditions. In the next two sections brief summaries of these two areas are presented.

[a] This work was supported by U. S. Public Health Grants MH-28849, MH-25642, and MH-08842; The Robert Alwin Hay Fund for Schizophrenia Research; the Abraham Ribicoff Research Facilities; and the State of Connecticut.

*Anatomy*

This chapter is limited solely to a discussion of the effects of ADs on central DA systems whose cell bodies are located in the midbrain.[1] Although several nomenclatures are in use, one of the easiest to understand describes midbrain DA systems as essentially being three in number. One of these systems is referred to as the nigro-striatal DA system because its cells are located primarily in the zona compacta (ZC) of the substantia nigra and project to the caudate–putamen nucleus. A second system is referred to as the mesolimbic system. Its cell bodies are located in the ventral tegmental area (VTA) and project to a variety of structures including the accumbens nucleus, central nucleus of the amygdala, lateral septal nucleus, and olfactory tubercles. The last system is referred to as the mesocortical system and consists of those DA cells in the VTA that project to the entorhinal, piriform, and prefrontal cortices. In addition, there are DA cells in the ZC that project to the cingulate cortex and are intermixed among those going to the striatum.

The function of two of these systems, the mesolimbic and mesocortical, is still unknown. Based on information concerning the areas that they project to it has been hypothesized that they are involved in mediating or modulating a variety of emotional and cognitive behaviors. On the other hand, the function of the nigro-striatal DA system is somewhat better understood due to its involvement in the etiology of Parkinson's disease. Thus, it is known that destruction of this pathway, which leads to a depletion of DA in the striatum, results in decreased motor activity (akinesia), rigidity, and tremor. There is also evidence that hyperfunctioning of this DA system results in abnormally increased motor activity. This has been observed in a variety of animal models and is thought to occur in human disorders such as Huntington's chorea, Gilles de la Tourette's disease, and tardive dyskinesia.

If we are to understand the observed effect of ADs on DA system functioning, it is necessary to know something about how DA cells behave under physiological conditions and what some of the mechanisms are that control their functioning.

## *Physiological Characteristics and Control of Activity*

DA cells have four activity states.[2,3,4] The first is an inactive state that intracellular recording has demonstrated to be due to hyperpolarization, the state that most cells in the brain are in when they are not firing. A small number of these inactive cells have been observed in every type of preparation examined to date. The second state is a spontaneously active one in which DA neurons fire in a slow (0.5–6 spikes per second) irregular pattern. The third state is also a spontaneously active one and consists of a very distinctive bursting pattern in which each subsequent action potential within the burst has a smaller amplitude and longer duration than the action potential immediately preceding it. This bursting pattern is also characterized by periods of total inactivity between bursts. Intracellular recordings from these cells demonstrate that part of the inactive period is due to a transient state of depolarization block. Most spontaneously active DA cells fire predominantly, but not exclusively, in one mode or the other. It is important to point out that both types of firing pattern have been observed in nondrugged, freely moving rats, and that a single cell has been observed to switch from a predominately single spiking mode to a bursting mode and back again.[5,6] The final state is an inactive one that is seen acutely only after the administration of certain peptides (e.g., cholecystokinin[7]) or after repeated administration of ADs.[8]

The latter state is discussed in detail in the section Effects of Repeated Antipsychotic Drug Administration.

Midbrain DA cell activity can be modulated by a variety of mechanisms. Two of the best characterized are often referred to as long-loop and short-loop feedback systems. Although most completely studied for the nigro-striatal system, more and more evidence is suggesting that similar control mechanisms are operative for most of the mesocortical and mesolimbic systems as well.

The long-loop system consists of feedback pathways from DA projection areas to the structures containing DA cell bodies. For example, it has been clearly demonstrated that there are striato-nigral feedback pathways that cannot only modulate DA cell activity but can also mediate some of the effects of DA agonists[9] and antagonists[10] on their functioning. These pathways are often referred to as being negative in character in that their effect on DA cell activity is to oppose changes in DA cell influence in the projection area. Thus, if there is increased release of DA, the feedback pathways tend to slow DA cells and vice versa.

The short-loop feedback system utilizes receptors for DA on the DA cells themselves (autoreceptors). It has been suggested that DA cells self-inhibit each other through dendrodendritic synapsis.[11] Evidence for this is perhaps strongest for DA neurons projecting to the nucleus accumbens.[12] It should be pointed out that many DA neurons also have the autoreceptors on their terminals that regulate DA synthesis and release.[13-15] However, not all DA cells appear to possess autoreceptors. Thus, DA neurons projecting to the prefrontal and cingulate cortices appear either to lack, or have a greatly diminished number of somatodendritic autoreceptors[16] and possess only release-regulating autoreceptors on their terminals.[17]

A third way DA cell activity is modulated may be through the release of cotransmitters. Thus, it has been demonstrated that some DA neurons contain CCK,[18,19] neurotensin (Seroogy and Fallon, personal communication), or both. A variety of studies have now shown CCK to be excitatory on some DA neurons at one dose[7,20] while potentiating the inhibitory effects of DA at the autoreceptor at another dose.[21] As yet, little is known about the role that these peptides may play in DA system functioning.

## ACUTE EFFECTS OF ANTIPSYCHOTIC DRUGS

### In Vivo *Studies*

Acutely, ADs change the functioning of midbrain DA neurons in a variety of ways. With the exception of ADs lacking Parkinson-like side effects (e.g., clozapine), all ADs increase the activity of both ZC and VTA neurons.[2,22] The degree to which they do this is dependent upon both the baseline rate of the individual cell being studied (i.e., the faster the baseline activity, the less increase in rate induced by an AD) and on the preparation used (e.g., anesthetics can have a marked effect on the responsivity of DA neurons to a wide variety of pharmacological agents). The increased activity induced by ADs in A9 DA cells has been demonstrated to be, at least in part, dependent upon intact striatonigral feedback pathways.[10,23] ADs have also been found to reverse the inhibition of ZC or VTA cells induced by direct- or indirect-acting DA agonists (e.g., apomorphine and d-amphetamine[2,22]). In most cases, reversal is to above baseline levels. However, the one exception again is clozapine, which even in high doses produces only a partial reversal of agonist-induced inhibition and never to above baseline levels.[22]

Clozapine has been observed to be different in other ways as well. For example, most ADs, when administered before a DA agonist, prevent its ability to induce inhibition of DA cells. However, clozapine in doses as high as 8 mg/kg iv fails to block apomorphine-induced inhibition. Interestingly, pretreatment with clozapine blocks the increase in DA cell activity normally induced by haloperidol.[24] Thus, clozapine appears to have a unique profile of effects on DA neuron functioning. One way that clozapine differs from other ADs is that it has higher anticholinergic activity. However, this cannot be the mechanism by which clozapine prevents haloperidol-induced activation of DA cells, because scopolamine (2 mg/kg, iv) by itself has no effect on DA cell activity and does not prevent activation by haloperidol.[24]

Another site at which ADs could act to affect the activity of DA cells is at the somatodendritic autoreceptor. The inhibition of these cells by microiontophoretic application of DA has been shown to be blocked by a variety of ADs, including iv haloperidol,[25,26] iv chlorpromazine,[25] and iontophoretically applied trifluoperazine.[26-28] On the other hand, trifluoperazine alone has no effect on DA cell discharge rate when administered locally to the cell recorded.[26-28] In contrast, the local infusion of haloperidol into the substantia nigra was reported to increase the firing rate of ZC cells.[11] The reason for the divergent results obtained with these two techniques remains unknown. Clozapine can also block DA-induced inhibition of DA cells when applied by means of iontophoresis. Thus 1 mg/kg iv decreases DA inhibitory effects by about 25%. However, it takes 25 mg/kg iv to produce an almost total blockade of DA-induced depression. Clozapine by itself has no effect on baseline firing rate.

DA antagonist blockade of DA autoreceptors can also affect the general responsiveness of DA neurons. For example, the postdischarge inhibitory period observed in the autocorrelation histograms of ZC DA neurons, thought by some to be due to self-inhibitory somatodendritic feedback mechanisms,[29,30] is dramatically shortened by the systemic administration of haloperidol.[31] Similarly, the inhibition observed in ZC cells after the invasion of the cell body region by a stimulus-elicited antidromic action potential (which is presumably releasing DA from the dendrites of DA neurons[32] and thereby stimulating local inhibitory autoreceptors) is shortened by both systemic haloperidol administration and microiontophoretically applied trifluoperazine.[33] In addition, antidromic activation of VTA neurons from the nucleus accumbens has been shown to inhibit the activity of these cells, presumably via similar inhibitory DA somatodendritic mechanisms.[34] This inhibitory effect is attenuated by the systemic administration of haloperidol. The fact that this effect is only moderately attenuated by ibotenic acid lesions of the nucleus accumbens further supports the notion that dendritic mechanisms may be important in regulating VTA DA neuronal activity.[12,34]

Activation of midbrain DA neurons by ADs is characterized not only by an increase in firing rate but by a change in firing pattern — from a predominately single spiking mode to a bursting mode. *In vivo* intracellular recording has demonstrated that iv haloperidol depolarizes the membrane of DA cells by 2 to 5 mV and increases their membrane input resistance 20–50%. This excitatory action of haloperidol may be due to the removal of an inhibitory GABAergic feedback input to DA cells, as the reversal potential of this haloperidol effect was similar to the GABA reversal potential.[35,36] Intravenous haloperidol also increases the rate of occurrence of fast potentials (thought to be due to electrotonic coupling between DA cells[37]) and causes these potentials to be observed where none had been present before. A similar phenomenon has been observed extracellularly. Lastly, acute AD administration appears to activate a population of "silent" hyperpolarized DA cells that have been found in every preparation studied to date.[3,38] When combined, the preceding results suggest that the effect of acute AD administration is a marked activation of midbrain DA systems.

## In Vitro *Studies*

The recently developed midbrain tissue slice preparation offers investigators a new approach to the study of neuronal function. Within the past five years a number of laboratories have adopted this preparation to study the electrophysiological and pharmacological properties of midbrain DA systems.

The mechanism of action of DA antagonists has been quantitatively evaluated by simultaneously perfusing slices with DA and ADs. In one study by Pinnock,[39] the effects of (-)-sulpiride, haloperidol, and *cis*-flupenthixol on DA dose-response curves were studied. The potencies of haloperidol and sulpiride were quite similar to those that have been described in binding studies. However, the potency of *cis*-flupenthixol was 100 times less than that found with binding and clinical efficacy studies. The reason for this discrepancy is unknown. In the presence of DA antagonists the dose-response curves for DA were shifted in parallel to the right. Schild plot analysis of these data suggests that because the slopes of the plots deviated from unity the antagonism is not competitive. This author cautioned that these experiments are tedious, requiring long recording periods and many perfusion medium changes, putting at risk the stability of the recording. Further, he suggested that Schild plot slopes might deviate from unity for reasons that were not addressed in these experiments. These technical problems need to be worked out to clarify the interpretation of future experiments. Recently, clozapine's ability to block DA-induced inhibition of ZC and VTA cells has been tested in the slice preparation.[40] Although some antagonism of the inhibition induced by DA was observed, it was relatively weak and variable. High doses (100 μM) were found to have a nonspecific depressant effect upon ZC DA cells. These findings somewhat resemble the *in vivo* data that demonstrated clozapine to be a relatively weak antagonist of DA-induced inhibition of ZC DA cells.

# EFFECTS OF REPEATED ANTIPSYCHOTIC DRUG ADMINISTRATION

When ADs are administered repeatedly (e.g., once a day for 21 days) their effect differs markedly from that observed after acute administration. The first studies (involving ZC DA cells exclusively) found that the great majority of midbrain DA neurons had become "silent" due to the induction of a tonic state of depolarization inactivation.[3] These findings were later confirmed and extended to A10 DA cells.[38,41,42] *In vivo* intracellular recording has recently verified that the inactivity is due to depolarization block.[43] Feedback pathways would appear to play a role in the development of AD-induced depolarization inactivation of both ZC and VTA neurons as destruction of the striato-nigral and pallido-nigral feedback pathways, prior to initiating repeated haloperidol administration, totally prevented the development of depolarization inactivation of ZC cells.[3] Prior lesioning of the nucleus accumbens produced similar results with VTA cells.[41] However, in accordance with the mounting evidence suggesting that autoreceptors play a more important role in regulating VTA DA cell activity than they do for ZC DA cells, acute knife cuts, which transected the midbrain, immediately reversed the depolarization inactivation of ZC but not VTA DA neurons induced by 21 days of repeated chlorpromazine treatment.[38] Further support for the possible importance of VTA DA cell autoreceptors in mediating AD-induced depolarization inactivation comes from the finding that there are two sets of midbrain DA cells that do not become inactivated by repeated AD administration: those DA neurons innervating the prefrontal and cingulate cortices,[38] both of which lack somatodendritic DA autoreceptors.[17]

Time course studies have demonstrated that two weeks of repeated AD administration are necessary to obtain maximal depolarization inactivation,[41] and that once obtained, it is still present after seven months of repeated treatment.[44] However, no permanent changes appear to have occurred, since after a two-week washout period (e.g., two weeks after discontinuing treatment) the number of DA cells firing in both the ZC and VTA areas has returned to control levels.

Not all ADs induce depolarization inactivation of ZC and VTA neurons. Those drugs that lack or have a markedly decreased incidence of Parkinson-like side effects and tardive dyskinesia (e.g., clozapine) induce depolarization inactivation only in VTA DA neurons.[38,42] On the other hand, drugs that possess extrapyramidal side effects but lack or have a low level of antipsychotic efficacy (e.g., metoclopramide) induce depolarization inactivation in ZC cells but not in VTA DA neurons.[42] Combined, these findings suggest that depolarization inactivation of DA neurons may be one of the mechanisms underlying both the time-dependent therapeutic and neurological side efects of these drugs.

What makes a drug like clozapine incapable of inducing depolarization inactivation of ZC neurons? In addition to its effects on DA systems, clozapine has at least two other actions in the brain: anticholinergic activity[45] and alpha noradrenergic receptor-blocking properties.[46-48] In an attempt to determine whether one or the other of these properties might be important in this regard, the number of spontaneously firing DA cells in the ZC and VTA areas was determined after 21 days of pretreatment with haloperidol and the anticholinergic drug trihexyphenidyl, haloperidol and the alpha-1 antagonist prazosin, or haloperidol and the alpha-2 antagonist idazoxan. The results were compared with clozapine or haloperidol treatment alone.[49] It was found that concomitant treatment with either trihexyphenidyl or prazosin, but not idazoxan, gave haloperidol a clozapine-like profile in terms of its effect on spontaneous ZC and VTA activity. Thus, when combined with an anticholinergic drug or an alpha-1 blocker, haloperidol no longer induced depolarization inactivation of ZC DA cells. The fact that the alpha-2 blocker did not have this effect ruled out the possibility that these were nonspecific results due to polypharmacy.

In another set of studies, 21 days of treatment with ip haloperidol was found to result in ZC DA cell autoreceptor supersensitivity seven days after cessation of treatment.[3,50] Furthermore, in a separate group of animals concurrent administration of lithium carbonate was found to prevent this change in receptor sensitivity.[50]

As so often happens in science a discovery like AD-induced depolarization inactivation of DA cells raises more questions than it answers. One such question is: What is the role of $D_1$ and $D_2$ receptors in mediating this effect and is it the same for all DA systems? As repeated administration of l-sulpiride, a selective $D_2$ antagonist, induced depolarization block in both ZC and VTA DA cells, it would appear that $D_2$ receptors are involved.[38] Preliminary studies, in which rats were treated for 21 days with the selective $D_1$ antagonist SCH 23390, suggest that $D_1$ receptor blockade does not play a role in AD-induced changes in ZC or VTA DA neuronal activity. Thus, repeated treatment with SCH 23390 did not decrease the number of spontaneously firing ZC or VTA DA cells (Esposito and Bunney, in preparation).

## SUMMARY AND CONCLUSIONS

The preceding data suggest that the primary effect of repeated AD administration on most midbrain DA neurons is inactivation. This depolarization-induced cessation of spontaneous activity would appear to have a marked effect on both basal and stimulated DA release from nerve terminals in that several studies, using voltametric techniques, have now demonstrated DA release to be diminished under these conditions.[51-53] These findings stand in marked contrast to the acute effects of ADs where biochemical techniques have been used to demonstrate a marked increase in the release of DA into projection areas.[53-55] The combined effects of acute and repeated AD administration on midbrain DA cell activity may explain the delay in onset of both their therapeutic and neurological side effects.[3,8,41]

## REFERENCES

1. BJORKLUND, A. & O. LINDVALL. 1984. Dopamine-containing systems in the CNS. *In* Classical Transmitters in the CNS, Part I. A. Bjorklund and T. Hokfelt, Eds.: 55–122. Elsevier, New York.
2. BUNNEY, B. S., J. R. WALTERS, R. H. ROTH & G. K. AGHAJANIAN. 1973. Dopaminergic neurons: Effect of antipsychotic drugs and amphetamine on single cell activity. J. Pharmacol. Exp. Ther. **185:** 560–571.
3. BUNNEY, B. S. & A. A. GRACE. 1978. Acute and chronic haloperidol treatment: Comparison of effects on nigral dopaminergic cell activity. Life Sci. **23:** 1715–1728.
4. GRACE, A. A. & B. S. BUNNEY. 1983. Intracellular and extracellular electrophysiology of nigral dopaminergic neurons—I. Identification and characterization. Neuroscience **10:** 301–315.
5. FREEMAN, A. S., L. T. MELTZER & B. S. BUNNEY. 1985. Firing properties of substantia nigra dopaminergic neurons in freely moving rats. Life Sci. **36:** 1983–1984.
6. FREEMAN, A. S. & B. S. BUNNEY. 1987. Activity of A9 and A10 dopaminergic neurons in unrestrained rats: Further characterization and effect of apomorphine and cholecystokinin. Brain Res. **405:** 46–55.
7. SKIRBOLL, L. R., A. A. GRACE, D. W. HOMER, J. REHFELD, M. GOLDSTEIN, T. HOKFELT & B. S. BUNNEY. 1981. Peptide-monoamine coexistance: Studies of cholecystokinin-like peptide action on midbrain dopamine neuron activity. Neuroscience **6:** 2111–2124.
8. BUNNEY, B. S. 1984. Antipsychotic drug effects on the electrical activity of dopaminergic neurons. Trends Neurosci. **7:** 212–215.
9. BUNNEY, B. S. & G. K. AGHAJANIAN. 1978. d-Amphetamine-induced depression of central dopaminergic neurons: Evidence for mediation by both autoreceptors and a striatonigral feedback pathway. N. S. Arch. Pharmacol. **304:** 255–261.
10. KONDO, Y. & K. IWATSUBO. 1980. Diminished response of nigral dopaminergic neurons to haloperidol and morphine following lesions in the striatum. Brain Res. **181:** 237–240.
11. GROVES, P. M., C. J. WILSON, S. J. YOUNG & G. V. REBEC. 1975. Self-inhibition by dopaminergic neurons. Science **190:** 522–529.
12. WANG, R. Y. 1981. Dopaminergic neurons in the rat ventral tegmental area. II. Evidence for autoregulation. Brain Res. **3:** 141–151.
13. KEHR, W., A. CARLSSON, M. LINDQVIST, T. MAGNUSSON & C. V. ATACK. 1972. Evidence for a receptor-mediated feedback control of striatal tyrosine hydroxylase activity. J. Pharm. Pharmacol. **24:** 744–747.
14. KEHR, W., A. CARLSSON & M. LINDQVIST. 1977. Catecholamine synthesis in rat brain after axotomy: Interaction between apomorphine and haloperidol. N. S. Arch Pharmacol. **297:** 111–117.
15. WOLF, M. E. & R. H. ROTH. 1987. Dopamine autoreceptors. *In* Structure and Function of Dopamine Receptors—Receptor Biochemistry and Methodology. I. Creese and C. M. Fraser, Eds. Alan Liss, New York. In Press.
16. CHIODO, L. A., M. J. BANNON, A. A. GRACE, R. H. ROTH & B. S. BUNNEY. 1984. Evidence for the absence of impulse-regulating somatodendritic and synthesis-modulating nerve terminal autoreceptors on subpopulations of mesocortical dopamine neurons. Neuroscience **12:** 1–16.
17. BANNON, M. J., R. L. MICHAUD & R. H. ROTH. 1980. Mesocortical dopamine neurons lack of autoreceptors modulating dopamine synthesis. Mol. Pharmacol. **19:** 270–275.

18. HOKFELT, T., J. F. REHFELD, L. SKIRBOLL, B. IVEMARK, M. GOLDSTEIN & K. MARKEY. 1980a. Evidence for coexistence of dopamine and CCK in mesolimbic neurons. Nature (London) 285: 476–478.

19. HOKFELT, T., L. SKIRBOLL, J. F. REHFELD, M. GOLDSTEIN, K. MARKEY & O. DANN. 1980. A subpopulation of mesoencephalic dopamine neurons projecting to limbic area contains a cholecystokinin-like peptide: Evidence from immunohistochemistry combined with retrograde tracing. Neuroscience 5: 2093–2124.

20. BUNNEY, B. S. 1987. Central dopamine-peptide interactions: Electrophysiological studies. Neuropharmacology 26: 1003–1009.

21. HOMMER, D. W. & L. R. SKIRBOLL. 1983. Cholecystokinin-like peptides potentiate apomorphine-induced inhibition of dopamine neurons. Eur. J. Pharmacol. 91: 151–152.

22. BUNNEY, B. S. & G. K. AGHAJANIAN. 1975. Antipsychotic drugs and central dopaminergic neurons: A model for predicting therapeutic efficacy and incidence of extrapyramidal side effects. In Predictability in Psychopharmacology: Preclinical and Clinical Correlations. A. Sudilovsky, S. Gershon, and B. Beer, Eds.: 225–245. Raven Press, New York.

23. HOMMER, D. W. & B. S. BUNNEY. 1980. Effect of sensory stimuli on the activity of dopaminergic neurons: Involvement of non-dopaminergic nigral neurons and striatonigral pathways. Life Sci. 27: 377–386.

24. BUNNEY, B. S. & G. K. AGHAJANIAN. 1975. The effect of antipsychotic drugs on the firing of dopaminergic neurons: A reappraisal. In Antipsychotic Drugs, Pharmacodynamics and Pharmacokinetics. G. Sedvall, Ed.: 305–318. Pergamon, New York.

25. AGHAJANIAN, G. K. & B. S. BUNNEY. 1974. Pre- and postsynaptic feedback mechanisms in central dopaminergic neurons. In Frontiers in Neurology and Neuroscience Research. P. Seeman and G. M. Brown, Eds.: 4–11. Univ. of Toronto Press, Toronto.

26. CHIODO, L. A. 1981. Studies on the regulation of the responsiveness of substantia nigra dopamine neurons to sensory stimuli. Ph.D. Dissertation. Univ. of Pittsburgh, Pittsburgh, Pa.

27. AGHAJANIAN, G. K. & B. S. BUNNEY. 1977. Dopamine "autoreceptors": Pharmacological characterization by microiontophoretic single cell recording studies. N. S. Arch. Pharmacol. 297: 1–7.

28. CHIODO, L. A. & B. S. BUNNEY. 1983. Electrophysiological studies on EMD 23 448, an indolyl-3-butylamine in the rat: A putative selective dopamine autoreceptor agonist. Neuropharmacology 22: 1087–1093.

29. GROVES, P. M., C. J. WILSON & R. J. MACGREGOR. 1977. Neuronal interactions in the substantia nigra revealed by statistical analysis of neuronal spike trains. In Interactions Among Putative Neurotransmitters in the Brain. S. Garattini, J. F. Pujol, and R. Samanin, Eds.: 191–215, New York.

30. WILSON, C. J., S. J. YOUNG & P. M. GROVES. 1977. Statistical properties of neuronal spike trains in the substantia nigra: Cell types and their interactions. Brain Res. 136: 243–260.

31. WILSON, C. J., G. A. FENSTER, S. J. YOUNG & P. M. GROVES. 1979. Haloperidol-induced alterations of post-firing inhibition in dopaminergic neurons of the rat striatum. Brain Res. 179: 165–170.

32. KORF, J., M. ZIELEMAN & B. H. C. WESTERINK. 1976. Dopamine release in substantia nigra? Nature 260: 257–258.

33. NAKAMURA, S., K. IWATSUTO, C. T. TSAI & K. IWAMA. 1979. Neuronal activity of the substantia nigra (pars compacta) after injection of kainic acid into the caudate nucleus. Exp. Neurol. 66: 682–691.

34. WANG, R. Y. 1981. Dopaminergic neurons in the rat ventral tegmental area. I. Identification and characterization. Brain Res. Rev. 3: 123–140.

35. GRACE, A. A. & B. S. BUNNEY. 1985. Opposing effects of striatonigral feedback pathways on midbrain dopamine cell activity. Brain Res. 333: 271–284.

36. BUNNEY, B. S. & A. A. GRACE. 1985. Depolarization inactivation of nigral dopamine neurons by repeated haloperidol administration: Analysis by in vivo intracellular recording. Neurosci. Abst. 311.15: 1076.

37. GRACE, A. A. & B. S. BUNNEY. 1983. Intracellular and extracellular electrophysiology of nigral dopaminergic neurons—3. Evidence for electrotonic coupling. Neuroscience 10: 333–348.

38. CHIODO, L. A. & B. S. BUNNEY. 1983. Typical and atypical neuroleptics: Differential effects of chronic administration on the activity of A9 and A10 midbrain dopaminergic neurons. J. Neurosci. **3:** 1607–1619.
39. PINNOCK, R. D. 1984. The actions of antipsychotic drugs on dopamine receptors in the rat substantia nigra. Brit. J. Pharmac. **81:** 631–635.
40. SUPPES, J. & R. D. PINNOCK. 1987. Sensitivity of neuronal dopamine response in the substantia nigra and ventral tegmentum to clozapine, metocloprimide and SCH 23390. Neuropharmacology **26:** 331–337.
41. WHITE, F. J. & R. Y. WANG. 1983. Comparison of the effects of chronic haloperidol treatment on A9 and A10 dopamine neurons in the rat. Life Sci. **32:** 983–993.
42. WHITE, F. J. & R. Y. WANG. 1983. Differential effects of classical and atypical antipsychotic drugs on A9 and A10 dopamine neurons. Science **221:** 1054–1057.
43. GRACE, A. A. & B. S. BUNNEY. 1986. Induction of depolarization block in midbrain dopamine neurons by repeated administration of haloperidol: Analysis using *in vivo* intracellular recording. J. Pharmacol. Exp. Ther. **238:** 1092–1100.
44. CHIODO, L. A. & B. S. BUNNEY. 1987. Population response of midbrain dopaminergic neurons to neuroleptics: Further studies on time course and nondopaminergic neuronal influences. J. Neurosci. **7:** 629–633.
45. SNYDER, S. H., S. P. BANERJEE, H. I. YAMAMURA & D. GREENBERG. 1974. Drugs, neurotransmitters and schizophrenia. Science **184:** 1243–1253.
46. BURKI, H. R., W. RUCH, H. ASPER, M. BEGGIOLINI & G. STILLE. 1974. Effect of single and repeated administration of clozapine on the metabolism of dopamine and noradrenaline in the brain of the rat. Eur. J. Pharmacol. **27:** 180–190.
47. MCMILLEN, B. A. & P. A. SHORE. 1978. Comparative effects of clozapine and alpha-adrenoceptor blocking drugs on regional noradrenaline metabolism in rat brain. Eur. J. Pharmacol. **52:** 225–230.
48. SOUTO, M., J. M. MONTI & H. ALTIER. 1978. Effects of clozapine on the activity of central dopaminergic and noradrenergic neurons. Pharmacol. Biochem. Behav. **10:** 5–9.
49. CHIODO, L. A. & B. S. BUNNEY. 1985. Possible mechanisms by which repeated clozapine administration differentially affects the activity of two subpopulations of midbrain dopamine neurons. J. Neurosci. **5:** 2539–2544.
50. GALLAGER, D. W., A. PERT & W. E. BUNNEY, JR. 1978. Haloperidol induced presynaptic dopamine supersensitivity is blocked by chronic lithium. Nature **273:** 309–312.
51. SCHENK, J. O. & B. S. BUNNEY. 1983. The effect of repeated haloperidol treatment on K⁺ stimulated "release" in the rat striatum measured by *in vivo* electrochemistry. Neurosci. Abst. **292.5.**
52. BUNNEY, B. S., L. A. CHIODO, A. A. GRACE & J. O. SCHENK. 1984. *In vivo* effects of acute and chronic antipsychotic drug administration on midbrain dopaminergic neuron activity. *In* Behavioral Pharmacology: Current Status. L. S. Seiden and R. L. Balsten, Eds.: 205–210. Alan Liss, New York.
53. BLAHA, C. D. & R. F. LANE. 1984. Direct *in vivo* electrochemical monitoring of dopamine release in response to neuroleptic drugs. Eur. J. Pharmacol. **98:** 113–117.
54. HUFF, R. M. & R. N. ADAMS. 1980. Dopamine release in N. accumbens and striatum by clozapine: Simultaneous monitoring by *in vivo* electrochemistry. Neuropharmacology **19:** 587–590.
55. IMPERATO, A. & G. DI CHIARA. 1984. Dopamine release and metabolism in awake rats after systemic neuroleptics as studied by trans-striatal dialysis. J. Neurosci. **5:** 297–306.

# Influence of Dopamine on Limbic Inputs to the Nucleus Accumbens

G. J. MOGENSON, C. R. YANG, AND C. Y. YIM

*Department of Physiology*
*University of Western Ontario*
*London, Ontario, Canada*

## INTRODUCTION

The nucleus accumbens of the basal forebrain, a major component of the ventral striatum, is rich in dopamine (DA). There is a good deal of clinical and experimental evidence that suggests that accumbens DA has functional significance. It has been implicated in locomotor activity,[1,2] in brain stimulation reward,[3] in self-administration of opiate drugs,[4] and in neurological and psychiatric disorders such as Parkinson's disease and schizophrenia.[5,6]

Anatomical connections of the accumbens place it strategically between limbic and motor structures.[7,8] Its nodal position suggests that the accumbens has a major role in the limbic-motor integration that underlies certain complex, adaptive behaviors.[9,10] DA, by altering in the accumbens the relay of limbic outputs to motor structures, may significantly modulate the influence that limbic structures exert on the extrapyramidal motor system. Our approach in the investigation of this possibility is to determine electrophysiologically how inputs to accumbens neurons are influenced by DA. This paper reviews some of the experimental findings from studies using this approach in rats under urethane anesthesia. The first section deals briefly with some empirical findings from early extracellular single-unit recording experiments and the second and third sections deal with more recent attempts to elucidate the mechanisms by which DA influences limbic inputs to accumbens neurons. In the last section, results from some behavioral experiments complementary to the electrophysiological findings are described. Results from the behavioral experiments are interpreted, along with those from electrophysiological experiments, to suggest an integrated hypothesis on possible functions of dopamine in the accumbens, especially its role in behavioral response initiation.

## NEUROMODULATORY ACTION OF DA IN THE NUCLEUS ACCUMBENS OBSERVED IN EXTRACELLULAR SINGLE-UNIT RECORDINGS

Our initial experimental approach was quite straightforward. The activity of accumbens neurons was sampled with standard extracellular electrophysiological recording techniques and the effect of ventral tegmental area (VTA) stimulation on these neurons was investigated. Early observations showed that although single-pulse VTA stimulation produced excitatory as well as inhibitory responses in the accumbens, they were not blocked by DA antagonists such as haloperidol or trifluoperazine. The responses to single-pulse stimulation of the VTA were later attributed to activation of non-dopaminergic projections to the accumbens.[11] Those experiments also showed that DA has a neuromodulatory, rather than a direct neuromediating, action in the accumbens. Our later experiments were therefore directed to investigating the interaction of DA with other synaptic inputs to the accumbens.[12,13]

Accumbens neurons were activated by single-pulse stimulation of the basolateral amygdala (see FIG. 1) or of the ventral subiculum of the hippocampus (see FIG. 2). Concomitant stimulation of the VTA at 10 Hz, but synchronized to be separated from single-pulse stimulations of the amygdala or hippocampus by at least 50 ms, produced substantial reduction of the excitatory response, often without significantly changing the baseline activity of the neuron (FIG. 1, left lower panel, and FIG. 2, right panel). This attenuating effect of VTA stimulation was independent of the response of the neuron to single-pulse stimulation of the VTA and was blocked by haloperidol and sulpiride. Iontophoretically applied DA mimicked the effect of VTA stimulation (FIG. 1, right lower panel) and suggested, along with the pharmacological blockade of the response by DA antagonists, that endogenously released DA from VTA stimulation had a neuromodulatory action in the accumbens.

These attenuating or modulating effects of DA have also been observed in the caudate nucleus. Excitatory responses of caudate neurons to electrical stimulation of the cerebral cortex are reduced by conditioning stimulation of the substantia nigra or by the iontophoretic application of DA.[14,15]

Early electrophysiological investigations of the action of dopamine in the striatum have focused on its postsynaptic effects. Most investigators reported predominantly

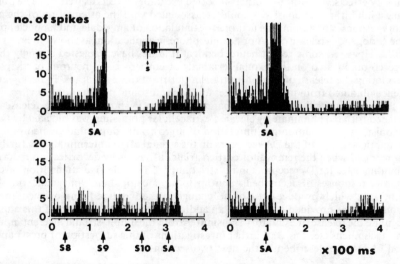

**FIGURE 1.** Peristimulus time histogram showing the excitatory responses of two neurons of the nucleus accumbens to single-pulse stimulation of the basolateral amygdala (SA). *Left upper panel*: normal response of first neuron (*inset* is single response photographed from oscilloscope). *Left lower panel*: excitatory response is reduced when conditioning stimulation to the VTA (train of 10 pulses, 300 µA, 0.15 ms at 10 Hz) precedes amygdala stimulation (SA). *Right upper panel*: normal response of second accumbens neuron to amygdala stimulation. *Right lower panel*: excitatory response is reduced when DA (10 nA) is applied iontophoretically to the accumbens neuron. (After Yim and Mogenson, 1982)

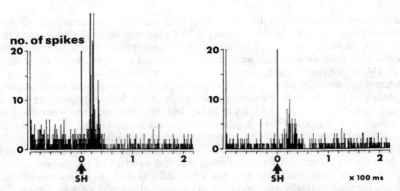

**FIGURE 2.** Peristimulus time histograms showing the excitatory response of an accumbens neuron to single-pulse stimulation of the ventral subiculum of the hippocampus. *Left panel*: excitatory response of an accumbens neuron to hippocampal stimulation (400 μA, 0.15 ms at 0.5 Hz) during application of Na$^+$ (20 nA) as a control. *Right panel*: attenuation of the excitatory response when 20-nA DA was applied iontophoretically to the accumbens neuron. A small but insignificant change in baseline firing of this neuron occurred during DA application. Conditioning stimulation of the VTA by trains of conditioning pulses delivered at 10 Hz also attenuated the excitatory response in a similar manner. All histograms were compiled from 150 sweeps. (After Yang and Mogenson.[13])

inhibitory effects,[16,17] although others reported excitatory effects as well.[18,19] The postsynaptic inhibitory action of DA could be associated with the attenuation of the excitatory responses of accumbens neurons to stimulation of amygdala and hippocampus by the endogenous release of DA or its iontophoretic application, as shown in FIGURES 1 and 2. However, some recent neurochemical findings have suggested strongly that DA receptors located on the axonal terminals of corticostriatal neurons participate in regulating the release of excitatory transmitter from these synapses. Experimental evidence obtained from rat striatal slices and synaptosomal preparations *in vitro*,[20,21] and from a push-pull perfusion preparation *in vivo*,[22] showed that the release of preloaded tritiated glutamate by elevated extracellular potassium was blocked by DA, its agonist, or by conditioning stimulation of nigrostriatal dopaminergic neurons. A presynaptic location of the DA receptors on the striatal afferent terminals was further demonstrated when the removal of corticostriatal afferents by decortication reduced the binding sites for D$_2$ receptors in rat striatum.[23,24] The selective attenuation of the excitatory responses of accumbens neurons to hippocampal and amygdala stimulation by DA, which produce little or no change in the baseline firing of accumbens neurons,[12,13] has provided evidence of an additional presynaptic action of this amine to regulate the release of excitatory transmitter from the limbic-striatal afferent inputs to the accumbens (see Fig. 3). Further investigations of this suggestion of presynaptic action of DA are described in the next two sections.

## PRESYNAPTIC ACTION OF DOPAMINE: A TEST OF THE EXCITABILITY OF THE AXONAL TERMINALS OF LIMBIC-STRIATAL AFFERENTS

The electrophysiological action of DA in modulating transmitter release from limbic afferent terminals to the accumbens was investigated by a test of the excitability of

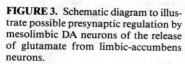

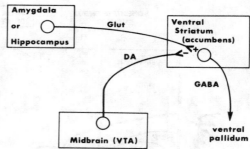

**FIGURE 3.** Schematic diagram to illustrate possible presynaptic regulation by mesolimbic DA neurons of the release of glutamate from limbic-accumbens neurons.

the axonal terminals of hippocampal–accumbens (HIPP-ACC) neurons.[25-27] This method enables the study of the influence of DA on the presynaptic terminals of afferent inputs dissociated from its postsynaptic actions (see FIG. 4 for the experimental setup).

The excitability of the axonal terminals of HIPP-ACC neurons, as reflected by the firing index, was abruptly enhanced by conditioning stimulation of the VTA (200–800 μA, 5–10 trains, 10 pulses/train delivered at 0.6 Hz). Iontophoretic application of DA (60–160 nA for 30–90 sec), a DA $D_2$ agonist, or potassium ions, but not a $D_1$ agonist, to the axonal terminals of HIPP-ACC neurons produced a gradual but prolonged increase of the firing index. In some of these neurons, there was an enhanced firing index with iontophoretic application of DA as well as with conditioning VTA stimulation (FIG. 5), even after ibotenic acid pretreatment in the accumbens (which ruled out the possibility of the dopaminergic effect being mediated indirectly by interneurons). Furthermore, if the accumbens stimulating current was adjusted to produce a baseline firing index near zero, conditioning stimulation of the VTA did not change the firing index. These observations suggest that DA did not tonically influence resting HIPP-ACC neurons, but enhanced their terminal excitability when the glutamatergic synapse was activated, for example, by a depolarizing current delivered to their terminals by the accumbens electrode. Therefore, it appears that some background activity in the terminals of HIPP-ACC neurons is necessary for the subsequent action of DA.[22,28]

The increase in firing index produced by conditioning VTA stimulation was reduced when sulpiride, a $D_2$ antagonist, was administered iontophoretically in the region of axonal terminals of HIPP-ACC neurons. When the conditioning VTA stimulation was repeated, the firing index gradually returned to the control level. In marked contrast, the enhanced firing index of HIPP-ACC neurons produced by conditioning VTA stimulation was not changed when SCH 23390, a selective DA $D_1$ antagonist, was injected intraperitoneally.[27] These results further support the presence of $D_2$ receptors on the axonal terminals of HIPP-ACC neurons.

The elevation by DA of the excitability of HIPP-ACC neurons may be due in part to its moderate depolarizing action on neuronal membranes.[29-31] It is known that moderate depolarization of the axonal terminals increases their excitability and reduces the quantal release of transmitter due to the associated reduction of the amplitude of subsequent action potentials invading the terminals.[32,33] The suggestion that dopamine increases the excitability of the HIPP-ACC afferent terminals by membrane depolarization is thus consistent with the pharmacological observation that dopamine reduces glutamate release in the striatum.[20-22] On the other hand, although dopamine is also known to regulate its own release by binding to $D_2$-type autoreceptors on the terminals of dopaminergic neurons, stimulation of these receptors by DA agonists tends

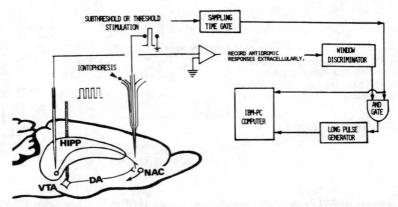

**FIGURE 4.** Block diagram to show the setup for the terminal excitability test. Antidromic responses of hippocampal neurons in the ventral subiculum region were evoked by single-pulse stimulation of the medial nucleus accumbens via the center barrel of multibarrel micropipette assemblies. The side barrels of the multibarrel micropipettes contained drugs and neurotransmitter substances used to characterize the DA receptors that mediate possible changes in terminal excitability. A stainless steel concentric bipolar electrode in the VTA was used to deliver conditioning pulses to activate the mesolimbic dopaminergic neurons. Each accumbens stimulation triggered a sampling gate, generating a pulse to start the computer, which registered the number of stimulations. When an antidromic response, isolated by a window discriminator, occurred during this preset gated interval, a long pulse was generated that triggered the computer to count the number of antidromic responses, and subsequently to compute the firing index. In a control trial, 6–8 antidromic responses of hippocampal neurons were recorded during a set of 20 stimuli delivered to the accumbens. Thus, a baseline firing index, reflecting the terminal excitability of the neuron, was tabulated continuously on-line by an IBM PC computer from the equation: (Number of antidromic responses/Number of stimulation trials) × 100. The baseline firing index was determined from at least 5–10 sets of test trials prior to further experimental treatments. (After Yang and Mogenson.[27])

to suppress the excitability of these terminals,[34,35] a phenomenon attributed to a hyperpolarizing action of DA shown in hippocampal pyramidal neurons.[36,37] These two seemingly contrasting findings indicate that changes in excitability of the presynaptic terminals in the accumbens by dopamine cannot simply be attributed to a change in membrane potential alone and that dopamine likely has multiple actions at different afferent $D_2$ binding sites in the accumbens.

## INTRACELLULAR RECORDING FROM ACCUMBENS NEURONS *IN SITU*: FURTHER CORROBORATIVE EVIDENCE OF A PRESYNAPTIC NEUROMODULATORY ACTION OF DOPAMINE IN THE ACCUMBENS

The previous section suggests that DA has a presynaptic action on nondopaminergic terminals in the accumbens. The function of that action is likely a modulation of transmitter release from these terminals as illustrated in pharmacological studies.[20-22] Results from extracellular recording experiments that showed that DA attenuated excitatory response of accumbens neurons to amygdala and hippocampal stimulation are consistent with the biochemical observations. Further illustration of the possible physiolog-

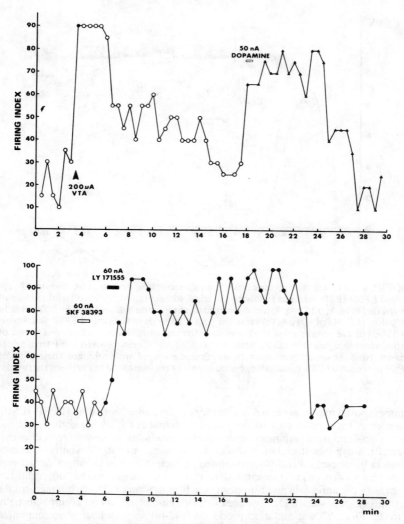

**FIGURE 5.** The firing index of two HIPP-ACC neurons was changed by conditioning VTA stimulation, iontophoretic application of DA, of a $D_1$ agonist SKF 38393, and of a $D_2$ agonist LY 171555. *Upper panel*: the firing index was increased by conditioning VTA stimulation (200 µA, 5 trains of 10-Hz pulses) and by the iontophoretic application of DA (50 nA). *Lower panel*: in another HIPP-ACC neuron, the firing index was not changed by the iontophoretic application of the $D_1$ agonist, SKF 38393 (60 nA), but the iontophoretic application of the $D_2$ agonist, LY 171555 (60 nA), produced a fourfold increase in the firing index. (After Yang and Mogenson.[27])

ical function of the presynaptic action of DA on nondopaminergic terminals in the accumbens was obtained from *in situ* intracellular recording experiments.[31]

Recordings made intracellularly from accumbens neurons *in situ* showed that stimulation of the amygdala or the hippocampus produced monosynaptically evoked ex-

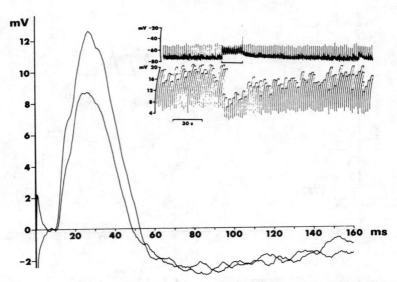

**FIGURE 6.** Intracellular recording made from an accumbens neuron *in situ* showing the typical evoked EPSP–IPSP sequence following electrical stimulation of the basolateral nucleus of the amygdala (400 µA, 0.15 ms). When the amygdala stimulation was preceded by VTA stimulation (10 pulses at 10 Hz of 600 µA, 0.15 ms), the peak amplitude of the evoked EPSP was attenuated by 32%, but the accompanied IPSP was not affected. *Inset* shows a continuous record of the resting membrane potential and the peak amplitude of the amygdala-evoked EPSP from a different neuron. Note the depolarization of the membrane potential and prolonged attenuation of the EPSP produced by VTA stimulation (period shown by the horizontal bar between the two traces).

citatory postsynaptic potential–inhibitory postsynaptic potential (EPSP–IPSP) sequences in the medial part of the nucleus accumbens (Fig. 6), comparable to the excitation–inhibition responses observed in extracellular single-unit recording experiments.[12] Amygdala stimulation tended to excite neurons in the ventral accumbens, whereas hippocampal stimulation tended to excite those in the more dorsal region. A number of neurons in the central part of the accumbens received converging inputs from both the amygdala and hippocampus. Stimulation of the ventral tegmental area in trains of pulses at 10 Hz produced three consistent effects on accumbens neurons (Fig. 6). First, VTA stimulation produced 3–12-mV depolarization accompanied by an increase in membrane conductance; second, a spontaneously occurring 0.8–1.0-Hz rhythmic oscillation of the membrane potential seen in over 80% of accumbens neurons was eliminated; third, EPSP but not the late IPSP evoked from either amygdala or hippocampal stimulation was attenuated. All of these effects produced by VTA stimulation were blocked by IP injection of haloperidol or sulpiride, indicating that the effects were at least in part mediated by release of endogenous DA.

The attenuation of the amygdala or hippocampal evoked EPSPs in accumbens neurons produced by VTA stimulation did not appear to be causally related to the concomitant membrane depolarization. This conclusion is suggested because similar depolarization produced by current injection through the recording electrode did not produce comparable attenuation of the EPSPs. Furthermore, the time course of recovery of the attenuation of the EPSPs and that of membrane depolarization were not always the same.[31] The implication from this conclusion is that DA released by VTA stimulation likely acts at different sites to produce these two effects. Membrane depolarization is likely due to a postsynaptic action of DA on the soma of the recorded accumbens neurons, and the preferential attenuation of evoked EPSPs could be the result of localized dendritic depolarization or presynaptic attenuation of transmitter release due to DA.

The hypothesis that VTA stimulation attenuates amygdala and hippocampal evoked EPSPs by a presynaptic action of dopamine is suggested for several reasons. First, it is consistent with the pharmacological finding that dopamine reduces glutamate release from cortical afferents to the striatum.[20-22] Second, the attenuated EPSPs often had similar half-amplitude decay times compared to the control,[31] indicating the absence of changes in the conductance of the postsynaptic membrane at the synapse.[38] Third, attenuation of the evoked EPSPs was always observed in the absence of comparable attenuation of the accompanied late IPSP. Furthermore, in neurons that receive converging inputs from both the amygdala and hippocampus, there was a preferential attenuation of the response to amygdala stimulation compared to the one produced by hippocampal stimulation.[39] These observations by themselves do not preclude an alternative interpretation, namely that endogenous dopamine released by VTA stimulation acts locally at restricted dendritic sites, but nevertheless, they are considered good corroborative evidence to suggest a presynaptic neuromodulatory action of dopamine in the accumbens.

Iontophoretically applied dopamine produced similar as well as different actions compared to VTA stimulation in the accumbens (FIG. 7). The resting membrane potential of the accumbens neuron was consistently depolarized, similarly to that observed in the caudate nucleus.[30,40] EPSPs evoked from amygdala or hippocampal stimulation were attenuated by iontophoretically applied dopamine, but whereas VTA stimulation did not attenuate the accompanied late IPSPs, exogenous dopamine attenuated both. Moreover, in those neurons that received converging inputs from the amygdala and hippocampus, and in which VTA stimulation produced a preferential attenuation of the amygdala-evoked response, iontophoretically applied dopamine did not show similar selectivity in its action. These findings suggest that the physiological action of endogenous dopamine in the accumbens, which may not be duplicated in iontophoresis studies, likely depends on its binding to restricted selective sites and also on the action of other neurotransmitters, such as cholecystokinin, that are normally coreleased with dopamine.[41]

## PHYSIOLOGICAL FUNCTION OF DOPAMINE IN THE NUCLEUS ACCUMBENS: IMPLICATIONS FROM ELECTROPHYSIOLOGICAL AND BEHAVIORAL OBSERVATIONS

The nucleus accumbens is a strategic target for a large number of limbic afferent inputs,[42] but sends efferents to only a small number of sites.[7] As shown by the electrophysiological findings, DA in the accumbens may have a role in regulating the transmission of the numerous incoming signals to the target sites of ventral striatal output neurons; for example, to the ventral pallidum. The behavioral implications of this dopaminergic mechanism as revealed by the electrophysiological observations were investigated in complementary behavioral experiments. A summary of the findings and an overview of possible functions of DA in the accumbens based on an integration of electrophysiological and behavioral observations are presented below.

Electrophysiological experiments showed that ventral pallidal neurons were inhibited

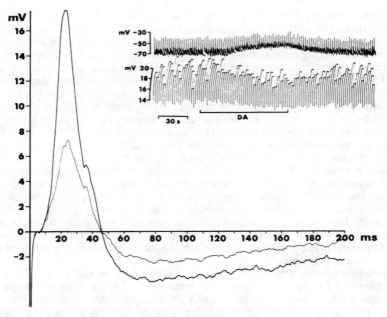

**FIGURE 7.** Extracellular iontophoretic application of dopamine (60 nA during period marked by the horizontal bar between the two traces in the inset) produced prolonged depolarization of the resting membrane potential of accumbens neurons. It also produced pronounced attenuation of the evoked EPSP from hippocampal stimulation; unlike the effect of VTA stimulation (see FIG. 6), iontophoretically applied dopamine typically attenuated both the EPSP and IPSP as shown in this figure.

by stimulation of the basolateral nucleus of the amygdala via a pathway through the nucleus accumbens.[43] Ventral pallidal neurons, on the other hand, project to the midbrain mesencephalic locomotor region[44] and GABAergic inhibition of neuronal activity in the ventral pallidum suppresses striatal–mediated locomotor activity.[45] Prediction from these observations is that the basolateral nucleus of the amygdala may have an inhibitory influence on ambulatory activity mediated by way of the projection to the accumbens and subsequently to the ventral pallidum. This suggestion is supported by reports in the literature that electrical stimulation of the amygdala in cats produces arrest of locomotion and general arousal and that lesions of the amygdala increase exploratory behavior in the rat.[46,47] In a recent behavioral study,[48] rats were placed in an experimental cage partitioned into three chambers with communicating holes between the chambers. Animals remain spontaneously active in the experimental cage for over 30 min, even for repeated trials. It was found that when N-methyl-D-aspartate (NMDA, an excitatory amino acid) was injected into the amygdala, this spontaneous exploratory behavior was significantly suppressed. Furthermore, the suppression of the exploratory behavior was enhanced by a small injection of nipecotic acid, a GABA uptake inhibitor, into the ventral pallidum, but was attenuated by injection of a low dose (5 µg) of dopamine into the accumbens that by itself did not enhance locomotor activity. These findings are not only consistent with the suggestion put forward but also illustrate a possible physiological function of DA in the accumbens. The amyg-

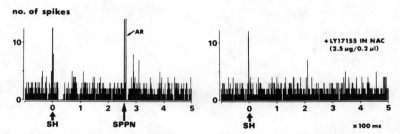

**FIGURE 8.** Peristimulus time histograms showing the effects of microinjection of LY 171555, a DA $D_2$ agonist, into the accumbens on the inhibitory response of an antidromically identified subpallidal–pedunculopontine nucleus (SP-PPN) neuron to hippocampal stimulation. *Left panel*: SH and SPPN indicate the time at which single-pulse stimulation was delivered to the hippocampus and to the pedunculopontine nucleus, respectively. AR indicates the short latency antidromic response of the subpallidal neuron to PPN stimulation. *Right panel*: 5 min after microinjection of LY 171555 (2 µg/0.2 µl) into the medial accumbens, the inhibitory response to hippocampal stimulation was reduced, suggesting a blockade of transmission of hippocampal signals to the subpallidal neuron by DA $D_2$ receptors in the accumbens. Only the response to hippocampal stimulation is shown in the right panel. (After Yang and Mogenson.[51])

dala, by way of the nucleus accumbens, may have a tonic or an acute inhibitory influence on the locomotor activity of the animal. Dopamine released in the accumbens, perhaps by other competing behavioral processes, can indirectly activate the motor system by suppressing the inhibition from the amygdala via a presynaptic modulatory action described in the previous sections.

The HIPP–ACC projection represents another major limbic input to the accumbens. Electrophysiological experiments showed that stimulation of the hippocampus: (1) excited accumbens output neurons (GABAergic or enkephalinergic),[49] which project directly to the ventral pallidum,[50] and (2) inhibited spontaneously active subpallidal (SP) neurons (including substantia innominata and lateral hypothalamus), which project directly to the midbrain mesencephalic locomotor region.[51] Microinjection of a DA $D_2$ agonist (LY 171555), but not a $D_1$ agonist (SKF 38393), into the medial accumbens attenuated the inhibitory response of these SP neurons to hippocampal stimulation (FIG. 8). The stimulation of $D_2$ receptors in the accumbens may thus inhibit the glutamatergic HIPP–ACC neurons from activating the accumbens–subpallidal neurons and consequently produce a blockade of the transmission of hippocampal signals to the subpallidal sites.

Many of the electrophysiological response of accumbens and subpallidal neurons are similar following stimulation of the hippocampus or the amygdala, suggesting that these limbic inputs share common pathways to the pallidal site. However, behavioral tests have shown that chemical activation of the hippocampus by microinjection of NMDA (0.5 µg/0.2 µl) into the ventral subiculum produced a marked increase in locomotor activity in the open field similar to the spatially oriented exploratory behavior typically mediated by the hippocampus.[52,53] Since reciprocal synaptic regulation of glutamatergic and dopaminergic neurons occurs in the striatum,[28] the NMDA-activation of the glutamatergic HIPP–ACC pathway may release DA from the VTA dopaminergic afferents to the accumbens and subsequently produce hyperkinetic responses indirectly via the action of DA on the accumbens output neurons.[54] Furthermore, injection of $D_2$ agonist (1–4 µg/0.2 µl) into the accumbens produced no effect on the baseline locomotor activity, but significantly reduced the hyperkinetic response induced by NMDA

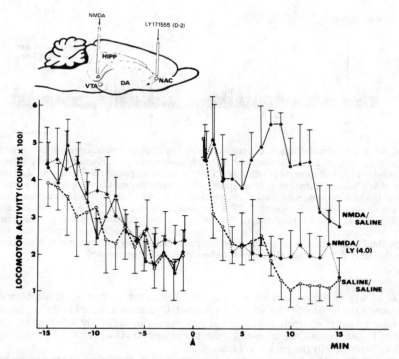

**FIGURE 9.** Effects on locomotor activity of microinjection of LY 171555, a DA D₂ agonist, into the nucleus accumbens induced by microinjection of NMDA into the ventral subiculum of the hippocampus. The locomotor response before and after drug injections into hippocampus and accumbens are shown. *Open circles*: mean locomotor activity recorded as photobeam interruptions before and after saline injection to both brain sites. *Solid circles*: locomotor activity before and after NMDA was injected into the hippocampus and saline solution injected into the accumbens. *Solid diamonds*: locomotor response before and after LY 171555 (4.0 µg/0.2 µl) was injected into the accumbens before NMDA was injected into the hippocampus. Mean and SEM are shown. *Arrow* indicates the time when drug injections were made. All injections were unilateral. *Inset*: diagram showing the injection sites in the hippocampus and the accumbens. (After Yang and Mogenson.[51])

injection into the hippocampus (Fig. 9). These behavioral observations thus suggest that: (1) via D₂ receptors, DA may inhibit presynaptically the glutamatergic HIPP–ACC neurons that mediate a hyperkinetic response in rats; (2) concurrent stimulation of D₂-type autoreceptors on the dopaminergic afferents in the accumbens reduce DA release[35] and, hence, minimize the release of DA by the NMDA-activated glutamatergic HIPP–ACC afferents. Consequently, an increase in locomotor responses by DA via this indirect action of the HIPP–ACC neurons on DA synapse is attenuated. Other parallel pathways beyond the pallidal site that may mediate this hyperkinetic response to hippocampal stimulation have been suggested elsewhere.[51] Nonetheless, behavioral observations indicate that the amygdala-mediated decreases and hippocampal-mediated increases in locomotor activities via the nucleus accumbens are reversed by DA or its

$D_2$ agonist in the accumbens, mediated in part by a presynaptic action on the limbic afferents.[48,51]

The functional significance of the presynaptic action of DA described in the electrophysiological and behavioral experiments are further considered below. A presynaptic action of DA, in contrast to a postsynaptic one, could exert a "focusing" or "selective" effect in the accumbens. Whereas postsynaptic actions of DA would influence all inputs to the accumbens neurons, presynaptic inhibition could reduce certain limbic or cortical inputs while transmission of other inputs through the ventral striatum are not inhibited indiscriminately. Such a "focusing" mechanism would not only allow the "selected" limbic structure to have the strongest modulation of the extrapyramidal system but also permit a switching between alternative types or sources of information.[55] This "focusing" or "selective" action of DA would be especially advantageous in the accumbens that receives multiple converging limbic inputs.[42] It would permit the expression of a particular behavioral act, associated with a certain pattern of limbic inputs, whereas other behavioral acts that are inappropriate or conflicting would be suppressed. For example, the selective attenuation of amygdala inputs to the accumbens by dopamine as previously mentioned enables accumbens output neurons to reflect the more predominant influence from other limbic structures, such as the hippocampus, that may bring about a different adaptive behavior according to specific environmental demands.

Besides a presynaptic action, DA has postsynaptic actions as well. At postsynaptic sites, DA may produce a general suppression of ventral striatal outputs to the subpallidum, the key target sites for striatal inhibitory GABAergic and enkephalinergic efferents.[49] The behavioral significance of this action is perhaps illustrated by the observation that dopamine injected into the accumbens has pronounced stimulatory effects on locomotor activity.[2] It is conceivable that nonselective postsynaptic inhibition of some striatal–pallidal neurons by DA leads to a disinhibition of pallidal neurons and the disinhibition of ventral pallidal neurons may cause the initiation of locomotor activity.

Another example of which correlation can be drawn between the electrophysiological and behavioral observations of the actions of DA in the accumbens was demonstrated by recent EEG recordings made from the nucleus accumbens of behaving rats. As mentioned in the preceding section, the resting membrane potential of accumbens neurons showed rhythmic oscillation of approximately 1 Hz and the oscillations were eliminated by DA.[31] Recently, it was shown that a rhythmic EEG of the same frequency could be recorded from the accumbens of behaving rats while the animals were immobile, but the EEG became desynchronized during periods of rearing or locomotion[56] (personal communication). The physiological significance of these observations is still not known, but the implication that DA, acting either presynaptically or postsynaptically, eliminates a synchronous oscillation of resting membrane potential of accumbens neurons as a prerequisite for behavioral initiation raises interesting questions and may provide further insights into the physiological function of DA in the accumbens.

We have tried to illustrate in this section how electrophysiological observations can be used to interpret behavioral observations in order to derive an integrated view of the functions of dopamine in the accumbens. The discussion, however, has been focused primarily on its locomotor effects. Dopamine nevertheless has other important behavioral roles as indicated earlier. A direct correlation between those behavioral and electrophysiological actions of DA remains to be investigated. As a general statement, however, it can be appreciated from neurochemical, electrophysiological, and behavioral evidence, that DA can regulate, as well as initiate, a variety of physiological responses by a complex combination of actions via activation of its receptors at multiple synaptic sites in the striatum. Experimentally, although some of these mechanisms are studied separately, they may operate physiologically all at the same time to produce appropriate behaviors according to the environmental demands.

## REFERENCES

1. MOGENSON, G. J., M. WU & S. K. MANCHANDA. 1979. Locomotor activity initiated by microinfusion of picrotoxin into the ventral tegmental area. Brain Res. **161:** 311-319.
2. PIJNENBERG, A. J. J. & J. M. VAN ROSSUM. 1973. Stimulation of locomotor activity following injection of dopamine into the nucleus accumbens. J. Pharm. Pharmacol. **25:** 1003-1005.
3. PHILLIPS, A. G. & H. C. FIBIGER. 1978. The role of dopamine in maintaining intracranial self-stimulation in the ventral tegmentum, nucleus accumbens, and medial prefrontal cortex. Can. J. Psychol. **32:** 58-66.
4. WISE, R. A. & M. A. BOZARTH. 1981. Brain substrates for reinforcement and drug self-administration. Prog. Neuropsychopharm. **5:** 467-474.
5. PRICE, K. S., I. J. FARLEY & O. HORNYKIEWICZ. 1978. Neurochemistry of Parkinson's disease: Relation between striatal and limbic dopamine. *In* Advances of Biochemical Psychopharmacology, Vol. 19. P. J. Roberts, G. N. Woodruff, and L. L. Iversen, Eds.: 293-300. Raven Press. New York.
6. MATHYSEE, S. 1981. Nucleus accumbens and schizophrenia. *In* The Neurobiology of the Nucleus Accumbens. R. B. Chronister and J. F. DeFrance, Eds.: 351-359. Haer Institute for Electrophysiological Research. Maine.
7. NAUTA, W. J. H., G. P. SMITH, R. L. M. FAULL & V. B. DOMESICK. 1978. Efferent connections and nigral afferents of the nucleus accumbens septi in the rat. Neurosci. **3:** 385-401.
8. MOGENSON, G. J., D. L. JONES & C. Y. YIM. 1980. From motivation to action: Functional interface between the limbic system and the motor system. Prog. Neurobiol. **14:** 69-97.
9. GRAYBIEL, A. M. 1984. Neurochemically specified subsystems in the basal ganglia. Presented at the CIBA Foundation Symposium.
10. MOGENSON, G. J. 1987. Limbic-motor integration. Prog. Psychobiol. Physiol. Psychol. **12:** 117-169.
11. MOGENSON, G. J. & C. Y. YIM. 1981. Electrophysiological and neuropharmacological-behavioral studies of the nucleus accumbens: Implications for its role as a limbic motor interface. *In* The Neurobiology of the Nucleus Accumbens. R. B. Chronister and J. F. DeFrance, Eds.: 210-229. Haer Institute for Electrophysiological Research. Maine.
12. YIM, C. Y. & G. J. MOGENSON. 1982. Responses of nucleus accumbens neurons to amygdala stimulation and its modification by dopamine. Brain Res. **239:** 401-405.
13. YANG, C. R. & G. J. MOGENSON. 1984. Electrophysiological responses of neurones in the nucleus accumbens to hippocampal stimulation and the attenuation of the excitatory responses by the mesolimbic dopaminergic system. Brain Res. **324:** 69-84.
14. HIRATA, K., C. Y. YIM & G. J. MOGENSON. 1984. Excitatory input from sensory motor cortex to neostriatum and its modification by conditioning stimulation of the substantia nigra. Brain Res. **321:** 1-8.
15. VIVES, F. & G. J. MOGENSON. 1986. Electrophysiological study of the effects of $D_1$ and $D_2$ dopamine antagonists on the interaction of converging inputs from the sensory motor cortex and substantia nigra neurons in the rat. Neuroscience **17:** 349-359.
16. CONNOR, J. D. 1970. Caudate nucleus neurons: Correlation of the effects of substantia nigra stimulation with iontophoretic dopamine. J. Physiol. **208:** 691-703.
17. MCCARTHY, P. S., R. J. WALKER & G. N. WOODRUFF. 1977. On the depressant action of dopamine in rat caudate nucleus and nucleus accumbens. Br. J. Pharmacol. **59:** 469-470.
18. YORK, D. H. 1979. The neurophysiology of dopamine receptors. *In* The Neurobiology of Dopamine, A. S. Horn, J. Korf, and B. H. C. Westerink, Eds.: 395-415. Academic Press. New York.
19. ASSAF, S. Y. & J. J. MILLER. 1977. Excitatory action of the mesolimbic dopamine system on septal neurons. Brain Res. **129:** 353-360.
20. ROWLAND, G. J. & P. J. ROBERTS. 1980. Activation of dopamine receptors inhibits calcium-

dependent glutamate release from corticostriatal terminals in vitro. Eur. J. Pharmacol. **62:** 241–242.

21. MITCHELL, P. R. & N. S. DOGGETT. 1980. Modulation of striatal $^3$H-glutamic acid release by dopaminergic drugs. Life Sci. **26:** 2073–2081.

22. GODUKHIN, O. V., A. D. ZHARIKOVA & A. YU BUDANTSEVG. 1984. Role of presynaptic dopamine receptors in regulation of the glutamatergic neurotransmission in rat neostriatum. Neuroscience **12:** 377–383.

23. SCHWARCZ, R., I. CREESE, J. T. COYLE & S. H. SNYDER. 1978. Dopamine receptors localized on cerebral cortical afferents to rat corpus striatum. Nature **271:** 766–768.

24. THEODOROU, A., C. REAVILL, P. JENNER & C. D. MARSDEN. 1981. Kainic acid lesions of striatum and decortication reduce specific $^3$H-sulpiride binding in rats, so D-2 receptors exist post-synaptically on corticostriate afferents and striatal neurones. J. Pharm. Pharmacol. **33:** 439–444.

25. CURTIS, D. R. & R. W. RYALL. 1966. Pharmacological studies upon spinal presynaptic fibres. Exp. Brain Res. **1:** 195–204.

26. WALL, P. D. Excitability changes in afferent fibre terminations and their relation to slow potentials. J. Physiol. (London) **142:** 1–21.

27. YANG, C. R. & G. J. MOGENSON. 1986. Dopamine enhances terminal excitability of hippocampal-accumbens neurones via D-2 receptor: Role of dopamine in presynaptic inhibition. J. Neurosci. **6:** 2470–2478.

28. NIEOULLON, A., L. KERKERIAN & N. DUSTICIER. 1983. Presynaptic controls in the neostratum: Reciprocal interactions between the nigrostriatal dopaminergic neurones and the corticostriatal glutamatergic pathway. Exp. Brain Res. Suppl. **7:** 54–65.

29. BERNARDI, G., M. G. MARCIANAI, C. MOROCUTTI, F. PAVONE & P. STANZIONE. 1978. The action of dopamine on rat caudate neurones intracellularly recorded. Neurosci. Lett. **8:** 235–240.

30. HERRLING, P. & C. D. HULL. 1980. Iontophoretically applied dopamine depolarizes and hyperpolarizes the membrane of cat caudate neurones. Brain Res. **192:** 441–462.

31. YIM, C. Y. & G. J. MOGENSON. 1986. Mesolimbic dopamine projection modulates amygdalaevoked EPSP in nucleus accumbens: An in vivo study. Brain Res. **369:** 347–352.

32. KUSANO, K., D. R. LIVENWOOD & R. WERMAN. 1967. Correlation of transmitter release with membrane properties of the presynaptic fibre of the squid giant synapse. J. Gen. Physiol. **50:** 2579–2601.

33. TAKEUCHI, A. & N. TAKEUCHI. 1962. Electrical changes in pre- and postsynaptic axons of giant synapse of Loligo. J. Gen. Physiol. **45:** 1181–1193.

34. TEPPER, J. M., S. NAKAMURA, S. I. YOUNG & P. M. GROVES. 1984. Autoreceptor-mediated changes in dopaminergic terminal excitability: Effects of striatal drug injections. Brain Res. **309:** 317–333.

35. MEREU, G., T. WESTFALL & R. Y. WANG. 1985. Modulation of terminal excitability of mesolimbic dopaminergic neurons by d-amphetamine and haloperidol. Brain Res. **358:** 110–121.

36. HERRLING, P. 1981. The membrane potential recorded in vivo displays four different reaction mechanisms to iontophoretically applied transmitter agonists. Brain Res. **212:** 331–343.

37. BERNARDO, L. S. & D. A. PRINCE. 1982. Dopamine modulates of calcium-activated potassium conductance in mammalian hippocampal pyramidal cells. Nature **297:** 76–79.

38. MILLER, M. W., H. PARNAS & I. PARNAS. 1985. Dopaminergic modulation of neuromuscular transmission in the prawn. J. Physiol. (London) **363:** 363–375.

39. YIM, C. Y., A. T. MADEJ & G. J. MOGENSON. 1986. Convergence of excitatory amygdala and hippocampal inputs to the nucleus accumbens and differential attenuation by VTA stimulation. Proc. Can. Fed. Biol. Soc. **29:** 111.

40. MERCURI, N., G. BERNARDI, P. CALABRESI, A. COTUGNO, G. LEVI & P. STAZIONE. 1985. Dopamine decreases cell excitability in rat striatal neurones by pre- and postsynaptic mechanisms. Brain Res. **358:** 110–121.

41. HOKFELT, T., J. F. REHFELD, L. SKIRBOLL, B. IVEMARK, M. GOLDSTEIN & K. MARLEY. 1980. Evidence for coexistence of dopamine and CCK in mesolimbic neurons. Nature **285:** 476–478.

42. PHILLIPSON, O. T. & A. C. GRIFFITHS. 1985. The topographic order of inputs to nucleus accumbens in the rat. Neuroscience 16: 275–296.
43. YIM, C. Y. & G. J. MOGENSON. 1983. Response of ventral pallidal neurons to amygdala stimulation and its modulation by dopamine projection to the nucleus accumbens. J. Neurophysiol. 50: 148–161.
44. SWANSON, L. W., G. J. MOGENSON, C. R. GERFEN & P. ROBINSON. 1984. Evidence for a projection from the lateral preoptic area and substantia innominata to the "mesencephalic locomotor region." Brain Res. 295: 161–178.
45. JONES, D. L. & G. J. MOGENSON. 1980. Nucleus accumbens to globus pallidus GABA projection subserving ambulatory activity. Am. J. Physiol. 238: R63–R69.
46. SCHWARTZBAUM, J. S. & P. E. GAY. 1966. Interacting behavioral effects of septal and amygdaloid lesions in the rat. J. Comput. Physiol. Psychol. 61: 59–65.
47. WHITE, N. & H. WEINGARTEN. 1976. Effects of amygdaloid lesions on exploration by rats. Physiol. Behav. 17: 73–79.
48. YIM, C. Y. & G. J. MOGENSON. 1987. NMDA stimulation of amygdala produced suppression of spontaneous locomotor activity in rats via the amygdala-nucleus accumbens-ventral pallidal pathway. Proc. Can. Fed. Biol. Soc. 30: 120.
49. STAINES, W. A., J. I. NAGY, S. R. VINCENT & H. C. FIBIGER. 1980. Neurotransmitters contained in the efferents of the striatum. 194: 391–402.
50. YANG, C. R. & G. J. MOGENSON. 1985. An electrophysiological study of the neural projection from the hippocampus to the ventral pallidum and the subpallidal areas by way of the nucleus accumbens. Neuroscience 15: 1015–1024.
51. YANG, C. R. & G. J. MOGENSON. 1987. Hippocampal signal transmission to the pedunculopontine nucleus and its regulation by dopamine D-2 receptors in the nucleus accumbens: An electrophysiological and behavioural study. Neuroscience. 23: 1041–1055.
52. O'KEEFE, J. & L. NADEL. 1978. The hippocampus as a cognitive map. Clarendon Press. Oxford, England.
53. MOGENSON, G. J. & M. A. NIELSEN. 1984. A study of the contribution of hippocampal-accumbens-subpallidal projections to locomotor activity. Behav. Neural Biol. 42: 38–51.
54. DONZANTI, B. A. & N. J. URETSKY. 1983. Effects of excitatory amino acid on locomotor activity after bilateral microinjection into the rat nucleus accumbens: Possible dependence on dopaminergic mechanisms. Neuropharmacol. 22: 971–981.
55. OADES, R. D. 1985. The role of noradrenaline in tuning and dopamine in switching between signals in the central nervous system. Neurosci. Biobehav. Rev. 9: 261–282.
56. LEUNG, L. W. S. & C. Y. YIM. 1987. Rhythmic delta activity in nucleus accumbens of behaving rats. Can. Fed. Biol. Soc. 30: 137.

# Influence of the Mesocortical/ Prefrontal Dopamine Neurons on Their Target Cells[a]

A. M. THIERRY,[b] J. MANTZ, C. MILLA,
AND J. GLOWINSKI

*Chaire de Neuropharmacologie*
*Collège de France (U. 114 INSERM)*
*11 Place Marcelin Berthelot*
*75231 Paris cedex 5, France*

## INTRODUCTION

Since the discovery of the cortical dopaminergic (DA) innervation,[1] converging efforts have been made in our laboratory to analyze the properties of the mesocortico–prefrontal DA neurons in the rat, using both biochemical and electrophysiological approaches.[2] The first indirect evidence for the existence of distinct DA cell groups within the ventral mesencephalic tegmentum (VMT) projecting either to the cerebral cortex or to different subcortical structures was obtained in functional studies. Indeed, stressful situations were found to activate selectively the mesocortical DA neurons as indicated by the enhanced rate of DA utilization,[3] an observation that has been confirmed by several groups.[2,4] Investigations on the effects of acute or chronic treatments with neuroleptics[5,6] and of lesions of specific pathways innervating the VMT on DA turnover in the prefrontal cortex and subcortical structures indicated also that DA cells projecting to the prefrontal cortex are submitted to regulations distinct from those intervening in the control of the activity of other DA cells.[7-9] The precise localization of the different DA cell groups within the VMT–substantia-nigra complex has been well defined in several anatomical studies.[10,11] Finally, the identification of DA cells by antidromic activation from several target areas indicated clearly that most cells innervating either the prefrontal cortex, the septum, or the nucleus accumbens, for example, were distinct cells.[12] This latter investigation revealed also that the VMT contains DA as well as non-DA cells [not affected by 6-hydroxydopamine (6-OHDA)] projecting to DA innervated areas, such as the prefrontal cortex, the septum, or the nucleus accumbens.[12,13] The non-DA cells can be distinguished from the DA ones by their higher conduction velocity.

In this review, we describe more recent electrophysiological studies in which attempts were made to (1) determine the influence of the mesocortico–prefrontal DA neurons on their target cells, and (2) compare the roles of these DA cells and of the noradrenergic (NA) neurons originating from the locus coeruleus in the regulation of the spontaneous or evoked activity of cortical cells. Finally, some of the properties

[a] This work was supported by grants from INSERM and Rhône-Poulenc Santé.
[b] To whom correspondence should be addressed.

101

of the prefronto–cortical efferent cells, particularly their extensive collateralization, will be discussed.

## INFLUENCE OF MESOCORTICO–PREFRONTAL DA NEURONS ON TARGET CELLS

As suggested first by Rose and Woolsey,[14] both in primate and nonprimate mammalian species, the prefrontal cortex can be defined as the projection area of the mediodorsal (MD) nucleus of the thalamus. In the rat, the medial pregenual region of the prefrontal cortex is reciprocally connected to the lateral part of the MD, while the medial part of the MD is reciprocally connected to the dorsal bank of the rhinal sulcus.[15,16] Both cortical areas defined by their thalamic afferents are innervated by mesocortical DA neurons.[17]

The effect of VMT stimulation on single-unit activity in the prefrontal cortex has been analyzed in ketamine anesthetized rats.[18] The electrical stimulation of the VMT (1 Hz) inhibited markedly the spontaneous activity (mean latency 17 ms, mean duration 109 ms) of a large majority of cells recorded in layers III to VI of the prefrontal cortex (85% of the cells), layers in which the DA nerve terminals are mainly distributed.[10,19] In few occasions only, this inhibition was preceded by an excitatory response. In some cases, the inhibitory response was followed by a rebound of discharge.

Several results suggest that the inhibitory influence evoked from the VMT upon cortical cells is mediated by the mesocortico–prefrontal DA neurons: (1) the iontophoretic application of DA on cortical neurons inhibits their spontaneous activity;[20] (2) the mean latency of the VMT-induced inhibition is compatible with the conduction velocity of the mesocortical DA neurons; and (3) as shown in FIGURE 1, the inhibitory responses are reduced markedly following the destruction of ascending DA and NA neurons (local injection of 6-OHDA into the medial forebrain bundle) or the depletion of catecholamines resulting from pretreatment of the animals with α-methyl-paratyrosine (α-MpT). Since the inhibitory responses evoked by the VMT stimulation still occur after lesion of the NA neurons alone (6-OHDA injections made lateral to the pedunculus cerebellaris), the DA neurons are indeed responsible for the observed inhibition of cells in the prefrontal cortex.

As shown by the measurement of DA-sensitive adenylate cyclase activity and by binding studies made with [$^3$H]SCH 23390, $D_1$ receptors are present in the prefrontal cortex.[21,22] In fact, a good correlation exists between the localization of these $D_1$ receptors and the distribution of the DA nerve terminals. Binding studies have also shown the existence of $D_2$ receptors in the prefrontal cortex.[23,24] Their distribution seems to differ from that of $D_1$ receptors. Neuroleptics, such as fluphenazine (2 mg/kg), spiroperidol (2 mg/kg), and sulpiride (100 mg/kg), administered intraperitoneally before the VMT electrical stimulation decreased markedly the inhibitory responses on cortical cells evoked from the VMT.[25] These results suggest that $D_2$ receptors are involved, since haloperidol in particular acts on $D_2$ but not on $D_1$ receptors. Surprisingly, haloperidol (at any dose tested 0.1 to 5 mg/kg iv or 0.5 to 5 mg/kg ip), levomepromazine (25 mg/kg ip), and the long-acting neuroleptic pipotiazine palmitic ester (32 mg/kg sc) failed to antagonize the inhibitory effect of the VMT stimulation on cells in the prefrontal cortex.[25] The lack of effect of haloperidol is particularly puzzling, since this butyrophenone acts on $D_2$ receptors and since haloperidol was found to block the inhibitory responses evoked in the nucleus accumbens by the electrical stimulation of the VMT.[26] Interestingly, other authors have also reported that haloperidol does not block the inhibitory responses evoked in the striatum either by activation of the nigro-striatal DA

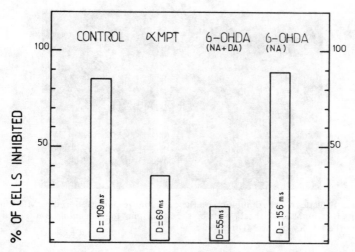

**FIGURE 1.** Effect of α-MpT or 6-OHDA pretreatment on the inhibitory responses induced by VMT stimulation on the spontaneous activity of prefrontal cortical cells. α-MpT: Animals were treated with α-MpT (200 mg/kg) 18 and 2 hours before the recording session. 6-OHDA (NA + DA): Animals in which DA and NA ascending bundles were lesioned by 6-OHDA microinjections. 6-OHDA (NA): Animals in which only an NA ascending bundle was lesioned by 6-OHDA microinjection into a brain site that left intact the DA ascending system. D: mean duration of the inhibitory responses.

neurons or local iontophoretic application of DA.[27,28] It should be added that levomepromazine and pipotiazine palmitic ester failed not only to block the inhibitory responses evoked from the VMT, but even increased their mean duration. The preferential effect of these neuroleptics on $D_1$ receptors or their action on α-NA receptors could be responsible for this phenomenon.

The electrical stimulation of the MD at a frequency of 5–10 Hz evokes a single spike or, in a few cases, two spike responses (with a mean latency of 16 ms) in 80% of the cells in the prefrontal cortex.[18] These excitatory responses mainly result from the activation of MD neurons, since the number of cortical neurons excited from the MD was reduced to 18% following destruction of MD neurons by a local microinjection of kainic acid. Most of the cortical cells inhibited by the VMT were excited by the MD stimulation. This allowed us to investigate the effect of the VMT stimulation on the excitatory responses evoked from the MD. In 75% of the cells tested the VMT stimulation applied before (3–45 ms) that of the MD (FIG. 2) blocked the excitatory responses evoked from the MD. This inhibitory effect was no longer observed following destruction of the ascending DA neurons or cortical DA depletion by α-methyl-paratyrosine pretreatment. The excitatory responses induced by the MD stimulation were also blocked by a microiontophoretic application of DA on cortical cells. Finally, the inhibitory effect of the VMT stimulation on excitatory responses of cortical cells evoked from the MD were antagonized by sulpiride. These results indicate that the mesocortico–prefrontal DA system is able to modulate signals delivered to cells in the prefrontal cortex by their main thalamic afferents.

Recently, we have been able to demonstrate that some cells in the prefrontal cortex

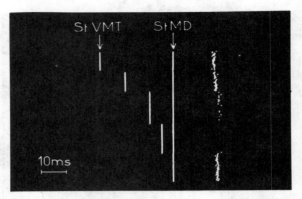

**FIGURE 2.** Effect of VMT stimulation on the excitatory response induced by MD stimulation (5 Hz) on a prefrontal cortical cell. Note by the dot display that the inhibition started with an increase in the latency of the MD response.

are activated by a noxious stimuli evoked by pressure on the tail. In fact, 26% of the cells tested in the prefrontal cortex ($n = 269$) were reproducibly activated by tail pinch (applied for 10 sec). A few cells (7%), however, were inhibited. As previously described, most of the recorded cells exhibited inhibitory responses under VMT electrical stimulation (1 Hz), and their spontaneous firing was completely blocked when the VMT stimulation was applied at a frequency of 10 Hz. In all cases (17 cells analyzed), the excitatory response evoked by the noxious stimuli was no longer observed when this peripheral stimuli was applied during the VMT electrical stimulation. Therefore, the mesocortico–prefrontal DA neurons seem to prevent the excitatory responses evoked by painful peripheral stimulation on cells of the prefrontal cortex.

## COMPARISON OF THE INFLUENCES OF ASCENDING DA AND NA NEURONS ON THE REGULATION OF THE ACTIVITY OF TARGET NEURONS IN THE PREFRONTAL CORTEX

As with other cortical areas, the prefrontal cortex is innervated by NA neurons originating from the locus coeruleus. Although the distribution of NA and DA nerve terminals is not identical,[29] microintophoretic studies have indicated that the activity of a population of cells in the prefrontal cortex is inhibited both by NA and DA.[20] An interaction of DA and NA ascending neurons on the cells of the prefrontal cortex is further suggested by results from our laboratory indicating that the NA neurons exert a permissive role on the denervation-induced supersensitivity of $D_1$ receptors in the prefrontal cortex.[30] This led us to investigate the effects of the electrical stimulation of the locus coeruleus on the spontaneous or evoked activity of cells in the prefrontal cortex and to compare them with those evoked from the VMT.

In contrast to the results obtained following electrical stimulation of the VMT (1 Hz) the electrical stimulation of the locus coeruleus (1 Hz) did not induce a consistent inhibitory response on cortical cells. However, a long-lasting poststimulus inhibition (mean duration 45 sec) was observed on 57% of the cortical cells tested following higher frequency stimulation of the locus coeruleus (20 Hz, 10 sec) (FIG. 3). The latter effect

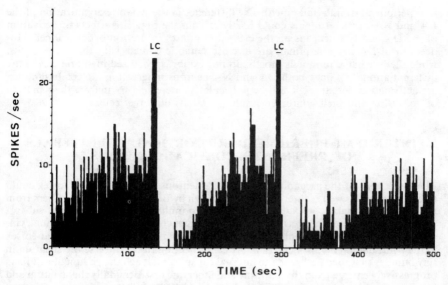

**FIGURE 3.** Inhibition of the firing rate of a prefrontal cortical neuron induced by locus coeruleus (LC) stimulation (20 Hz, 10 sec). The periods of stimulation are indicated by horizontal bars and the concomitant peaks correspond to the stimulus artefacts. Note the long lasting poststimulus inhibition and the progressive recovery of the spontaneous firing.

was not seen again following the specific destruction of the dorsal ascending NA pathway (local 6-OHDA injection near the pedunculus cerebellaris) or depletion of catecholamines induced by α-methylparatyrosine pretreatment. Our results agree with those of other authors who have observed a long-lasting inhibition of the spontaneous firing of cells located either in the cingulate or in the sensory motor cortex following electrical stimulation of the locus coeruleus.[31,32]

As previously indicated, the electrical stimulation of the VMT inhibits the excitatory responses of prefronto–cortical cells evoked from the MD (5–10 Hz) or those induced by peripheral painful stimuli (tail pinch). This was not the case following the activation of NA neurons, since both types of excitatory responses on prefronto–cortical cells were still observed when these responses were evoked during the locus coeruleus poststimulus period. In fact, the stimulation of the locus coeruleus induced a marked poststimulus depression of the spontaneous firing of the cells (background firing), while leaving intact the excitatory responses evoked either by the MD stimulation or the noxious tail-pinch stimuli, thus increasing the signal/noise ratio. Such a phenomenon has already been described by other workers in structures other than the prefrontal cortex.[33]

In conclusion, the mesocortical DA and locus coeruleus NA neurons can influence the activity of cells in the rat medial prefrontal cortex. However, these regulatory neuronal systems exert distinct modalities of action in the transfer of information from prefronto–cortical cells. While the activation of the DA system induces a tonic inhibition of both the spontaneous and the evoked firing of the cortical cells, the activation of the dorsal NA system that induces a long-lasting inhibition of the basal activity does not affect either the responses evoked from the MD or those produced by noxious peripheral stimuli (tail pinch). The difference in the synaptic organization of the DA and NA nerve terminals could partly explain the opposite effects of activation of the DA and NA neurons on the evoked responses in prefronto–cortical cells. Indeed, most DA nerve terminals are in close synaptic contact with their target cells, while the NA nerve terminals mostly do not exhibit specialized membrane synaptic differentiation.[34,35] Since both DA and NA neurons innervating the cerebral cortex are activated under stress, it will be particularly interesting to analyze their pattern of activation and their combined resulting actions on target cells.


## INTERHEMISPHERIC AND SUBCORTICAL COLLATERALS OF PREFRONTO–CORTICAL NEURONS

The target cells of the ascending DA and NA neurons in the prefrontal cortex could be efferent cells as well as interneurons. As shown by Beckstead,[36] efferent fibers from the medial prefrontal cortex in the rat project to multiple cortical areas and subcortical structures. Thus, the prefronto–cortical efferent cells innervate the perirhinal, cingulate, restrosplenial, and entorhinal cortex, as well as the medial prefrontal cortex in the contralateral hemisphere. Subcortical projecting fibers traverse the striatum in tiny bundles that then gather in the internal capsule and reach the pedunculus. Fibers progressively emerge from this pathway and innervate rostrocaudally the striatum and basal forebrain nuclei, the midline thalamic nuclei (the MD receiving an important innervation), the lateral hypothalamic area, and mesencephalic structures (such as the VMT, the substantia nigra, the superior colliculus, or the central gray). Further, caudally, fibers enter the midline pontine nuclei, and a few of them continue in the pyramidal tract. The majority of these cortical efferents project ipsilaterally, but a large contingent of them also projects contralaterally. On the other hand, as early as 1894, Ramon y Cajal[37] and later on Lorente de No[38] described the existence of cortical pyramidal neurons that project to the ipsilateral striatum but also send an axonal branch across the corpus callosum. Finally, it should also be said that the superficial (II–III) versus deep (V–VI) layer dissociation of cortically and subcortically projecting cells does not seem to occur in the rat.[39]

This complex organization of the efferent projections from the rat prefrontal cortex led us to determine whether the prefronto–cortical neurons project via axonal branches to contralateral cortical and to ipsi- and/or contralateral subcortical structures.[40] For this purpose, the antidromic stimulation method coupled with the reciprocal collision test was used (FIG. 4). Cortical cells could be antidromically driven from the homotypic contralateral prefrontal cortex as well as from the ipsi- or contralateral efferent subcortical pathways (the antidromic stimulation being made at the level of the medial striatum). Indeed, among 282 cells stimulated antidromically from a given site, 35% of them were also antidromically driven from one or two of the other stimulation sites. Since the reciprocal collision test was always positive, it was concluded that these cortical neurons send distinct axonal branches to the different areas from which antidromic spikes are evoked (FIG. 5). All types of branching patterns were found; that is, ipsi- and contralateral striatum, ipsilateral striatum, contralateral prefrontal cortex, and ipsi- and contralateral striatum–contralateral prefrontal cortex. A large proportion (35%) of the prefronto–cortical cells projecting to ipsilateral subcortical structures were also found to send axon collaterals to contralateral subcortical areas. In addition, an important proportion of prefronto–cortical cells (55%) innervating the homotypic contralateral area were also found to project to subcortical structures. Further, caudally, we could also demonstrate that cortical efferents may send axonal collaterals to dien-

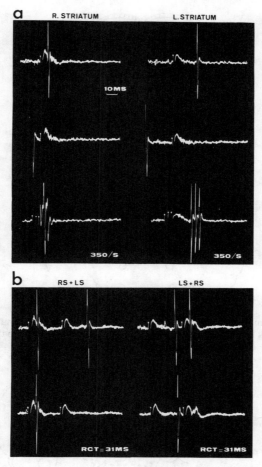

**FIGURE 4.** Demonstration of axonal branching of a prefrontal cortical neuron antidromically activated by stimulation of the right striatum (RS) and left striatum (LS). (a) Characterization of the antidromic response. *From top to bottom,* for each site of stimulation: fixity of latency, collision with a spontaneous spike, ability to follow high-frequency stimulation. (b) Determination of reciprocal collision times (RCT). RCT is the largest interval between the two stimulations at which blockade of the second antidromic spike is obtained (*bottom traces*). This cell sends axon collaterals to RS and LS, since the RCT was greater (31 ms) than the difference in the latencies (13 ms) of the two antidromic responses plus the refactory period of the axon at the second site stimulated. (RP = 2 and 2.1 ms for RS and LS, respectively.)

cephalic (MD or habenula) and/or distinct mesencephalic structures, such as the VMT, substantia nigra, grisea centralis, or superior colliculus[41] (FIG. 6).

In these studies, a widespread distribution of the latency of the antidromic responses was observed (2–32 ms). However, the mean conduction time of the fibers was of the same order of magnitude (7–12 ms) for the various structures analyzed. It should be

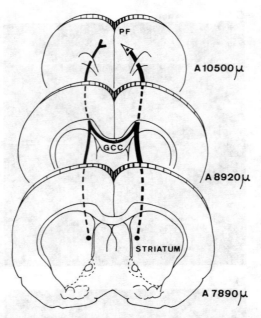

**FIGURE 5.** Schematic representation of axonal branching of efferent prefrontal cortical (PF) neurons projecting to the homotypic contralateral prefrontal cortex and to the ipsi- and/or contralateral striatum (or subcortical areas).

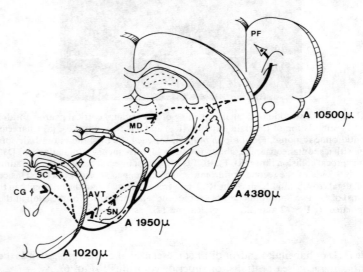

**FIGURE 6.** Schematic representation of axonal branching of efferent prefrontal cortical neurons (PF) projecting to ipsilateral diencephalic (MD: mediodorsal nucleus of the thalamus) or mesencephalic structures (SN: substantia nigra: AVT: ventral tegmental area; CG: central gray; SC: superior colliculus). Cortical neurons projecting to two or three of these structures could be identified and all possible branching patterns were demonstrated.

added that the estimated conduction velocity of the prefronto–cortical efferent fibers is particularly slow since its mean value varied from 0.6 to 1.9 m/sec when calculated from the various cortical and subcortical structures investigated.

Although a systematic analysis was not made, in several cases the spontaneous activity of prefronto–cortical cells antidromically driven from subcortical structures was inhibited by electrical stimulation of the VMT. This was shown in particular for cortical cells innervating the MD or the VMT. A cortico–VMT projection exerting a stimulatory effect on cells projecting either to the septum or the nucleus accumbens was also demonstrated.[42]

The functional significance of a large number of prefrontal cortical neurons with divergent axon collaterals is not yet known. However, it can be suggested that such a pattern of organization may contribute to a well-coordinated transfer of information in time and space in several target structures both ipsi- and contralaterally. There is little doubt that a large proportion of the cells that receive signals from different structures, and particularly the MD of the thalamus (lateral part), are under the control of the mesocortico–prefrontal DA neurons and the NA neurons originating from the locus coeruleus, as discussed extensively in the present review. Experiments are in progress to also determine the influence of the serotoninergic neurons originating from the dorsal raphe in their regulation.

# REFERENCES

1. THIERRY, A. M., G. BLANC, A. SOBEL, L. STINUS & J. GLOWINSKI. 1973. Dopaminergic terminals in the rat cortex. Science **182:** 499–501.
2. THIERRY, A. M., J. P. TASSIN & J. GLOWINSKI. 1984. Biochemical and electrophysiological studies of the mesocortical dopamine system. *In* Monoamine Innervation of Cerebral Cortex. L. Descarries, T. R. Reader, and H. H. Jasper, Eds.: 233–261. Alan Liss, New York.
3. THIERRY, A. M., J. P. TASSIN, G. BLANC & J. GLOWINSKI. 1976. Selective activation of the meso-cortical DA system by stress. Nature **263:** 242–244.
4. BANNON, J. M. & R. H. ROTH. 1983. Pharmacology of mesocortical dopamine neurons. Pharmacol. Rev. **35:** 53–68.
5. SCATTON, B., J. GLOWINSKI & L. JULOU. 1976. Dopamine metabolism in the mesolimbic and mesocortical dopaminergic systems after single or repeated administration of neuroleptics. Brain Res. **109:** 184–189.
6. SCATTON, B., A. BOIREAU, C. GARRET, J. GLOWINSKI & L. JULOU. 1977. Action of palmitic ester of pipotiazine on dopamine metabolism in the nigro-striatal, mesolimbic and mesocortical systems. Naunyn Schmiedeberg Arch. Pharmacol. **296:** 169–175.
7. HERVÉ, D., G. BLANC, J. GLOWINSKI & J. P. TASSIN. 1982. Reduction of dopamine utilization in the prefrontal cortex but not in the nucleus accumbens after selective destruction of noradrenergic fibers innervating the ventral tegmental area in the rat. Brain Res. **237:** 510–516.
8. HERVÉ, D., H. SIMON, G. BLANC, M. LE MOAL, J. GLOWINSKI & J. P. TASSIN. 1981. Opposite changes in dopamine utilization in the nucleus accumbens and the frontal cortex after electrolytic lesion of the median raphe in the rat. Brain Res. **216:** 422–428.
9. HERVÉ, D., H. SIMON, G. BLANC, A. LISOPRAWSKI, M. LE MOAL, J. GLOWINSKI & J. P. TASSIN. 1979. Increased utilization of dopamine in the nucleus accumbens but not in the cerebral cortex after dorsal raphe lesion in the rat. Neurosci. Lett. **15:** 127–133.
10. LINDVALL, O. & A. BJORKLUND. 1974. The organization of the ascending catecholamine neuron systems in the rat brain as revealed by the glyoxylic acid method. Acta Physiol. Scand. Suppl. **412:** 1–48.
11. SWANSON, L. W. 1982. The projections of the ventral tegmental area and adjacent regions: A combined fluorescent retrograde tracer and immunofluoresence study in the rat. Brain Res. Bull. **9:** 321–353.
12. DENIAU, J. M., A. M. THIERRY & J. FÉGER. 1980. Electrophysiological identification of

mesencephalic ventromedial tegmental (VMT) neurons projecting to the frontal cortex, septum and nucleus accumbens. Brain Res. **189:** 315–326.

13. THIERRY, A. M., J. M. DENIAU, D. HERVÉ & G. CHEVALIER. 1980. Electrophysiological evidence for non-dopaminergic mesocortical and mesolimbic neurons in the rat. Brain Res. **201:** 210–214.

14. ROSE, J. E. & C. N. WOOLSEY. 1948. The orbitofrontal cortex and its connections with the mediodorsal nucleus in rabbit, sheep and cat. Res. Publ. Assoc. Nerv. Ment. Dis. **27:** 210–232.

15. LEONARD, C. M. 1969. The prefrontal cortex of the rat. I. Cortical projection of the mediodorsal nucleus. II. Efferent connections. Brain Res. **12:** 321–334.

16. KRETTEK, J. E. & S. L. PRICE. 1977. Cortical projections of the mediodorsal nucleus and adjacent thalamic nuclei in the rat. J. Comp. Neurol. **171:** 157–192.

17. DIVAC, I., A. BJÖRKLUND, O. LINDVALL & R. E. PASSINGHAM. 1978. Converging projections from the medio-dorsal thalamic nucleus and mesencephalic dopaminergic neurons to the neocortex in three species. J. Comp. Neurol. **180:** 59–72.

18. FERRON, A., A. M. THIERRY, C. LE DOUARIN & J. GLOWINSKI. 1984. Inhibitory influence of the mesocortical dopaminergic system on spontaneous activity or excitatory response induced from the thalamic medio-dorsal nucleus in the rat medial prefrontal cortex. Brain Res. **302:** 257–265.

19. BERGER, B., A. M. THIERRY, J. P. TASSIN & M. A. MOYNE. 1976. Dopaminergic innervation of the rat prefrontal cortex: A fluorescence histochemical study. Brain Res. **106:** 133–145.

20. BUNNEY, B. S. & G. K. AGHAJANIAN. 1976. Dopamine and norepinephrine innervated cells in the rat prefrontal cortex: Pharmacological differentiation using microiontophoretic techniques. Life Sci. **19:** 1783–1792.

21. TASSIN, J. P., J. BOCKAERT, G. BLANC, L. STINUS, A. M. THIERRY, S. LAVIELLE, J. PRÉMONT & J. GLOWINSKI. 1978. Topographical distribution of dopaminergic innervation and dopaminergic receptors of the anterior cerebral cortex of the rat. Brain Res. **154:** 241–251.

22. SAVASTA, H., D. A. DUBOIS & B. SCATTON. 1986. Autoradiographic localization of D1 dopamine receptors in the rat brain with ($^3$H)SCH 23390. Brain Res. **375:** 291–301.

23. MARCHAIS, D., J. P. TASSIN & J. BOCKAERT. 1980. Dopaminergic component of ($^3$H)spiroperidol binding in the rat anterior cerebral cortex. Brain Res. **183:** 235–240.

24. BOUTHENET, M. L., M. P. MARTRES, N. SALES & J. C. SCHWARTZ. 1987. A detailed mapping of dopamine D2 receptors in rat central nervous system by autoradiography with ($^{125}$I) Iodosulpiride. Neuroscience **20:** 117–155.

25. THIERRY, A. M., C. LE DOUARIN, J. PENIT, A. FERRON & J. GLOWINSKI. 1986. Variation in the ability of neuroleptics to block the inhibitory influence of dopaminergic neurons on the activity of cells in the rat prefrontal cortex. Brain Res. Bull. **16:** 155–160.

26. LE DOUARIN, C., J. PENIT, J. GLOWINSKI & A. M. THIERRY. 1986. Effect of ventro-medial mesencephalic tegmentum (VMT) stimulation on the spontaneous activity of nucleus accumbens neurons: Influence of the dopamine system. Brain Res. **363:** 290–298.

27. ZARZECKI, P., D. J. BLAKE & G. G. SOMJEN. 1977. Neurological disturbances, nigrostriate synapses and iontophoretic dopamine and apomorphine after haloperidol. Exp. Neurol. **57:** 956–970.

28. SKIRBOLL, L. R. & B. S. BUNNEY. 1979. The effects of acute and chronic haloperidol treatment on spontaneously firing neurons in the caudate nucleus of the rat. Life Sci. **25:** 1419–1434.

29. LINDVALL, O. & A. BJÖRKLUND. 1984. General organization of cortical monamine systems. In Monoamine Innervation of Cerebral Cortex. L. Descarries, T. R. Reader, and H. H. Jasper, Eds.: 9–40. Alan Liss. New York.

30. TASSIN, J. P., J. M. STUDLER, D. HERVÉ, G. BLANC & J. GLOWINSKI. 1986. Contribution of noradrenergic neurons to the regulation of dopaminergic (D1) receptor denervation supersensitivity in rat prefrontal cortex. J. Neurochem. **46:** 243–248.

31. DILLIER, N., J. LASZLO, B. MULLER, W. P. KOELLA & H. R. OLPE. 1978. Activation of an inhibitory noradrenergic pathway projecting from the locus coeruleus to the cingulate cortex of the rat. Brain Res. **154:** 61–68.

32. PHILLIS, J. N. & G. K. KOSTOPOULOS. 1977. Activation of a noradrenergic pathway from the brain stem to rat cerebral cortex. Gen. Pharmacol. **8:** 207–211.
33. WOODWARD, D. J., H. C. MOISES, B. D. WATERHOUSE, B. J. HOFFER & R. FREEDMAN. 1979. Modulatory actions of norepinephrine in the central nervous system. Fed. Proc., Fed. Am. Soc. Exp. Biol. **38:** 2109–2116.
34. SEGUELA, P., K. C. WATKINS & L. DESCARRIES. 1986. Preliminary data on the ultrastructural features of dopamine terminals in adult rat cerebral cortex. Soc. Neurosci. Abst. **12:** 770.
35. DESCARRIES, L., K. C. WATKINS & Y. LAPIERRE. 1977. Noradrenergic axon terminals in the cerebral cortex of rat. III. Topometric ultrastructural analysis. Brain Res. **133:** 197–122.
36. BECKSTEAD, R. M. 1979. An autoradiographic examination of cortico-cortical and subcortical projections of the mediodorsal-projection (prefrontal) cortex in the rat. J. Comp. Neurol. **184:** 43–62.
37. RAMON Y CAJAL, S. 1984. Les nouvelles idées sur la structure du système nerveaux chez l'homme et chez les vertébrés. Reinvald. Paris.
38. LORENTE DE NO, R. 1922. La corteza cerebral del raton. Trab. Inst. Cajal. Invest. Biol. **20:** 41–78.
39. JONES, E. G. 1981. Anatomy of cerebral cortex: Columnar input-output organization. *In* The Organization of Cerebral Cortex. F. O. Schmitt, F. G. Worden, S. G. Dennis, and G. Andelman, Eds.: 199–235. MIT Press. Cambridge, Mass.
40. FERINO, F., A. M. THIERRY, M. SAFFROY & J. GLOWINSKI. 1987. Interhemispheric and subcortical collaterals of medial prefrontal cortical neurons in the rat. Brain Res. **417:** 257–266.
41. THIERRY, A. M., G. CHEVALIER, A. FERRON & J. GLOWINSKI. 1983. Diencephalic and mesencephalic efferents of the medial prefrontal cortex in the rat: Electrophysiological evidence for the existence of branched axons. Exp. Brain Res. **50:** 275–282.
42. THIERRY, A. M., J. M. DENIAU & J. FEGÉR. 1979. Effects of stimulation of the frontal cortex on identified output VMT cells in the rat. Neurosci. Lett. **15:** 103–107.

# Heterologous Regulation of Receptors on Target Cells of Dopamine Neurons in the Prefrontal Cortex, Nucleus Accumbens, and Striatum

J. GLOWINSKI,[a] D. HERVÉ, AND J. P. TASSIN

*Chaire de Neuropharmacologie*
*Collège de France (U. 114 INSERM)*
*11 Place Marcelin Berthelot*
*75231 Paris cedex 5, France*

## INTRODUCTION

The numerous dopaminergic (DA) cells distributed in the ventral mesencephalic tegmentum (VMT)–substantia nigra (SN) complex are segregated in several groups of cells that give rise to the different ascending DA systems innervating several cortical areas or subcortical structures (for review, see reference 1). These DA cell groups can be distinguished not only by their target areas but also by their afferent pathways.[2-4] In addition, in some cases they differ also in their morphological aspects or in the identity of their co-transmitter (either neurotensin of cholecystokinin).[5-7]

In most areas innervated by DA neurons, binding studies on membranes[8,9] or autoradiographic analysis on slices[10-12] made with selective ligands have allowed the existence of $D_1$ and $D_2$ receptors to be demonstrated. Slight differences can be seen in the precise distribution of these two types of receptors within a given structure, as seen particularly in the prefrontal cortex[13] or the striatum.[14] The distribution of $D_1$ receptors, which are coupled positively to adenylate cyclase, was first described in species like the rat by measuring DA-sensitive adenylate cyclase on homogenates prepared from microdiscs of tissues punched out from frozen serial coronal slices.[15] Studies made in our laboratory have demonstrated the existence of a DA-sensitive adenylate cyclase ($D_1$ receptors) on neurons in primary cultures originating either from the cerebral cortex or from the striatum of mouse embryos.[16,17] In agreement with results obtained on the pituitary,[18] striatal $D_2$ receptors in adult tissues are coupled negatively to adenylate cyclase,[19] and this inhibitory effect on the enzyme activity can be observed as well on striatal neurons of mouse embryos in primary cultures.[20]

Although for many years, the function of the $D_1$ receptor has been questioned by several workers, this is no longer the case. Thanks to the discovery of the potent selective $D_1$ antagonist SCH 23390,[21] it could be demonstrated that some behavioral responses induced either by DA or by some of its agonists are mediated through $D_1$

---

[a] To whom correspondence should be addressed.

receptors.[22,23] The elegant investigations performed by Greengard and his colleagues have revealed the existence of a specific protein, DARPP 32, that is distributed in target areas of ascending DA neurons.[24] Through protein kinase A, DARPP 32 can be phosphorylated, as a result of the interaction of DA with $D_1$ receptors and the subsequent activation of adenylate cyclase and production of cyclic AMP. Once phosphorylated DARPP 32 acts as a potent inhibitor of protein phosphatase 1, which has a broad spectrum of action.[25] Therefore, by its action on $D_1$ receptors, DA can contribute to the heteroregulation of signals delivered through other receptors coupled or not to adenylate cyclase. By this type of mechanism or others, heteroregulations of $D_1$ receptors may occur as well.

We summarize the results of studies on the long-term heteroregulation of $D_1$ receptors in the prefrontal cortex, nucleus accumbens, and striatum of the rat resulting from the destruction (or changes in activity) of neuronal pathways innervating DA target areas. These heteroregulations were demonstrated by analyzing modifications in the development of the classical denervation-induced supersensitivity of $D_1$ receptors. We also provide some indication about the effects of DA denervation and of prolonged blockade of DA transmission on the heteroregulation of neurotensin binding sites in DA innervated areas.

## HETEROREGULATION OF $D_1$ RECEPTORS IN THE PREFRONTAL CORTEX BY NORADRENERGIC NEURONS ORIGINATING IN THE LOCUS COERULEUS

Bilateral electrolytic lesions of the VMT that destroy the ascending DA neurons innervating the prefrontal cortex and several subcortical limbic structures induce the expected denervation supersensitivity of $D_1$ receptors in the prefrontal cortex[26] (FIG. 1). This effect was shown by measuring DA-sensitive adenylate cyclase in homogenates from microdiscs of tissues punched out in the medial prefrontal cortex where the highest concentrations of DA nerve terminals and $D_1$ receptors are found. Analyzed four to six weeks after the lesions, this enhanced DA-sensitive adenylate cyclase activity results both from a change in the number of $D_1$ receptors and from a slight increase in the apparent affinity of these receptors for DA. In addition, it is proportional to the extent of DA denervation, but also to some extent to the precise location of the lesion within the VMT. Although this effect is linked to the destruction of the DA neurons, we cannot exclude the possibility that other neuronal systems originating or passing through the VMT, which are destroyed by the lesions and which project to the prefrontal cortex, are also involved in the regulation of $D_1$ receptors.

Surprisingly, bilateral chemical lesions made by local microinjections of 6-hydroxydopamine (6-OHDA) into the VMT that destroy ascending DA neurons in the VMT did not induce the expected denervation supersensitivity of the $D_1$ receptors[26] (FIG. 1). Since electrolytic lesions preserve the cortical NA innervation and that 6-OHDA lesions affect ascending NA fibers that pass near the location of the DA cells, the destruction of the cortical NA innervation could be responsible for the lack of development of denervation-induced supersensitivity of the $D_1$ receptors. A good correlation was found between the extent of damage of the NA fibers and the reduction of the expected denervation supersensitivity of the $D_1$ receptors (estimated in electrolytically lesioned rats). This permissive role of ascending NA fibers originating in the locus coeruleus for the appearance of denervation-induced supersensitivity of $D_1$ receptors was also supported by experiments on rats with bilateral electrolytic lesions of the VMT and bilateral 6-OHDA lesions of the dorsal NA bundle (made near the pedunculus

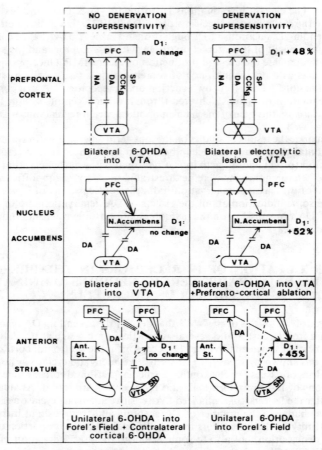

**FIGURE 1.** Effects of different types of lesions on the development of denervation-supersensitivity of $D_1$ receptors in the prefrontal cortex, nucleus accumbens, and striatum of rats. Animals were sacrificed four to six weeks after the lesions. DA-sensitive adenylate cyclase ($D_1$ receptors) was estimated on homogenates from microdiscs of tissues punched out either from the prefrontal cortex (PFC), the nucleus accumbens (N. accumbens), or the anterior part of the striatum (Ant. St.). Bilateral 6-OHDA or electrolytic lesions were made into the VTA. Unilateral 6-OHDA lesions were made into Forel's field or the prefrontal cortex. Changes in DA-sensitive adenylate cyclase activity are expressed in percentage of control values.

cerebellaris superior). No significant change in DA-sensitive adenylate cyclase activity was found in the prefrontal cortex of rats with the two types of lesions, although lesions of NA neurons alone were without effect on the enzyme activity.[27]

Recent experiments made with Drs. Taghzouti, Simon, and Le Moal have revealed that the NA neurons also play a permissive role in the expression of two behavioral deficits induced by bilateral electrolytic lesions of the VMT.[28] Such lesioned rats exhibit an increased nocturnal locomotor activity and a reduced spontaneous alternation behavior, two deficits of the complex "VMT syndrome" that has been studied extensively by Le Moal *et al.*[29] No significant changes in nocturnal locomotor activity or in spontaneous alternations were seen in rats with bilateral electrolytic VMT lesions and bilateral 6-OHDA lesions of the dorsal NA bundle when compared to sham-operated rats. Therefore, the concomitant destruction of the NA neurons and of the VMT DA neurons reduced markedly the deficits observed in rats with electrolytic VMT lesions. This functional recovery indicates that deficits induced by a given lesion can be abolished by another type of lesion and provides new insights on the antagonistic properties of ascending DA and NA neurons. However, a functional hierarchy exists between these systems since no significant increase in the mean nocturnal locomotor activity or decrease in spontaneous alternations was observed in rats with lesions of the NA neurons alone (except a greater variability in individual responses). These results could explain why numerous deficits of the VMT syndrome are more pronounced in rats with electrolytic lesions than in animals with 6-OHDA lesions.[30] These biochemical results and the electrophysiological data reported by A. M. Thierry during the Conference on the Mesocorticolimbic Dopamine System also suggest that the functional antagonism previously described occurs at the level of the prefrontal cortex. However, the possibility that subcortical structures innervated both by DA and NA neurons and connected by prefrontal cortical efferents might also be involved cannot be ruled out.

## HETEROREGULATION OF $D_1$ RECEPTORS IN THE NUCLEUS ACCUMBENS AND THE STRIATUM BY CORTICAL EFFERENTS

### *Nucleus Accumbens*

In contrast to the results obtained in the medial prefrontal cortex, the expected denervation-induced supersensitivity of $D_1$ receptors in the nucleus accumbens did not occur four to six weeks after bilateral electrolytic lesions of the VMT, in spite of very pronounced destruction of the DA innervation[26] (FIG. 1). Similar negative effects were seen in rats with 6-OHDA VMT lesions (FIG. 1). This lack of denervation-induced supersensitivity of $D_1$ receptors in the nucleus accumbens cannot be related to the combined destruction of the DA and NA innervations, since this phenomenon is observed in VMT lesioned rats in which the ascending NA fibers are preserved. These data led us to suspect that changes in the activity of prefronto–cortical nucleus accumbens neurons linked to the destruction of the cortical DA innervation might contribute to the regulation of $D_1$ receptors in the nucleus accumbens.

A projection from the prefrontal cortex to the nucleus accumbens has been well established on the basis of morphological data.[31] A marked reduction in the high-affinity uptake of $^3$H-glutamate is observed in synaptosomes from the nucleus accumbens of rats with bilateral ablation of the prefrontal cortex[32] (FIG. 1). This suggests further that the cortical neurons that innervate this subcortical structure are glutamatergic. In fact, a great majority of efferent prefrontal cortical neurons are branched neurons that innervate several subcortical structures ipsi- and contralaterally, as well as the contralateral homotypic cortical area (reference 33; see also reference 34).

A slight but significant increased activation of the DA-sensitive adenylate cyclase was observed in the nucleus accumbens of rats with bilateral ablation of the prefrontal cortex.[32] This activation was much more pronounced in animals with cortical lesions and bilateral 6-OHDA VMT lesions (FIG. 1) and resulted both from an increased number and a slightly enhanced apparent affinity of the $D_1$ receptors.[32] Therefore, the "denervation-induced supersensitivity of $D_1$ receptors" in the nucleus accumbens seems to appear only when signals from the prefrontal cortex (likely transferred by the cortico-nucleus accumbens projection) are suppressed or eliminated. Such an effect was not observed following destruction of the glutamatergic fibers originating from the hippocampus, another structure that innervates the nucleus accumbens. This provides some information about the specificity of prefronto–cortical efferent neurons in the regulation of the nucleus accumbens $D_1$ receptors.

The DA-sensitive adenylate cyclase activity was also increased in the nucleus accumbens of rats with VMT 6-OHDA lesions made in the presence of desmethylimipramine, a procedure that partially preserves the cortical DA innervation but allows the complete destruction of the DA innervation in the nucleus accumbens.[26,35] These results confirm that a tonic regulation of the prefronto–cortical efferent cells by the mesocortico–prefrontal DA neurons is required for the appearance of the denervation-induced supersensitivity of $D_1$ receptors in the nucleus accumbens. Since the prefronto–cortical efferent cells are inhibited following electrical stimulation of afferent DA neurons,[36] a prolonged disinhibition of the spontaneous or evoked activity of these cells may occur following 6-OHDA VMT lesions that destroy all ascending DA neurons (including those projecting to the prefrontal cortex and the nucleus accumbens). Such a phenomenon may be responsible for the lack of denervation-induced supersensitivity of $D_1$ receptors in the nucleus accumbens. Recordings of the prefronto–cortical cells innervating subcortical structures in rats with 6-OHDA VMT lesions are necessary to further substantiate this hypothesis.

### Striatum

The striatum is not only innervated by the nigro-striatal DA neurons but also by VMT DA cells that innervate predominantly the anteromedial part of the striatum.[37,38] A good correlation exists between the distributions of DA nerve terminals and $D_1$ receptors that are more abundant in the anterior part of the striatum.[39] It is also well established that the striatum is innervated by cells from all cortical areas.[40] The prefronto–cortical cells project preferentially into the anteromedial part of the striatum, while its laterodorsal part is innervated predominantly by fibers originating from the sensory-motor cortex.[31,40] These projections are bilateral, but the contralateral projection originating from the prefrontal cortex is much more important than that from the sensory-motor cortex.[41] Several workers have attempted to demonstrate denervation-induced supersensitivity of $D_1$ receptors in the rat striatum. Contradictory results were obtained and when positive effects were found, variations in their amplitude were seen from one study to another.[42-45] On the basis of results obtained either in the prefrontal cortex or in the nucleus accumbens, these variations could be attributed to: (1) the type of lesions made in order to destroy the ascending DA neurons; (2) the time at which the DA-sensitive adenylate cyclase activity was estimated after the lesions; and (3) to the existence of complex heteroregulations of the $D_1$ receptors by cortico-striatal glutamatergic neurons.

In order to completely destroy the striatal DA innervation, unilateral local 6-OHDA lesions were made into the Forel's field, a site through which all ascending DA fibers (including those innervating the ipsilateral frontal cortex) and NA fibers pass. This lesion induced the expected denervation-induced supersensitivity of $D_1$ receptors in the anteromedial and laterodorsal parts of the striatum (FIG. 1). However, the increased DA-sensitive adenylate cyclase activity was more pronounced in the anteromedial than in the laterodorsal part, the maximal responses occurring three weeks after the lesion.[46]

When experiments were made six weeks after the lesion, the denervation-induced supersensitivity of $D_1$ receptors was still observed in the anteromedial part (about 45%) but not in the laterodorsal part of the striatum. This suggests that different heteroregulations of $D_1$ receptors by afferent fibers on DA target cells could be involved in distinct striatal areas. In this context, Savasta *et al.* have reported recently that the denervation-induced supersensitivity of $D_2$ receptors (visualized by autoradiographic studies) is more pronounced in the laterodorsal part than in the anteromedial part of the striatum.[47]

The results obtained in the striatum differ from those found in the nucleus accumbens in that no change in DA-sensitive adenylate cyclase activity was observed in the latter structure six weeks after 6-OHDA VMT lesions of the ascending DA neurons. However, in this case, the lesions made were bilateral. Therefore, the sustained denervation-induced supersensitivity of $D_1$ receptors in the anteromedial part of the striatum seen in rats with unilateral 6-OHDA lesions of the Forel's field could be related to the preserved DA innervation in the contralateral prefrontal cortex and thus to the unaffected activity of the contralateral prefronto–cortical cells that innervate both striata.

In agreement with this hypothesis, the denervation-induced supersensitivity of the $D_1$ receptors in the anteromedial part of the striatum was no longer observed in rats with both a unilateral 6-OHDA lesion made in the Forel's field and a 6-OHDA lesion made locally into the contralateral prefrontal cortex (experiments made six weeks after the lesions)[46] (FIG. 1).

The lack of $D_1$ receptor supersensitivity in the anterior part of the striatum of rats, with both a unilateral 6-OHDA lesion in Forel's field and a 6-OHDA lesion in the contralateral prefrontal cortex, is reminiscent of results obtained in the nucleus accumbens following bilateral 6-OHDA lesions of the VMT that destroy the DA and NA nerve terminals bilaterally in the prefrontal cortex as well. Therefore, it can be suggested that long changes in the regulation of the prefronto–cortical cells in both hemispheres linked to the ipsi- and contralateral catecholaminergic denervation may be responsible for the lack of denervation-induced supersensitivity of the striatal $D_1$ receptors. Although the respective roles of the cortical DA and NA innervation in this process have still to be demonstrated, from the results obtained in the nucleus accumbens following selective destruction of the cortical NA innervation, it can be suggested that the destruction of the DA innervation is of major importance. Preliminary experiments indicate that the denervation-induced supersensitivity of $D_1$ receptors in the anteromedial part of the striatum still occurs in rats with a unilateral 6-OHDA lesion of Forel's field and bilateral ablation of the prefrontal cortex. It remains to be determined whether lesions of cortical cells projecting to the laterodorsal part of the striatum will enable the detection of sustained denervation supersensitivity of $D_1$ receptors in this striatal area. This could confirm further the role of the corticostriatal glutamatergic neurons in the heteroregulation of striatal $D_1$ receptors. Such a role is supported by morphological data that indicate that both the corticostriatal fibers and the nigro-striatal DA neurons innervate the dendritic spines of the spiny medium-size neurons that project to the SN.[48,49] It has also been shown that $D_1$ receptors are localized on these spiny medium-size neurons (which in their great majority are GABAergic).[50]

## HETEROREGULATION OF NEUROTENSIN RECEPTORS IN DA TARGET AREAS BY AFFERENT DA NEURONS

Heterologous fibers (containing either NA or glutamate) can contribute to the regulation of $D_1$ receptors in the prefrontal cortex and in subcortical structures such as the nucleus accumbens and the striatum. Reciprocally, DA neurons could regulate the sensitivity of receptors other than DA receptors in DA-innervated areas. For example, using striatal neurons from the mouse embryo in primary cultures, we have shown that the inhibitory effect of somatostatin on adenylate cyclase activity is modified in the presence of DA.[51] Several DA-innervated areas in the rat are rich in neurotensin immunoreactive fibers.[52] Such fibers are seen particularly in the nucleus accumbens and the striatum and to a lesser extent in the prefrontal cortex. Therefore, in collaboration with Drs. Kitabgi, Rostene, Dana, and Vincent, we have examined whether the destruction of ascending DA neurons or the prolonged blockade of DA transmission by a neuroleptic could affect the binding of $^{125}$I-neurotensin in DA target areas.[53]

This investigation was also stimulated by studies indicating that: (1) neurotensin is co-localized with DA in several cells of the VMT–SN complex and that neurotensin-containing fibers are present in the mesencephalic area;[6] (2) $^3$H-neurotensin binding sites are present on DA neurons;[54,55] and (3) neurotensin in the VMT–SN complex can stimulate the activity of ascending DA neurons.[56]

As indicated by autoradiographic analysis, the bilateral destruction of ascending DA neurons (and of NA fibers as well) by local microinjections of 6-OHDA made into the VMT resulted six weeks later in large decreases in the number of $^{125}$I-neurotensin binding sites in the mesencephalon and in the striatum.[53] These results confirmed those of other workers who concluded that $^{125}$I-neurotensin binding sites are present on DA neurons.[54,55] In contrast, these lesions produce an increase in the number of $^{125}$I-neurotensin binding sites in the lateral part of the prefrontal cortex, despite a large decrease in cortical DA levels. This is in favor of a heteroregulation of these binding sites by DA neurons. The denervation of the DA neurons could also induce a modification of the density of $^{125}$I-neurotensin binding sites on target cells of DA neurons in other structures of the brain. However, this effect may be masked by the presence of a larger proportion of $^{125}$I-neurotensin binding sites on DA nerve terminals. Supporting this hypothesis, a significant increase in the number of $^{125}$I-neurotensin binding sites occurred not only in the lateral part of the prefrontal cortex but also in its medial part as well as in the enthorinal cortex, the nucleus accumbens, and the central part of the striatum following chronic treatment with a long-acting neuroleptic, the pipothiazine palmitate (three subcutaneous injections made 40, 20, and 5 days before sacrifice, 32 mg/kg).[53] Although the effect was more pronounced in cortical areas than in subcortical structures, these results clearly indicate that the prolonged blockade of DA transmission is responsible for a heteroregulation of $^{125}$I-neurotensin binding sites in several DA-innervated areas. Interestingly, neither the bilateral VMT 6-OHDA lesions, nor the long-term treatment with pipothiazine palmitate significantly affected the binding of $^{125}$I-neurotensin in structures not innervated by DA neurons.

Three mechanisms at least could be responsible for the heteroregulation of $^{125}$I-neurotensin binding sites by DA neurons.

(1) The influence of DA neurons on postsynaptic $^{125}$I-neurotensin binding sites could be indirect and mediated by local circuits. DA could act on DA receptors located on neurotensin-containing neurons or nerve terminals. In this case, the increase in $^{125}$I-neurotensin binding could result from prolonged modifications of neurotensin release. Supporting this hypothesis, chronic treatment with neuroleptics have been shown to enhance neurotensin levels in some cerebral areas innervated by DA neurons in the rat brain.[57,58]

(2) DA and neurotensin receptors could be located on similar target cells innervated by distinct DA- and neurotensin-containing fibers, and the prolonged interruption of DA transmission could lead to a heteroregulation of the density of $^{125}$I-

neurotensin binding sites. Experiments on cortical neurons in primary cultures are in progress to determine whether these receptors can be co-localized on similar cells and whether they can be subjected to heteroregulation.

(3) DA and neurotensin receptors could be located on similar target cells inner-vated by mixed neurotensin–DA fibers. This would explain easily the increased regula-tion of neurotensin receptors seen in the lateral prefrontal cortex following destruc-tion of the ascending DA fibers. A change in neurotensin release (decrease) or a heteroregulation of the neurotensin receptors following blockade of DA receptors could thus explain the increased number of $^{125}$I-neurotensin binding sites seen following long-term treatment with the pipothiazine palmitate. Recent results obtained in collabora-tion with G. Tramu and P. Kitabgi (reported by J. P. Tassin during the Conference) have demonstrated the existence of mixed neurotensin-DA fibers innervating the prefrontal cortex but not the other DA-innervated areas investigated (nucleus accumbens-striatum).[64] However, since an increase in the number of $^{125}$I-neurotensin binding sites is also observed following prolonged blockade of DA transmission in structures not innervated by mixed neurotensin–DA fibers, mechanisms distinct from those inter-vening in the prefrontal cortex could be involved in the heteroregulation of $^{125}$I-neuro-tensin binding sites in other DA innervated structures. In this context, it can be re-called that the heteroregulation of $D_1$ receptors by cholecystokinin differs in areas of the nucleus accumbens innervated either by distinct DA and cholecystokinin fibers or by mixed DA–cholecystokinin fibers.[59] Cholecystokinin potentiates the increase in cyclic-AMP production induced by DA in the posterior part of the nucleus accumbens, which is innervated by mixed cholecystokinin–DA fibers, while the opposite is observed in the anterior part innervated by distinct DA and cholecystokinin fibers.

## CONCLUDING REMARKS

Several remarks can be made on the basis of results described in the present article.

(1) The discrepancies found concerning denervation-induced supersensitivity of receptors could be linked to the type and/or specificity of the lesions made and to heteroregulation of the density or sensitivity of the receptors. Indeed, they could be related to the concomitant destruction or dysregulation of other neuronal pathways.

(2) Observations made at the cortical level emphasize the role of the NA neurons in regulating cortical $D_1$ receptors. Since several types of interaction exist between NA and serotoninergic neurons and since these aminergic systems exert antagonistic ef-fects in several cases,[60,61] experiments are being made to determine whether or not the selective destruction of serotoninergic neurons originating from the dorsal raphe in-duce similar or opposite effects on $D_1$ receptors when compared to those seen fol-lowing the destruction of the NA neurons.

(3) Several interactions between the cortico-striatal glutamatergic neurons and the nigro-striatal DA neurons have been described. Indeed, the glutamatergic fibers seem to control presynaptically the release of DA and vice versa.[62,63] The present data dem-onstrate an additional role for the glutamatergic neurons in control of responses medi-ated by the DA neurons on target cells not only in the striatum but also in the nucleus accumbens.

(4) The DA neurons seem to be implicated in the heteroregulation of neurotensin

receptors on target cells. It remains to be determined whether other types of receptors may also be affected following destruction of the ascending DA neurons.

(5) Finally, the analysis of long-term heteroregulation of receptors in abnormal situations (lesions) provides information on interactions between different pathways of a complex neuronal network. Such interactions may intervene in physiological states. Therefore, this approach seems to be of heuristic value for determining the respective roles of identified neuronal pathways in cerebral functions.

## REFERENCES

1. BJÖRKLUND, A. & O. LINDVALL. 1978. The mesotelencephalic dopamine neuron system: A review of its anatomy. In Limbic Systems. K. E. Livingston & O. Hornykiewicz, Eds.: 297–331. Plenum. New York.

2. HERVÉ, D., G. BLANC, J. GLOWINSKI & J. P. TASSIN. 1982. Reduction of dopamine utilization in the prefrontal cortex but not in the nucleus accumbens after selective destruction of noradrenergic fibers innervating the ventral tegmental area in the rat. Brain Res. 237: 510–516.

3. LISOPRAWSKI, A., D. HERVÉ, G. BLANC, J. GLOWINSKI & J. P. TASSIN. 1980. Selective activation of the mesocortico-frontal dopaminergic neurons induced by lesion of the habenula in the rat. Brain Res. 183: 229–234.

4. HERVÉ, D., H. SIMON, G. BLANC, M. LE MOAL, J. GLOWINSKI & J. P. TASSIN. 1981. Opposite changes in dopamine utilization in the nucleus accumbens and the frontal cortex after electrolytic lesion of the median raphe in the rat. Brain Res. 216: 422–428.

5. HÖKFELT, T., B. J. EVERITT, E. THEODORSSON-NORHEIM & M. GOLDSTEIN. 1984. Occurrence of neurotensin-like immunoreactivity in subpopulations of hypothalamic, mesencephalic and medullary catecholamine neurons. J. Comp. Neurol. 222: 543–559.

6. HÖKFELT, T., L. SKIRBOLL, J. F. REHFELD, M. GOLDSTEIN, K. MARKEY & O. DANN. 1980. A subpopulation of mesencephalic dopamine neurons projecting to limbic areas contains a cholecystokinin-like peptide: Evidence from immunocytochemistry combined with retrograde tracing. Neuroscience 5: 2093–2124.

7. STUDLER, J. M., H. SIMON, F. CESSELIN, J. C. LEGRAND, J. GLOWINSKI & J. P. TASSIN. 1981. Biochemical investigation on the localization of the cholecystokinin octapeptide in dopaminergic neurons originating from the ventral tegmental area of the rat. Neuropeptides 2: 131–139.

8. SEEMAN, P. 1980. Brain dopamine receptors. Pharmacol. Rev. 32: 229–313.

9. BILLARD, W., V. RUPERTO, G. CROSBY, L. C. IORIO & A. BARNETT. 1984. Characterization of the binding of ($^3$H)SCH 23390, a selective D1 receptor antagonist ligand, in rat striatum. Life Sci. 35: 1885–1893.

10. SAVASTA, M., A. DUBOIS & B. SCATTON. 1986. Autoradiographic localization of D1 dopamine receptors in the rat brain with ($^3$H)SCH 23390. Brain Res. 375: 291–301.

11. PALACIOS, J. M., D. L. NIEHOFF & M. J. KUHAR. 1981. ($^3$H)Spiperone binding sites in brain: Autoradiographic localization of multiple receptors. Brain Res. 213: 277–289.

12. BOUTHENET, M. L., M. P. MARTRES, N. SALES & J. C. SCHWARTZ. 1987. A detailed mapping of D2 receptors in rat central nervous system by autoradiography with ($^{125}$I)iodosulpride. Neuroscience 20: 117–155.

13. MARCHAIS, D., J. P. TASSIN & J. BOCKAERT. 1980. Dopaminergic component of ($^3$H) spiroperidol binding in the rat anterior cerebral cortex. Brain Res. 183: 235–240.

14. BOYSON, S. J., P. McGONIGLE & P. B. MOLINOFF. 1986. Quantitative autoradiographic localization of the D1 and D2 subtypes of dopamine receptors in rat brain. J. Neurosci. 6: 3177–3188.

15. TASSIN, J. P., J. BOCKAERT, G. BLANC, L. STINUS, A. M. THIERRY, S. LAVIELLE, J. PRÉMONT & J. GLOWINSKI. 1978. Topographical distribution of dopaminergic innervation and dopaminergic receptors of the anterior cerebral cortex of the rat. Brain Res. 154: 241–251.

16. PRÉMONT, J., M. C. DAGUET DE MONTETY, A. HERBET, J. GLOWINSKI, J. BOCKAERT &

A. PROCHIANTZ. 1983. Biogenic amines and adenosine-sensitive adenylate cyclases on striatal neurons. Dev. Brain Res. **9:** 53–61.

17. CHNEIWEISS, H., J. GLOWINSKI & J. PRÉMONT. 1985. VIP receptors linked to an adenylate cyclase and their relationship with biogenic amines and somatostatin sensitive adenylate cyclase on central neuronal and glial cells in primary cultures. J. Neurochem. **44:** 779–786.

18. ENJALBERT, A. & J. BOCKAERT. 1983. Pharmacological characterization of the D2 dopamine receptor negatively coupled with adenylate cyclase in rat anterior pituitary. Mol. Pharmacol. **23:** 576–584.

19. ONALI, P. L., M. C. OLIANAS & G. L. GESSA. 1985. Characterization of dopamine receptors mediating inhibition of adenylate cyclase activity of rat striatum. Mol. Pharmacol. **28:** 138–145.

20. WEISS, S., M. SEBBEN, A. J. GARCIA-SAINZ & J. BOCKAERT. 1985. D2-dopamine receptor-mediated inhibition of cyclic AMP formation in striatal neurons in primary culture. Mol. Pharmacol. **27:** 595–599.

21. IORIO, L. C., A. BARNETT, F. H. LEITZ, V. P. HOUSER & C. A. KORDUBA. 1983. SCH 23390, a potential benzazepine antipsychotic with unique interactions on dopaminergic systems. J. Pharmacol. Exp. Ther. **226:** 462–468.

22. CHRISTENSEN, A. V., J. ARNT, J. HYTTEL, J. J. LARSEN & O. SVENDSEN. 1984. Pharmacological effects of a specific dopamine D1 antagonist SCH 23390 in comparison with neuroleptics. Life Sci. **34:** 1529–1540.

23. ARNT, J. 1985. Behavioural stimulation is induced by separate dopamine D1 and D2 receptor sites in reserpine-pretreated but not in normal rats. Eur. J. Pharmacol. **113:** 79–88.

24. WALAAS, S. I., D. W. ASWAD & P. GREENGARD. 1983. A dopamine- and cyclic AMP-regulated phosphoprotein enriched in dopamine-innervated brain regions. Nature **301:** 69–71.

25. NESTLER, E. J., S. I. WALAAS & P. GREENGARD. 1984. Neuronal phosphoproteins: Physiological and clinical implications. Science **225:** 1357–1364.

26. TASSIN, J. P., H. SIMON, D. HERVÉ, G. BLANC, M. LE MOAL, J. GLOWINSKI & J. BOCKAERT. 1982. Non-dopaminergic fibres may regulate dopamine-sensitive adenylate cyclase in the prefrontal cortex and nucleus accumbens. Nature **295:** 696–698.

27. TASSIN, J. P., J. M. STUDLER, D. HERVÉ, G. BLANC & J. GLOWINSKI. 1986. Contribution of noradrenergic neurons to the regulation of dopaminergic (D1) receptor denervation supersensitivity in rat prefrontal cortex. J. Neurochem. **46:** 243–248.

28. TAGHZOUTI, K., H. SIMON, D. HERVÉ, G. BLANC, J. M. STUDLER, J. GLOWINSKI, M. LE MOAL & J. P. TASSIN. 1988. Behavioural deficits induced by an electrolytic lesion of the rat ventral mesencephalic tegmentum are corrected by a superimposed lesion of the dorsal noradrenergic system. Brain Res. **440:** 172–176.

29. LE MOAL, M., L. STINUS & D. GALEY. 1976. Radiofrequency lesion of the ventral mesencephalic tegmentum: Neurological and behavioural considerations. Exp. Neurol. **50:** 521–535.

30. GALEY, D., H. SIMON & M. LE MOAL. 1977. Behavioral effects of lesions in the A10 dopaminergic area of the rat. Brain Res. **124:** 83–97.

31. BECKSTEAD, R. M. 1979. An autoradiographic examination of cortico-cortical and subcortical projections of the medio-dorsal projection (prefrontal) cortex in the rat. J. Comp. Neurol. **18:** 43–62.

32. REIBAUD, M., G. BLANC, J. M. STUDLER, J. GLÓWINSKI & J. P. TASSIN. 1984. Non-DA prefronto-cortical efferents modulate D1 receptors in the nucleus accumbens. Brain Res. **305:** 43–50.

33. FERINO, F., A. M. THIERRY, M. SAFFROY & J. GLOWINSKI. 1987. Interhemispheric and subcortical collaterals of medial prefrontal cortical neurons in the rat. Brain Res. In press.

34. THIERRY, A. M., J. MANTZ, C. MILLA & J. GLOWINSKI. 1988. Influence of the mesocortical/prefrontal dopamine neurons on their target cells. This volume.

35. HERVÉ, D., J. M. STUDLER, G. BLANC, J. GLOWINSKI & J. P. TASSIN. 1986. Partial protection by desmethylimipramine of the mesocortical DA neurons from the neurotoxic effect of 6-OHDA injected in ventral mesencephalic tegmentum. The role of noradrenergic innervation. Brain Res. **383:** 47–53.

36. FERRON, A., A. M. THIERRY, C. LE DOUARIN & J. GLOWINSKI. 1984. Inhibitory influence of the mesocortical dopaminergic system on spontaneous activity or excitatory response

induced from the thalamic medio-dorsal nucleus in the rat medial prefrontal cortex. Brain Res. **302:** 257–265.

37. TASSIN, J. P., A. CHERAMY, G. BLANC, A. M. THIERRY & J. GLOWINSKI. 1986. Topographical distribution of dopaminergic innervation and of dopaminergic receptors in the rat striatum. I. Microestimations of ($^3$H)dopamine uptake and dopamine content in mocrodiscs. Brain Res. **107:** 291–301.

38. FALLON, J. H. & R. Y. MOORE. 1978. Catecholaminergic innervation of the basal forebrain. IV. Topography of the dopamine projection of the basal forebrain and neostriatum. J. Comp. Neurol. **180:** 545–580.

39. BOCKAERT, J., J. PRÉMONT, J. GLOWINSKI, A. M. THIERRY & J. P. TASSIN. 1976. Topographical distribution of dopaminergic innervation and of dopaminergic receptors in the rat striatum. II. Distribution and characteristics of dopamine adenylate cyclase. Interaction of D-LSD with dopaminergic receptors. Brain Res. **107:** 303–315.

40. HEIMER, L., G. F. ALHEID & L. ZABORSKY. 1985. Basal ganglia. In The Rat Nervous System, Vol. 2: G. Paxinos, Ed.: 37–86. Academic Press. New York/Sydney.

41. DONOGHUE, J. P. & M. HERKENHAM. 1986. Neostriatal projection from individual cortical fields conform to histochemically distinct striatal compartments in the rat. Brain Res. **365:** 397–403.

42. VON VOIGTLANDER, P. F., S. J. BOUKMA & S. JOHNSON. 1973. Dopaminergic denervation supersensitivity and dopamine stimulated adenyl cyclase activity. Neuropharmacology. **12:** 1081–1086.

43. MISHRA, R. K., E. L. GARDNER, R. KATZMAN & M. H. MAKMAN. 1974. Enhancement of dopamine-stimulated adenylate cyclase activity in rat caudate after lesions in substantia nigra: Evidence for denervation supersensitivity. Proc. Natl. Acad. Sci. U.S.A. **71:** 3883–3887.

44. PRÉMONT, J., J. P. TASSIN, A. M. THIERRY & J. GLOWINSKI. 1975. Supersensitivity of dopaminergic and β-adrenergic receptors of rat caudate nucleus and cerebral cortex. Exp. Brain Res. (Suppl.) **23:** 165.

45. STAUNTON, D. A., B. B. WOLFE, P. M. GROVES & P. B. MOLINOFF. 1981. Dopamine receptor changes following destruction of the nigro-striatal pathway: Lack of relationship to rotational behaviour. Brain Res. **211:** 315–327.

46. TASSIN, J. P., D. HERVÉ, G. BLANC, A. M. THIERRY & J. GLOWINSKI. 1987. Functional significance of long-term receptor hetero-regulation. Further evidence for cortico-subcortical relationships. (Abst.). In Proc. 7th European Winter Conf. on Brain Research. Val Thorens, France. 72. March 1987.

47. SAVASTA, M., A. DUBOIS, C. FEUERSTEIN, M. MANIER & B. SCATTON. 1987. Denervation supersensitivity of striatal D2-dopamine receptors is restricted to the ventro- and dorsolateral regions of the striatum. Neurosci. Lett. **74:** 180–186.

48. SOMOGYI, P., J. P. BOLAM & A. D. SMITH. 1981. Monosynaptic cortical input and local axon collaterals of identified striatonigral neurons. A light and electron microscopic study using the Golgi-peroxidase transport degeneration procedure. J. Comp. Neurol. **195:** 567–584.

49. FREUND, T. F., J. F. POWELL & A. D. SMITH. 1984. Tyrosine hydroxylase-immunoreactive boutons in synaptic contact with identified striato-nigral neurons with particular reference to dendritic spine. Neuroscience **13:** 1189–1215.

50. OUIMET, C. C., P. E. MILLER, H. C. HEMMINGS, JR, S. I. WALAAS & P. GREENGARD. 1984. DARPP-32, a dopamine- and adenosine 3′:5′-monophosphate-regulated phosphoprotein enriched in dopamine-innervated brain regions. III: Immunocytochemical localization. J. Neurosci. **4:** 111–124.

51. CHNEIWEISS, H., J. GLOWINSKI & J. PRÉMONT. 1985. Modulation by monoamines of somatostatin-sensitive adenylate cyclase on neuronal and glial cells from the mouse brain in primary cultures. J. Neurochem. **44:** 1825–1831.

52. JENNES, L., W. E. STUMPF & P. W. KALIVAS. 1982. Neurotensin: Topographical distribution in rat brain by immunohistochemistry. J. Comp. Neurol. **210:** 211–224.

53. HERVÉ, D., J. P. TASSIN, J. M. STUDLER, C. DANA, P. KITABGI, J. P. VINCENT, J. GLOWINSKI & W. ROSTENE. 1986. Dopaminergic control of $^{125}$I-labeled neurotensin binding site density in corticolimbic structures of the rat brain. Proc. Natl. Acad. Sci. U.S.A. **83:** 6203–6207.

54. PALACIOS, J. M. & M. J. KUHAR. 1981. Neurotensin receptors are located on dopamine-containing neurons in rat midbrain. Nature **294:** 587–589.
55. QUIRION, R., C. C. CHIUEH, H. D. EVERIST & A. PERT. 1985. Comparative localization of neurotensin receptors on nigro-striatal and mesolimbic dopaminergic terminals. Brain Res. **327:** 385–389.
56. NEMEROFF, C. B., D. LUTTINGER, D. E. HERNANDEZ, R. B. MAILMAN, G. A. MASON, S. D. DAVIS, E. WIDERLOV, G. D. FRYE, C. A. KILTS, K. BEAUMONT, G. R. BREESE & A. J. PRANGE, JR. 1983. Interactions of neurotensin with brain dopamine systems: Biochemical and behavioral studies. J. Pharmacol. Exp. Ther. **225:** 337–345.
57. GOVONI, S., J. S. HONG, H. Y. T. YANG & E. COSTA. 1980. Increase of neurotensin content elicited by neuroleptics in nucleus accumbens. J. Pharmacol. Exp. Ther. **215:** 455–474.
58. GOEDERT, M., S. D. IVERSEN & P. C. EMSON. 1985. The effects of chronic neuroleptic treatment on neurotensin-like immunoreactivity in the rat central nervous system. Brain Res. **335:** 334–336.
59. STUDLER, J. M., M. REIBAUD, D. HERVÉ, G. BLANC, J. GLOWINSKI & J. P. TASSIN. 1986. Opposite effects of sulfated cholecystokinin on DA-sensitive adenylate cyclase in two areas of the rat nucleus accumbens. Eur. J. Pharmacol. **126:** 125–128.
60. BARBACCIA, M. L., N. BRUNELLO, D. M. CHUANG & E. COSTA. 1983. On the mode of action of imipramine: Relationship between serotonergic axon terminal function and down-regulation of β-adrenergic receptors. Neuropharmacology **22:** 373–383.
61. COSTALL, B., D. FORTUNE, R. J. NAYLOR, C. D. MARSDEN & C. J. PYCOCK. 1975. Serotonergic involvement with neuroleptic catalepsy. Neuropharmacology **14:** 859–868.
62. CHESSELET, M. F. 1984. Presynaptic regulation of neurotransmitter release in the brain. Neuroscience **12:** 347–375.
63. CHÉRAMY, A., R. ROMO, G. GODEHEU, P. BARUCH & J. GLOWINSKI. 1986. In vivo presynaptic control of dopamine release in the cat caudate nucleus. II. Facilitatory or inhibitory influence of L-glutamate. Neuroscience **19:** 1081–1090.
64. STUDLER, J. M., P. KITABGI, G. TRAMU, D. HERVÉ, J. GLOWINSKI & J. P. TASSIN. 1988. Extensive co-localization of neurotensin with dopamine in rat meso-cortico-frontal dopaminergic neurons. Neuropeptides **11:** 95–100.

# An *in Vivo* Voltammetric Study of the Response of Mesocortical and Mesoaccumbens Dopaminergic Neurons to Environmental Stimuli in Strains of Rats with Differing Levels of Emotionality

BERNARD SCATTON,[a,c] MAGALI D'ANGIO,[a] PETER DRISCOLL,[b] AND ANDRÉ SERRANO[a]

[a]*Laboratoires d'Etudes et de Recherches Synthélabo*
*Biochemical Pharmacology Group*
*31 Avenue Paul Vaillant Couturier*
*92220 Bagneux, France*

[b]*Institut für Verhaltenswissenschaft*
*Eidgenössische Technische Hochschule, Zürich*
*8092 Zürich, Switzerland*

## INTRODUCTION

A host of evidence has suggested that the mesocorticolimbic dopaminergic neurons which originate in the A10 mesencephalic dopaminergic cell group are implicated in the control of cognitive processes and emotional behavior. Thus, electrolytic or neurotoxic (6-hydroxydopamine) lesions of the ventral tegmental area in the rat lead to deficits in basic behaviors required for survival (such as maternal, hoarding, and social behavior), to hypoemotivity, difficulties in suppressing previously learned responses or in tolerating frustrating situations, and to exploratory and locomotor disturbances.[23,24,36-38] Deficits in cognitive functions have also been observed after specific lesions of the dopaminergic terminals in the prefrontal cortex of both rats[37,38] and monkeys;[1] the animals showed retention impairments in a delayed alternation task that is considered to be a sensitive and selective test for frontal cortical function. Also, lesions of dopaminergic terminals in the septum lead to increased emotional reactivity evidenced by enhanced sensitivity to frustrative effects.[28,40] Finally, lesion of the dopaminergic afferents to the nucleus accumbens causes deficits in the initiation of behavioral responses.[36,39]

Our understanding of the nature and type of information received by mesocorticolimbic dopaminergic neurons or of their reactivity to changes in the external environment is as yet relatively scant. Electrophysiological studies have shown that mesen-

[c] To whom correspondence should be addressed.

124

cephalic dopaminergic neurons can be activated by simple sensory stimuli.[2,29] Moreover, dopamine metabolism in the nucleus accumbens is increased in response to arousing (tail pinch) and complex environmental (social interaction) stimuli.[4,27] Exposure of BALB/C mice to a novel environment for 2 min has been reported to cause an increase in prefrontal cortical dopamine metabolism.[19,42] Stressful environmental stimuli are also known to be associated with an increased dopamine metabolism in the prefrontal cortex.[3,6,9,15,22,44]

These results indicate that mesocorticolimbic dopaminergic pathways are activated in response to environmental stimuli. It is conceivable that when there is a change in the animal's environment, the stimulation of sensory afferents leads to stimulation of the ascending reticular system, which then directly or indirectly activates ascending mesocorticolimbic dopaminergic pathways. However, it is not yet clear whether all mesocorticolimbic dopaminergic neurons are activated in response to environmental stimuli or whether different dopaminergic pathways can be recruited according to the nature (sensory modality) of the stimulus. Another important, but as yet unsolved question concerns the significance of the specific activation of mesocorticolimbic dopaminergic neurons induced by stressful stimuli. This increase in cortical dopamine metabolism may be viewed as a biochemical manifestation of anxiety or fear caused by the aversive nature of the stimulus or else may reflect coping of the animal with the stressor.

In the present paper, we have attempted to address these various questions. To this end, we have studied initially the influence of two environmental stimuli differing in their sensory modalities — tail pinch (a widely used arousing stimulus) and short-lasting immobilization — on dopamine metabolism in both nucleus accumbens and the prefrontal cortex of Sprague-Dawley rats. Second, to investigate further the involvement of mesocortical and mesoaccumbens dopaminergic systems in emotional and anxious states, we have studied the effects of an anxiogenic agent (methyl-β-carboline carboxylate, β-CCM) on dopamine metabolism in the frontal cortex and nucleus accumbens of Sprague-Dawley rats. In this series of experiments, the effects of anxiolytic agents on tail-pinch-, immobilization- and β-CCM-induced increases in dopamine metabolism in these brain regions have also been evaluated. Finally, to address the problem of the significance of the increase in cortical dopamine metabolism induced by stressful environmental stimuli, we have investigated the effects of selected biologically relevant stimuli on dopamine metabolism in the prefrontal cortex of genetically distinct strains of rats differing in emotionality.

In this study, dopamine metabolism has been assessed in the frontal cortex and nucleus accumbens of freely moving rats by measuring extracellular levels of 3,4-dihydroxyphenylacetic acid (DOPAC) through the use of *in vivo* voltammetry with electrochemically pretreated carbon fiber electrodes[12,13,35] implanted with a micromanipulator.[26] Currently, *in vivo* voltammetry enables direct and continuous measurement of the levels of the major dopamine metabolite DOPAC *in vivo* in discrete brain areas of conscious freely moving rats.

## EXPERIMENTAL PROCEDURES

Male Sprague-Dawley rats (COBS CD strain from Charles River, France) weighing 250–300 g and experimentally naive male RHA/Verh (300-g) and RLA/Verh (280-g) Wistar-derived rats were used. Rats were housed in individual home cages and had free access to food and water.

Voltammetric measurements were performed on unrestrained awake animals using a classical 3-electrode system with working carbon fiber, reference and auxiliary electrodes, and a PRG5 polarograph (Tacussel, France). Working electrodes made from three pyrrolytic carbon fibers (diameter 8 μm, length 500 μm each) were electrochemically pretreated before use by applying a triangular wave potential of +1.5 V for 20 sec as described previously.[13,35] The carbon fiber electrode was positioned in the brain areas through the use of a newly designed micromanipulator[26-28] implanted stereotaxically a few days prior to the voltammetric recordings under chloral hydrate (400-mg/kg ip) anaesthesia. The stereotaxic coordinates (atlas of Paxinos and Watson[31]) were the following: frontal cortex, 2.7 mm anterior to bregma, 0.7 mm lateral to the midline, 5 mm below the cortex surface; nucleus accumbens 2.2 mm, 1.5 mm, and 6 mm, respectively. The micromanipulator was cemented to the skull surface using four stainless steel screws and acrylic dental cement. The reference electrode (Ag/AgCl-coated silver wire) was placed between the dura mater and the skull, while the auxiliary platinum electrode was soldered to a stainless steel screw implanted in the skull bone. The working, auxiliary, and reference electrodes were connected to a small 3-pin plug that was cemented to the skull. The animals were allowed one week to recover before being submitted to the experimental sessions.

For voltammetric recordings, the electrochemically pretreated working electrode was positioned using the electrode holder, and the plug was connected to the polarograph through a flexible cable and swivel connector. The following recording parameters were used: ramp potential from −200 mV to +400 mV; scan rate 10 mV/sec; pulse modulation of a square wave form (pulse amplitude 50 mV, pulse period 0.2 sec, pulse duration 48 msec). Differential pulse voltammograms were recorded every 2 min. Before and after each experiment, carbon fiber electrodes were calibrated in a 20-μM DOPAC/200-μM ascorbic acid/20-μM 5-HIAA solution in 0.1-M phosphate buffer, pH 7.4. Electrochemical signals were quantified automatically by measuring the height of the oxidation peaks recorded at −100 mV (ascorbic acid), +100 mV (DOPAC), and +300 mV (5-HIAA) using a SP 4100 computer integrator (Spectra Physics). The *in vivo* voltammetric data were expressed as follows: for each individual animal, the mean of the heights of the electrochemical signals measured during the period preceding the experimental procedure was used as a control value and individual data were expressed as percentages of this baseline period. The means with SEM of results obtained on five to six rats were calculated using corresponding periods.

In all experimental situations, the voltammetric recordings were performed every 2 min. The different experimental situations studied were the following:

- *Unfamiliar environment (Y-maze)*: Rats were placed in a novel Y-maze and allowed to explore for 30 min before being returned to their home cages.

- *Loud-noise application*: Rats were subjected to a high-intensity noise (by using a radio and emitting continuously varying frequencies) for 30 min in their home cage.

- *Tail-pinch stress*: A mild tail pressure was administered with sponge-padded forceps for 8 min, 2 cm from the tip of the tail. Animals were tested in their home cages. Food pellets were available during the tail-pinch situation.

- *Immobilization*: In the experiments performed with Sprague-Dawley rats, the animals were restrained for 4 min in the hands of the experimenter. In the experiments performed with RHA/Verh and RLA/Verh rats, the animals were placed in a restraint box for 20 min and then returned to their home cages.

# EFFECTS OF ENVIRONMENTAL STIMULI WITH DIFFERENT SENSORY MODALITIES ON DOPAMINE METABOLISM IN THE FRONTAL CORTEX AND NUCLEUS ACCUMBENS OF SPRAGUE-DAWLEY RATS

A variety of environmental stimuli have previously been shown to increase dopamine metabolism in the mesocortical dopaminergic system of the rat (see the Introduction). To investigate whether the activity of dopaminergic neurons projecting to the nucleus accumbens or prefrontal cortex can be selectively affected depending upon the nature of the environmental stimulus, we have studied the effects of tail pinch, a mild arousing stimulus, and of physical immobilization for a short time (4 min) on extracellular DOPAC levels in these two brain structures in freely moving Sprague-Dawley rats. These stimuli were sufficiently different in nature to enhance the probability of producing stimulus-specific response patterns.

Under our experimental conditions, three oxidation peaks corresponding to the oxidation of ascorbic acid (peak 1), DOPAC (peak 2), and 5-HIAA (peak 3) were recorded at $-100$ and $+100$ mV, respectively, in the nucleus accumbens and anteromedial prefrontal cortex of freely moving rats (FIG. 1). Previous pharmacological studies performed on immobilized or anesthetized rats have clearly established the identity of peak 2 with DOPAC and that extracellular DOPAC recorded in the prefrontal cortex originates from dopaminergic and not noradrenergic neurons.[35] The amplitude of the DOPAC peak recorded from the nucleus accumbens was greater than that recorded from the prefrontal cortex.

**FIGURE 1.** Typical voltammograms recorded from the anteromedial prefrontal cortex of freely moving rats. *In vitro* recordings were performed using a 200-µM ascorbic acid/20-µM DOPAC/20-µM 5-HIAA solution in 0.1-M sodium phosphate buffer, pH 7.4.

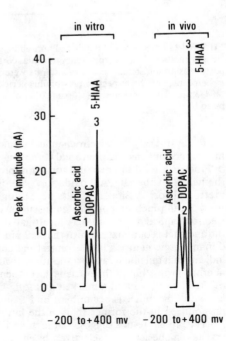

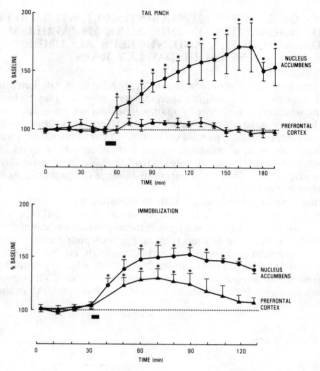

**FIGURE 2.** Effects of tail pinch and immobilization on extracellular DOPAC levels in the nucleus accumbens and anteromedial prefrontal cortex of freely moving Sprague-Dawley rats. Tail pinch was administered for 8 min and rats were immobilized for 4 min. Results are expressed as percentage of the respective prestimulus periods and are means with SEM of data obtained on 4–5 rats. The *bar* represents the time of application of the stimulus. * $p < 0.05$ vs. the control period.

In control rats, the electrochemical signal recorded at $+100$ mV (DOPAC) in both nucleus accumbens and prefrontal cortex was stable over at least a 4-h period. As shown in FIGURE 2, mild tail pressure for 8 min provoked a large and prolonged increase in the height of the DOPAC oxidation peak in the nucleus accumbens but not in the prefrontal cortex. Similar results were found in parallel experiments in which the effects of tail pinch on postmortem tissue levels of DOPAC (measured by HPLC with electrochemical detection) were investigated.[4] Previous electrophysiological studies in the anesthetized rat have shown that tail pinch increases the firing rate of presumptive dopaminergic neurons in the ventral mesencephalic region.[29] These data altogether indicate that tail pinch causes a specific activation of those mesencephalic dopaminergic neurons projecting to the nucleus accumbens. In contrast, immobilization for 4 min of the animals, caused a marked and long-lasting elevation of extracellular DOPAC levels in both nucleus accumbens and frontal cortex, the effect being slightly more pronounced in the former than in the latter brain region (FIG. 2).

The present results suggest that mesocortical and/or mesoaccumbens dopaminergic systems can be activated selectively by environmental stimuli, depending on the nature (possibly sensory modality) of the applied stimulus. It is conceivable that different populations of dopamine-containing cells in the ventral tegmental area are activated selectively in response to differing stimuli. Electrophysiological studies have indeed indicated that those mesocortical prefrontal dopaminergic neurons originating in the ventral tegmental area are distinct from those innervating the nucleus accumbens, the septum, or the head of the striatum.[5,43] Moreover, dopamine-containing cells innervating the prefrontal cortex and the nucleus accumbens are controlled by different afferent pathways. Thus, a bilateral habenula lesion causes an increase in dopamine utilization in the prefrontal cortex but not in the nucleus accumbens of the rat.[25] Conversely, neurons originating in the dorsal raphe regulate the activity of the mesoaccumbens but not the activity of the mesocortical dopaminergic neurons.[18] Electrolytic lesion of the median raphe induces opposite short-lasting changes in the rate of dopamine utilization in the prefrontal cortex and nucleus accumbens in the rat.[17] Finally, selective destruction of noradrenergic fibers that innervate the ventral tegmental area reduces dopamine utilization in the prefrontal cortex but not in the nucleus accumbens of the rat.[16] These data altogether are consistent with the view that the populations of dopamine-containing cells in the ventral tegmental area, which project to the prefrontal cortex or nucleus accumbens, are submitted to distinct interneuronal regulatory processes. Raphe neurons and ascending noradrenergic neurons could possibly serve as relay stations in translating the changes in the animal's environment into changes in the activity of specific dopaminergic cell groups.

We observed that in the environmental situations investigated, the increase in extracellular DOPAC levels in the nucleus accumbens and/or prefrontal cortex persisted long after cessation of the stimulus. This would suggest that a short-lasting environmental stimulus is able to induce a sustained activation of mesocorticolimbic dopaminergic neurons. However, care should be exercised when interpreting data obtained by measurement of dopamine metabolites, since previous *in vivo* dialysis studies have revealed that enhanced extracellular DOPAC levels do not necessarily reflect augmented dopamine release, but may rather index increased dopamine synthesis.[20] The persistence of the elevation of extracellular DOPAC concentrations long after tail pinch or immobilization were initiated may thus reflect an increase in tyrosine hydroxylase activity and a subsequent breakdown and spillover of intraneuronal dopamine.

## EMOTIONAL/ANXIOUS STATES AND MESOCORTICOLIMBIC DOPAMINERGIC SYSTEMS

Several studies have demonstrated that the mesocortical dopaminergic neurons projecting to the prefrontal cortex are specifically activated during stress; the extent of activation being dependent on the amount of physical stress.[6,9,22,44] Recent work has also shown that these neurons are activated by exposure to an environmental stimulus associated previously with inescapable footshock,[15] thus suggesting that the prefrontal dopaminergic system is involved in fear or anxiety. The fact that anxiolytic agents of various chemical classes antagonize, in nonsedative doses, the electric footshock stress-induced augmentation of prefrontal cortical DOPAC in the rat and mouse[3,9,22] adds further support to this view.

It is generally accepted that the pharmacological effects of the anxiolytic benzodiazepines are mediated via specific receptors in the CNS.[14,30] The β-carbolines, β-CCM, and ethyl-β-carboline carboxylate (β-CCE) have been shown to possess actions opposite to those of the benzodiazepines in animal models used to measure anxiety.[10,33] These behavioral effects of the β-carbolines have been interpreted as being due to in-

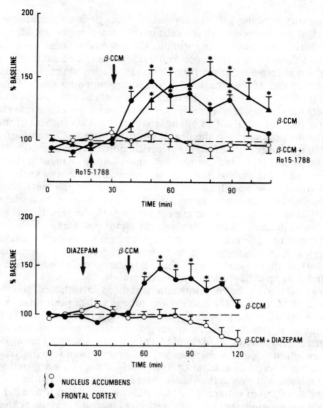

**FIGURE 3.** Effects of β-CCM (10-mg/kg sc) alone or in combination with Ro 15-1788 (30-mg/kg ip) or diazepam (2-mg/kg ip) on extracellular DOPAC levels in the nucleus accumbens and prefrontal cortex of freely moving Sprague-Dawley rats. Ro 15-1788 and diazepam were injected 10 and 30 min, respectively, before the injection of β-CCM. Results are expressed as a percentage of the prestimulus period, and represent means with SEM of data obtained on 4–5 rats per group. *Arrows* indicate the time of administration of the pharmacological agents. * $p < 0.01$ vs. the saline-treated rats.

creased anxiety, and one of these β-carbolines (FG 7142) has indeed been claimed to be anxiogenic in humans.[7] In order to investigate further the involvement of mesocorticolimbic dopaminergic neurons in emotional states, we have studied the effects of the anxiogenic β-carboline, β-CCM on dopamine metabolism in the frontal cortex and/or nucleus accumbens of Sprague-Dawley rats. We have also compared the ability of anxiolytic agents to prevent an environmental aversive stimulus- and the β-CCM-induced alterations in dopamine metabolism in these brain regions.

As shown in FIGURE 3, similarly to immobilization, β-CCM (10-mg/kg sc) caused a marked increase in extracellular DOPAC levels in both nucleus accumbens and prefrontal cortex of freely moving Sprague-Dawley rats, the effect being similar in magnitude in both regions. This effect was of short duration and has disappeared at 80 min postinjection. This is in contrast with immobilization or tail-pinch stresses for which increased DA metabolism was seen long after cessation of the stimulus (cf. Fig. 2). This difference may be ascribed to a short duration of action of the β-CCM.

The stimulating effect of β-CCM on extracellular DOPAC levels in the nucleus accumbens was antagonized by pretreatment of the animals with the benzodiazepine receptor antagonist Ro 15-1788 (30-mg/kg ip) or with diazepam (2-mg/kg ip) (Fig. 3). Ro 15-1788 or diazepam on their own did not affect extracellular DOPAC levels (data not shown).

Similarly, pretreatment with diazepam (2-mg/kg ip) prevented the rise in extracellular DOPAC concentrations observed in the nucleus accumbens after a short-lasting (4-min) immobilization or tail pinch (Fig. 4). Diazepam also antagonized the tail-pinch-induced increase in extracellular DOPAC in the nucleus accumbens when given shortly after cessation of the stimulus (Fig. 4).

The present results indicate that, like stressful external stimuli, a pharmacologically induced anxiogenic stimulus produced by systemic administration of β-CCM is associated with an activation of dopamine metabolism in both nucleus accumbens and frontal cortex. Previous reports have similarly shown that systemic administration of β-CCM, β-CCE, or FG 7142 increases postmortem tissue levels of DOPAC in the rat frontal cortex.[3,41] The blockade by Ro 15-1788 of the activating effect of β-CCM on dopamine metabolism suggests that it is mediated by a benzodiazepine receptor. The β-CCM-induced increase in extracellular DOPAC concentrations in the nucleus accumbens most likely results from its anxiety-promoting action as it was antagonized by pretreatment with a nonsedative dose of diazepam. These results together with the fact that diazepam also antagonized the immobilization-induced increase in dopamine metabolism add further weight to the current view that the mesocorticolimbic dopaminergic system is involved in anxiety.

Not only preventive but also curative treatment with diazepam antagonized the stress-induced alterations in dopamine metabolism in the nucleus accumbens. This suggests that anxiolytic agents do not impair the perception of the stressful stimulus, but rather act at a more integrative level.

On the basis of previous studies dealing with the effects of electric footshocks on dopamine metabolism in a variety of dopamine-rich brain areas in the rat, it has been claimed that the mesocortical dopaminergic system projecting to the prefrontal cortex is *selectively* activated by stress.[22,34,44] The present results, however, indicate that anxiogenic agents (e.g., β-CCM) activate *both* mesolimbic and mesocortical dopaminergic systems. We have also seen in the preceding section that stressful environmental stimuli (e.g., immobilization) cause an activation of dopamine metabolism not only in the frontal cortex but also in the nucleus accumbens. Moreover, in complementary experiments, we have observed that a short-lasting handling (5 sec) or conditioned fear (exposure to an environmental stimulus previously associated with inescapable electric footshocks) are able to increase significantly extracellular DOPAC levels in the nucleus accumbens of freely moving Sprague-Dawley rats (unpublished data). Therefore, it appears that not only the mesocortical but also the mesoaccumbens dopaminergic system is activated by stress. As discussed in the preceding section, the specific activation of either of these dopaminergic systems is likely to be determined primarily by the sensory modality of the acute stressor, although other mechanisms cannot be ruled out. A difference in the nature (sensory modality) of the acute stressor would thus account for the apparent discrepancy observed between our results and those of others concerning the influence of stress on dopamine metabolism in the nucleus accumbens.

Mesolimbic dopaminergic neurons projecting to the nucleus accumbens are known to play a key role in the control of locomotor activity in the rodent.[21,32] The increase in extracellular DOPAC levels seen in the nucleus accumbens after systemic injection of β-CCM (or stress) may thus conceivably be connected to an alteration of the level

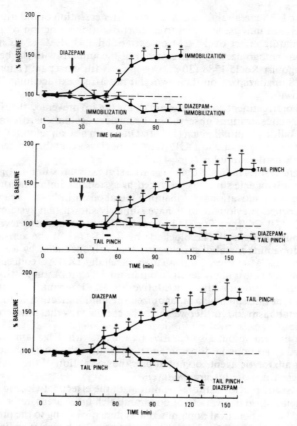

**FIGURE 4.** Antagonism by preventive or curative treatment with diazepam (2-mg/kg ip) of immobilization and tail-pinch-induced increases in extracellular DOPAC levels in the nucleus accumbens of Sprague-Dawley rats. Rats were immobilized for 4 min and tail pinch was administered for 8 min. Diazepam was injected 30 min before initiation of immobilization and 20 min before initiation or 5 min after cessation of tail pinch. Results are expressed as a percentage of the prestimulus period and represent means with SEM of data obtained on 4 rats per group. *Arrows* indicate ip administration of diazepam. * $p < 0.01$ vs. the respective saline-treated controls.

of activity of the animals. However, this hypothesis is highly unlikely, as (1) high doses of anxiogenic β-carbolines do not increase, but rather decrease, locomotor activity in the rodent, (2) similarly to β-CCM, immobilization stress enhances dopamine metabolism in the nucleus accumbens.

## EFFECTS OF ENVIRONMENTAL STIMULI ON DOPAMINE METABOLISM IN THE FRONTAL CORTEX OF ROMAN HIGH- AND LOW-AVOIDANCE RATS

From previous and the present studies, it appears that anxiogenic environmental or pharmacological stimuli cause an activation of mesocorticolimbic dopaminergic neurons projecting to the prefrontal cortex and/or to the nucleus accumbens. The significance of the stress-induced activation of these neurons is, however, not yet clear. By analogy with the hormonal changes (e.g., increase in plasma corticosterone) caused by stress, the augmentation of cortical dopamine metabolism could be viewed as a biochemical manifestation of the emotional reaction provoked by the stressor whose extent is dependent on the amount of physical stress. An alternative, though speculative, explanation would be that this biochemical response reflects heightened attention of the animal in an attempt to cope with the stressor. In order to gain an insight into this problem, the effects of various environmental (stressful) situations (unfamiliar environment, loud noise, immobilization) on extracellular levels of DOPAC in the prefrontal cortex have been compared in the Roman high (RHA/Verh) and low (RLA/Verh) avoidance lines of rats, which differ drastically in their level of emotionality (see reference 8 for a review). RHA/Verh and RLA/Verh rats are selected and bred for the rapid acquisition versus the nonacquisition, respectively, of a two-way active avoidance response. On the basis of many physiological and behavioral parameters, RLA/Verh rats are considered as more "emotional," or anxious, than RHA/Verh rats.[8,11] For instance, RLA/Verh rats show freezing behavior and increased defecation in a shuttle box and an open-field, and show more maternal behavior than RHA/Verh rats. Moreover, RLA/Verh rats show a higher elevation of plasma corticosterone than RHA/Verh rats when placed in an open-field.

When chronically implanted, freely moving RHA/Verh and RLA/Verh rats were placed in an unfamiliar environment (Y-maze) for 30 min, there was an increase in the amplitude of the cortical DOPAC oxidation peak in the former but not in the latter strain of rats (FIG. 5). Similarly, application of a high-intensity loud noise for 30 min to the animals caused an elevation of the amplitude of the cortical DOPAC oxidation peak in RHA/Verh but not in RLA/Verh rats (FIG. 5). In both of these experimental situations, cortical DOPAC levels in RHA/Verh rats returned to baseline within 30 min after cessation of the stimulus. Finally, immobilization for 20 min of the animals induced a progressive and marked increase in extracellular DOPAC levels in the frontal cortex of RHA/Verh but not of RLA/Verh rats (FIG. 5). The DOPAC peak remained elevated for at least 50 min after cessation of the stress.

The present results indicate that, similar to what has been observed in Sprague-Dawley rats, stressful stimuli (with different sensory modalities) are able to increase cortical dopamine metabolism in Wistar-derived Roman rats. In all experimental situations, an increased cortical dopamine metabolism was observed exclusively in the strain of rats showing the lower emotionality (RHA/Verh). These data therefore suggest that the stress-induced increase in cortical DOPAC is unlikely to represent a direct biochemical manifestation of fear or anxiety caused by the stressor.

RHA/Verh rats have been shown to be more active than RLA/Verh rats in several test situations, including operant conditioning for food reward, the aquatic Hebb-Williams maze, the open field , and labyrinth exploration, and some of the stress situations tested (e.g., Y-maze) produced an increased exploratory behavior in RHA/Verh rats only.[8] It could thus be argued that the stress-induced augmentation of cortical dopamine metabolism observed in RHA/Verh rats is connected to an alteration of their level of activity. However, this possibility can be dismissed, as immobilization also caused an increase of extracellular cortical DOPAC levels in RHA/Verh rats. Moreover, in complementary experiments in which RLA/Verh rats were forced to run on a rotarod (D'Angio *et al.*, in preparation) there was no appreciable increase in extracellular DOPAC levels in the frontal cortex of this line of rat.

On the other hand, since RLA/Verh rats are more emotional than RHA/Verh rats, the lack of stress-induced increase in cortical DOPAC in this line may be due to the development of an habituation to stress. However, this is highly unlikely, as in all stressful situations tested so far, RLA/Verh rats showed clear signs of emotional response (e.g.,

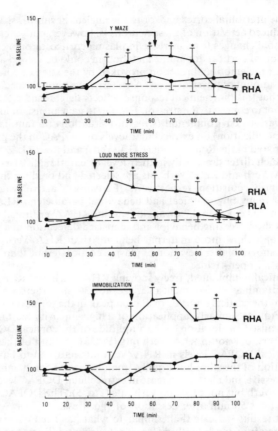

**FIGURE 5.** Effects of various environmental stressful stimuli on extracellular DOPAC levels in the prefrontal cortex of freely moving RHA/Verh and RLA/Verh rats. Rats were placed in an unfamiliar environment (Y-maze) for 30 min, subjected to a high-intensity loud noise for 30 min, or placed in a restraint box for 20 min. *Arrows* indicate the times of onset and cessation of the stimulus. Results are expressed as a percentage of the prestimulus period and represent means with SEM of data obtained on 5 rats per group. * $p < 0.01$ vs. the respective prestimulus period.

defecation, freezing, and self-grooming). Moreover, in contrast to the stressful situations tested, social interaction with an intruder male Wistar rat for 30 min provoked an increase in extracellular DOPAC levels in the prefrontal cortex of RLA/Verh rats (D'Angio *et al.*, in preparation), which shows that the mesocortical dopaminergic system in these animals can be activated under certain circumstances.

A number of experiments have shown that biochemical, physiological, and/or pathological changes in an organism in response to stress do not seem to be caused by the aversive or anxious nature of the stressor but by the ability or inability of the organism to deal with this stressor (see reference 45). It is thus tempting to suggest that the increased cortical DA metabolism induced by stress may reflect heightened attention of the animal in an attempt to cope with the stressor. This hypothesis is supported by our recent demonstration that cortical endogenous DOPAC levels (as measured by HPLC) are increased in RHA/Verh rats submitted to inescapable footshocks, but are normal in those RHA/Verh rats that are allowed to terminate the same shocks (and are thus able to cope with the stressor) (Driscoll *et al.*, in preparation). Such an explanation would also be consistent with the role played by the prefrontal cortical dopaminergic pathway in attentional and cognitive processes.

## REFERENCES

1. BROZOSKI, T. J., R. M. BROWN, H. E. ROSVOLD & P. S. GOLDMAN. 1979. Cognitive deficit caused by regional depletion of dopamine in prefrontal cortex of rhesus monkey. Science **205:** 929–932.
2. CHIODO, L. A., S. M. ANTELMAN, A. R. CAGGIULA & C. G. LINEBERRY. 1980. Sensory stimuli alter the discharge rate of dopamine (DA) neurons: Evidence for two functional types of DA cells in the substantia nigra. Brain Res. **189:** 544–549.
3. CLAUSTRE, Y., J. P. RIVY, T. DENNIS & B. SCATTON. 1986. Pharmacological studies on stress-induced increase in frontal cortical dopamine metabolism in the rat. J. Pharmacol. Exp. Ther. **238:** 693–700.
4. D'ANGIO, M., A. SERRANO, J. P. RIVY & B. SCATTON. 1987. Tail-pinch stress increases extracellular DOPAC levels (as measured by in vivo voltammetry) in the rat nucleus accumbens but not frontal cortex: Antagonism by diazepam and zolpidem. Brain Res. **409:** 169–174.
5. DENIAU, J. M., A. M. THIERRY & J. FEGER. 1980. Electrophysiological identification of mesencephalic ventro-medial tegmental (VMT) neurons projecting to the frontal cortex, septum and nucleus accumbens. Brain Res. **189:** 315–326.
6. DEUTCH, A. Y., S. Y. TAM & R. H. ROTH. 1985. Footshock and conditioned stress increase 3,4-dihydroxyphenylacetic acid (DOPAC) in the ventral tegmental area but not substantia nigra. Brain Res. **333:** 143–146.
7. DOROW, R., R. HOROWSKI, G. PASCHELKE, M. AMIN & C. BRAESTRUP. 1983. Severe anxiety induced by FG 7142, a β-carboline ligand for benzodiazepine receptors. Lancet. **ii:** 98–99.
8. DRISCOLL, P. & K. BATTIG. 1982. Behavioral, emotional and neurochemical profiles of rats selected for extreme differences in active, two-way avoidance performance. *In* Genetics of the Brain. I. Lieblich, Ed.: 96–123. Elsevier, Amsterdam/New York.
9. FADDA, F., A. ARGIOLAS, M. R. MELIS, A. H. TISSARI, P. C. ONALI & G. L. GESSA. 1978. Stress-induced increase in 3,4-dihydroxyphenylacetic acid (DOPAC) levels in the cerebral cortex and in nucleus accumbens: Reversal by diazepam. Life Sci. **23:** 2219–2224.
10. FILE, S. E., R. G. LISTER, R. MANINOV & J. C. TUCKER. 1984. Intrinsic behavioral actions of propyl-β-carboline-3-carboxylate. Neuropharmacology **23:** 463–466.
11. GENTSCH, C., M. LICHTSTEINER, P. DRISCOLL & H. FEER. 1982. Differential hormonal and physiological responses to stress in Roman high- and low-avoidance rats. Physiol. Behav. **28:** 259–263.
12. GONON, F., M. BUDA, R. CESPUGLIO, M. JOUVET & J. F. PUJOL. 1980. In vivo electrochemical detection of catechols in the neostriatum of anaesthetized rats: Dopamine or DOPAC? Nature (London) **286:** 902–904.
13. GONON, F., C. FOMBARLET, M. BUDA & J. F. PUJOL. 1981. Improvement of pyrolytic carbon fiber electrodes by electrochemical treatments. Anal. Biochem. **53:** 1386–1389.
14. HAEFELY, W. 1984. Benzodiazepine interactions with GABA receptors. Neurosci. Lett. **47:** 201–206.
15. HERMAN, J. P., D. GUILLONNEAU, R. DANTZER, B. SCATTON, L. SEMERDJIAN-ROUQUIER & M. LE MOAL. 1982. Differential effects of inescapable footshocks on dopamine turnover in cortical and limbic areas of the rat. Life Sci. **30:** 2207–2214.
16. HERVE, D., G. BLANC, J. GLOWINSKI & J. P. TASSIN. 1982. Reduction of dopamine utiliza-

tion in the prefrontal cortex but not in the nucleus accumbens after selective destruction of noradrenergic fibers innervating the ventral tegmental area. Brain Res. **237:** 510–516.

17. HERVE, D., H. SIMON, G. BLANC, M. LE MOAL, J. GLOWINSKI & J. P. TASSIN. 1981. Opposite changes in dopamine utilization in the nucleus accumbens and the frontal cortex after electrolytic lesion of the median raphe in the rat. Brain Res. **216:** 422–428.

18. HERVE, D., H. SIMON, G. BLANC, A. LISOPRAWSKI, M. LE MOAL, J. GLOWINSKI & J. P. TASSIN. 1979. Increased utilization of dopamine in the nucleus accumbens but not in the cerebral cortex after dorsal lesion in the rat. Neurosci. Lett. **15:** 127–133.

19. HERVE, D., J. P. TASSIN, C. BARTHELEMY, G. BLANC, S. LAVIELLE & J. GLOWINSKI. 1979. Difference in the reactivity of the mesocortical dopaminergic neurons to stress in the BALB/C and C57 BL/6 mice. Life Sci. **25:** 1659–1664.

20. IMPERATO, A. & G. DI CHIARA. 1985. Dopamine release and metabolism in awake rats after systemic neuroleptics as studied by trans-striatal dialysis. J. Neurosci. **5:** 297–306.

21. KELLY, P.H., P. W. SEVIOUR & S. D. IVERSEN. 1975. Amphetamine and apomorphine responses in the rat following 6-OHDA lesions of the nucleus accumbens septi and corpus striatum. Brain Res. **94:** 507–522.

22. LAVIELLE, S., J. P. TASSIN, A. M. THIERRY, G. BLANC, D. HERVE, C. BERTHELEMY & J. GLOWINSKI. 1978. Blockade by benzodiazepines of the selective high increase in dopamine turnover induced by stress in mesocortical dopaminergic neurons of the rat. Brain Res. **168:** 585–594.

23. LE MOAL, M., B. CARDO & L. STINUS. 1969. Influence of ventral mesencephalic lesions on various spontaneous and conditional behaviours in the rat. Physiol. Behav. **4:** 567–574.

24. LE MOAL, M., D. GALEY & B. CARDO. 1975. Behavioral effects of local injection of 6-hydroxydopamine in the medial ventral tegmentum in the rat. Possible role of the mesolimbic dopaminergic system. Brain Res. **88:** 190–194.

25. LISOPRAWSKI, A., D. HERVE, G. BLANC, J. GLOWINSKI & J. P. TASSIN. 1980. Selective activation of the mesocortico-frontal dopaminergic neurons induced by lesion of the habenula in the rat. Brain Res. **183:** 229–234.

26. LOUILOT, A., M. BUDA, F. GONON, H. SIMON, M. LE MOAL & J. F. PUJOL. 1985. Effect of haloperidol and sulpiride on dopamine metabolism in nucleus accumbens and olfactory tubercle: A study by in vivo voltammetry. Neuroscience **14:** 775–782.

27. LOUILOT, A., M. LE MOAL & H. SIMON. 1986. Differential reactivity of dopaminergic neurons in the nucleus accumbens in response to different behavioral situations. An in vivo voltammetric study in free moving rats. Brain Res. **397:** 395–400.

28. LOUILOT, A., K. TAGHZOUTI, J. M. DEMINIERE, H. SIMON & M. LE MOAL. 1987. Dopamine and behavior: Functional and theoretical considerations. *In* Neurotransmitters Interactions in the Basal Ganglia. M. Sandler, C. Feuerstein, and B. Scatton, Eds.: 193–204. Raven Press, New York.

29. MAEDA, H. & G. J. MOGENSON. 1982. Effects of peripheral stimulation on the activity of neurons in the ventral tegmental area, substantia nigra and midbrain reticular formation of rats. Brain Res. Bull. **8:** 7–14.

30. MOHLER, H. & G. RICHARDS. 1983. Receptors for anxiolytic drugs. *In* Neurochemical, Behavioral and Clinical Perspectives. J. B. Molick, S. J. Enna, and H. I. Yamamura, Eds.: 15–40. Raven Press, New York.

31. PAXINOS, G. & C. WATSON. 1982. The Rat Brain in Stereotaxic Coordinates. Academic Press, New York.

32. PIJNENBURG, A. J. J., W. M. M. HONIG, J. A. M. VAN DER HEYDEN & J. M. VAN ROSSUM. 1976. Effects of chemical stimulation of the mesolimbic dopamine system upon locomotor activity. Eur. J. Pharmacol. **3:** 45–58.

33. PRADO DE CARVALHO, L., G. GRECKSCH, G. CHAPOUTHIER & J. ROSSIER. 1983. Anxiogenic and non-anxiogenic benzodiazepine antagonists. Nature (London) **301:** 64–66.

34. REINHARD, JR., J. R., M. J. BANNON & R. H. ROTH. 1982. Acceleration by stress of dopamine synthesis and metabolism in prefrontal cortex: Antagonism by diazepam. Naunyn Schmiedeberg's Arch. Pharmacol. **308:** 374–377.

35. SERRANO, A., M. D'ANGIO & B. SCATTON. 1986. In vivo voltammetric measurement of extracellular DOPAC levels in the anteromedial prefrontal cortex of the rat. Brain Res. **378:** 191–196.

36. SIMON, H. 1981. Neurones dopaminergiques A10 et système frontal. J. Physiol. **77**: 81–85.
37. SIMON, H., B. SCATTON & M. LE MOAL. 1979. Definitive disruption of spatial delayed alternation in rats after lesions in the ventral mesencephalic tegmentum. Neurosci. Lett. **15**: 319–324.
38. SIMON, H., B. SCATTON & M. LE MOAL. 1980. Dopaminergic A10 neurones are involved in cognitive functions. Nature (London) **286**: 150–151.
39. TAGHZOUTI, K., H. SIMON, A. LOUILOT, J. P. HERMAN & M. LE MOAL. 1985. Behavioral study after local injection of 6-hydroxydopamine into the nucleus accumbens in the rat. Brain Res. **344**: 9–20.
40. TAGHZOUTI, K., M. LE MOAL & H. SIMON. 1985. Enhanced frustrative nonreward effect following 6-hydroxydopamine lesions of the lateral septum in the rat. Behav. Neurosci. **99**: 1066–1073.
41. TAM, S. Y. & R. H. ROTH. 1985. Selective increase in dopamine metabolism in the prefrontal cortex by the anxiogenic beta-carboline FG 7142. Biochem. Pharmacol. **34**: 1595–1598.
42. TASSIN, J. P., D. HERVE, G. BLANC & J. GLOWINSKI. 1980. Differential effects of a two minute open-field session on dopamine utilization in the frontal cortices of BALBC and C57 BL/6 mice. Neurosci. Lett. **17**: 67–71.
43. THIERRY, A. M., J. M. DENIAU, D. HERVE & G. CHEVALIER. 1980. Electrophysiological evidence for non-dopaminergic mesocortical and mesolimbic neurons in the rat. Brain Res. **201**: 210–214.
44. THIERRY, A. M., J. P. TASSIN, G. BLANC & J. GLOWINSKI. 1976. Selective activation of the mesocortical dopaminergic system by stress. Nature (London) **263**: 242–244.
45. VOGEL, W. H. 1985. Coping, stress, stressors and health consequences. Neuropsychobiology **13**: 129–135.

# Stress and the Mesocorticolimbic Dopamine Systems[a]

ROBERT H. ROTH, SEE-YING TAM, YOSHISHIGE IDA,
JING-XIA YANG, AND ARIEL Y. DEUTCH

*Departments of Pharmacology and Psychiatry*
*Yale University School of Medicine*
*New Haven, Connecticut 06510*

## INTRODUCTION

It has been appreciated for many years that exposure to various forms of stress may result in a metabolic activation of central catecholamine-containing neurons. Although stressful events provoke a number of neurochemical and hormonal effects and influence a variety of neurotransmitter systems, certain stressors, such as low-intensity, short-duration footshock,[1] conditioned fear,[2,3] and exposure to a novel environment,[4] appear to selectively influence those dopamine (DA) neurons innervating the medial prefrontal cortex, a brain region believed to be involved in anticipatory phenomena and cognitive function.[5] This report is focused on a characterization of the effects elicited by experimental stress paradigms and related pharmacological treatments that result in a robust and fairly selective activation of the subset of midbrain DA neurons projecting to the prefrontal cortex.

Several years after the discovery of the mesocortical DA projections it began to be appreciated that midbrain DA neurons were not as homogenous as once believed, and that they possessed a number of different biochemical, physiological, and pharmacological properties. The first evidence indicating that certain mesocortical DA neurons may be functionally different from those of the mesolimbic and other midbrain DA systems was provided by examination of the effect of stress on these systems. DA utilization was found to be markedly increased in the prefrontal cortex but only slightly (nucleus accumbens) or not affected at all (olfactory tubercle, septum, amygdala, and striatum) in subcortical structures of rat brain following short periods (20 min) of intermittent footshock stress.[1] The high and selective reactivity of the mesoprefrontal DA neurons to intermittent footshock stress has since been confirmed by a number of other groups, although there are some reported inconsistencies concerning the responsiveness of other mesocortical DA systems[3,6–8] that are probably related to differences in the stress paradigms employed. Extensive evidence has also demonstrated that the mesoprefrontal DA system possesses other distinct characteristics as compared to its mesocortical, mesolimbic, and nigrostriatal counterparts.[9,10] It has been suggested that many of these unique characteristics may be attributed to distinct control mechanisms regulating these mesoprefrontal DA neurons. Some of these unique characteristics, which are listed below, appear to be the consequence of the lack of impulse-regulating somatodendritic and synthesis-modulating nerve terminal DA autoreceptors on these neurons.[11]

[a] This work was supported in part by grants from the U.S. Public Health Service, MH-14092, and the State of Connecticut.

1. A higher rate of physiological activity (firing) and a different pattern of activity (more bursting).
2. A higher turnover rate of transmitter.
3. Greatly diminished biochemical and electrophysiological responsiveness to dopamine agonists and antagonists.
4. Lack of tolerance development following chronic antipsychotic drug administration.
5. Resistance to the development of depolarization-induced inactivation following chronic treatment with antipsychotic drugs.
6. Transmitter synthesis more readily influenced by altered availability of precursor tyrosine.

However, it was initially unclear whether the preferential responsiveness of the mesoprefrontal DA system to stress was related to the absence of functional somatodendritic and synthesis-modulating nerve terminal autoreceptors or to other regulatory controls. The experiments described below indicate that the absence of functional autoreceptors does not appear to be the major critical determinant in the enhanced responsiveness of the mesoprefrontal DA neurons to stress, since other mesocortical DA neurons that lack functional autoreceptors are nonresponsive.

## METHODS

Male Sprague-Dawley rats (Camm) were used in all experiments. Initial studies were directed at selection of an appropriate mild footshock paradigm that would result in a robust and reproducible metabolic activation of the DA neurons in the prefrontal cortex. Pilot experiments revealed that the stimulation threshold for eliciting an increase in DA metabolite levels in the prefrontal cortex within 20 min was approximately 0.15 mA. Shock intensities were calibrated with an oscilloscope across a 101-kΩ resistor connected between adjacent grid bars in the shock box as previously described.[3] Stimulation intensities of less than 0.15 mA were ineffective. Intermittent stimulations slightly above threshold at an intensity of 0.2 mA (160-msec duration, with 320-msec intervals), were observed to elicit a robust and reproducible increase in DA metabolites in the prefrontal cortex. Increasing the stimulation intensity to 0.3–0.4 mA led to jumping behavior and vocalization, but did not result in a further significant increase in prefrontal levels of 3,4-dihydroxyphenylacetic acid (DOPAC). For subsequent studies we therefore selected the lowest current intensity (0.2 mA) that elicited a reproducible activation of the prefrontal cortex; under these experimental conditions no overt escape behavior or vocalization were noted.

Rats were killed by decapitation, the brain removed and dissected into discrete regions as previously described.[3] DOPAC and DA levels were determined by high-performance liquid chromatography (HPLC) coupled with electrochemical detection.[12] Homovanillic acid (HVA) when measured was determined by a gas-chromatography mass-spectrometric method.[13]

## RESULTS

Mild-intensity intermittent footshock for 20 min significantly increased DOPAC and HVA levels in the prefrontal cortex. Significant changes in DOPAC were not observed in other mesotelencephalic dopamine projections (FIG. 1). including other mesocor-

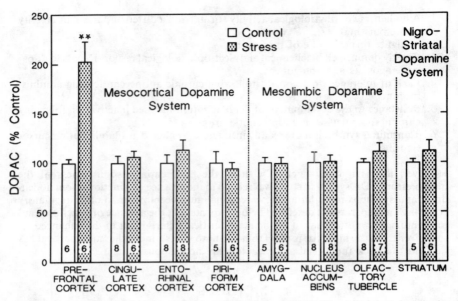

**FIGURE 1.** Effects of mild intermittent footshock stress on DOPAC levels in selected midbrain dopamine projection fields. Rats were subjected to a 20-min period of mild electric footshock (0.2-mA, 160-msec duration, 320-msec interval) and killed immediately after stress. Values are expressed as the mean percentage of unstressed control DOPAC levels ± SEM. ** Differs significantly from unstressed controls ($p < 0.01$).

tical and mesolimbic projection fields examined. Exposure to this stress paradigm did not significantly alter levels of the noradrenergic metabolites, 3-methoxy-4-hydroxyphenylethylene glycol (MHPG) and dihydroxyphenylglycol (DHPG) in the prefrontal cortex, parietal cortex, or hippocampus; a small but significant increase in DHPG was observed in the hypothalamus. In the DA cell body-enriched areas of the ventral tegmentum (VTA) and substantia-nigra, increases in DOPAC were only observed in the VTA.

As previously observed by our laboratory and others, the stress-induced changes in DA metabolites could be reversed by benzodiazepine and nonbenzodiazepine anxiolytics, including even those anxiolytic agents with minimal sedative properties (FIG. 2).[14-16] In addition, the inhibitory effects of the anxiolytic benzodiazepines could be totally nullified by administration of benzodiazepine antagonists, implicating the involvement of benzodiazepine/GABA receptors in the mediation of the activation of the mesoprefrontal DA neurons by stress (FIG. 3).

Since one of the main characteristics of emotional states is that they are subject to conditioning and thus can be elicited by presentation of a neutral stimulus that has been previously paired with an adversive stimulus, we sought to determine whether a specific activation of the mesoprefrontal DA system could also be elicited by a conditioned fear paradigm. We observed that conditioned fear resulted in a selective activation of the mesoprefrontal DA neurons as reflected by an increase in DOPAC levels, thus confirming a previous report.[2] We also observed an increase in metabolite levels in the VTA.[3]

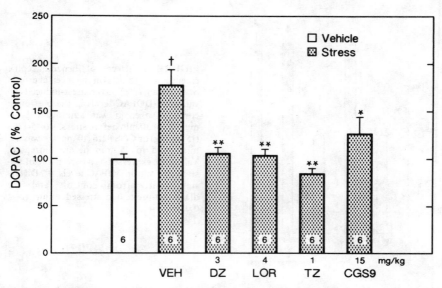

**FIGURE 2.** Reversal of the stress-induced increase in prefrontal DOPAC levels by anxiolytic benzodiazepines. Diazepam (DZ), lorazepam (LOR), triazolam (TZ), CGS9 (CGS 9896), or saline vehicle was administered at doses indicated 30 min before stress. Rats were stressed for 20 min and killed immediately after stress. Values are expressed as the mean percentage of DOPAC levels in the prefrontal cortex of unstressed vehicle-treated control rats ± SEM. + Differs significantly from unstressed vechicle controls ($p < 0.01$); ** differs significantly from the stressed vehicle-treated group ($p < 0.01$); * differs significantly from the stressed vehicle-treated group ($p < 0.05$).

In addition to conditioned fear, the effects of two other nonpainful stress paradigms, immobilization and swim stress, were evaluated.[17,18] Both stressors resulted in an increase in dopamine metabolites in the prefrontal cortex. However, the specificity in the DA metabolite changes was related to the duration of the stress. Swim stress for periods of 5 to 15 min resulted in an increase in DOPAC levels in the prefrontal cortex, while DA metabolite levels in other midbrain DA systems were unaffected. Immobilization produced a time-dependent increase in DOPAC levels in both the prefrontal cortex and nucleus accumbens. The DOPAC increase was apparent in the prefrontal cortex within 5 min, maximal within 30 min, and dissipated during continued restraint within 60–90 min. In the nucleus accumbens a significant increase in DOPAC was observed within 30 min and this increase was maintained throughout the two-hour period of restraint (FIG. 4). Thus, the response of the mesoprefrontal DA system is not only more rapid in onset than that observed in the mesoaccumbens DA system, but appears to develop tolerance even during the continued presence of the stressor.

The restraint-induced increase in DOPAC in the prefrontal cortex and nucleus accumbens was prevented by pretreatment with anxiolytic benzodiazepines; furthermore, the inhibitory effects of these agents could be nullified by administration of a benzodiazepine antagonist, for example, Ro 15-1788 (FIG. 5). It was of interest that administration of the benzodiazepine antagonist alone potentiated the stress-induced increase in DOPAC in the prefrontal cortex. This finding is consistent with the possibility

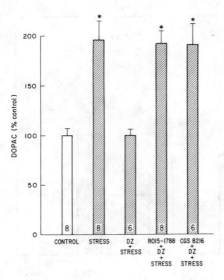

**FIGURE 3.** Effects of benzodiazepine receptor antagonists on the reversal effects of diazepam (DZ) on the stress-induced elevation of DOPAC levels in the prefrontal cortex. Diazepam was administered (5-mg/kg ip) 30 min before stress. Ro 15-1788 (15 mg/kg) or CGS 8216 (10 mg/kg) was administered ip 15 min before diazepam. Values are expressed as a percentage of unstressed control DOPAC levels. ** Differs significantly from controls and the diazepam-pretreated stressed group ($p <$ 0.01).

that prolonged stress may elicit the release of an endogenous substance with benzodiazepine agonist properties that suppresses the stress-induced activation of the prefrontal cortex. However, numerous other plausible mechanisms could be responsible for this adaptive response of the prefrontal cortex.

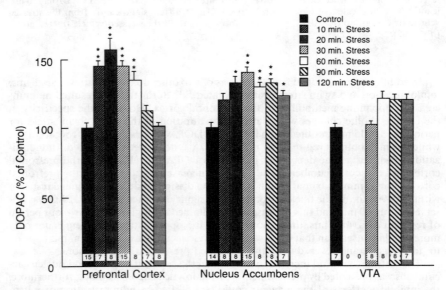

**FIGURE 4.** Time course of the effects of immobilization stress on DOPAC levels in prefrontal cortex, nucleus accumbens, and VTA. Each *bar* represents the mean ± SEM DOPAC level expressed as a percentage of the respective control nonstressed levels. The numbers in the bars indicate the number of animals. Significantly different from control * $p < 0.05$; ** $p < 0.01$.

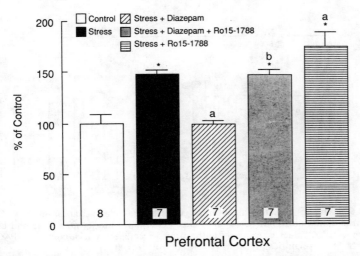

**FIGURE 5.** Reversal of the immobilization stress-induced increase in prefrontal DOPAC by diazepam and its antagonism by benzodiazepine antagonists. Diazepam (2-mg/kg ip) and/or Ro 15-1788 (5-mg/kg ip) were administered 10 min and/or 20 min, respectively, before the initiation of the stress. After drug treatment rats were exposed to immobilization stress for 10 min and were killed by decapitation immediately after the end of the stress period. The *vertical bars* represent the mean DOPA levels expressed as a percentage of control values ± SEM. The numbers in the bars indicate the number of experiments. * $p < 0.05$: significantly different from control group; b $p < 0.05$: significantly different from stress + diazepam group; a $p < 0.05$: significantly different from stress group.

## SELECTIVE ACTIVATION OF MESOPREFRONTAL DA NEURONS BY ANXIOGENIC BETA-CARBOLINES

It is now generally accepted that the pharmacological effects of the anxiolytic benzodiazepines are mediated through specific receptors in the CNS. Beta-carboline carboxylate esters are specific benzodiazepine receptor ligands that antagonize the various central effects of the benzodiazepines. Some of the beta-carbolines have been found to be anxiogenic in animals and humans. We have examined the influence of several of these anxiogenic beta-carbolines on midbrain DA systems. One of these agents, FG-7142 (methyl-beta-carboline-3-carboxamide), has been studied in detail. This agent produces a dose-dependent increase in DA metabolism in the prefrontal cortex of the rat, without causing any significant increase in DA metabolism in other cortical, limbic, or striatal DA projection fields[19] (FIG. 6). A significant decrease in DOPAC is observed in the striatum which is probably a reflection of an activation of the reticulata cells that exert a tonic inhibitory effect on the DA neurons in the pars compacta. This decrease in the concentration of DOPAC in the striatum is paralleled by a decrease in DOPAC levels in the substantia nigra. Likewise, the increase observed in dopamine metabolite levels in the prefrontal cortex is paralleled by an increase in the DA cell body region of the VTA. This selective increase in DA metabolism induced in the

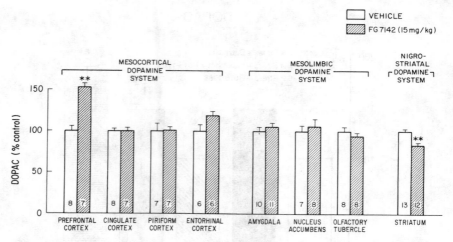

**FIGURE 6.** Effects of FG-7142 (anxiogenic beta-carboline) administration on DOPAC levels in selected midbrain dopamine projection fields. FG-7142 (15-mg/kg ip) was administered 30 min before sacrifice. Values are expressed as the mean percentage of vehicle control DOPAC levels ± SEM. ** Differs significantly from vehicle controls ($p < 0.01$).

mesoprefrontal DA neurons by FG-7142 is prevented by pretreatment with anxiolytic benzodiazepines (i.e., diazepam, lorazepam) or benzodiazepine antagonists, such as Ro 15-1788 or CGS 8216[20] (FIG. 7). Similar results have recently been reported by others.[16] These data are consistent with a benzodiazepine-GABA receptor modulation of the mesoprefrontal cortical subset of VTA DA neurons.

## DIFFERENTIAL AFFERENT CONTROL OF VENTRAL TEGMENTAL NEURONS

The preceding data generated with several different stress paradigms were not consistent with the earlier speculation that the lack of somatodendritic impulse modulating and nerve terminal synthesis modulating autoreceptors accounts for the unique responsiveness of the prefrontal cortex to mild stress.[5] Since regions such as the cingulate cortex (that lack autoreceptors) do not respond to stress, these data suggest that other mechanisms play a role in the stress-elicited metabolic activation of the prefrontal cortex.

The VTA is controlled by a wide range of extrinsic regulatory influences. Among these extrinsic controls may be distinct afferent inputs that regulate VTA DA neurons in a regionally selective manner. The tachykinins appear to be intricately involved in the response of the prefrontal cortical DA system to certain types of stress. Exposure to footshock stress selectively activates the mesoprefrontal DA system and results in a concomitant decrease in levels of substance P (SP) in the VTA.[21,22] This peptidergic involvement in the response of the mesoprefrontal DA neurons to footshock stress appears to be critical, since immunoneutralization of VTA SP prevents the stress-induced mesocortical DA activation.[8] However, the lack of effect of SP antibody infusion on basal mesolimbic or mesocortical DA metabolite levels appears to argue against a normal

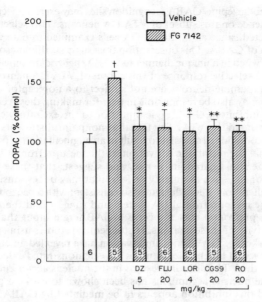

**FIGURE 7.** Effects of benzodiazepine receptor agonists and antagonists on the activating effects of FG-7142 on prefrontal DOPAC levels. Diazepam (DZ), flurazepam (FLU), lorazepam (LOR), CGS 9896 (CGS9), and Ro 15-1788 (RO) were administered at the indicated dosage 30 min before FG-7142 (15-mg/kg) treatment. Rats were killed 30 min after FG-7142 administration. Values are expressed as a percentage of the vehicle control DOPAC levels ± SEM. + Differs significantly from vehicle controls ($p < 0.01$); * differs significantly from the FG-7142-treated group ($p < 0.05$); ** differs significantly from the FG-7142-treated group ($p < 0.01$).

tonic excitatory effect of SP on A10 DA neurons. The precise identity of the VTA neurons innervated by SP afferents remains to be determined.

Although SP levels decline in the VTA following mild footshock stress, the levels of the aliphatic tachykinin, substance K (SK) do not correspondingly decrease.[22] In addition, the levels of SP are not altered in the VTA by short periods of swim or restraint stress or by administration of the beta-carboline, FG-7142.[20] These findings suggest that the mechanisms responsible for the activation of mesoprefrontal DA by various stressors may differ and may not in all cases be related to an activation of the SP input to the VTA.

The finding that a number of stress paradigms, as well as pharmacological manipulations that produce anxiety states in man, are all able to selectively activate the mesoprefrontal DA neurons in rodents suggests that this cortical projection may be involved. Furthermore, the observation that anxiolytic benzodiazepines block both stress and beta-carboline-induced activation of the mesoprefrontal DA neurons suggests that a benzodiazepine/GABA receptor may mediate this activation. In addition, the finding that the antagonism of the stress-induced activation by benzodiazepines can be nullified by administration of benzodiazepine antagonists argues in favor of a critical role for benzodiazepine/GABA receptors in the stress-induced activation of the mesoprefrontal DA neurons. The selective activation of mesoprefrontal DA neurons produced by systemic administration of the inverse benzodiazepine agonist, FG-7142, suggests that benzodiazepine/GABA recognition sites may exert a selective and powerful modulatory influence on this subset of VTA DA neurons. This selective effect of FG-7142 was unexpected, since all midbrain DA cells examined to date were inhibited by direct application of GABA. This observation thus suggests that mesoprefrontal dopamine cells may be wired in a unique manner to GABA/benzodiazepine-dependent mechanisms, allowing a selective response of this subset of VTA DA neurons. The fact that mesoprefrontal dopamine neurons are not subject to autoreceptor-mediated regulation of firing rate may also be responsible in part for making these cells more sensitive to control by the inhibitory GABAergic inputs or to the excitatory effects exerted by other afferent inputs to the VTA. The fact that nonpainful stressors (swim stress, restraint stress, and conditioned stress) also result in an augmentation in prefrontal DOPAC levels indicates that the metabolic activation of the mesoprefrontal DA neurons does not depend on the stress paradigm per se, and suggests that these paradigms share a common component, such as anxiety or fear, that may be responsible for initiating this biochemical alteration. These data are also consistent with a benzodiazepine receptor modulation of the mesoprefrontal DA system and suggest that the A10 DA neurons projecting to the prefrontal cortex receive a GABAergic input that plays a role in regulating the activity of these neurons. Histochemical studies using glutamate decarboxylase as a marker for GABAergic innervation have revealed an enrichment of this enzyme in the VTA and biochemical studies have demonstrated a decrease in the ventromedial part of the VTA following lesions in the nucleus accumbens.[23] In addition, stimulation of the nucleus accumbens has been shown to evoke a potent inhibition of VTA cells, and this inhibition appears to be mediated by GABA.[24] However, it is still unclear whether mesoprefrontal DA neurons are under an inhibitory control by a specific GABAergic pathway, since GABAergic modulation of the A10 DA cells could be achieved by interneurons in the VTA rather than by a long axon pathway.

Recent immunohistochemical studies using monoclonal antibodies directed against purified benzodiazepine/GABA receptors have revealed that VTA neurons in rodents, nonhuman primates, and in man, possess benzodiazepine/GABA receptors (Deutch and Roth, unpublished data). The biochemical studies previously described, together with this new anatomical data, are consistent with a key role for benzodiazepine/GABA receptors in the VTA in mediating the biochemical activation of A10 DA neurons by stress and/or following beta-carboline administration. The immunohistochemical studies also add support to the speculation that benzodiazepine/GABA receptors in the VTA may be involved in the control of mesocorticolimbic function in man.

## ACKNOWLEDGMENTS

The authors thank Ms. Ewa Beckman for her excellent assistance in the preparation of this manuscript.

### REFERENCES

1. THIERRY, A. M., J. P. TASSIN, G. BLANC & J. GLOWINSKI. 1976. Selective activation of the mesocortical DA system by stress. Nature. 263: 242–244.
2. HERMAN, J. P., D. GUILLONNEAU, R. DANTZER, B. SCATTON, L. SEMERDJAN-ROUQUIER & M. LE MOAL. 1982. Differential effects of inescapable foot-shocks and of stimuli previously paired with inescapable foot-shocks on dopamine turnover in cortical and limbic areas of the rat. Life Sci. 30: 2207–2214.
3. DEUTCH, A. Y., S.-Y. TAM & R. H. ROTH. 1985. Footshock and conditioned stress increase 3,4-dihydroxyphenylacetic acid (DOPAC) in the ventral tegmental area but not substantia nigra. Brain Res. 333: 143–146.

4. TASSIN, J. P., D. HERVE, G. BLANC & J. GLOWINSKI. 1980. Differential effects of a two-minute open field session on dopamine utilization in the frontal cortices of BALB/C and C57 BL/6 mice. Neurosci. Lett. **17:** 67–71.
5. BANNON, M. J. & R. H. ROTH. 1983. Pharmacology of mesocortical dopamine neurons. Pharmacol. Rev. **35:** 53–68.
6. LAVIELLE, S., J. P. TASSIN, A. M. THIERRY, G. BLANC, D. HERVE, C. BATHELEMY & J. GLOWINSKI. 1978. Blockade by benzodiazepines of the selective high increase in dopamine turnover induced by stress in mesocortical dopaminergic neurons of the rat. Brain Res. **168:** 585–594.
7. FADDA, F., A. ARGIOLAS, M. R. MELIS, A. TISSARI, P. ONALI & G. L. GESSA. 1978. Stress-induced increase in 3,4-dihydroxyphenylacetic acid (DOPAC) levels in the cerebral cortex and in N. accumbens: Reversal by diazepam. Life Sci. **23:** 2219–2224.
8. BANNON, M. J., P. J. ELLIOT, J. E. ALPERT, M. GOEDERT, S. D. IVERSON & L. L. IVERSON. 1983a. Selective activation of mesocortical dopamine neurons by stress: The role of substance P afferents demonstrated using *in vivo* application of substance P monoclonal antibody. Nature **306:** 791–792.
9. BANNON, M. J., M. E. WOLF & R. H. ROTH. 1983b. Pharmacology of dopamine neurons innervating the prefrontal, cingulate and piriform cortices. Eur. J. Pharmacol. **91:** 119–125.
10. ROTH, R. H. 1984. CNS dopamine autoreceptors: Distribution pharmacology and function. Ann. N.Y. Acad. Sci. **430:** 27–53.
11. CHIODO, L. A., M. J. BANNON, A. A. GRACE, R. H. ROTH & B. S. BUNNEY. 1984. Evidence for the absence of impulse regulating somatodendritic and synthesis-modulating nerve terminal autoreceptors on subpopulations of mesocortical dopamine neurons. Neuroscience **12:** 1–16.
12. MICHAUD, R. L., M. J. BANNON & R. H. ROTH. 1981. The use of C8-octyl columns for the analysis of catecholamines by ion-pair reversed-phase liquid chromatography with amperometric detection. J. Chromatogr. **225:** 335–345.
13. BACAPOULOS, N. G., G. BUSTOS, D. E. REDMOND, JR., J. BAULU & R. H. ROTH. 1978. Regional sensitivity of primate brain dopaminergic neurons to haloperidol: Alterations following chronic treatment. Brain Res. **157:** 396–401.
14. TAM, S.-Y. 1986. Mesoprefrontal dopamine neurons: Studies on their regulatory control. Ph.D. Dissertation. Yale University. New Haven, Conn.
15. ONEL, K. K., S.-Y. TAM. & R. H. ROTH. 1984. Benzodiazepine receptor modulation of stress-induced activation of prefrontal dopamine neurons. Soc. Neurosci. Abst. **10:** 881.
16. CLAUSTRE, Y., J. P. RIVY, T. DENNIS & B. SCATTON. 1986. Pharmacological studies on stress-induced increase in frontal cortical dopamine metabolism in the rat. J. Pharmacol. Exp. Ther. **238:** 693–700.
17. KNORR, A. M., M. P. GALLOWAY & R. H. ROTH. 1984. Swim stress selectively increases norepinephrine metabolism in rat hypothalamus. Fed. Proc., Fed. Am. Soc. Exp. Biol. **43:** 745.
18. YANG, J.-X., A. M. KNORR, K. ONEL, S.-Y. TAM, A. Y. DEUTCH, L. LUBICH & R. H. ROTH. 1985. Effect of different stress paradigms on central dopamine and norepinephrine metabolism. Soc. Neurosci. Abstr., Part 2. **11:** 1210.
19. TAM, S.-Y. & R. H. ROTH. 1985. Selective increase in dopamine metabolism in the prefrontal cortex by the anxiogenic beta-carboline FG 7142. Biochem. Pharm. **34:** 1595–1598.
20. TAM, S.-Y. & R. H. ROTH. 1986. Pharmacological characterization of stress and beta-carboline induced activation of mesoprefrontal dopamine neurons. Soc. Neurosci. Abst. **12:** 247.
21. LISOPRAWSKI, A., G. BLANC & J. GLOWINSKI. 1981. Activation by stress of the habenulo-interpeduncular substance P neurons in the rat. Neurosci. Lett. **25:** 47–51.
22. BANNON, M. J., A. Y. DEUTCH, S.-Y. TAM, N. ZAMIR, J.-M. LEE, J. E. MAGGIO, R. ESKAY & R. H. ROTH. 1986. Mild footshock stress dissociates substance P from substance K and dynorphin from met- and leu-enkephalin. Brain Res. **381:** 393–396.
23. WALAAS, I. & F. FONNUM. 1980. Biochemical evidence for gamma-aminobutyrate containing fibers from the nucleus accumbens to the substantia nigra and ventral tegmental area in the rat. Neuroscience **5:** 63–72.
24. WOLF, P., H. R. OLPE, D. ARVITH & H. L. HAAS. 1978. GABAergic inhibition of neurons in the ventral tegmental area. Experientia **34:** 73–74.

# Intracerebral Transplantation of Dopamine Neurons: Understanding the Functional Role of the Mesolimbocortical Dopamine System and Developing a Therapy for Parkinson's Disease[a]

P. BRUNDIN,[b,e] R. E. STRECKER,[c]
F. H. GAGE,[d] O. LINDVALL,[b] AND A. BJÖRKLUND[b]

[b] Department of Medical Cell Research
University of Lund
Biskopsgatan 5
S-223 62 Lund, Sweden

[c] Hana Biologics Inc.
850 Marina Village Parkway
Alameda, California 94501

[d] Department of Neurosciences
University of California at San Diego
La Jolla, California 92093

## INTRODUCTION

The first reports of successful neural grafting to the mammalian brain originate from the turn of the century.[1] However, the field never gained much attention until the 1970s when the first reports appeared showing that grafted neurons could affect the behavior of the recipient mammal and reduce the neurological symptoms induced by a prior lesion of the host brain.[2,3] These findings stimulated an almost explosive interest in the field of neural grafting and led to the engagement of several diverse disciplines of the neurosciences that have, using a multidisciplinary approach, contributed to an increased understanding of the capacity and limitations of grafted neurons. In many respects, experiments involving grafts of fetal dopamine (DA) neurons have come to

[a] This work was supported by grants from the Swedish MRC (04X-3874), Thorsten and Elsa Segerfalk's Foundation, and Riksbankens Jubileumsfond. Cyclosporin A was supplied by Sandoz Ltd., Täby, Sweden.
[e] To whom correspondence should be addressed.

play a central role in the understanding of the functional characteristics of neural grafts and their clinical potential. The pioneering role of DA grafts in neural transplantation research is partly due to the fact that the very first reports of functional effects of neural grafts in the mammalian brain came from experiments conducted within the DA system of the rat.[2,3] In addition, DA graft research has been aided by the vast knowledge existing on the pharmacology and functional role of DA, by the large number of methodological tools available for morphological and behavioral studies on DA neurons, and finally, by the exciting goal of developing a new therapy for Parkinson's disease (PD).

The objectives of the present review are twofold: first, to summarize experimental data on the functional capacity of DA neuron grafts placed in the limbic forebrain; and second, to describe morphological and functional characteristics of human fetal DA neurons grafted to a rat model of PD. Most of the grafting to the limbic system reported here has been performed to the nucleus-accumbens-septi region (NAS). The DA projection to this nucleus has classically been referred to as part of the mesolimbic DA system.[4] However, since it is now generally agreed that the NAS is part of the ventral striatum,[5] it seems most logical to include its DA input within the mesostriatal DA system.[6] The ventral striatum that is innervated by DA neurons mainly located in the ventral tegmental area (VTA), receives afferents from limbic cortical and subcortical areas.[6] NAS seems therefore to be a highly suitable region for studying the effects of DA neuron grafts on limbic function, as opposed to those parts of the dorsal striatum that are nonlimbic in their connectivity and innervated by more laterally located DA neurons found in the substantia nigra pars compacta.[6]

## BEHAVIORAL EFFECTS OF DOPAMINE NEURONS GRAFTED IN THE NIGROSTRIATAL SYSTEM

The most extensively used animal model in DA graft research has been the rat with a uni- or bilateral 6-hydroxydopamine (6-OHDA) lesion of the ascending nigrostriatal pathway. The focus of attention in these studies has been the functions that are classically considered to be attributable to DA activity in those striatal regions that are innervated by the substantia nigra (A9 of Dahlström and Fuxe[7]). In the rat with a unilateral 6-OHDA lesion of the nigrostriatal pathway, it has been possible to reverse drug-induced circling, sensory inattention, and to ameliorate deficits in conditioned turning (for a review, see reference 8). Rats with bilateral 6-OHDA lesions have shown improvement of sensorimotor and akinetic impairments after the grafting of DA neurons to the caudate–putamen,[9,10] and in aged rats, grafts of DA neurons to the caudate–putamen have been found to reduce deficits in motor coordination.[11] These studies in rodents have recently been extended to primates where fetal mesencephalic tissue has been reported to survive grafting to the striatum[12,13] and give rise to some functional effects[14] in monkeys treated with DA neurotoxin MPTP.

## THE ROLE OF THE MESOLIMBIC DA NEURONS IN BEHAVIOR

The functional role of DA in the mesolimbocortical system has been explored extensively in studies involving specific 6-OHDA lesions of DA projections and in experiments with intracerebral injections of drugs. The putative functional role of DA in the NAS has been described as modulating the relay link between classic motor regions, such as the striatum, and limbic structures, such as the amygdala and the hippocampus.[15] Rats with lesions of mesolimbic DA neurons (in many studies, specifically the DA input to the NAS) display a series of deficits in locomotor behavior, such as decreased spontaneous locomotion and exploration, diminished locomotor response to amphetamine, and increased locomotor response to low doses of apomorphine.[16-19] These data are in good agreement with earlier studies showing that DA injected directly into the NAS elicits an increase in locomotion and that similar injections of DA receptor antagonists can block the locomotor response induced by systemic administration of amphetamine.[20,21] Furthermore, lesions in the mesolimbocortical DA system can result in, for example, disruption of hoarding behavior, impaired learning, hypoexploration and failure to inhibit response strategies.[19,22] In summary, the mesolimbocortical DA system, together with the projection to the NAS, is implicated in a series of locomotor behaviors and may play an important part in aspects of cognition.

## EFFECTS OF DOPAMINE NEURONS GRAFTED IN THE MESOLIMBOCORTICAL SYSTEM

### Drug-Induced and Spontaneous Locomotor Behavior

In rats with bilateral local 6-OHDA lesions of the DA terminals in the NAS, bilateral implants of fetal DA neuron-rich tissue into the NAS have been found to reverse the locomotor hyporesponsiveness to amphetamine caused by the lesion.[23-26] More recently, we have found that the implantation of DA neurons into the NAS on only *one* side is sufficient to reinstate a locomotor response to amphetamine in a similar behavioral model.[27] In the same study we also observed that the hyperresponsiveness to apomorphine was eliminated by the unilateral DA grafts. Similar findings have been reported in rats with 6-OHDA lesions of the DA cell bodies in the VTA.[28] DA neurons implanted into the NAS and prefrontal cortex of such animals not only normalized changes in amphetamine and apomorphine-induced activity, but also increased spontaneous daytime activity above both control and lesion levels.[28]

In summary, these findings support previous data emphasizing the importance of DA in the performance of locomotion. Moreover, the findings suggest that the functional role of DA in the NAS during *locomotion* may not be dependent on an intricate afferent input to the cell body of the DA neuron, since grafted DA neurons ectopically placed in the NAS seem to subserve the function equally as well as the mesencephalic DA neurons of the normal projection system.

### Circling Behavior

Kelly and Moore have hypothesized that DA release in the NAS does not influence the direction of turning in circling behavior, but plays an important role in amplifying the body asymmetry caused by an imbalance in DA neurotransmission in the caudate–putamen.[29] This hypothesis is derived from experiments with specific combined 6-OHDA lesions in the NAS bilaterally and the caudate–putamen unilaterally that show that 6-OHDA lesions of the DA input to the NAS reduce the speed of amphetamine-induced turning in rats with unilateral 6-OHDA lesions in caudate–putamen.[30] We recently studied the validity of this hypothesis in rats that received a unilateral 6-OHDA lesion of the nigrostriatal pathway, causing them to turn ipsilaterally in response to amphetamine, followed by bilateral local 6-OHDA lesions of the DA inner-

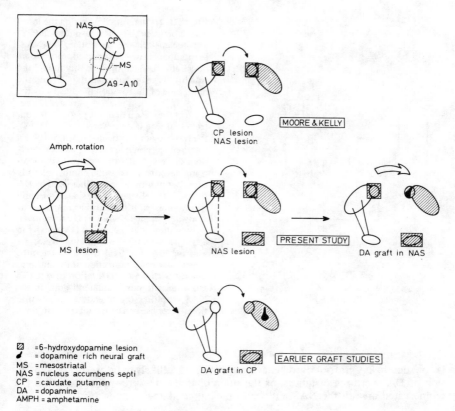

**FIGURE 1.** The diagram illustrates the design and result of the experiment in reference 27 and previous studies (see references 8 and 30). A unilateral DA graft in the NAS was found to amplify amphetamine-induced rotation in rats with a unilateral lesion of the mesostriatal DA pathway (ipsilateral to the graft in the NAS) and bilateral 6-OHDA lesion of the NAS.

vation in the NAS (see Fig. 1 for experimental design). In agreement with previous work, the second series of 6-OHDA lesions caused a marked reduction in the magnitude of amphetamine-induced circling and locomotor activity (Fig. 1). We subsequently grafted DA neurons to the NAS on the side ipsilateral to the initial mesostrital 6-OHDA lesion, with the hypothesis that if the NAS only plays an amplifying function in circling behavior, the DA graft should, although it reinnervates the NAS on the side with a totally DA-depleted striatal complex, give rise to an *increase* in the magnitude of circling. Indeed, the results confirmed this hypothesis[27] and also extended previous findings of a functional heterogeneity within the striatal complex (Fig. 2) as well as of the regional specificity of graft-derived effects. It should be noted that previous studies have demonstrated that when a DA graft is placed in the caudate–putamen on the side of a nigrostriatal 6-OHDA lesion, amphetamine-induced rotation asymmetry is *decreased* or abolished[8] (Fig. 1). The results of our recent study also show that, although there presumably is a massive release of DA under amphetamine stimu-

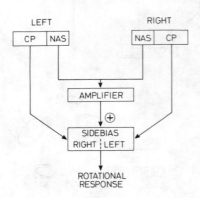

**FIGURE 2.** Diagram illustrating the interaction between the caudate–putamen (CP) and nucleus-accumbens-septi region (NAS) in rotational behavior (adapted from Moore and Kelly[29]). According to this model the side bias is governed from the CP, and the amplitude of the rotational behavior by the NAS. If there is a relatively greater DA release in the CP on one side (e.g., if the contralateral side is denervated by 6-OHDA), the resulting motor behavior will involve a rotational response in the contralateral direction. The magnitude or intensity of this rotational response, that is the number of body turns per unit time, can be increased by DA release in the NAS on either side of the brain (the "amplifier" function). The results of the study in reference 27 conform to this model, as they show that increasing DA activity in a single 6-OHDA denervated NAS, by grafting DA-rich fetal tissue unilaterally, does not affect the direction of the side bias in a rat with a 6-OHDA lesion of one CP. However, the same unilateral graft in the NAS amplifies the already existing rotational response and causes an increase in the speed of turning.

lation, neural DA graft-derived behavioral effects are unlikely to be exerted by a diffusion of DA over long distances, as the functional effects were well localized to the reinnervated area in the NAS and ventromedial caudate–putamen (FIG. 3).[27]

### Hoarding Behavior

Normal rats that are maintained on a restricted diet will display a distinct hoarding behavior when presented with food pellets in an open arena. In rats with lesions of the DA system originating in the VTA this behavior is disrupted and the lesioned rats fail to collect food pellets to the same extent as normal rats.[25] Herman and co-workers[25] have found that bilateral DA grafts to the NAS can restore hoarding behavior in rats with bilateral 6-OHDA lesions of the NAS, but only if the rats are given a low dose of amphetamine prior to the test. These data can suggest that the integrity of a normal afferent input to the DA neurons is necessary for the activation of the DA system in hoarding behavior, and that if ectopically grafted DA neurons fail to establish such an input, they will therefore require pharmacological activation in order to perform their permissive role in hoarding behavior.

### Conditioned Behavior

In a recent study, we investigated the importance of the mesotelencephalic DA system in the performance of a conditioned learning paradigm. We utilized the conditioned

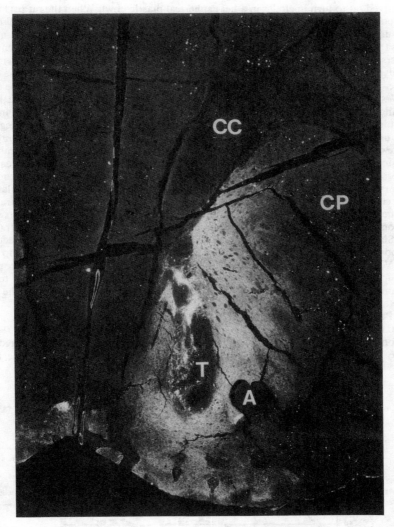

**FIGURE 3.** Catecholamine histofluorescence photomicrograph showing a coronal section at the level of the NAS through the brain of a rat (from the study in reference 27) that received a unilateral implant of mesencephalic DA neurons in the right NAS. As a consequence of the nigrostriatal lesion, there is an absence of DA innervation in the dorsolateral caudate–putamen (CP). A 6-OHDA injection was also given in the NAS region, but the DA innervation has now been restored by the DA neurons in the cell suspension transplant (T). However, as the graft-derived DA fibers do not reach the dorsolateral CP, this region remains denervated. CC = corpus callosum forceps minor, A = anterior commissure. (The photograph was taken by Ragnar Martensson using a newly developed automated dark-field condensor scanner equipment)

turning task developed by Freed and Yamamoto,[31] which involves teaching a water-deprived rat to turn in circles in a hemispherical plastic bowl. When the rat performs a body turn in the desired direction, it is given a reward, consisting of a small drop of sucrose-water delivered through a hole in the wall of the training bowl. We trained rats that had received 6-OHDA injections close to the VTA, damaging the ascending fibers of the mesotelencephalic DA system. In a previous postmortem biochemical study[32] we found that the same type of lesion produces a depletion of DA in the caudate–putamen, and the nucleus accumbens–olfactory tubercle–septum to more than 90%. However, the rats were neither markedly akinetic, nor aphagic or adipsic, indicating that the DA depletion in the caudate–putamen was subtotal.[33] After an initial shaping period of 3 to 10 days, when the rats were given sucrose-water rewards regardless of the direction in which they turned, the rats that had reached a criterion number of rewards in a training session were then trained to perform left turns during 15 training sessions. Normal rats gradually acquired this behavior and reached a group mean of approximately 7 full left turns per minute (FIG. 4). A group of VTA lesion control animals and in addition, a group of VTA lesioned rats that had received large bilateral DA cell suspension grafts in the NAS and the head of the caudate–putamen were trained in the conditioned turning task. Both the grafted and nongrafted groups of rats with lesions of the VTA were significantly impaired in the rewarded turning to the left (FIG. 4). Similarly, when the rats were subsequently trained to circle in the right direction, opposite to the direction previously rewarded, the VTA lesioned grafted group and the VTA lesioned group were markedly impaired in comparison to the normal control group. Interestingly, this particular group of grafted rats had previously been tested in amphetamine-induced locomotion and displayed a complete recovery of the amphetamine locomotor response.

Previous studies have indicated that the DA in the caudate–putamen plays an essential role in the initiation of conditioned turning.[34] If rats are subjected to 6-OHDA lesions of the nigrostriatal pathway, they are unable to learn to circle in the direction away from the lesion, whereas they can learn to circle toward the lesioned side, sug-

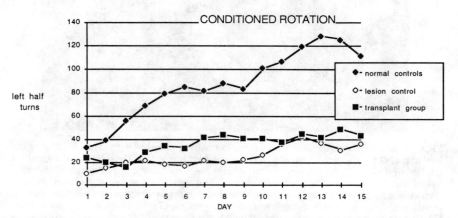

**FIGURE 4.** Results from the conditioned rotation experiment discussed in the text. Normal rats learn to turn significantly faster than rats with bilateral 6-OHDA lesions of the ventral mesencephalic DA neurons (lesion control). Rats with bilateral DA grafts in the caudate–putamen and the NAS (transplant group) showed no amelioration of this lesion-induced deficit, although the same rats were found to have a complete restoration of amphetamine-induced locomotion.

gesting that the deficit is mainly one of motor initiation. Unlike our findings, a recent study has shown that DA grafts reinnervating the caudate–putamen can ameliorate the unilateral lesion-induced deficit in turning.[35] In our study there were large surviving grafts in the caudate–putamen, but the lesion also markedly depleted DA in the NAS, which may be important in driving the circling behavior. Although the NAS was also reinnervated by the DA cell suspension implants, leading to reinstatement of amphetamine-induced locomotor response, it is possible that, in agreement with the aforementioned studies of hoarding behavior,[25] the DA neurons grafted to the NAS were not able to drive a complex behavior, that is, conditioned turning, without pharmacological stimulation.

## THE POSSIBLE APPLICATION OF THE NEURAL GRAFTING TECHNIQUE IN PATIENTS WITH PARKINSON'S DISEASE

In PD there is a progressive degeneration of mesencephalic DA neurons,[36] which leads to a widespread deficiency of DA transmission in both the striatal and limbocortical forebrain regions.[37,38] The reduction of DA levels has been reported to be most pronounced in the putamen (up to 95%), and more moderate in the caudate nucleus and nucleus accumbens.[37] The cortical DA projections seem to be less severely affected. Patients with PD differ with respect to symptomatology, which probably reflects individual patterns of degeneration in the DA terminal areas. In the clinical trials performed so far (cf. below) the catecholamine-producing tissue, that is, adrenal medullary cells, has been implanted unilaterally either in the putamen or caudate nucleus. In view of the role of the NAS in initiating locomotor responses, as observed in animal experiments, it seems probable that optimal relief in a PD patient with pronounced gait akinesia may require graft placement also in this region. Ideally the number and placements of grafts should be decided on the basis of a careful analysis of the symptomatology of each individual patient. Computerized movement analysis promises to be of great value for this purpose, since it seems to distinguish between groups of PD patients with characteristic patterns of locomotor and postural dysfunction.[39]

There are already in the literature reports of at least six cases in which autologous grafts of adrenal medulla have been made to the caudate nucleus or putamen of patients with PD,[40–42] and a large number of studies are underway. In four of the patients the implantations were made stereotaxically either into the caudate nucleus or the putamen, but the patients exhibited only a small and transient improvement in motor function, probably due to poor survival of the grafts.[40,41] In contrast, in two relatively young PD patients, where an open microsurgical technique was used to introduce adrenal medullary tissue into the caudate nucleus, marked beneficial effects were reported. Most surprisingly there has been a progressive improvement in these two patients leading to a near normalization of motor function after grafting. These results appear to contrast both with the time-course and degree of functional recovery observed in animal experiments.[43] The findings in the two young patients remain preliminary and should preferably be verified in older PD patients with a more typical history of the disorder, and with quantified neurological assessment both prior to and after grafting, before making any definite evaluation of the approach. However, the results from the clinical trials with adrenal medullary grafts seem to support the idea that implantation of catecholamine-producing tissue into the basal ganglia could be a valuable therapeutic strategy in PD. From the available animal experiments it seems clear, though, that grafts of fetal DA neurons possess a much greater functional potential than do adrenal medullary grafts (for comparison, see reference 44).

The Swedish Society for Medicine has recently adopted provisional ethical guidelines for the use of fetal tissue from induced abortions in transplantation (c.f. reference 44). According to their guidelines it has been found acceptable from the ethical point of view to use fetal DA neurons from induced abortions in Sweden for the development of a transplantation therapy in patients with severe PD. On this basis we are performng a series of experiments with grafting of human fetal DA neurons to the rat model of PD in order to elucidate some critical issues of direct importance for future clinical trials, for example, optimal donor age, survival, growth, and functional capacity of grafted cells and the necessity for immunosuppression.

## ESTABLISHING OPTIMAL PARAMETERS FOR HUMAN DA-RICH DONOR TISSUE

Animal experiments have shown that the donor DA neurons have to be of fetal age,[8] in order to survive grafting with the dissociated tissue technique. Therefore, we have explored the possibility of using brain cells from aborted human fetuses as donor tissue. Specifically, we have xenografted human fetal DA neurons to the DA denervated striatum of immunosuppressed rats and studied the survival rate of DA neurons of different donor ages, their growth properties and functional capacity and, finally, the immunological constraints. In our initial study we grafted human fetal mesencephalic tissue from donors of ages between 9 and 19 weeks postconception to the 6-OHDA denervated striatum of rats immunosuppressed with cyclosporin A.[45] We have previously observed that mouse DA neurons can be xenografted to rat striatum with a survivability comparable to syngeneic rat grafts if the recipients are chronically treated with cyclosporin A.[46,47] Good graft survival, with up to 1800 DA neurons per host, was obtained in rats receiving grafts from the 9-week-old donor. The grafted human DA neurons exhibited an extensive DA fiber outgrowth throughout the whole host striatum. In addition, they often had long, coarse processes resembling dendrites that also extended into the host striatum. The cell bodies of the grafted human DA neurons were sometimes up to 50-μm along their major axis, which is clearly larger than grafted rat DA neurons. Recently we have tested the importance of immunosuppression for the survival of human fetal DA neurons grafted to the rat model. Nineteen to 20 weeks after grafting we found surviving grafts in all seven recipients that were immunosuppressed with cyclosporin A, whereas no surviving grafts were detected in nonimmunosuppressed rats.[48] These results are consistent with studies of xenografted mouse DA neurons[46,47] and suggest that immunosuppression will probably be necessary in a clinical setting where the donor and recipient inevitably will be genetically dissimilar.

## FUNCTIONAL PROPERTIES OF GRAFTED HUMAN FETAL DA NEURONS

The functional capacity of intrastriatal implants of human fetal DA neurons has been examined in the 6-OHDA denervated rat striatum. Substantial functional effects have only been monitored from grafts prepared from 9-week-old, or younger, donors, which as previously discussed, are the donor ages that have reliably yielded good graft survival. Rats receiving such implants show the first signs of behavioral compensation in the amphetamine-induced rotation test around 12 weeks after grafting[45] (FIG. 5). This reduction in amphetamine-induced rotation asymmetry progressively becomes more pronounced up to 18–20 weeks after grafting, when a large proportion of the

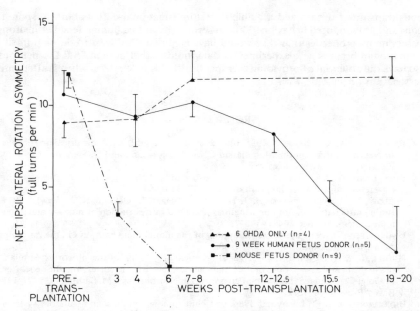

**FIGURE 5.** Time course of the reduction in amphetamine-induced rotation asymmetry in rats with unilateral mesostriatal 6-OHDA lesions after intrastriatal grafting of ventral mesencephalic tissue obtained either from mouse fetuses (dash-dotted line) or an aborted human fetus (9 weeks postconception: solid line). Data from references 45 and 46.

graft recipients show a complete reversal of the circling behavior. The results on amphetamine-induced rotation essentially resemble those obtained when grafting cell suspensions of fetal rat or mouse mesencephalic tissue, with the one exception that the onset of the functional effects of human fetal DA grafts occurs much later (12–15 weeks post grafting) than for grafts of rodent donor tissue, which usually exhibit functional effects on amphetamine-induced rotation 2–4 weeks post-transplantation[8,45,46] (FIG. 5). In a recent study we have also observed a reduction in apomorphine-induced rotation, which is considered to reflect DA receptor supersensitivity in the striatum,[49] in rats receiving DA neurons from an 8-week-old donor,[48] which resembles findings with intracortically placed solid human fetal nigral grafts.[50] Moreover, 18 weeks after grafting we found a significant normalization of spontaneous side bias when the rats were tested overnight in a rotation bowl, suggesting that the grafted human DA neurons are also able to compensate for deficits in spontaneous, non-drug-induced behavior.[48] A similar restoration of spontaneous rotation side bias in rats with unilateral 6-OHDA lesions has been reported to occur also after grafting rat mesencephalic tissue.[51]

Studies on grafted rat DA neurons have shown that they can exhibit spontaneous firing[52] and, with the intracerebral microdialysis technique it has been possible to monitor spontaneous DA release from intrastriatal implants of rat DA neurons.[53,54] Recently we have found, using the same microdialysis technique, that human fetal DA neurons also possess a high degree of spontaneous DA release when grafted to the rat striatum.[48]

In summary, grafted human fetal DA neurons are able to reinnervate the striatum in immunosuppressed rats and seem to retain their intrinsic slow human rate of maturation and development. Moreover, grafted human fetal DA neurons show sponta-

neous transmitter release and are able to restore functional deficits both in spontaneous and drug-induced behaviors. Thus, it seems that grafted human fetal DA neurons
possess many properties that they would have acquired if allowed to develop in situ
in the human brain. These experimental data indicate that human fetal DA neurons
also have the potential of providing therapeutically valuable effects when grafted into
the striatum of patients with PD.

## REFERENCES

1. BJÖRKLUND, A. & U. STENEVI. 1985. Intracerebral neural grafting: A historical perspective.
   *In* Neural Grafting in the Mammalian CNS. A. Björklund and U. Stenevi, Eds.: 3–14.
   Elsevier, Amsterdam/New York.
2. BJÖRKLUND, A. & U. STENEVI. 1979. Reconstruction of the nigrostriatal pathway by intracerebral nigral transplants. Brain Res. **177**: 555–560.
3. PERLOW, M. J., W. J. FREED, B. J. HOFFER, Å. Seiger, L. Olson & R. J. WYATT. 1979.
   Brain grafts reduce motor abnormalities produced by destruction of nigrostriatal dopamine system. Science **204**: 643–647.
4. UNGERSTEDT, U. 1971. Stereotaxic mapping of the monoamine pathways in the rat brain.
   Acta Physiol. Scand. Suppl. **367**: 1–48.
5. HEIMER, L. & R. D. WILSON. 1975. The subcortical projections of the allocortex: Similarities in the neural associations of the hippocampus, the piriform cortex, and the neocortex.
   *In* Golgi Centennial Symposium: Perspectives in Neurobiology. M. Santini, Ed.: 177–193.
   Raven Press, New York.
6. BJÖRKLUND, A. & O. LINDVALL. 1986. Catecholaminergic brain stem regulatory systems.
   *In* Handbook of Physiology: The Nervous System, Vol. 4, Intrinsic Regulatory Systems
   in the Brain. F. E. Bloom, Ed.: 155–235. American Physiological Society. Bethesda, Md.
7. DAHLSTRÖM, A. & K. FUXE. 1964. Evidence for the existence of monoamine neurons in
   the central nervous system. I. Demonstration of monoamines in the cell bodies of brain
   stem neurons. Acta Physiol. Scand. Suppl. **232**: 1–55.
8. BRUNDIN, P. & A. BJÖRKLUND. 1987. Survival, growth and function of dopaminergic neurons
   grafted to the brain. *In* Neural Regeneration. F. J. Seil, E. Herbet, and B. M. Carlson,
   Eds.: Prog. Brain Res. **71**: 293–308. Elsevier, Amsterdam/New York.
9. DUNNETT, S. B., A. BJÖRKLUND, U. STENEVI & S. D. IVERSEN. 1981. Behavioural recovery
   following transplantation of substantia nigra in rats subject to 6-OHDA lesions of the
   nigrostriatal pathway. II. Bilateral lesions. Brain Res. **229**: 457–470.
10. DUNNETT, S. B., A. BJÖRKLUND, R. H. SCHMIDT, U. STENEVI & S. D. IVERSEN. 1983. In-
    tracerebral grafting of neuronal cell suspensions. V. Behavioural recovery in rats with
    bilateral 6-OHDA lesions following implantation of nigral cell suspensions. Acta Physiol.
    Scand. Suppl. **522**: 39–47.
11. GAGE, F. H., S. B. DUNNETT, U. STENEVI & A. BJÖRKLUND. 1983. Aged rats: Recovery
    of motor impairments by intrastriatal nigral grafts. Science **221**: 966–969.
12. BAKAY, R. A. E., M. FIANDACA, D. L. BARROW, A. SCHIFF & D. C. COLLINS. 1985. Prelim-
    inary report on the use of fetal tissue transplantation to correct of MPTP-induced
    Parkinson-like syndrome in primates. Appl. Neurophysiol. **48**: 358–361.
13. SLADEK, JR., J. R., T. J. COLLIER, S. N. HABER, R. H. ROTH & D. E. REDMOND, JR. 1986.
    Survival and growth of fetal catecholamine neurons grafted into primate brain. Brain
    Res. Bull. **1**: 809–818.
14. REDMOND, D. E., J. R. SLADEK, JR., R. H. ROTH, T. J. COLLIER, J. D. ELSWORTH, J. D.
    DEUTCH & S. HABER. 1986. Fetal neuronal grafts in monkeys given methylphenyltetra-
    hydropyridine. Lancet **I**: 1125–1127.
15. MOGENSEN, G. J., D. L. JONES & C. Y. YIM. 1980. From motivation to action: Functional
    interface between the limbic system and the motor system. Prog. Neurobiol. **14**: 69–97.
16. KOOB, G. F., L. STINUS & M. LE MOAL. 1981. Hyperactivity and hypoactivity produced
    by lesions to the mesolimbic dopamine system. Behav. Brain Res. **3**: 341–359.
17. KELLY, P. H. & D. C. S. ROBERTS. 1983. Effects of amphetamine and apomorphine on

locomotor activity after 6-OHDA and electrolytic lesions of the nucleus accumbens septi. Pharmacol. Biochem. Behav. **19:** 137-143.
18. KOOB, G. F. & N. R. SWERDLOW. 1988. The functional output of the mesolimbic dopamine system. This volume.
19. SIMON, H. & M. LE MOAL. Mesencephalic dopaminergic neurons. Role in the general economy of the brain. This volume.
20. PIJNENBURG, A. J. J. & J. M. VAN ROSSUM. 1973. Stimulation of locomotor activity following injection of dopamine into the nucleus accumbens. J. Pharm. Pharmac. **25:** 1003-1005.
21. PIJNENBURG, A. J. J., W. M. M. HONIG & J. M. VAN ROSSUM. 1975. Inhibition of d-amphetamine-induced locomotor activity by injection of haloperidol into the nucleus accumbens of the rat. Psychopharmacolgia (Berlin) **41:** 87-95.
22. TAGHZOUTI, K., H. SIMON, A. LOUILOT, J. P. HERMAN & M. LE MOAL. 1985. Behavioral study after local injection of 6-hydroxydopamine into the nucleus accumbens in the rat. Brain Res. **344:** 9-20.
23. NADAUD, D., J. P. HERMAN, H. SIMON & M. LE MOAL. 1984. Functional recovery following transplantation of ventral mesencephalic cells in rats subjected to 6-OHDA lesions of the mesolimbic dopaminergic neurons. Brain Res. **304:** 137-141.
24. HERMAN, J-P., K. CHOULLI & M. LE MOAL. 1985. Hyper-reactivity to amphetamine in rats with dopaminergic grafts. Exp. Brain Res. **60:** 521-526.
25. HERMAN, J-P., K. CHOULLI, M. GEFFARD, D. NADAUD, K. TAGHZOUTI & M. LE MOAL. 1986. Reinnervation of the nucleus accumbens and frontal cortex of the rat by dopaminergic grafts and effects on hoarding behavior. Brain Res. **372:** 210-216.
26. CHOULLI, K., J. P. HERMAN, J. M. RIVET, H. SIMON & M. LE MOAL. 1987. Spontaneous and graft-induced behavioral recovery after 6-OHDA lesions of the nucleus accumbens in the rat. Brain Res. **407:** 376-380.
27. BRUNDIN, P., R. E. STRECKER, E. LONDOS & A. BJÖRKLUND. 1987. Dopamine neurons grafted unilaterally to the nucleus accumbens affect drug-induced circling and locomotion. Exp. Brain Res. **69:** 183-194.
28. DUNNETT, S. B., S. T. BUNCH, F. H. GAGE & A. BJÖRKLUND. 1984. Dopamine-rich transplants in rats with 6-OHDA lesions of the ventral tegmental area: Effects on spontaneous and drug-induced locomotor activity. Behav. Brain Res. **13:** 71-82.
29. MOORE, K. E. & P. H. KELLY. 1978. Biochemical pharmacology of mesolimbic and mesocortical dopaminergic neurons. *In* Psychopharmacology: A Generation of Progress. M. A. Lipton, A. Di Mascio, and K. F. Killam, Eds.: 221-234. Raven Press, New York.
30. KELLY, P. H. & K. E. MOORE. 1976. Mesolimbic dopaminergic neurones in the rotational model of nigrostriatal function. Nature **263:** 695-696.
31. YAMAMOTO, B. K. & C. FREED. 1982. The trained circling rat: A model for inducing unilateral caudate dopamine metabolism. Nature (London) **298:** 467-468.
32. BRUNDIN, P., F. H. GAGE, S. B. DUNNETT & A. BJÖRKLUND. 1985. Ventral tegmental area dopamine system: Locomotor and cognitive performance following 6-hydroxydopamine-induced damage. Soc. Neurosci. Abstr. 212.4.
33. UNGERSTEDT, U. 1971. Aphagia and adipsia after 6-hydroxy-dopamine induced degeneration of the nigro-striatal dopamine system. Acta Physiol. Scand. Suppl. **367:** 95-1224.
34. DUNNETT, S. B. & A. BJÖRKLUND. 1983. Conditioned turning in rats: Dopaminergic involvement in the initiation of movement rather than the movement itself. Neurosci. Lett. **41:** 173-178.
35. DUNNETT, S. B., I. Q. WHISAW, G. H. JONES & O. ISACSON. 1986. Effects of dopamine-rich grafts on conditioned rotation in rats with unilateral 6-OHDA lesions. Neurosci. Lett. **68:** 127-133.
36. FORNO, L. S. 1982. Pathology of Parkinson's disease. *In* Movement Disorders. C. D. Marsden and S. Fahn, Eds.: 25-40. Butterworths. London.
37. NYBERG, P., A. NORDBERG, P. WESTER & B. WINBLAD. 1983. Dopaminergic deficiency is more pronounced in putamen than in nucleus caudatus in Parkinson's disease. Neurochem. Pathol. **1:** 193-202.
38. SCATTON, B., F. JAVOY-AGID, J. C. MONTFORT & Y. AGID. 1984. Neurochemistry of monoaminergic neurons in Parkinson's disease. *In* Catecholamines Part C: Neurophar-

macology and Central Nervous System – Therapeutic Aspects. E. Usidin, A. Dahlström, and J. Engel, Eds.: 43–52, Alan Liss. New York.

39. JOHNELS, B., P. INGVARSSON, U. RYDGREN, M. THORSELIUS & G. STEG. 1987. Measuring motor function in Parkinson's disease. In Motor Disturbances II. C. D. Marsden, B. Conrad, and R. Benecke, Eds.: 131–144. Academic Press. London.

40. BACKLUND, E.-O., P.-O. GRANBERG, B. HAMBERGER, E. KNUTSSON, A. MÅRTENSSON, G. SEDVALL, Å. SEIGER & L. OLSON. 1985. Transplantation of adrenal medullary tissue to striatum in Parkinsonism. First clinical trials. J. Neurosurg. 62: 169–173.

41. LINDVALL, O., BACKLUND, E.-O., L. FARDE, G. SEDVALL, R. FREEDMAN, B. HOFFER, A. NOBIN, Å. SEIGER & L. OLSON. 1987. Transplantation in Parkinson's disease: Two cases of adrenal medullary grafts to putamen. Ann. Neurol. 22: 457–468.

42. MADRAZO, I., R. DRÜCKER-COLIN, V. DIAZ, J. MARTINEZ-MARTA, C. TORRES & J. J. BECERRIL. 1987. Open microsurgical autograft of adrenal medulla to the right caudate nucleus in Parkinson's disease: A report of two cases. New Eng. J. Med. 326: 831–834.

43. STRÖMBERG, I., M. HERRERA-MARSCHITZ, U. UNGERSTEDT, T. EBENDAL & L. OLSON. 1985. Chronic implants of chromaffin tissue into the dopamine-denervated striatum. Effects of NGF on graft survival, fiber growth and rotational behavior. Exp. Brain Res. 60: 335–349.

44. LINDVALL, O., S. B. DUNNETT, P. BRUNDIN & A. BJÖRKLUND. 1987. Transplantation of catecholamine-producing cells to the basal ganglia in Parkinson's disease: Experimental and clinical studies. In Parkinson's Disease: Clinical and Experimental Advances. C. Rose, Ed: 189–206. John Libbey. London.

45. BRUNDIN, P., O. G. NILSSON, R. E. STRECKER, O. LINDVALL, B. Åstedt & A. BJÖRKLUND. 1986. Behavioural effects of human fetal dopamine neurons grafted in a rat model of Parkinson's disease. Exp. Brain Res. 65: 235–240.

46. BRUNDIN, P., O. G. NILSSON, F. H. GAGE & A. BJÖRKLUND. 1985. Cyclosporin A increases survival of cross-species intrastriatal grafts of embryonic dopamine-containing neurons. Exp. Brain Res. 60: 204–208.

47. BRUNDIN, P., R. E. STRECKER, O. LINDVALL, O. ISACSON, O. G. NILSSON, G. BARBIN, A. PROCHIANTZ, C. FORNI, A. NIEOULLON, H. WIDNER, F. H. GAGE & A. BJÖRKLUND. 1987. Intracerebral grafting of dopamine neurons: Experimental basis for a clinical application in patients with Parkinson's disease. Ann. NY Acad. Sci. 495: 473–496.

48. BRUNDIN, P., R. E. STRECKER, H. WIDNER, D. J. CLARKE, O. G. NILSSON, B. Åstedt, O. Lindvall & A. BJÖRKLUND. 1987. Human fetal dopamine neurons grafted in a rat model of Parkinson's disease: Immunological aspects, spontaneous and drug-induced behaviour and dopamine release. Exp. Brain Res. 70: 192–208.

49. UNGERSTEDT, U. 1971. Post-synaptic supersensitivity after 6-hydroxydopamine induced degeneration of the nigro-striatal dopamine system. Acta Physiol. Scand., Suppl. 367: 49–68.

50. STRÖMBERG, I., M. BYGDEMAN, M. GOLDSTEIN, Å. Seiger & L. OLSON. 1986. Human fetal substantia nigra grafted to the dopamine denervated striatum of immunosuppressed rats: Evidence for functional reinnervation. Neurosci. Lett. 71: 271–276.

51. DUNNETT, S. B., I. Q. WHISAW, D. RODGERS & G. H. JONES. 1987. Dopamine rich grafts ameliorate whole body motor asymmetry and sensory neglect but not independent limb use in rats with 6-hydroxydopamine lesions. Brain Res. 415: 63–87.

52. WUERTHELE, S. M., W. J. FREED, L. OLSON, J. MORIHISA, L. SPOOR, R. J. WYATT & B. J. HOFFER. 1981. Effect of dopamine agonists and antagonists on the electrical activity of substantia nigra neurons transplanted into the lateral ventricle of the rat. Exp. Brain Res. 44: 1–10.

53. ZETTERSTRÖM, T., P. BRUNDIN, F. H. GAGE, T. SHARP, O. ISACSON, S. B. DUNNETT, U. UNGERSTEDT & A. BJÖRKLUND. 1986. In vivo measurement of spontaneous release and metabolism of dopamine from intrastriatal nigral grafts using intracerebral dialysis. Brain Res. 362: 344–349.

54. STRECKER, R. E., T. SHARP, P. BRUNDIN, T. ZETTERSTRÖM, U. UNGERSTEDT & A. BJORKLUND. 1987. Autoregulation of dopamine release and metabolism by intrastriatal nigral grafts as revealed by intracerebral dialysis. Neuroscience. 22: 169–178.

# Neurotoxicity in Dopamine and 5-Hydroxytryptamine Terminal Fields: A Regional Analysis in Nigrostriatal and Mesolimbic Projections

L. S. SEIDEN,[a] D. L. COMMINS, G. VOSMER,

K. AXT, AND G. MAREK

*Department of Pharmacological and Physiological Sciences*
*The University of Chicago*
*947 East 58th Street*
*Chicago, Illinois 60637*

## INTRODUCTION

Methamphetamine (MA), *d-N*-methyl-β-phenylisopropylamine, is a potent indirectly acting amine; it enhances the release of dopamine (DA), norepinephrine (NE), and 5-hydroxytryptamine (5-HT) from synaptosomes. The physiological and behavioral effects of MA have been well characterized. MA effects on the autonomic nervous system include cardiovascular stimulation, bronchodilation, mydriasis, and other effects mediated by alpha and beta noradrenergic receptors.[1] MA effects on the central nervous system include psychomotor stimulation and anorexia, and thus has been widely used to suppress food intake and increase mental alertness and physical endurance. In addition, the central effects of MA and related compounds include hypodipsia, respiratory stimulation, and hyperthermia. MA increases responding on several schedules of reinforcement and can lead to increased aggressive behavior in rats and pigeons.[2,3]

Probably due to its mood-elevation and antifatigue effects, MA is self-administered by humans as well as by a number of animal species in experimental models.[4] Self-administration by these species has led to the definition of MA as a positively reinforcing drug. The positive reinforcing effects of MA have contributed to the high abuse liability of MA and its congeners as evidenced by epidemics of MA abuse that have occurred between 1950 and 1970 in Japan, Great Britain, Sweden, and the United States. It was during this time that undesirable side effects occurring from the continuous use of MA and related amphetamine compounds were recognized. An acute complication is a psychosis that can include paranoid delusions, disordered thought, inappropriate aggressive behavior, and hallucinations.[5] The high abuse liability and undesirable side effects led to an effort to determine whether or not MA and related compounds produced long-lasting effects on the central nervous system.[6-9]

The behavioral effects of the amphetamines are mediated by DA, NE, and 5-HT transmitter systems in the brain.[10-13] Amphetamine (AMPH) and MA have similar mechanisms of action, but AMPH has been studied more than MA. Both compounds

---

[a] To whom correspondence should be addressed.

161

block reuptake and promote release of the monoaminergic transmitters. Furthermore, AMPH releases DA from cytoplasmic rather than granular pools in the DA nerve ending, and the released DA is transported from cytoplasm to extracellular space by a carrier system that is sodium-dependent and calcium-independent. This same carrier-mediated transport is involved in the reuptake of DA.[14,15] Since the psychomotor stimulants have a range of pharmacological effects that are mediated in part by monoamines, neurotoxicological studies began with examining the monamine system.

This paper reviews data collected over the last 10 years indicating that MA and some related drugs including amphetamine exert toxic effects on brain DA and/or 5-HT. We cite evidence that MA-induced depletion of DA and 5-HT is a general phenomenon occurring in several species of animals; we also consider the mechanism by which MA toxicity occurs and how different regions of the brain are differentially affected by MA.

We have specified criteria that would demonstrate neurotoxicity as follows.

- First, the levels of the transmitter must be reduced for two weeks or more after the drug has been discontinued.

- Second, the number of uptake sites must also be reduced without a change in the affinity constant ($K_m$) for uptake. Where nerve cells are actually undergoing degeneration, one would expect that there would be a decrease in the concentration of uptake sites and thus a decrease in $V_{max}$.

- Third, the enzyme that is rate-limiting for the synthesis of the relevant transmitter must be reduced (decreased $V_{max}$).

- Fourth, one must see evidence of morphological changes that would be consistent with degenerating nerve cells.

The morphological evidence is sometimes difficult to obtain; therefore, a presumption of neurotoxicity is made when only the first three criteria are met.

## NEUROTOXICITY OF MA

Early work revealed that AMPH in relatively low doses (those used to achieve an anorectic or a slight stimulant effect) did not produce toxic reactions in monoamine-containing fibers. However, parachloroamphetamine (PCA) at doses that were in the same range as those used to elicit behavioral changes with substituted phenethylamines produced a marked reduction in levels of brain 5-HT and 5-HT metabolites, as well as a decrease in the number of 5-HT reuptake sites.[16-19] It was later concluded by several investigators that the neurochemical deficits produced by PCA were due to nerve terminal degeneration.[11,18,20,21] The possibility that AMPH and related compounds might also be toxic seemed to have been discarded because the dose of AMPH normally used in animal studies did not produce comparable 5-HT deficits. However, reports that administration of higher doses of MA for several days causes a decrease in neostriatal tyrosine hydroxylase activity for as long as a week beyond the period of drug administration suggested that MA may be toxic to DA fibers.[22,23] We observed that rhesus monkeys given MA in large doses (3.5–6 mg/kg/every 3 hours, administered iv with the total daily dose between 28 and 48 mg/kg/day for 90–180 days) showed a profound depletion of DA in the striatum when sacrificed 3–6 months after the last injection.[24] Such long-lasting DA depletions (3–6 months) strongly suggest that the changes in DA levels were permanent. In subsequent work, it was discovered that it was unnecessary to administer MA for as long as 3–6 months in order to produce the DA depletions. A period of two weeks of MA administration was sufficient to cause the reduction in DA when measured two weeks after the last injection.[24]

Since MA is metabolized differently between species, it was important to determine whether MA toxicity generalized across species. In particular, the metabolism of MA in rhesus monkeys differs from that in humans, and administration of MA might have different consequences if a metabolite of MA was involved in the toxicity. The MA-induced neurotoxicity to DA and 5-HT fibers was demonstrated in rats, mice and cats.[25-29] In addition, guinea pigs, which metabolize MA in the same way as humans, also showed MA-induced neurotoxicity.[30] The fact that MA can induce toxicity in dopaminergic and serotonergic neurons in five species suggests that this drug may have similar effects in humans. It is important to note that doses observed to induce neurotoxicity are 25- to 100-fold higher than doses generally used to produce physiological or behavioral effects. Therefore, one would not expect to see neurotoxic effects at doses used to achieve anorexia or reduce fatigue (10–50 mg/day). However, an AMPH or MA abuser may use up to 1 or 2 grams over a 24- to 48-hour period. These doses would be comparable to the doses that engendered neurotoxic effects in the animal studies.

We have found that the number of reuptake sites for DA ($V_{max}$) was reduced by 50% by MA treatment. In these experiments MA was given to rats eight times over a period of four days at a dose of 50 mg/kg injection. Two weeks later the rats were sacrificed and synaptosomal membranes from striatum were prepared in a sucrose medium. The synaptosomes were incubated in a buffered medium with varying concentrations of $^3$H-DA.[31] Appropriate $K_m$ values of $12 \times 10^{-8}$ M were found in both control and MA-treated animals. In contrast, the $V_{max}$ (expressed as $^3$HDPM $^3$HDA/mg protein) was $7.9 \times 10^3$ for control animals and $5.4 \times 10^3$ for MA-treated animals, indicating a loss of DA uptake sites. The reduction in the number of reuptake sites is consistent with the notion that MA may cause the death of nerve terminals. AMPH also reduces the number of uptake sites for DA. Compounds that are structurally similar to MA, such as methylenedioxyamphetamine (MDA),[32] methylenedioxymethylamphetamine (MDMA),[33] and fenfluramine, cause long-term reduction in 5-HT and in the number of 5-HT uptake sites.[11,34] In contrast, when we examined DA binding sites using $^3$H-spiroperidol, no differences in the affinity or the number of binding sites were found.[25]

Biochemical evidence suggests that striatal nerve terminals degenerate in rats after MA administration, but confirmation of this hypothesis requires one to observe neurotoxicity on a morphological basis. The altered chemistry of the brain could be explained on a pharmacokinetic basis by postulating down-regulation of rate-limiting enzymes and reuptake sites. Lesion experiments demonstrate that the postoperative period during which optimal silver impregnation of degenerating structures can be obtained with the Fink–Heimer method[35] depends on the neural system under study and is transient. Although the neurochemical deficits produced by MA are long-lasting, MA-induced degeneration is detected by the Fink–Heimer method for only a limited time, shortly after drug administration. To maximize our ability to see degeneration with the Fink–Heimer method, a single, very high dose of MA was used rather than lower, repeated doses, and the subjects were sacrificed two days after drug treatment. We found that a single injection of 100 mg/kg caused a 50% depletion of DA and of DA reuptake sites when measured two weeks later. Rats that were sacrificed 48 hours after this same drug treatment showed silver impregnation of degenerating terminals in the striatum.[36-38] The results clearly show that degeneration occurs in the striatum, but does not prove that the fibers are dopaminergic, although this would be consistent with biochemical measures suggesting that MA is toxic to DA nerve terminals.[38–42]

In addition, degenerating neurons were observed in layers III–IV of the somatosensory cortex.[36] This observation concerning the somatosensory cortex may be related to the fact that chronic MA users often have somatosensory abnormalities that result in lesions to the skin from excessive scratching or picking. It is also of interest that the degeneration of cortical cells may be secondary to the degeneration of 5-HT terminals localized in the same layer of the somatosensory cortex. We have also seen degenerating terminals in the hippocampus and degenerating neuronal perikarya in somatosensory cortex following administration of MDA[32] and MDMA,[33] respectively.

## PROPOSED MECHANISM BY WHICH MA IS NEUROTOXIC

We have hypothesized that MA exerts its toxic effects on DA and 5-HT neurons by causing conversion of DA to 6-hydroxydopamine (6-OHDA) and 5-HT to 5,6-dihydroxytryptamine (5,6-DHT), compounds that are known to be neurotoxic to the DA and 5-HT systems, respectively. This hypothesis is based upon the following convergent findings. We have observed that α-methyl-$p$-tyrosine (AMT), a competitive inhibitor of tyrosine hydroxylase, the rate-limiting enzyme for DA synthesis, can block the neurotoxic effects of MA.[43] Reserpine, on the other hand, potentiates the effects of MA.[43] It has been suggested that MA preferentially releases DA from cytoplasmic binding sites by reversing the direction of the high-affinity transport system, as demonstrated by Raiteri et al.[14] and Liang and Rutledge.[15] Reserpine enhancement and AMT-induced blockade support the theory that MA-induced toxicity is dependent upon cytoplasmically stored DA. Therefore, it is reasonable to hypothesize that the massive release of DA from the cytoplasmic pool induced by MA may in some way be neurotoxic.

In 1959, Senoh and Witkop[44] and Senoh et al.[45] showed that DA could be nonenzymatically converted to trihydroxyphenethylamines such as 2,4,5-trihydroxyphenethylamine (6-hydroxydopamine, 6-OHDA). If DA is released by MA and MA also blocks both DA reuptake and monoamine oxidase[46] the amount of unbound DA present following MA administration would be large and a significant amount of oxidative products might be formed. To test this hypothesis, male rats were injected with 100 mg/kg of MA and sacrificed after a time interval of either 20 or 30 minutes, 1, 2, 4, 8, or 16 hours. We found that 6-OHDA was formed in the striatum between 30 minutes and 2 hours.[47] The amount of 6-OHDA detected was approximately 5% of normal DA levels. We infused into the ventricles of a rat a dose of 6-OHDA that produces depletions of DA comparable to those produced by 100 mg/kg of MA and found that the levels of 6-OHDA in striatum one-half to 2 hours after infusion were at least roughly comparable to the levels of 6-OHDA formed after MA administration. In a similar experiment, we administered the same 100 mg/kg dose of MA and were able to detect 5,6-DHT in the hippocampus.[48] Since 6-OHDA and 5,6-DHT are neurotoxic to the DA and 5-HT systems, respectively, we reasoned that the formation of these toxins after MA may be responsible for effects of MA on the DA and 5-HT systems. These experiments are difficult to perform because the levels of toxin found are low and their formation is not detectable in every MA-treated rat. Our current research involves trying to determine the causes of this variability to see if it is a matter of differences in the postinjection sacrifice time, in the sensitivity of our assay, or known differences in the sensitivities of different rats to the DA and 5-HT depleting effects of MA. This situation needs to be clarified before our hypothesis that 6-OHDA and 5,6-DHT mediate the neurotoxic effects of MA becomes firm. There are alternative hypotheses that may account for the neurotoxicity. For example, the 5,6-DHT and 6-OHDA formed may be markers for the MA-induced formation of hydroxy radicals that are also toxic to nerve cells, but are nonspecific, unlike 6-OHDA and 5,6-DHT. However, if this were the case, it would not explain why MA effects are so specific to DA and 5-HT cells.

## COMPARISON OF NEUROTOXICITY IN NIGROSTRIATAL AND MESOLIMBIC REGIONS OF THE BRAIN

In summary, the data presented so far indicate that MA causes degeneration in DA- and 5-HT-containing neurons. We have proposed that the administration of MA causes the release of DA or 5-HT from cytoplasmically bound storage pools and that the DA or 5-HT is oxidized to form 6-OHDA or 5,6-DHT, respectively, which then act as neurotoxins. In view of the fact that in the early studies DA and 5-HT were examined in only a few regions of the brain, it was of interest to determine if indeed there was uniform neural toxicity across different brain regions. Therefore, we decided to examine areas of the brain that received their primary dopaminergic innervation from the substantia nigra as opposed to areas that received their primary dopaminergic innervation from the DA mesencephalic cell body cluster in the ventral tegmental area (VTA).

The aim of the following study was to determine the relative depletion of DA and 5-HT in the nigro-striatal terminal fields and to compare them with depletions of DA and/or 5-HT in the mesolimbic terminal fields. The corpus striatum was taken as the tissue receiving a DA projection primarily from the substantia nigra; the nucleus accumbens, septum, amygdala, frontal cortex, and olfactory tubercle were taken as tissues representing primarily mesocortical terminal fields. The rats in this study were injected either with a single dose of MA (50 or 100 mg/kg) or eight injections of 50 mg/kg, injected 12 hours apart for four days. Our results indicate that the DA and 5-HT depletions induced by MA in the various terminal fields did not depend on whether the terminal field had its origin in the substantia nigra or VTA.

The DA depletions observed in the mesolimbic terminal fields following MA administration were comparable in some cases to the DA depletions in nigro-striatal terminal fields. Striatal DA was depleted between 50 and 70%, but there was not a systematic difference based on the dosing regimen (FIG. 1). MA-induced depletions in mesolimbic terminal fields varied. Neither the olfactory tubercle or the septum showed any depletion of DA (FIG. 2). The frontal cortex showed a relatively small depletion at the 100-mg/kg single dose and a larger depletion with the 8- × 50-mg/kg dosing regimen (FIG. 2). The amygdala, frontal cortex, and the nucleus accumbens were depleted of DA by the same amount as the striatum (see FIGS. 1 and 2). Thus, some of the mesolimbic structures are depleted to the same extent as the striatum while others are not. DA was not depleted in the hypothalamus, a brain region where the source of DA is largely intrinsic (FIG. 2). Similarly, DA in the brain stem was unaffected by any of the doses of MA (FIG. 1).

In contrast to the regionally specific depletion of DA produced by MA, 5-HT was depleted in all brain regions examined, although not always to the same extent. Depletion of 5-HT in the striatum was observed for all of the dosing procedures. (FIG. 3). Both the olfactory tubercle and the septum were depleted of 5-HT (FIG. 4), but not of DA (FIG. 2). The olfactory tubercle and septum had lower levels of 5-HT after the multiple-injection regimen of MA than after the single-dose regimen. The frontal cortex, the amygdala, and hypothalamus showed depletions of both DA and 5-HT, but the 5-HT depletions were larger in each of these regions. Brain stem 5-HT (FIG. 3), but

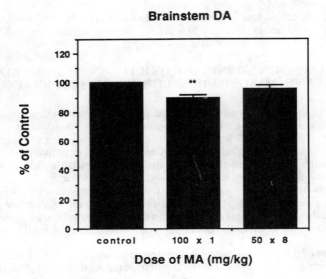

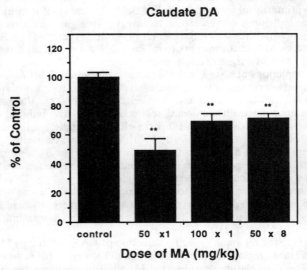

**FIGURE 1.** Levels of DA expressed as percentage of control, in brain stem and caudate nucleus, 2 weeks after various doses of MA administered subcutaneously. Control levels, expressed as ng DA/mg tissue, were brain stem: $0.094 \pm 0.002$ and caudate nucleus: $9.52 \pm 0.35$. All n's were at least 7, $**p < 0.01$.

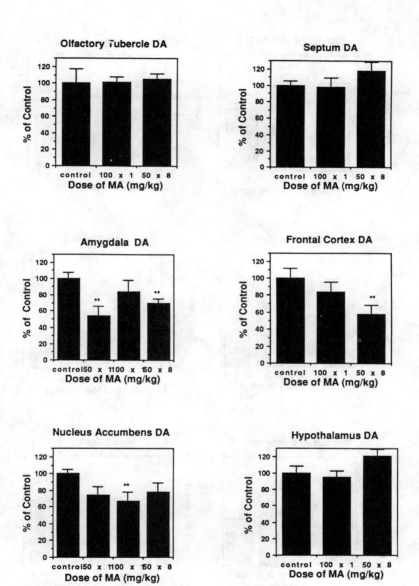

**FIGURE 2.** Levels of DA expressed as percentage of control, in olfactory tubercle (OT), septum (S), amygdala (A), frontal cortex (FC), nucleus accumbens (NA), and hypothalamus (H) 2 weeks after various doses of MA administered subcutaneously. Control levels, expressed as ng DA/mg tissue, were OT: $4.69 \pm 0.16$; S: $0.567 \pm 0.031$; A: $0.307 \pm 0.022$; FC: $0.107 \pm 0.012$; NA: $6.52 \pm 0.35$; H: $0.240 \pm 0.018$. All n's were at least 7, $**p < 0.01$.

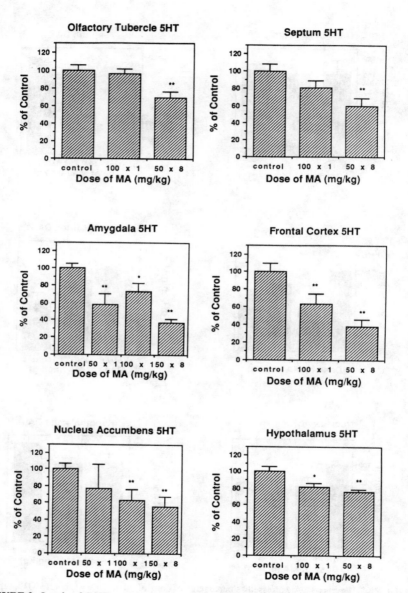

**FIGURE 3.** Levels of 5-HT expressed as percentage of control, in brain stem (B), caudate nucleus (C), and hippocampus (HI) 2 weeks after various doses of MA administered subcutaneously. Control levels, expressed as ng 5-HT/mg tissue, were B: 0.484 ± 0.22; C: 0.357 ± 0.036; HI: 0.258 ± 0.012. All n's were at least 7, *$p < 0.05$, ** $p < 0.01$.

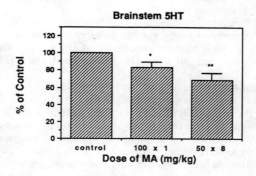

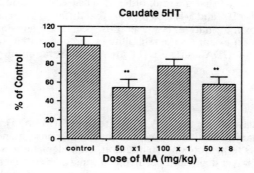

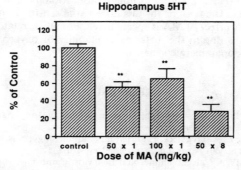

**FIGURE 4.** Levels of 5-HT expressed as percentage of control, in olfactory tubercle (OT), septum (S), amygdala (A), frontal cortex (FC), nucleus accumbens (NA), and hypothalamus (H) 2 weeks after various doses of MA administered subcutaneously. Control levels, expressed as ng 5-HT/mg tissue, were OT: 0.758 ± 0.048; S: 0.443 ± 0.037; A: 0.419 ± 0.022; FC: 0.220 ± 0.010; NA: 0.627 ± 0.042; H: 0.564 ± 0.032. All n's were at least 7, $*p < 0.05$, $** p < 0.01$.

not DA (FIG. 1), was depleted by MA administration. In addition, 5-HT was severely depleted in the hippocampus (FIG. 3).

Overall, 5-HT terminal fields seemed more susceptible to the neurotoxic effects of MA than the DA terminal fields. For the different brain regions examined, depletions of DA and 5-HT were proportional, that is, if DA was not depleted, 5-HT was depleted by a small amount, but when DA was depleted, the 5-HT depletions were greater.

The mechanisms that would account for DA or 5-HT depletions in various brain structures may be related to the mechanism we have proposed for MA-induced neurotoxicity, that is, the conversion of neurotransmitters to neurotoxins after the release of the transmitter by MA. Using this framework as an explanation, and assuming equal distribution of MA throughout the brain, one would have to assume that 5-HT is more readily converted to 5,6-DHT than DA is converted to 6-OHDA. In addition, some brain areas must form the toxins more readily than others, perhaps because of an increase in the availability of superoxides, or a decrease in endogenous compounds that detoxify the superoxides such as cysteine or ascorbic acid. The data that support this speculation are the fact that the rank order of sensitivity to toxic effects in different areas is the same for DA and 5-HT, suggesting that different brain areas have differing capabilities for toxin formation. However, this speculation remains to be tested, and it depends to a great extent on the reliability of the observation that DA and 5-HT are converted to 6-OHDA and 5,6-DHT after administration of MA.

## SUMMARY

In summary, we have shown that MA is toxic to both 5-HT and DA cells and we have proposed a mechanism that would account for this response, namely, the conversion of the transmitters to neurotoxins. In addition, brain depletions of DA seem regionally specific with larger depletions occurring in some areas than in others. The depletions, however, do not seem to depend entirely on the nuclei of origin, that is, substantia nigra versus VTA. 5-HT was depleted by different amounts in the various regions examined and the 5-HT depletions, although proportional to the DA depletions, were consistently greater. The reasons for this differential sensitivity of the 5-HT and DA systems to the toxic effect of MA is speculative, but may be related to the differential formation of toxins due to the differing availability of oxygen and superoxides at serotonergic and dopaminergic synapses.

### REFERENCES

1. LEWANDER, T. 1977. Effects of amphetamine in animals. *In* Drug Addiction II. W. R. Martin, Ed.: 18–33. Springer-Verlag. New York.
2. SEIDEN, L. S. & L. A. DYKSTRA. 1977. Psychopharmacology: A Behavioral and Biochemical Approach. Van Nostrand–Reinhold. New York.
3. MASON, S. T. 1984. Catecholamines and Behavior. Cambridge Univ. Press. Cambridge, England.
4. SCHUSTER, C. R. 1981. The behavioral pharmacology of psychomotor stimulant drugs. *In* Handbook of Experimental Pharmacology. F. Hoffmeister and G. Stille, Eds.: 587–605. Springer-Verlag. Berlin/Heidelberg.
5. ELLINWOOD, E. H. 1969. Amphetamine psychosis: A multidimensional process. Semin. Psychiatry 1: 208–226.
6. BUENING, M. K. & J. W. GIBB. 1974. Influence of methamphetamine and neuroleptic drugs on tyrosine hydroxylase activity. Eur. J. Pharmacol. 26: 30–34.

7. JONSSON, L. & L. GUNNE. 1970. Clinical studies of amphetamine psychosis. *In* Int. Symp. on Amphetamines and Related Compounds. E. Costa and S. Garattini, Eds.: 929–936. Raven Press. New York.

8. KILOH, L. A. & S. BRANDON. 1962. Habituation and addiction to amphetamines. Br. Med. J. **2:** 40–43.

9. KOGAN, J. F., W. K. NICHOLS & J. W. GIBB. 1976. Influence of methamphetamine on nigral and striatal tyrosine hydroxylase activity and on striatal dopamine levels. Eur. J. Pharmacol. **36:** 363–371.

10. MOORE, K. E., L. A. CARR & J. A. DOMINIC. 1970. Functional significance of amphetamine-induced release of brain catecholamines. *In* Amphetamines and Related Compounds: Proc. Mario Negri Institute for Pharmacological Research. E. Costa and S. Garattini, Eds.: 371–384. Raven Press. New York.

11. HARVEY, J. A. 1978. Neurotoxic action of halogenated amphetamines. Ann. N.Y. Acad. Sci. **305:** 289–305.

12. MABRY, P. D. & B. A. CAMPBELL. 1973. Serotonergic inhibition of catecholamine-induced behavioral arousal. Brain Res. **49:** 381–391.

13. CREESE, I. & S. IVERSEN. 1975. Behavioral sequelae of dopaminergic degeneration: Postsynaptic supersensitivity in pre- and postsynaptic receptors. *In* Proc. 13th Annual Meeting of the College of Neuropsychopharmacology. E. Usdin and W. Bunney, Eds.: 171–177.

14. RAITERI, M., F. CERITO, A. M. CERVONI & G. LEVI. 1979. Dopamine can be released by two mechanisms differentially affected by the dopamine transport inhibitor nomifensine. J. Pharmacol. Exp. Ther. **208:** 195–202.

15. LIANG, N. Y. & C. O. RUTLEDGE. 1982. Evidence for carrier-mediated efflux of dopamine from corpus striatum. Biochem. Pharmacol. **30:** 2479–2484.

16. FULLER, R. W. & J. C. BAKER. 1974. Long-lasting reduction of brain 5-hydroxytryptamine concentration by 3-chloroamphetamine and 4-chloroamphetamine in iprindole-treated rats. J. Pharmacol. Exp. **26:** 912–914.

17. FULLER, R. W. & K. W. PERRY. 1974. Long-lasting depletion of brain serotonin by 4-chloroamphetamine in guinea pigs. Brain Res. **82:** 383–385.

18. SANDERS-BUSH, E., J. A. BUSHING & F. SULSER. 1972. Long-term effects of p-chloroamphetamine on tryptophan hydroxylase activity and on the levels of 5-hydroxytryptamine and 5-hydroxyindole acetic acid in brain. Eur. J. Pharmacol. **20:** 385–388.

19. SANDERS-BUSH, E., J. A. BUSHING & F. SULSER. 1975. Long-term effects of p-chloroamphetamine and related drugs on central serotonergic mechanisms. J. Pharmacol. Exp. Ther. **192:** 33–41.

20. FULLER, R. W. 1978. Neurochemical effects of serotonin neurotoxins: An introduction. Ann. N.Y. Acad. Sci. **305:** 178–201.

21. SANDERS-BUSH, E. & L. R. STERANKA. 1978. Immediate and long-term effects of p-chloroamphetamine on brain amines. Ann. N.Y. Acad. Sci. **305:** 208–221.

22. KODA, L. Y. & J. W. GIBB. 1973. Adrenal and striatal tyrosine hydroxylase activity after methamphetamine. J. Pharmacol. Exp. Ther. **185:** 42–48.

23. COE, B. K. & A. WEISSMAN. 1966. p-Chlorophenylalanine: A specific depletor of brain serotonin. J. Pharmacol. Exp. Ther. **154:** 499–516.

24. SEIDEN, L. S., M. W. FISCHMAN & C. R. SCHUSTER. 1975/76. Long-term methamphetamine changes in brain catecholamines in tolerant rhesus monkeys. Drug Alcohol Depend. **1:** 215–219.

25. RICAURTE, G. A., C. R. SCHUSTER & L. S. SEIDEN. 1980. Long-lasting effects of repeated methamphetamine administration on dopamine and serotinin neurons in the rat brain: A regional study. Brain Res. **193:** 153–160.

26. WAGNER, G. C., G. A. RICAURTE, L. S. SEIDEN, C. R. SCHUSTER, R. J. MILLER & J. WESTLEY. 1980. Long-lasting depletions of striatal dopamine and loss of dopamine uptake sites following repeated administration of methamphetamine. Brain Res. **181:** 151–160.

27. WAGNER, G. C., C. R. SCHUSTER & L. S. SEIDEN. 1981. Neurochemical consequences following administration of CNS stimulants to the neonatal rat. Pharmacol. Biochem. Behav. **14:** 117–119.

28. LEVINE, M. S., C. D. HULL, E. GARCIA-RILL, L. ERINOFF, N. A. BUCHWALD & A. HELLER. 1980. Long-term decreases in spontaneous firing of caudate neurons induced by amphetamine in cats. Brain Res. **194:** 263–268.

29. SEIDEN, L. S. & G. A. RICAURTE. 1987. Neurotoxicity of methamphetamine and related drugs. *In* Psychopharmacology: A Third Generation of Progress. H. Y. Meltzer, Ed.: 359–366. Raven Press. New York.

30. WAGNER, G. C., C. R. SCHUSTER & L. S. SEIDEN. 1979. Methamphetamine induced changes in brain catecholamines in rats and guinea pigs. Drug Alcohol Depend. **4:** 435–438.

31. SNYDER, S. H. & J. T. COYLE. 1968. Regional differences in 3H-norepinephrine and 3H-dopamine uptake in rat brain homogenates. J. Pharmacol. Exp. Ther. **165:** 78–86.

32. RICAURTE, G. A., L. S. SEIDEN & C. R. SCHUSTER. 1985. Hallucinogenic amphetamine selectively destroys brain serotonin nerve terminals: Neurochemical and anatomical evidence. Science **229:** 986–988.

33. COMMINS, D. L., G. VOSMER, R. VIRUS, W. WOOLVERTON, C. R. SCHUSTER & L. S. SEIDEN. 1987. Biochemical and histological evidence that methylenedioxymethylamphetamine (MDMA) is toxic to neurons in the rat brain. J. Pharmacol. Exp. Ther. **241:** 338–345.

34. SCHUSTER, C. R., M. LEWIS & L. S. SEIDEN. 1986. Fenfluramine neurotoxicity. Psychopharm. Bull. **22:** 148–151.

35. HEIMER, L. 1978. Selective silver-impregnation of degenerating axoplasm. *In* Contemporary Research Methods in Neuroanatomy. W. J. H. Nauta and S. O. E. Ebbesson, Eds.: 106–131. Springer-Verlag. New York.

36. COMMINS, D. L. & L. S. SEIDEN. 1986. Alpha methyl para tyrosine blocks methamphetamine-induced degeneration in the rat somatosensory cortex. Brain Res. **365:** 15–20.

37. RICAURTE, G. A., R. W. GUILLERY, L. S. SEIDEN & C. R. SCHUSTER. 1982. Dopamine nerve terminal degeneration produced by high doses of methylamphetamine in the rat brain. Brain Res. **235:** 93–103.

38. RICAURTE, G. A., R. W. GUILLERY, L. S. SEIDEN & C. R. SCHUSTER. 1984. Nerve terminal degeneration after a single injection of d-amphetamine in iprindole treated rats: Relation to selective long-lasting dopamine depletion. Brain Res. **291:** 378–382.

39. MAREK, G. & L. S. SEIDEN. 1985. Dopamine uptake inhibitors and methamphetamine neurotoxicity. Soc. Neurosci. Abstr. **11:** 1194.

40. SCHMIDT, C. J. & J. W. GIBB. 1985. Role of the dopamine uptake carrier in the neurochemical response to methamphetamine: Effects of amfonelic acid. Eur. J. Pharmacol. **109:** 73–80.

41. FULLER, R. W. & S. HEMRICK-LUECKE. 1980. Long-lasting depletion of striatal dopamine by a single injection of amphetamine in iprindole-treated rats. Science **209:** 305–307.

42. STERANKA, L. R. 1982. Long-term decreases in striatal dopamine, 3,4-dihydroxyphenylacetic acid and homovanillic acid after a single injection of amphetamine in iprindole-treated rats: Time course and time-dependent interactions with amfonelic acid. Brain Res. **234:** 123–136.

43. WAGNER, G. C., J. B. LUCOT, C. R. SCHUSTER & L. S. SEIDEN. 1983. Alpha methyltyrosine attenuates and reserpine increases methamphetamine-induced neuronal changes. Brain Res. **270:** 285–288.

44. SENOH, S. & B. WITKOP. 1959. Non-enzymatic conversions of dopamine to norepinephrine and trihydroxyphenylethyl amines. J. Am. Chem. Soc. **81:** 6222–6235.

45. SENOH, S., B. WITKOP, C. CREVELING & S. UDENFRIEND. 1959. Chemical, enzymatic and metabolic studies on the mechanism of oxidation of dopamine. J. Am. Chem. Soc. **81:** 1768–1771.

46. SUZUKI, O., H. HATTORI, M. ASANO, M. OYA & Y. KATSUMATA. 1980. Inhibition of monoamine oxidase by d-methamphetamine. Biochem. Pharmacol. **29:** 2071–2073.

47. SEIDEN, L. S. & G. VOSMER. 1984. Formation of 6-hydroxydopamine in caudate nucleus of rat brain after a single large dose of methamphetamine. Pharmacol. Biochem. Behav. **21:** 29–31.

48. COMMINS, D. L., K. A. AXT & L. S. SEIDEN. 1987. 5,6-Dihydroxytryptamine, a serotonergic neurotoxin is formed endogenously in the rat brain. Brain Res. **403:** 7–14.

# The Biochemistry and Pharmacology of Mesoamygdaloid Dopamine Neurons[a]

CLINTON D. KILTS,[b,c] CARL M. ANDERSON,[b]
TIMOTHY D. ELY,[b] AND RICHARD B. MAILMAN[d]

*Departments of Psychiatry[b] and Pharmacology[c]*
*Duke University Medical Center*
*Durham, North Carolina 27710*

[d] *Departments of Psychiatry and Pharmacology*
*Biological Sciences Research Center*
*University of North Carolina*
*Chapel Hill, North Carolina 27514*

## INTRODUCTION

The amygdala is a phylogenetically old brain structure central to every definition of the anatomical and functional organization of the limbic system. The amygdala is critically involved in a diverse array of complex functions, including emotion, memory, the perception of and appropriate reaction to stimuli, regulation of neuroendocrine secretion, and the autonomic nervous system, as well as other functions subserving the preservation of self and species. [1-5] The amygdala is not a homogenous structure, but is rather an assembly of heterogenous nuclear groups differing in their cytoarchitecture,[6] biochemistry[7,8] function,[9] and afferent and efferent neuronal projections.[10,11] We now list the considerable evidence that has accumulated in support of a neurotransmitter or neuromodulator role for dopamine (DA) in the amygdala:

- Demonstrated DA innervation from cell bodies located in the ventral mesencephalon.[51,13]

- DA is well represented and unevenly distributed in the amygdaloid complex.[7,15]

- DA produces a neuroleptic-reversible inhibition of spontaneously firing and glutamate-activated cells in the amygdala.[52]

- Presence of a responsive mechanism for neuronal DA release.[53]

- Presence of presynaptic sites for DA uptake.[54,55]

- Presence of enzymatic machinery for DA synthesis and catabolism.[56,57]

- Presence of DA receptors defined by binding sites labeled by radioactive DA ligands.[32,58]

- Presence of a *d*opamine- and cyclic *A*MP-*r*egulated *p*hosphoprotein (32,000 MW; DARPP-32), a postulated intracellular transducer of DA receptor (D$_1$ subtype) occupancy.[59]

[a] This work was supported by National Institute of Mental Health Grant MH-39967.

173

Despite anatomical and neurophysiological evidence and the presence of biochemical and molecular markers of DA synapses, little is known concerning the role of DA neurotransmission in modulating the functional output of the amygdaloid complex. This discussion will focus on the mechanisms of regulation and signal transduction and the physiology and pharmacology of mesoamygdaloid DA neurons at a level of anatomical resolution (i.e., discrete component nuclei) commensurate with the functional organization of the amygdaloid complex. Based upon these endpoints, the collective findings of these studies support (1) the distinction of mesoamygdaloid DA neurons from other mesotelencephalic DA systems, (2) the delineation of mesoamygdaloid DA neurons into distinct populations innervating discrete nuclei, and (3) the parceling of DA function in the limbic system into many more neuronal systems or subsystems than previously proposed based upon anatomical comparisons.

## THE DISTRIBUTION AND DYNAMICS OF DA IN THE AMYGDALOID COMPLEX

Histofluorescent mapping of DA in the amygdaloid complex indicated a nonuniform density of DA innervation of component nuclear groups.[12,13] The results of the combined application of micropunch dissection and either radioenzymatic[7,14] or high-performance liquid-chromatography–electrochemical detection[15] assays corroborate the heterogeneous distribution of DA in the amygdala; a striking 75-fold gradient in DA concentration exists between adjacent amygdaloid nuclei (TABLE 1). Dopamine is particularly well represented in the central and lateral amygdaloid nuclei where concentrations are one-third that of the DA-rich projections in the olfactory tubercle and nucleus accumbens. Relative to DA, concentrations of norepinephrine are more evenly distributed across the amygdaloid nuclei examined.[15]

The uneven distribution of DA among the amygdaloid nuclei typifies their biochemical heterogeneity and suggests that the functional significance of DA neurotransmission in the amygdala would vary between its component nuclei. However, concentration is but one factor in estimating the functional significance of a neurotransmitter in a given brain region. An important functional variable is the rate at which neurons utilize or renovate their neurotransmitter content as a function of impulse-coupled release and metabolism. This rate of turnover in populations of mesoamygdaloid DA neurons was estimated by calculating the rate of depletion of the DA content of discrete amygdaloid nuclei following the administration of the tyrosine hydroxylase inhibitor α-methyltyrosine (α-MT).[16] The rates of α-MT-induced depletion, expressed as rate constants ($k$, $h^{-1}$), of DA and the estimated rate of DA synthesis in amygdaloid and other brain nuclei or areas (for purposes of comparison) are summarized in TABLE 1. A comparison of the rate constants for the decline of DA indicated a wide-ranging gradient of estimated activity of populations of mesoamygdaloid DA neurons, with the slowest rate of turnover observed in the central and medially aligned amygdaloid nuclei. The low rate of impulse activity of DA neurons projecting to the central nucleus relative to other amygdaloid nuclei, as inferred from their turnover rates, is reinforced by the observation that the ratio of the concentration of homovanillic acid (HVA) to that of DA, and index of impulse-coupled DA release, in this nucleus is lower than that of any other amygdaloid nucleus (TABLE 1). The rate constant for DA decline in the lateral amygdaloid nucleus was similar to that of the medial prefrontal cortex and other mesocortical projection fields of DA neurons with a high estimated activity. In general, the estimated activity of mesoamygdaloid DA neurons exceeded that of DA projections to the caudate nucleus, nucleus accumbens, olfactory tubercle, and me-

**TABLE 1.** Distribution, Turnover Rate, and Metabolism of Dopamine in Discrete Brain Nuclei

| Brain Nuclei | Dopamine | | | HVA Concentration | HVA/DA |
| --- | --- | --- | --- | --- | --- |
| | Concentration | Rate Constant ($k$) (1/h)[a] | Synthesis Rate[b] | | |
| Amygdaloid | | | | | |
| Central | 23.9 ± 1.5 | −0.399 ± 0.059 | 9.5 | 0.79 ± 0.07 | 0.033 |
| Lateral | 14.5 ± 2.3 | −1.029 ± 0.247 | 14.9 | 1.2 ± 0.09 | 0.083 |
| Basal | 3.5 ± 0.21 | −0.771 ± 0.076 | 2.7 | 0.44 ± 0.04 | 0.13 |
| Medial | 0.26 ± 0.03 | −0.506 ± 0.092 | 0.13 | 0.11 ± 0.01 | 0.42 |
| Cortical | 1.3 ± 0.14 | −0.899 ± 0.093 | 1.15 | 0.57 ± 0.06 | 0.44 |
| Intercalated cell group | | | | | |
| anterior | 15.9 ± 2.4 | — | — | 2.0 ± 0.12 | 0.13 |
| posterior | 2.2 ± 0.25 | — | — | 0.30 ± 0.04 | 0.14 |
| Posterior | 0.53 ± 0.06 | −0.673 ± 0.099 | 0.36 | 0.24 ± 0.04 | 0.45 |
| Medial posterior | 0.39 ± 0.03 | −0.443 ± 0.092 | 0.17 | 0.15 ± 0.03 | 0.38 |
| Basal posterior | 2.1 ± 0.22 | −0.804 ± 0.110 | 1.66 | 0.25 ± 0.02 | 0.12 |
| Anterior | | | | | |
| amygdaloid area | 1.6 ± 0.26 | — | — | 1.5 ± 0.08 | 0.94 |
| Medial prefrontal cortex | 0.36 ± 0.04 | −1.221 ± 0.120 | 0.44 | 0.36 ± 0.03 | 1.0 |
| Olfactory tubercle | 47.6 ± 3.1 | −0.290 ± 0.058 | 13.8 | 4.5 ± 0.32 | 0.095 |
| Caudate nucleus | 89.6 ± 7.9 | −0.382 ± 0.059 | 33.8 | 7.9 ± 0.34 | 0.09 |

NOTE: Groups of rats were sacrificed 0, 30, 60, or 90 min following α-MT (250 mg/kg, ip). Dopamine and HVA concentrations are ng/mg protein.
[a] $k$ ($x$ ± S.E.E.) was calculated by computing a least squares regression analysis of the common logarithm of the dopamine concentration against time following α-MT.
[b] Synthesis rate (ng/mg protein/hr) was calculated by multiplying $k$ by the endogenous (time 0) dopamine concentration.

dian eminence. The varying estimated activity of populations of DA neurons inner-vating discrete amygdaloid nuclei suggests the differential involvement of autoregula-tory or transsynaptic regulatory mechanisms in controlling their basal activity. Regardless of the underlying mechanisms these results reinforce the functional heterogeneity of the amygdaloid nuclei and suggest a focal role for DA in modulating the output of the amygdaloid complex.

## ABSENCE OF DA SYNTHESIS-MODULATING NERVE TERMINAL AUTORECEPTORS ON MESOAMYGDALOID DA NEURONS

The availability of DA for neuronal release is regulated by the tonic inhibitory influence of DA synthesis-modulating nerve terminal autoreceptors. This autoregulatory mech-anism is inequivalently expressed in different DA systems with a subset of meso-cortical[17,18] and hypothalamic[19] DA neuronal populations postulated to be pharmaco-logically and functionally unique as a result of a lack of this modulatory mechanism. Dopamine nerve terminals possessing tonically inhibitory synthesis-regulating autore-ceptors typically respond to a diminished synaptic cleft content of DA, secondary to a cessation of impulse activity, with an increased rate of DA synthesis.[20] Such a dis-inhibition resulting from a diminished autoreceptor occupancy is consistently observed for DA projections in the caudate nucleus, nucleus accumbens, and olfactory tubercle following the administration of gammabutyrolactone (GBL).[21-23] In contrast, the ac-cumulation of 3,4-dihydroxyphenylalanine (DOPA) following decarboxylase inhibi-tion, an *in vivo* estimate of tyrosine hydroxylase activity,[24] was not increased by GBL in any of the amygdaloid nuclei examined and in fact was significantly decreased in the central and basal amygdaloid nuclei (Table 2). Since the estimated rate of DA syn-thesis in the amygdaloid nuclei is not increased by a diminished synaptic cleft content of DA, it would appear that mesoamygdaloid DA neurons lack tonically inhibitory terminal autoreceptors regulating neuronal DA synthesis. Similar results were obtained following surgical axotomy,[25] thereby supporting the contention that the failure of GBL to evoke an increased DA synthesis in the amygdaloid complex is not attributable to an inability of GBL to produce a cessation of impulse flow in mesoamygdaloid DA neurons.

The attenuation of the GBL-induced increase in DA synthesis by apomorphine is often offered as evidence supporting the diminished activation of presynaptic DA receptors in mediating the effects of GBL[20] and in establishing the relative sensitivity of autoreceptor populations.[22] Apomorphine administration blocked the GBL-induced increase in DOPA accumulation in the caudate nucleus, nucleus accumbens, and ol-factory tubercle (Table 3). Pretreatment with apomorphine either decreased or did not affect the rate of DOPA accumulation in the amygdaloid nuclei relative to animals receiving only GBL. In terms of the autoregulation of DA synthesis by presynaptic receptors, mesoamygdaloid DA neurons resemble mesocortical DA projections to the medial prefrontal cortex and tuberoinfundibular DA projections to the median emi-nence, and are distinct from other mesotelencephalic DA projection fields in the cau-date nucleus, nucleus accumbens, and olfactory tubercle.

The uniform absence of synthesis-modulating autoreceptors on terminals of popu-lations of mesoamygdaloid DA neurons would appear to be causally unrelated to their differential rates of biochemically estimated impulse activity (*vide supra*), an associa-tion postulated for mesocortical DA neuronal populations.[17] Nor does the uniform absence of such autoreceptors parallel the widely varying degree of tolerance observed

**TABLE 2.** Effect of Gammabutyrolactone (GBL) Administration Alone or in Animals Pretreated with Apomorphine on the Rate of DOPA Accumulation in Discrete Amygdaloid Nuclei or Other Brain Nuclei or Areas

| Brain Nuclei or Area | DOPA Concentration (ng/mg Protein) | | |
|---|---|---|---|
| | Vehicle-Treated | GBL-Treated | Vehicle/GBL-Treated |
| Amygdaloid | | | |
| Central | $6.6 \pm 0.36$ | $4.9 \pm 0.13^a$ | $2.5 \pm 0.18^b$ |
| Lateral | $5.9 \pm 0.25$ | $5.5 \pm 0.49$ | $2.4 \pm 0.19^b$ |
| Basal | $3.7 \pm 0.18$ | $2.4 \pm 0.26^a$ | $1.8 \pm 0.11$ |
| Medial | $2.6 \pm 0.20$ | $3.5 \pm 0.52$ | $2.6 \pm 0.43$ |
| Cortical | $2.5 \pm 0.30$ | $2.2 \pm 0.28$ | $1.6 \pm 0.23$ |
| Posterior | $1.9 \pm 0.07$ | $1.9 \pm 0.20$ | $1.4 \pm 0.19$ |
| Medial posterior | $1.1 \pm 0.04$ | $1.3 \pm 0.14$ | $1.0 \pm 0.11$ |
| Basal posterior | $3.1 \pm 0.25$ | $2.5 \pm 0.41$ | $1.9 \pm 0.29$ |
| Anterior amygdaloid area | $3.7 \pm 0.28$ | $3.1 \pm 0.19$ | $1.6 \pm 0.23^b$ |
| Caudate nucleus | $18.4 \pm 0.98$ | $58.4 \pm 3.2^a$ | $11.6 \pm 0.79^b$ |
| Nucleus accumbens | $19.8 \pm 2.9$ | $43.6 \pm 3.0^a$ | $8.4 \pm 0.67^b$ |
| Olfactory tubercle | $16.3 \pm 0.88$ | $37.2 \pm 4.2^a$ | $9.8 \pm 1.7^b$ |
| Medial prefrontal cortex | $1.7 \pm 0.26$ | $1.6 \pm 0.10$ | $1.4 \pm 0.19$ |
| Median eminence | $9.1 \pm 1.4$ | $8.2 \pm 1.2$ | $5.0 \pm 0.42^b$ |

NOTE: Animals were sacrificed 45 min following apomorphine (1 mg/kg, sc), 35 min following GBL (750 mg/kg, ip) or vehicle (0.9% saline, 1 ml/kg, ip), and 30 min after NSD-1015 (100 mg/kg, ip). Values represent the mean $\pm$ SEM of $4-7$ determinations.

[a] Significantly different ($p < 0.05$) from vehicle-treated animals.
[b] Significantly different ($p < 0.05$) from GBL-treated animals.

in the response of populations of mesoamygdaloid DA neurons to haloperidol following chronic drug administration (*vide infra*). Therefore the significance of the absence of this receptor-mediated autoinhibition of DA synthesis to the physiology and pharmacology of mesoamygdaloid DA neurons is currently unknown.

## SIGNAL TRANSDUCTION AND MESOAMYGDALOID DA NEURONS: NONASSOCIATION WITH A DA-MODULATED ADENYLATE CYCLASE

The adenylate cyclase system is a multicomponent complex that transduces the occupancy of coupled receptors to alterations in the formation of the putative second messenger, cyclic adenosine monophosphate (AMP).[26] This signal transduction mechanism is closely associated with DA neurons in the CNS such that demonstration of this couple fulfills a major criterion supporting a neurotransmitter role for DA and represents the major point of distinction between DA receptor subtypes.[27,28] Initial studies of the presence of DA-stimulated adenylate cyclase activity in homogenates of the rat amygdala, dissected *in toto*, yielded contradictory findings.[29,30] The initial goal of this study was to determine if the distribution of a DA-modulated adenylate cyclase in the amygdaloid complex exhibited a pattern of internuclear distribution paralleling the heterogeneous distribution of its affector, DA. Such a covarying distribution of DA-stimulated adenylate cyclase activity and DA content has been demonstrated among subdivisions of the cerebral cortex.[31] That the distribution of DA-

**TABLE 3.** Comparative Effects of $D_1$ Receptor Ligands, $Mg^{2+}$, GTP, and Forskolin on Adenylate Cyclase Activity in the Microdissected Caudate Nucleus and Central Amygdaloid Nucleus

| | Adenylate Cyclase Activity Cyclic AMP Formation (pmoles/min/mg protein) | |
|---|---|---|
| Addition[a] | Dorsolateral Caudate | Central Amygdaloid Nucleus |
| Homogenate[b] ($N$ = 3) | | |
| (2 mM $Mg^{2+}$, 3 µM GTP) | | |
|   None | $75 \pm 1$ | $232 \pm 6$ |
|   Fenoldopam (10) | $132 \pm 6^d$ | $205 \pm 19$ |
|   None | $55 \pm 1$ | $187 \pm 18$ |
|   DA (100) | $126 \pm 4^d$ | $178 \pm 6$ |
|   SCH 23390 (1) | $52 \pm 2$ | $174 \pm 4$ |
|   DA (100) + SCH 23390 (1) | $54 \pm 1$ | $171 \pm 7$ |
| Particulate Membrane Preparation[c] ($N$ = 4) | | |
|   None | $42 \pm 1$ | $65 \pm 1$ |
|   DA (10) | $42 \pm 4$ | $62 \pm 5$ |
|   Mg (2) | $122 \pm 4$ | $247 \pm 8$ |
|   Mg (2) + DA (10) | $148 \pm 6^d$ | $260 \pm 6$ |
|   Mg (2) + GTP (3) | $170 \pm 4$ | $715 \pm 19$ |
|   Mg (2) + GTP (3) + DA (10) | $300 \pm 6^d$ | $706 \pm 20$ |
|   Mg (2) + GTP (3) + Forskolin (10) | $2423 \pm 90$ | $1463 \pm 140$ |

[a] Numbers in parentheses indicate reaction mixture concentrations in µM, except for $Mg^{2+}$ (mM).

[b] Homogenates were prepared according to the procedure of Schulz and Mailman.[36]

[c] Membrane preparations were prepared according to the procedure of Gnegy and Treisman[41] except no GTP or $Mg^{2+}$ was included in the 0.75-mM EGTA buffer used for final resuspension.

[d] $p < 0.01$ (two-tailed Students' t-test).

stimulated adenylate cyclase activity in the amygdala varies between its component nuclei is suggested by recent light-microscopic quantitative autoradiography results demonstrating a widely varying distribution of binding sites for the $D_1$ receptor-selective antagonist SCH 23390 in the amygdaloid complex.[32]

Using a radiometric assay, the basal adenylate cyclase activity of discrete amygdaloid nuclei, particularly the central amygdaloid nucleus, was found to be greater than that of DA-rich projection fields in the olfactory tubercle, caudate nucleus, and nucleus accumbens (FIG. 1). Dopamine produced a concentration-dependent stimulation of cyclic AMP synthesis in homogenates of the caudate nucleus and nucleus accumbens; a DA concentration of 100 µM more than doubled the basal rate in both brain regions. In striking contrast, neither of the incubation media concentrations of DA examined significantly increased adenylate cyclase activity in homogenates of any of the amygdaloid nuclei (FIG. 1). The caudate–putamen sampled immediately dorsal to the central and lateral amygdaloid nuclei exhibited a relatively low rate of estimated enzyme activity that was stimulated by DA in a concentration-dependent manner. The lack of effect of DA in the amygdaloid complex is therefore not an artifact of the micropunch dissection technique used as a consistent and robust DA stimulation was observed in other DA projection fields dissected by the same technique at the same

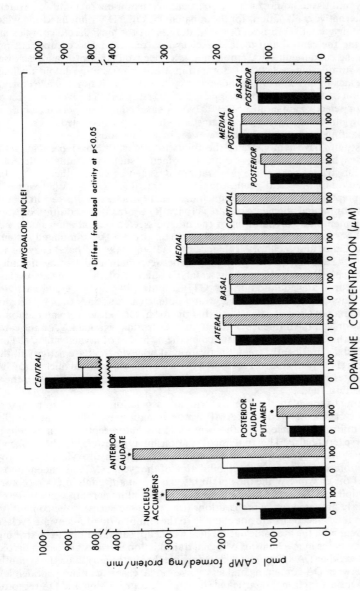

**FIGURE 1.** Basal and dopamine-responsive adenylate cyclase activity in homogenates of amygdaloid and other brain nuclei. Values represent results of one of three experiments yielding similar results with each dopamine concentration examined in triplicate. Enzyme activity measured by the formation of [$^{32}$P] cyclic AMP from [$^{32}$P] ATP. Standard error of the mean was less than 8% of mean value in all cases and are not shown.

time. Dopamine was similarly without effect on cyclic AMP formation in homogenates of the unfrozen, macrodissected amygdala. Subsequent experiments using a nonradiometric assay and tissue homogenates or particulate membrane preparations sought to examine alternative explanations for the apparent lack of a DA-stimulated adenylate cyclase in the amygdaloid complex (TABLE 3). Results for the amygdaloid complex are illustrated using the central amygdaloid nucleus as a representative component nucleus. Unlike the caudate nucleus, fenoldopam, a selective $D_1$ receptor agonist[33] was ineffective in stimulating cyclic AMP formation in the central amygdaloid nucleus. Therefore the lack of effect of DA on adenylate cyclase activity is not due to a concurrent stimulation of functionally opposing $D_1$ and $D_2$ receptors. The lack of effect of the $D_1$ receptor-selective antagonist SCH 23390 on basal adenylate cyclase activity in the central amygdaloid nucleus argues against a high affinity of coupled receptors for DA and a resulting maximal enzyme activation by endogenous DA.

Previous studies have demonstrated the ability to reconstitute both basal and DA-stimulated adenylate cyclase by the addition of cofactors such as guanine nucleotides and $Mg^{2+}$ to rat striatal particulate preparations depleted of such cofactors.[34,35] Indeed, the addition of $Mg^{2+}$ and guanosine triphosphate (GTP), but neither alone, to a membrane preparation of the micropunch dissected caudate nucleus restored both basal and DA-stimulated adenylate cyclase activity. By contrast, the addition of $Mg^{2+}$ and GTP to a membrane preparation of the microdissected central amygdaloid nucleus restored basal enzyme activity, but did not constitute a DA-stimulated system. The interdependence and facilitory influence of GTP and $Mg^{2+}$ on basal enzyme activity supports the absence of a coupling defect between guanyl nucleotide–liganded regulatory proteins ($N_S$ and $N_i$) and the catalytic subunit of the adenylate cyclase system in the central amygdaloid nucleus. GTP stimulated adenylate cyclase activity in the central amygdaloid nucleus with a greater potency and efficacy than in the caudate nucleus (data not shown), suggesting that the former has either a greater amount of available $N_S$ or that the influence of the guanyl nucleotide–liganded $N_S$ on the catalytic subunit in this nucleus is not countered by the influence of an activated $N_i$. Forskolin produced a significantly greater activation of adenylate cyclase activity in the caudate nucleus (1430% of control) compared to the central amygdaloid nucleus (595% of control) suggesting differences in the amount of catalytic subunits between these two DA projection fields.

It is tempting to speculate that the uniform nonassociation between DA receptors and adenylate cyclase-catalyzed cyclic AMP synthesis in the amygdala may be causally related to the uniform absence of synthesis-modulating autoreceptors on mesoamygdaloid DA nerve terminals.[25] This functional relationship is plausible, as El Mestikawy and co-workers[37] have reported that the regulation of tyrosine hydroxylase activity by presynaptic autoreceptors may involve modulation of the cyclic AMP-dependent phosphorylation of the enzyme. While the possibility exists that amygdaloid DA receptors are loosely coupled to the adenylate cyclase system, a coupling perhaps demonstrated in less rigorously prepared tissue preparations (e.g., perfused slices),[28] the contention that amygdaloid DA receptors are not coupled to the stimulation of adenylate cyclase is most consistent with the available data. There would appear, therefore, to be striking qualitative differences in mechanisms of signal transduction between mesoamygdaloid DA neurons and other DA systems. It is thus feasible that in the amygdala the synaptic contacts are between DA-containing and less conventional cells (e.g., neuropeptidergic), and further that the functional significance of synaptic transmission and DA receptor blockade at these sites would differ markedly from the synapses of other DA systems in the CNS. Whether amygdaloid DA receptors are coupled to the inhibition of adenylate cyclase activity remains to be systematically examined.

These findings form a function-based map of the distribution of $D_1$ receptors in the amygdaloid nuclear complex that is in poor agreement with the internuclear distribution of $D_1$ receptors defined by radioligand binding site analysis.[32,38,39] This apparent mismatch is consistent with the existence of subpopulations of $D_1$ receptors in the CNS with one subtype mediating a stimulation of cyclic AMP synthesis and another mediating cyclic AMP-independent effects.[40]

## EFFECTS OF HALOPERIDOL AND APOMORPHINE ON THE BIOCHEMICALLY ESTIMATED ACTIVITY OF POPULATIONS OF MESOAMYGDALOID DA NEURONS

Further comparisons of the mechanisms of regulation of populations of mesoamygdaloid DA neurons relative to other DA systems were addressed by mapping the pharmacological responses to the acute administration of prototypal DA receptor antagonists and agonists. The impulse activity and synthesis of DA in populations of DA neurons innervating the caudate nucleus, nucleus accumbens, olfactory tubercle, posterior pituitary, and cerebral cortex appear to be regulated by postsynaptic DA receptors that activate neuronal feedback loops.[19,17] Such long-loop negative feedback mechanisms, in concert with autoreceptor-mediated regulatory mechanisms, underly the reflex response of DA neurons to the administration of DA receptor agonists and antagonists. Consistent with previous reports,[19,17] the administration of the DA antagonist haloperidol markedly increased NSD-1015-induced DOPA accumulation in the caudate nucleus and nucleus accumbens while producing a much smaller effect in the medial prefrontal cortex (FIG. 2). Haloperidol produced an increase in DOPA accumulation in discrete amygdaloid nuclei that was significantly less than that observed in the caudate nucleus and nucleus accumbens, yet greater than that in the medial prefrontal cortex. The lesser response of mesoamygdaloid DA neurons relative to those projecting to the caudate nucleus or nucleus accumbens reflects the differing contribution of noradrenergic neurons to basal tyrosine hydroxylase activity and the distinct role of DA synthesis-modulating nerve terminal autoreceptors (*vida supra*) in the integrated response to DA receptor blockade. The administration of the DA agonist apomorphine significantly decreased DOPA accumulation in the caudate nucleus, nucleus accumbens, medial prefrontal cortex, and amygdaloid nuclei (FIG. 2). These results suggest that the synthesis of DA in mesoamygdaloid DA neurons is under the regulatory influence of receptor-mediated negative neuronal feedback, and thus resembles mesotelencephalic DA neurons in general. While these findings are consistent with the involvement of long-loop neuronal feedback, the indirect, and perhaps neuronal population-variable, contribution of DA release-regulating nerve terminal autoreceptors in the response to apomorphine is probable.[42]

The acute administration of antipsychotic drugs results in a reflex activation of all studied populations of mesotelencephalic DA neurons (*vide supra*).[43,44] However, populations of mesotelencephalic DA neurons differ greatly in their adaptive response to the chronic administration of antipsychotic drugs with biochemically estimated activity exhibiting either a sustained or variably attenuated reflex response following prolonged drug administration.[45,46,18,43] The effect of a challenge dose (0.3 mg/kg) of haloperidol on DA metabolism in discrete projection fields was compared in groups of animals receiving either 28 consecutive daily injections of haloperidol (0.3 mg/kg) or drug vehicle relative to animals receiving chronic vehicle injections and subsequent vehicle challenge. The results for selected amygdaloid nuclei and other brain nuclei

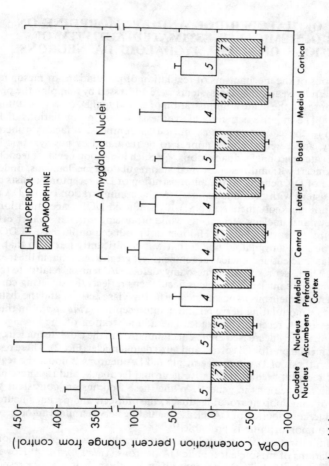

**FIGURE 2.** Effects of haloperidol or apomorphine on the NSD-1015-induced accumulation of DOPA in amygdaloid and other brain nuclei or areas. Haloperidol (1 mg/kg, ip) or apomorphine (1 mg/kg, sc) was administered 60 or 35 min prior to sacrifice, respectively. Values (means ± SEM) are expressed as a percent of the DOPA concentration of vehicle-injected controls. All subjects received NSD-1015 (100 mg/kg, ip) 30 min prior to sacrifice. Numbers at base of each histobar represent number of determinations per group.

or areas (for comparison) are illustrated in FIGURE 3. Consistent with previous reports,[43,18] the haloperidol-induced increase in HVA concentration in the caudate nucleus and nucleus accumbens is moderately attenuated following chronic haloperidol administration. The relatively small response of mesoprefrontal cortex DA neurons to haloperidol is also similarly attenuated by chronic drug treatment. Four weeks of repeated daily haloperidol administration resulted in profound tolerance development in the central and lateral amygdaloid nuclei; HVA concentrations in animals receiving chronic haloperidol treatment and subsequent haloperidol challenge (i.e., Hal/Hal) did not differ significantly from subjects receiving only vehicle injections (i.e., Veh/Veh). In contrast, little evidence for tolerance development was observed in the cortical amygdaloid nucleus. This delineation of adaptive drug response adds a pharmacological dimension to the heterogeneity of DA neuronal projection fields in the amygdaloid complex.

Recent electrophysiological[47,48] and clinical biochemistry[49] findings suggest that a diminished, rather than sustained, compensatory response of DA neurons to prolonged antipsychotic drug administration is causally related to therapeutic efficacy. Such a scenario would result in a progressively decreased physiological antagonism (by neuronal DA release) of pharmacological DA receptor blockade and is consistent with overwhelming evidence indicating that DA receptor blockade is critical to antipsychotic drug action. Extending this logic, that subset of DA neurons that exhibit a maximal degree of tolerance development at a rate paralleling the gradual development of clinical benefit and that innervate brain structures that subserve functions disordered in schizophrenia would represent the critical substrates of the therapeutic action of antipsychotic drugs. The present findings and our developing understanding of the role of the amygdaloid complex in the perception of and reaction to the environment[50,3] suggest that populations of mesoamygdaloid DA neurons innervating the central and lateral amygdaloid nuclei represent strong candidates for this role.

# SUMMARY

Populations of DA neurons innervating the component nuclei of the amygdaloid complex differ in their inferred density of innervation, estimated rate of impulse activity, and adaptive response to the prolonged administration of antipsychotic drugs. Mesoamygdaloid DA neurons have in common the absence of tonically inhibitory, nerve terminal autoreceptors regulating DA synthesis, the nonassociation with a DA-stimulated adenylate cyclase, and the regulation of DA synthesis by receptor-mediated neuronal feedback mechanisms and end-product inhibition. The output of the amygdaloid complex appears to be organized into distinct functions subserved by component nuclei. The present findings suggest a differing role for DA afferents in modulating the functional output of discrete nuclei. The significance of this focal influence will be speculative pending a more complete understanding of the physiology of DA neurotransmission in the amygdaloid complex.

Populations of DA neurons innervating discrete amygdaloid nuclei exhibit a composite of mechanisms of regulation and signal transduction and pharmacology that differ from that of other mesotelencephalic DA systems. These comparisons highlight the fact that the nucleus accumbens and olfactory tubercle do not represent or reflect DA neurotransmission in the limbic system. The study of the physiology, pharmacology, and pathology of mesolimbic DA neurons can and should extend beyond the nucleus accumbens and olfactory tubercle to the amygdala and other brain structures central to the organization of the limbic system. It is our opinion that the term "mesolimbic"

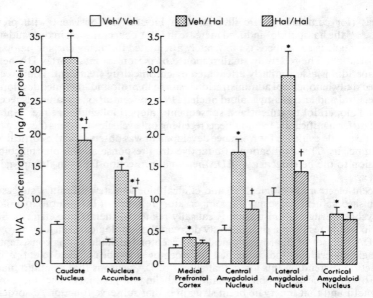

**FIGURE 3.** Effect of acute or chronic administration of haloperidol on the homovanillic acid (HVA) concentration of amygdaloid and other brain nuclei or areas. Groups of rats (5–7/group) received daily doses (ip) of vehicle (0.3% tartaric acid, 1 ml/kg) or haloperidol (0.3 mg/kg) for 28 days, and an additional group of vehicle-treated rats was challenged with haloperidol on day 28 (Veh/Hal). Subjects were sacrificed 2 hr following the last injection. $*p < 0.05$ compared to vehicle-injected controls; $\dagger\, p < 0.05$ compared to vehicle-injected/haloperidol-challenged subjects.

DA system has purely anatomical connotations and that a more specific terminology (e.g., meso-central amygdaloid nuclear) would express the functional organization of this system more accurately.

## REFERENCES

1.  MOGENSON, G. J. & F. R. CALARESU. 1973. Cardiovascular responses to electrical stimulation of the amygdala in the rat. Exp. Neurol. **49:** 166–180.
2.  HALGREN, E. 1981. The amygdala contribution to emotion and memory: Current studies in humans. *In* The Amygdaloid Complex. Y. Ben-Ari, Ed.: 395–408. Elsevier/North-Holland Biomedical Press, Amsterdam. The Netherlands.
3.  AGGLETON, J. P. & M. MISHKIN. 1986. The amygdala: Sensory gateway to the emotions. *In* Emotion: Theory, Research and Experience, Vol. 3: 281–299.
4.  GLOOR, P. 1960. Amygdala. *In* Handbook of Physiology. Sect. 1 Neurophysiology. J. Field, H. W. Magoun, and V. E. Hall, Eds. Vol. II.: 1395–1420. American Physiological Society. Washington, D.C.
5.  BEAULIEU, S., T. DI PAOLO, J. COTE & N. BARDEN. 1987. Participation of the central amygdaloid nucleus in the response of adrenocorticotropin secretion to immobilization stress: Opposing roles of the noradrenergic and dopaminergic systems. Neuroendocrinology **45:** 37–46.
6.  MILLHOUSE, O. E. & J. DEOLMOS. 1981. Aspects of the neuronal organization of the amygdala. *In* The Amygdaloid Complex, INSERM Symposium, Y. Ben-Ari, Ed. No. 20:33–43. Elsevier/North-Holland Biomedical Press. New York.

7. BROWNSTEIN, M., J. M. SAAVEDRA & M. PALKOVITS. 1974. Norepinephrine and dopamine in the limbic system of the rat. Brain Res. **79:** 431–436.

8. ROBERTS, G. W., P. L. WOODHAMS, J. M. POLAK & T. J. CROW. 1982. Distribution of neuropeptides in the limbic system of the rat: The amygdaloid complex. Neuroscience **7:** 91–131.

9. SIEGEL, A. 1984. Anatomical and functional differentiation within the amygdala–behavioral state modulation. *In* Modulation of Sensorimotor Activity During Alterations in Behavioral States. R. Bandler, Ed.: 299–323, Alan Liss. New York.

10. OTTERSEN, O. P. 1980. Afferent connections to the amygdaloid complex of the rat and cat: II. Afferents from the hypothalamus and the basal telencephalon. J. Comp. Neurol. **194:** 267–289.

11. OTTERSEN, O. P. 1981. Afferent connections to the amygdaloid complex of the rat with some observations in the cat. III. Afferents from the lower brain stem. J. Comp. Neurol. **202:** 335–356.

12. UNGERSTEDT, U. 1971. Stereotaxic mapping of the monoamine pathways in the rat brain. Acta Physiol. Scand. Suppl. **367:** 1–48.

13. FALLON, J. H., D. A. KOZIELL & R. Y. MOORE. 1978. Catecholamine innervation of the basal forebrain. II. Amygdala, suprarhinal cortex and entorhinal cortex. J. Comp. Neurol. **180:** 509–532.

14. BEN-ARI, Y., R. E. ZIGMOND & K. E. MOORE. 1975. Regional distribution of tyrosine hydroxylase, norepinephrine and dopamine within the amygdaloid complex of the rat. Brain Res. **87:** 96–101.

15. KILTS, C. D. & C. M. ANDERSON. 1986. The simultaneous quantification of dopamine, norepinephrine and epinephrine in micropunched rat brain nuclei by on-line trace enrichment HPLC with electrochemical detection: Distribution of catecholamines in the limbic system. Neurochem. Int. **9:** 437–445.

16. BRODIE, B. B., E. COSTA, A. DLABAC, N. H. NEFF & H. H. SMOOKLER. 1966. Application of steady state kinetics to the estimation of synthesis rate and turnover time of tissue catecholamines. J. Pharmacol. Exp. Ther. **154:** 493–498.

17. BANNON, M. J., R. L. MICHAUD & R. H. ROTH. 1981. Mesocortical dopamine neurons: Lack of autoreceptors modulating dopamine synthesis. Mol. Pharmacol. **19:** 270–275.

18. BANNON, M. J., J. R. REINHARD, JR., E. B. BUNNEY & R. H. ROTH. 1982. Unique response to antipsychotic drugs is due to absence of terminal autoreceptors in mesocortical dopamine neurones. Nature **296:** 444–446.

19. DEMAREST, K. T. & K. E. MOORE. 1979. Comparison of dopamine synthesis regulation in the terminals of nigrostriatal, mesolimbic, tuberoinfundibular and tuberohypophyseal neurons. J. Neural Trans. **46:** 263–277.

20. WALTERS, J. R. & R. H. ROTH. 1976. Dopaminergic neurons: An in vivo system for measuring drug interactions with presynaptic receptors. Naunyn-Schmiedeberg's Arch Pharmacol. **296:** 5–14.

21. NOWYCKY, M. C. & R. H. ROTH. 1978. Dopaminergic neurons: Role of presynaptic receptors in the regulation of transmitter biosynthesis. Prog. Neuropsychopharmacol. **2:** 139–158.

22. DEMAREST, K. T., K. L. LAWSON-WENDLING & K. E. MOORE. 1983. D-amphetamine and γ-butyrolactone alteration of dopamine synthesis in the terminals of nigrostriatal and mesolimbic neurons. Possible role of various autoreceptor sensitivities. Biochem. Pharmacol. **32:** 691–697.

23. ANDEN, N.-E., M. GRABOWSKA-ANDEN & B. LILJENBERG. 1983. Demonstration of autoreceptors on dopamine neurons in different brain regions of rats treated with gammabutyrolactone. J. Neural Trans. **58:** 143–152.

24. CARLSSON, A., J. N. DAVIS, W. KEHR, M. LINDQVIST & C. V. ATACK. 1972. Simultaneous measurement of tyrosine and tryptophan hydroxylase activities in brain *in vivo* using an inhibitor of the aromatic amino acid decarboxylase. Naunyn-Schmiedeberg's Arch. Pharmacol. **275:** 153–168.

25. KILTS, C. D., C. M. ANDERSON, T. D. ELY & J. K. NISHITA. 1987. Absence of synthesis-modulating nerve terminal autoreceptors on mesoamygdaloid and other mesolimbic dopamine neuronal populations. J. Neurosci. **7:** 3961–3975.

26. BIRNBAUMER, L., J. CODINA, R. MATTERA, R. A. CERIONE, J. D. HILDERBRANDT, T. SUNYER, F. J. ROJAS, M. G. CARON, R. J. LEFKOWITZ & R. IYENGAR. 1985. Structural basis of

adenylate cyclase stimulation and inhibition by distinct guanine nucleotide regulatory proteins. *In* Molecular Mechanisms of Transmembrane Signalling. Cohen and Houslay, Eds.: 131–192. Elsevier Science Publishers, Biomedical Division. Amsterdam. The Netherlands.

27.  KEBABIAN, J. W. & D. B. CALNE. 1979. Multiple receptors for dopamine. Nature **277**: 93–96.

28.  STOOF, J. C. & J. W. KEBABIAN. 1981. Opposing roles for D-1 and D-2 dopamine receptors in efflux of cyclic AMP from rat neostriatum. Nature **294**: 366–368.

29.  CLEMENT-CORMIER, Y. C. & G. A. ROBISON. 1977. Adenylate cyclase from various dopaminergic areas of the brain and the action of antipsychotic drugs. Biochem. Pharmacol. **26**: 1719–1722.

30.  RACAGNI, G. & A. CARENZI. 1976. The anterior amygdala dopamine sensitive adenylate cyclase: Point of action of antipsychotic drugs. Pharmacol. Res. Comm. **8**: 149–157.

31.  TASSIN, J. P., M. REIBAUD, G. BLANC, J. M. STUDLER & J. GLOWINSKI. 1984. Regulation of the sensitivity of $D_1$ receptors in the prefrontal cortex and the nucleus accumbens by nondopaminergic pathways. *In* Catecholamines: Neuropharmacology and Central Nervous System – Theoretical Aspects. 103–111. Alan Liss. New York.

32.  DAWSON, T. M., D. R. GEHLERT, R. T. McCABE, A. BARNETT & J. K. WAMSLEY. 1986. D-1 dopamine receptors in the rat brain: A quantitative autoradiographic analysis. J. Neurosci. **6**: 2352–2365.

33.  FLAIM, K. E., G. W. GESSNER, S. T. CROOKE, H. M. SARAU & J. WEINSTOCK. 1985. Binding of a novel dopaminergic agonist radioligand [$^3$H]-fendolopam (SKF 82526) to D-1 dopamine receptors in rat striatum. Life Sci. **36**: 1427–1436.

34.  KEBABIAN, J. W., T. C. CHEN & T. E. COTE. 1979. Endogenous guanyl nucleotides: Components of the striatum which confer dopamine-sensitivity to adenylate cyclase. Comm. Psychopharmacol. **3**: 421–428.

35.  CLEMENT-CORMIER, Y. C. & G. A. ROBISON. 1977. Adenylate cyclase from various dopaminergic areas of the brain and the action of antipsychotic drugs. Biochem. Pharmacol. **26**: 1719–1722.

36.  SCHULTZ, D. W. & R. B. MAILMAN. 1984. An improved, automated adenylate cyclase assay utilizing preparative HPLC: Effects of phosphodiesterase inhibitors. J. Neurochem. **42**: 764–774.

37.  EL MESTIKAWY, S., J. GLOWINSKI & M. HAMON. 1986. Presynaptic dopamine autoreceptors control tyrosine hydroxylase activation in depolarized striatal dopaminergic terminals. J. Neurochem. **46**: 12–22.

38.  DUBOIS, A., M. SAVASTA, O. CURET & B. SCATTON. 1986. Autoradiographic distribution of the $D_1$ agonist [$^3$H]SKF 38393, in the rat brain and spinal cord. Comparison with the distribution of $D_2$ dopamine receptors. Neuroscience **19**: 125–137.

39.  BOYSON, S. J., P. McGONIGLE & P. B. MOLINOFF. 1986. Quantitative autoradiographic localization of the $D_1$ and $D_2$ subtypes of dopamine receptors in rat brain. J. Neurosci. **6**: 3177–3188.

40.  MAILMAN, R. B., D. W. SCHULZ, C. D. KILTS, M. H. LEWIS, H. ROLLEMA & S. WYRICK. 1986. Biochemical and functional studies of D-1 dopamine receptors. Psychopharmacol. Bull. **22**: 593–598.

41.  GNEGY, M. & G. TREISMAN. 1981. Effect of calmodulin on dopamine-sensitive adenylate cyclase activity in rat striatal membranes. Mol. Pharmacol. **19**: 256–263.

42.  GALLOWAY, M. P., M. E. WOLF & R. H. ROTH. 1986. Regulation of dopamine synthesis in the medial prefrontal cortex is mediated by release modulating autoreceptors: Studies *in vivo*. J. Pharmacol. Exp. Ther. **236**: 689–698.

43.  MATSUMOTO, T., H. UCHIMURA, M. HIRANO, J. S. KIM, H. YOKOO, M. SHIMOMURA, T. NAKAHARA, K. INOUE & K. OOMAGARI. 1983. Differential effects of acute and chronic administration of haloperidol on homovanillic acid levels in discrete dopaminergic areas of rat brain. Eur. J. Pharmacol. **89**: 27–33.

44.  BANNON, M. J., E. WOLF & R. H. ROTH. 1983. Pharmacology of dopamine neurons innervating the prefrontal, cingulate and piriform cortices. Eur. J. Pharmacol. **91**: 119–125.

45.  SCATTON, B. 1977. Differential regional development of tolerance to increase in dopamine turnover upon repeated neuroleptic administration. Eur. J. Pharmacol. **46**: 363–369.

46.  SCATTON, B. 1981. Differential changes in DOPAC levels in the hippocampal formation,

septum and striatum of the rat induced by acute and repeated neuroleptic treatment. Eur. J. Pharmacol. **71:** 499–503.

47. CHIODO, L. A. & B. S. BUNNEY. 1983. Typical and atypical neuroleptics: Differential effects of chronic administration on the activity of A9 and A10 midbrain dopaminergic neurons. J. Neurosci. **3(8):** 1607–1619.

48. WHITE, F. J. & R. Y. WANG. 1983. Differential effects of classical and atypical antipsychotic drugs on A9 and A10 dopamine neurons. Science **221:** 1054–1057.

49. PICKAR, D., R. LABARCA, A. R. DORAN, O. M. WOLKOWITZ, A. ROY, A. BREIER, M. LINNOILA & S. M. PAUL. 1986. Longitudinal measurement of plasma homovanillic acid levels in schizophrenic patients. Arch. Gen. Psychiat. **43:** 669–676.

50. GLOOR, P., A. OLIVIER, L. F. QUESNEY, F. ANDERMANN & S. HOROWITZ. 1982. The role of the limbic system in experiential phenomena of temporal lobe epilepsy. Ann. Neurol. **12:** 129–144.

51. UNGERSTEDT, U. 1971. Stereotaxic mapping of the monoamine pathways in the rat brain. Acta Physiol. Scand. Suppl. **367:** 1–48.

52. BEN-ARI, Y. & J. S. KELLY. 1976. Dopamine evoked inhibition of single cells of the feline putamen and basolateral amygdala. J. Physiol. **256:** 1–21.

53. CHARRIERE, B., F. DAUDET, B. GUIBERT, C. BARBERIS & V. LEVIEL. 1983. "In situ" release of dopamine in the nucleus amygdalodeus centralis. Brain Res. **271:** 386–387.

54. SCATTON, B., A. DUBOIS, M. L. DUBOCOVICH, N. R. ZAHNISER & D. FAGE. 1985. Quantitative autoradiography of $^3$H-nomifensine binding sites in rat brain. Life Sci. **36:** 815–822.

55. JAVITCH, J. A., S. M. STRITTMATTER & S. H. SNYDER. 1985. Differential visualization of dopamine and norepinephrine uptake sites in rat brain using [$^3$H]mazindol autoradiography. J. Neurosci. **5:** 1513–1521.

56. SAAVEDRA, J. M. & J. ZIVIN. 1976. Tyrosine hydroxylase and dopamine-β-hydroxylase: Distribution in discrete areas of the rat limbic system. Brain Res. **105:** 517–524.

57. HIRANO, M., J. S. KIM, M. SAITO, H. UCHIMURA, M. ITO & T. NAKAHARA. 1978. Monoamine oxidase activities for serotonin and tyramine in individual limbic and lower brain stem nuclei of the rat. J. Neurochem. **30:** 263–267.

58. DUBOIS, A., M. SAVASTA, O. CURET & B. SCATTON. 1986. Autoradiographic distribution of the $D_1$ agonist [$^3$H]SKF 38393, in the rat brain and spinal cord. Comparison with the distribution of $D_2$ dopamine receptors. Neuroscience **19:** 125–137.

59. OUIMET, C. C., P. E. MILLER, H. C. HEMMINGS, JR., S. I. WALLAS & P. GREENGARD. 1984. Darpp-32, a dopamine- and adenosine 3′:5′-monophosphate-regulated phosphoprotein enriched in dopamine-innervated brain regions. J. Neurosci. **4:** 111–124.

# Stress-Related Activation of Cerebral Dopaminergic Systems[a]

ADRIAN J. DUNN

*Department of Neuroscience*
*University of Florida College of Medicine*
*Gainesville, Florida 32610*

## INTRODUCTION

An activation of peripheral (autonomic) catecholaminergic systems during stress has long been known,[1] but more recently it has been determined that cerebral catecholamine-containing neurons are also affected.[2-6] The emphasis has been on noradrenergic neurons,[7] with relatively few reports of effects on dopaminergic neurons.[3,4] However, Thierry *et al.*[8] reported that a series of footshocks greatly accelerated the rate of decline of dopamine (DA) in the rat prefrontal cortex following blockade of synthesis with α-methyl-*p*-tyrosine (αMPT). A lesser effect was observed in nucleus accumbens, but no significant changes were observed in the striatum or olfactory tubercle. Subsequently, Lavielle *et al.*[9] showed that footshock treatment increased the contents of the DA catabolite, DOPAC, in the prefrontal and cingulate cortices, but not in the nucleus accumbens, amygdala, septum, or striatum. Increases in prefrontal cortex DOPAC or DOPAC:DA ratios following footshock have now been confirmed by many.[10-17] In most of these reports the effects were largely confined to the mesocortical or mesolimbic DA systems, but there are reports of effects of stress on DA metabolism in other regions.[17-20]

In the studies described below, we have measured the content of the major catecholamines and their catabolites using high-performance liquid chromatography (HPLC) with electrochemical detection in several brain regions. We have performed this analysis after a variety of stressors. The results indicate that stressors such as footshock and restraint can activate DA metabolism as assessed by the DOPAC:DA and HVA:DA ratios in most brain regions, to parallel the activation of noradrenergic systems.

## MATERIALS AND METHODS

Male CD-1 mice (25–35 g) were obtained from Charles River (Wilmington, Massachusetts). They were housed in individual cages with free access to food and water on a 12–12-hr light–dark cycle (lights on 7 a.m.) for three days before the commencement of experimental manipulations. All experimental manipulations were performed between 8 a.m. and 2 p.m. (except the experiments with Newcastle disease virus, which were performed between 1 and 4 p.m.).

[a] This work was supported by U.S. National Institute of Mental Health Grant MH 25486 and by Office of Naval Research Grant N0001-4-85K-0300.

## Neurochemistry

Animals were killed by decapitation and trunk blood was collected into heparinized 1.5-ml Eppendorf tubes. The brain was rapidly excised, chilled, and dissected into the required regions as rapidly as possible.[21] Tissue samples were promptly weighed in tared 1.5-ml Eppendorf tubes and frozen on dry ice within 5 min of death. They were homogenized within 24 hr by brief ultrasonication in 0.4–0.5 ml of 0.1 M $HClO_4$ containing 0.1 mM EDTA and an internal standard of N-methyldopamine (NMDA, 10–100 ng). The homogenates were frozen and stored at $-50°$ until HPLC-EC analysis. Immediately before analysis the samples were thawed, centrifuged, and samples of the supernatant were applied directly to the HPLC system.

The HPLC system was that described elsewhere.[21,50] The reverse phase (ODS C18) chromatography column was eluted with a mobile phase of 0.05 sodium phosphate–0.05 M citrate buffer (about pH 3.2), 0.1 mM EDTA, 0.2–0.4 mM sodium octylsulfonate, containing 5–12% methanol. The precise concentrations of octylsulfonate and methanol, and the precise pH and column temperature were adjusted to achieve optimal separation of (in order of elution) uric acid, norepinephrine (NE), epinephrine, normetanephrine (NM), dihydroxphenylacetic acid (DOPA), 3-methoxy,4-hydroxyphenyleneglycol (MHPG), dopamine (DA), 3,4-dihydroxyphenylacetic acid (DOPAC), NMDA, tyramine, 5-hydroxyindoleacetic acid (5-HIAA), serotonin (5-HT), 3-methoxytyramine (3-MT), homovanillic acid (HVA), and tryptophan (Trp).

Plasma corticosterone was determined by radioimmunoassay after extraction of plasma with methylene chloride.[22,23]

# RESULTS AND DISCUSSION

For most of our experiments we have used mice, but our major findings have been confirmed in rats. In the mouse, as opposed to the rat and man, MHPG and other catecholamine catabolites are largely unsulfated.[24] Thus it is not necessary to hydrolyze samples before determining catabolite concentrations, a great technical advantage because manipulations of the extracts cause degradation of the metabolites and problems with the HPLC separations.

In our first experiments we examined the concentrations of catecholamines, indoleamines and their catabolites in various brain regions immediately following a series of 20–22 1-sec footshocks of 0.18 mA given in a period of 15 min. Because ratios of the catabolite to the parent amine have been proposed as a "utilization index" for the amine,[9] we have expressed the results in this form. A typical set of results for the DA catabolite ratios is shown in FIGURE 1. Footshock treatment consistently elevated DOPAC:DA ratios in the prefrontal cortex. We also observed a statistically significant increase of DOPAC/DA in the brain stem, and have frequently observed a similar increase in the hypothalamus, although that did not occur in this particular experiment. No statistically significant changes were observed in olfactory tubercle, nucleus accumbens, or caudate–putamen. These changes were caused primarily by significant increases in DOPAC, because the DA contents were not significantly altered. FIGURE 1 also shows that HVA/DA was elevated in the prefrontal cortex, but this change was not statistically significant.

To determine whether these changes were specific for footshock, we tested another stressor, restraint. Mice were restrained [17,50] for 30 min, and brain samples taken immediately after this. The results (FIG. 2) showed significantly elevated DOPAC:DA ratios in all regions studied, including, prefrontal cortex, nucleus accumbens, cau-

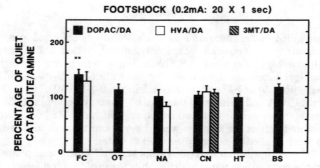

**FIGURE 1.** The effect of footshock treatment of mice on the DOPAC:DA, HVA:DA, and 3-MT:DA ratios of various brain regions (prefrontal cortex, FC; olfactory tubercle, OT; nucleus accumbens, NA; caudate–putamen, CN; hypothalamus, HT; brain stem, BS). Mice received 20–22 footshocks of 0.18 mA (1 sec) during 15 min. The contents of dihydroxyphenylacetic acid (DOPAC), dopamine (DA), homovanillic acid (HVA), and 3-methoxytyramine (3-MT) were measured by HPLC with electrochemical detection. Metabolite contents of quiet mice were: DA: FC, 0.06; OT, 7.5; NA, 5.9; CN, 10.9; HT, 0.45; BS, 0.12; DOPAC: FC, 0.058; OT, 4.0; NA 3.7; CN, 1.7; HT, 0.27; BS, 0.09; HVA: FC, 0.04; NA, 0.93; CN, 0.52; 3-MT: CN, 0.76; all in ng/mg tissue. *Significantly different from quiet mice (Student's $t$-test: $p < 0.05$; **$2p < 0.01$, $n = 8$).

date–putamen, hypothalamus, and brain stem. Significant elevations in HVA:DA ratios were also observed in nucleus accumbens, caudate–putamen, and hypothalamus. There were no statistically significant changes of 3-MT or 3-MT:DA ratios in nucleus accumbens or caudate–putamen, the only regions in which 3-MT was measurable. These changes in DA metabolism following restraint confirm the observations of others.[18,19,25-30]

These results posed the question whether the response to restraint was qualitatively different from that produced by footshock, or whether our chosen parameters for restraint constituted a more potent stressor. Thus we repeated our experiments with footshock using the same number of shocks over the same time period, but at a higher current level (0.45 mA). The results were qualitatively rather similar to those obtained

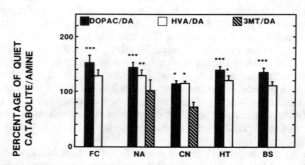

**FIGURE 2.** The effect of 30 min restraint on the DOPAC:DA, HVA:DA, and 3-MT:DA ratios of various brain regions (see FIG. 1). *Significantly different from quiet mice (Student's $t$-test; $2p < 0.05$, **$2p < 0.01$, ***$2p < 0.001$; $n = 10$).

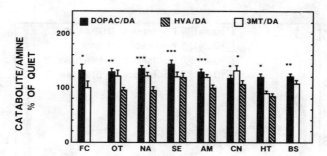

**FIGURE 3.** The effect of footshock treatment of mice on the DOPAC:DA, HVA:DA, and 3-MT:DA ratios of various brain regions (see FIG. 1; septum, SE; amygdala, AM). Mice received 20–22 footshocks of 0.45 mA (1 sec) during 15 min. *Significantly different from quiet mice (Student's $t$-test: $2p < 0.05$, **$2p < 0.01$, ***$2p < 0.001$, $n = 10$).

with restraint. DOPAC:DA ratios were elevated in all regions studied, including prefrontal cortex, olfactory tubercle, nucleus accumbens, septum, amygdala, caudate–putamen, hypothalamus, and brain stem (FIG. 3). HVA:DA ratios were also elevated in most brain regions, but this effect was statistically significant only in nucleus accumbens and caudate–putamen. No significant changes were observed in 3-MT:DA ratios in regions in which they were measurable. The stressful treatments also altered NE metabolism as determined by the production of MHPG. MHPG:NE ratios were increased by either footshock or restraint in most regions of the brain.[15,17,50]

The lack of changes in 3-MT is almost certainly because comparison of concentrations of this metabolite following microwave fixation with those obtained from unfixed tissue have suggested that there is a rapid postmortem increase in 3-MT.[31-35] Thus any differences in the *in vivo* concentrations of this metabolite were probably obscured by postmortem increases. Some oxidation of 3-MT to HVA may also have occurred, which may explain why changes in the latter appear to reflect, but are smaller than the changes in DOPAC.[34,35] Similar problems occur with the NE catabolite, NM,[34,36] thus we will not include data for NM or 3-MT in subsequent figures.

FIGURE 4 shows the results from one experiment, summarizing the catabolite changes we observe following footshock in the prefrontal cortex, hypothalamus, and brain stem. DOPAC:DA ratios are consistently increased in the prefrontal cortex and brain stem. Statistically significant changes in this index are less reliable in the hypothalamus (probably because the change is smaller), but do occur in this and all other regions measured when the footshock period is prolonged beyond 15 min or is of greater intensity. MHPG:NE ratios are consistently increased in all regions where MHPG is measurable. Unfortunately, MHPG is present in low concentrations, is relatively labile to oxidation, produces a proportionately smaller signal on the electrochemical detector, and runs in a crowded region of the chromatogram, so that accurate determinations of this catabolite are not always possible. The 5-HIAA:5-HT ratios are not significantly altered by mild stressors such as 15-min footshock, but do increase following longer periods of footshock or restraint. The changes are in all cases primarily due to increases of the catabolites. We have observed no consistent changes in DA or 5-HT, but have on occasion observed small but statistically significant reductions in NE in the hypothalamus or brain stem, particularly after more intense stress, or during passive avoidance behavior. However, the increases in MHPG:NE ratios were primarily due to increases in MHPG. Free tryptophan is consistently increased in all brain regions

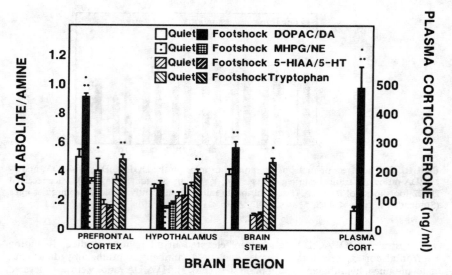

**FIGURE 4.** The effect of footshock treatment of mice on the DOPAC:DA, MHPG:NE, and 5-HIAA:5-HT ratios, and the tryptophan content of prefrontal cortex, hypothalamus, and brain stem. Data for plasma corticosterone are also included. Mice were treated as in the experiment of FIGURE 1, but with 0.3-mA footshocks. *Significantly different from quiet mice (Student's $t$-test $2p < 0.05$. **$2p < 0.01$, ***$2p < 0.001$: $n = 6$).

by footshock or restraint, confirming the results of Curzon *et al.*[37] This effect is accompanied by small changes in the total plasma tryptophan concentration.[37a] Plasma corticosterone is consistently increased by all stressful treatments.

We have observed effects very similar to these in rats subjected to 30 min of electric footshock (40 1-sec shocks at 0.5 mA) or restraint (Dunn and Koppenaal, unpublished).

The rather global anatomical changes in DOPAC:DA ratios prompted us to perform a more discrete anatomical analysis. FIGURE 5 shows that all three subdivisions of the prefrontal cortex DA projection, medial, sulcal, and cingulate cortex[38] show similar responses of DOPAC:DA ratios to 30-min footshock. In our experience, however, the changes in the medial division are larger and more consistent than those in the sulcal division and the cingulate cortex. Surprisingly, the general activation of DA systems was also found when we subdivided the hypothalamus into a preoptic region, a medial basal hypothalamic region containing the median eminence, and the remainder. MHPG:NE ratios were also elevated in the subdivisions of both prefrontal cortex and hypothalamus (FIG. 6). The increase in DOPAC:DA ratios in the medial basal hypothalamus is surprising because it is well established that prolactin secretion is increased during stress,[39] and that the release of prolactin in the median eminence is under inhibitory control of tuberoinfundibular DA neurons.[40] Moreover, Fuxe *et al.*[41] reported changes in catecholamine fluorescence in the median eminence consistent with decreases of DA release, and Demarest *et al.*[42] found changes in measures of DA synthesis and release in rat median eminence during restraint stress. However, subsequent studies found the latter effects only in female and not in male rats.[42] Thus there may not be a conflict between these studies and our findings in male mice.

The increases in DOPAC:DA ratios disappeared relatively rapidly following a period

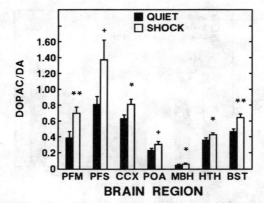

**FIGURE 5.** The effect of footshock treatment of mice on the DOPAC:DA ratios of various brain regions. Mice were footshocked as in the experiment of FIGURE 1, but for 30 min at 0.25 mA. PFM: prefrontal medial cortex; PFS: sulcal cortex; CCX: cingulate cortex; POA: preoptic area; MBH: medial basal hypothalamus (including the median eminence region); HTH: the remainder of hypothalamus; BST: brain stem. *Significantly different from quiet mice ($2p < 0.05$, **$2p < 0.01$, $^+2p < 0.1$: $n = 10$).

of footshock, and were absent in prefrontal cortex 30 min, 1 hr, or 1 day following 15-min footshock, although in the hypothalamus there was still a statistically significant increase at 30 min. When the footshock treatment was repeated daily, similar increases in DOPAC:DA and MHPG:NE ratios were observed in the prefrontal cortex, hypothalamus, and brain stem after 5, 8, or 10 days. But after 10 days, the DOPAC:DA ratio was decreased relative to that after 1 day in the medial prefrontal cortex, but not in the hypothalamus and brain stem (FIG. 7). After this same time period there was also a small, but statistically significant decline in the response of brain stem MHPG:NE ratio relative to that after 1 day (FIG. 8). No significant changes were observed 24 hours after the tenth day of footshock (data not shown).

Interestingly, similar results were observed when the stressor was a conditioned

**FIGURE 6.** The effect of footshock treatment of mice on the MHPG:NE ratios of various brain regions. The same experiment as in FIGURE 5. *Significantly different from quiet mice ($2p < 0.05$, **$2p < 0.01$, ***$2p < 0.001$).

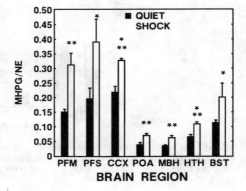

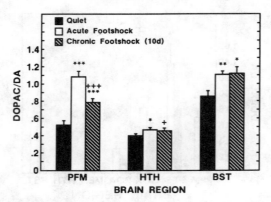

**FIGURE 7.** The effects of acute (1 day) or chronic (10 days) footshock treatment of mice on the DOPAC:DA ratios of various brain regions. Mice were footshocked as in the experiment of FIGURES 5 and 6, but for one or ten successive days. *Significantly different from quiet mice ($2p < 0.05$, **$2p < 0.01$, ***$2p < 0.001$, $p < 0.05$). ⁺⁺⁺Significantly different from 1 day footshock ($2p < 0.001$: $n = 8$).

one. If mice are merely replaced in an apparatus in which they received footshock on the previous day, they show brain catecholamine responses indistinguishable from those that occur in naive animals after receiving footshock. This is true for both DOPAC:DA ratios (FIG. 9) and also MHPG:NE ratios. This result is consistent with the reports of others.[38,44,45] Because our measures appeared to be very sensitive to stressful treatments in mice, we decided to study even weaker stressors in a more behavioral context, passive avoidance training. FIGURE 10 shows that significant increases in prefrontal cortex and brain stem DOPAC:DA ratios were observed 10 min after a single footshock during training in one-trial passive avoidance.[21] This was accompanied by increases in MHPG:NE, decreases in NE in the hypothalamus, and increases in plasma

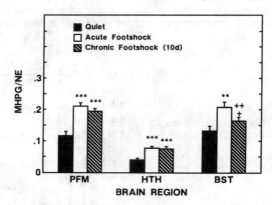

**FIGURE 8.** The effects of acute (1 day) or chronic (10 days) footshock treatment of mice on the MHPG:NE ratios of various brain regions. The same experiment as in FIGURE 7. **Significantly different from quiet mice ($2p < 0.01$, ***$2p < 0.001$). ⁺⁺⁺Significantly different from 1 day footshock ($2p < 0.001$: $n = 8$).

**FIGURE 9.** The effects of conditioned footshock on DOPAC:DA ratios of the prefrontal cortex (PFC), hypothalamus, and brain stem of mice. Mice were shocked as in the experiment of FIGURE 1. On the next day, half of the mice were shocked, and the other half were replaced in the apparatus but with the shock turned off. QQ: mice left quietly in their home cages on both days 1 and 2; QS: mice shocked only on day 2; SS: mice shocked on both days; SAE: mice shocked on day 1, but merely exposed to the apparatus on day 2. *Significantly different from quiet mice ($2p < 0.05$; **$2p < 0.01$; ***$2p < 0.001$: $n = 8$).

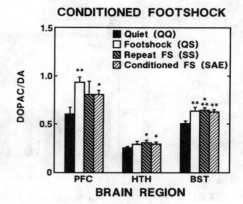

corticosterone. Some similar changes occurred on testing for the performance of the passive avoidance learning (FIG. 11). Increases in prefrontal cortex DOPAC:DA and in hypothalamic and brain stem MHPG:NE were observed in trained, but not in untrained mice. These increases were accompanied by increases in plasma corticosterone that were related to the performance of the animals. (See reference 21 for a fuller discussion of these data.)

A possible complication in conditioning experiments is evident from the results shown in FIGURE 12. In this experiment one group of mice was left quiet, one group was footshocked with the standard procedure ($20 \times 1$ sec at 0.2 mA in 15 min), and a third group was placed in the same boxes in which the second group was shocked, but without cleaning the boxes. The results indicated that mere exposure to a box in

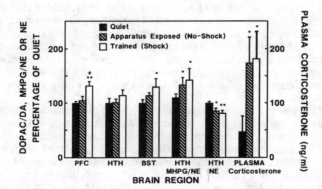

**FIGURE 10.** Responses of DOPAC:DA ratios in the prefrontal cortex, hypothalamus, and brain stem, and of MHPG:NE and NE in the hypothalamus of mice 10 min after passive avoidance training. Data for plasma corticosterone are also included. *Solid bars*: quiet mice left undisturbed until just before decapitation; *hatched bars*: mice placed in the behavioral apparatus, but without footshock; *open bars*: mice trained with one 2-sec footshock (0.35 mA). *Significantly different from quiet mice ($2p < 0.05$, **$2p < 0.01$: $n = 6$). ⁺Significantly different from mice exposed to the apparatus but not shocked ($2p < 0.05$). (For full details, see reference 21 from which this figure is reproduced with permission.)

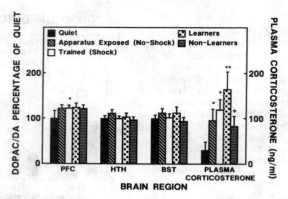

**FIGURE 11.** Responses of DOPAC:DA ratios in the prefrontal cortex, hypothalamus, and brain stem of mice 10 min after performance of passive avoidance behavior. Data for plasma corticosterone are also included. *Solid bars*: quiet mice left undisturbed until just before decapitation ($n = 6$); *hatched bars*: mice placed in the behavioral apparatus on the first and second days, but without footshock ($n = 7$); *open bars*: mice trained with one 2-sec footshock (0.35 mA) on the first day, and tested 24 hr later ($n = 18$); *spotted bars* (learners): mice in the trained group that exhibited step-through latencies on the retention test $> 50$ sec ($n = 8$); *striped bars* (non-learners): mice in the (last) trained group that exhibited step-through latencies on the retention test $< 50$ sec ($n = 10$). *Significantly different from quiet mice ($2p < 0.05$, **$2p < 0.01$). +Significantly different from mice that learned the task ($2p < 0.05$). (For full details, see reference 21 from which this figure is reproduced with permission.)

which another animal had recently been subjected to footshock was sufficient to trigger changes in DOPAC:DA ratios, MHPG:NE ratios, and plasma corticosterone similar to those observed in the shocked animals. We have found this to be a reproducible finding that substantiates the folklore of experimental psychology that fear can be smelled. We do not yet know the mechanism of this effect, but we suspect the involvement of an olfactory cue, because when the boxes are cleaned with ethanol–water mixtures and allowed to dry between animals, we do not observe such clear-cut effects, although we do observe small changes in the amine catabolites and plasma corticosterone associated with the handling (see, for example, FIGS. 10 and 11). We note that Tassin *et al.*[46] reported responses of prefrontal cortex DOPAC in mice after only 2 min in an open field.

It was of interest to examine the response to a rather different kind of stressor (one to which humans can relate), a virus infection. We injected mice with Newcastle disease virus (NDV), a chicken virus that does not reproduce in mice, but which causes a temporary fever (approximately 2°) peaking at 2 hr, and a delayed increase in plasma corticosterone.[47,48] At the peak of the plasma corticosterone response, 8 hr after injection, we found significant changes in biogenic amine catabolites that resembled those we observed following footshock or restraint. DOPAC:DA and HVA:DA ratios in the brain stem were significantly increased (FIG. 13). MHPG:NE ratios were also increased in the hypothalamus and brain stem. Tryptophan was significantly increased in all three brain regions. Interestingly, there were no statistically significant changes of DOPAC, MHPG, or 5-HIAA in the prefrontal cortex. This may indicate the absence of a classical sensory component to the stress. However, an alternative explanation is that changes in the prefrontal cortex may have occurred at an earlier time point, which we have not yet tested. These changes in brain biogenic amine metabolism indicate clearly that

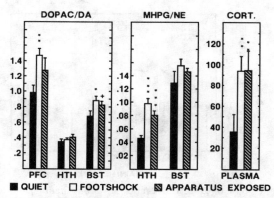

**FIGURE 12.** Responses of DOPAC:DA and MHPG:NE ratios and plasma corticosterone (CORT ng/ml) of mice exposed to an apparatus in which mice had previously been shocked. Mice were shocked as in the experiment of FIGURE 1, and a second group of mice was placed in the shock boxes shortly after this, but without cleaning the boxes. *Solid bars*: quiet mice; *open bars*: mice footshocked as in FIGURE 1; *shaded bars*: mice placed in the apparatus without shock. *Significantly different from quiet mice ($p < 0.05$; **$2p < 0.01$; ***$2p < 0.001$; $^{+}2p < 0.1$: $n = 6$).

events in the periphery involving the immune system are communicated to the brain. We believe that the mechanism involves a polypeptide produced by immune cells, interleukin-1 (IL-1), which is known to be synthesized and secreted following NDV infection, and which is believed to be involved in the production of fever.[49]

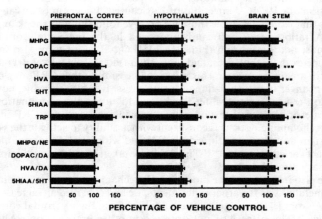

**FIGURE 13.** Responses of biogenic amines and catabolites to injection of Newcastle disease virus (NDV). Mice were injected ip with 0.3 ml (750 HA units) of NDV or allantoic fluid (vehicle) and brain samples collected 8 hr later. The data are combined results of 7 separate experiments involving intact and hypophysectomized mice. *Significantly different from vehicle (ANOVA $p < 0.05$, **$p < 0.01$, ***$p < 0.001$, $^{+}p < 0.1$). In intact animals alone, there were also statistically significant increases in MHPG in prefrontal cortex, DOPAC:DA, HVA:DA, and 5-HIAA:5-HT ratios in hypotholamus, and 5-HIAA:5-HT ratios in brain stem. (For full details, see reference 48 from which these data are derived.)

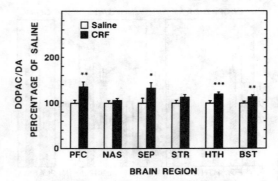

**FIGURE 14.** The response of DOPAC:DA ratios in various brain regions to the injection of CRF. Human/rat CRF (1 μg) or saline was injected ICV into mice and brain regions sampled 30 min later. The combined results of three separate experiments. *Significantly different from saline ($p < 0.05$, **$p < 0.01$, ***$p < 0.001$, ANOVA). (For full details, see reference 51 from which this figure is reproduced with permission.)

We have also investigated potential endocrine mediation of the cerebral catecholamine changes. We have observed no changes of biogenic amines or catabolites following injections of corticosterone (0.5–2.0 mg/kg SC), and the changes in tryptophan or catecholamine catabolites observed following footshock or restraint are not altered in adrenalectomized animals.[16,50] We have also not observed significant changes following peripheral injections of ACTH (0.1–0.5 μg/g ACTH $_{1-24}$ SC), although there were some small changes following intracerebroventricular (ICV) injections that we are continuing to investigate. However, there appear to be substantial changes following administration of CRF. ICV injections of 1 μg caused changes in brain catecholamine metabolites that closely resemble those we observe following footshock or restraint.[51] DOPAC:DA ratios were significantly increased in the prefrontal cortex, septum, hypothalamus, and brain stem (FIG. 14); MHPG:NE ratios were also increased in prefrontal cortex, hypothalamus, and brain stem (FIG. 15). However, tryptophan was not altered in any brain region. This raises the possibility that CRF may mediate intracerebral changes in catecholamines during stress. It is also possible, however, that the activation reflects a positive feedback loop to ensure the coordination of endocrine and catecholaminergic responses in stress.[5] Such a role for CRF in activating cerebral catecholamine systems is consistent with its ability to activate the sympathetic nervous system and the adrenal medulla,[52,53] and with its ability to mimic stresslike behaviors in a variety of tasks.[54-57] This evidence taken together could implicate CRF as the primary stress hormone.

We have also investigated the biochemical mechanisms of the effect on prefrontal cortex DA metabolism. In earlier experiments, we had observed an increase in the synthesis of DA from [³H]tyrosine in slices obtained from the prefrontal cortex of footshocked mice.[14] This effect was not observed in other brain regions. Although our preliminary investigations (like those of others[11,27]) did not reveal an effect on tyrosine hydroxylase (TH), we had studied this enzyme under assay conditions that might not have revealed an activation of the enzyme. Thus we reexamined TH, taking care to ensure that the assay conditions would reveal an activation of the enzyme by phosphorylation.[58] These precautions included performing the assay within a very short time after excision of the tissue, and including pyrophosphate in the homogenization buffer to inhibit protein phosphatases.[59] Under these conditions we found that a single

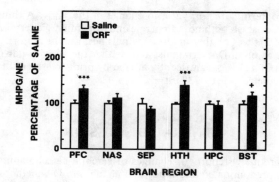

**FIGURE 15.** The response of MHPG:NE ratios in various brain regions to the injection of CRF. Human/rat CRF (1 µg) or saline was injected ICV into mice and brain regions sampled 30 min later. The same experiments as in FIGURE 14. *** Significantly different from saline ($p < 0.001$, $^+p < 0.1$: ANOVA). (For full details, see reference 51 from which this figure is reproduced with permission.)

period of footshock treatment increased the activity of TH from prefrontal cortex (FIG. 16). This effect was statistically significant only in the prefrontal cortex (and the hippocampus), although small increases also occurred in the nucleus accumbens and caudate–putamen.[58] It is interesting, nevertheless, that the magnitudes of the effects on TH in the major DA terminal regions paralleled those on DOPAC:DA ratios, perhaps suggesting a coupling between release and TH activation. The effect was also observed in rats, and with restraint stress in mice. If pyrophosphate was not included in the homogenized buffer or the homogenate was preincubated (permitting dephosphorylation), no increase in activity was detected. The characteristics of the activated enzyme indicated that the major change was an increase in the affinity of the enzyme

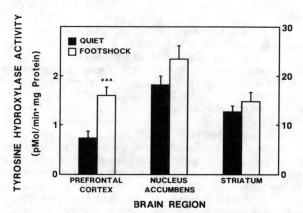

**FIGURE 16.** The effect of footshock on tyrosine hydroxylase (TH) activity in the prefrontal cortex, nucleus accumbens, and caudate–putamen. Mice were footshocked as in the experiment of FIGURE 5. TH was assayed under conditions of suboptimal tetrahydropterin cofactor, and in the presence of pyrophosphate. ***Significantly different from the quiet group (Student's $t$-test: $p < 0.001$: $n = 10$). (For full details, see reference 58 from which these data are derived.)

for its tetrahydropterin cofactor, with no change in the $V_{max}$. Although TH in the prefrontal cortex exists in both noradrenergic and dopaminergic terminals, we believe that the major effect was on that in DA terminals because the majority of TH in this region is known to be in DA terminals, and neither the activity nor the magnitude of the activation of TH was significantly altered by prior treatment of the mice with DSP-4, which depleted NE by 73%.[58]

## GENERAL DISCUSSION

Whereas there are many reports of changes of cerebral catecholamine metabolism, data on NE has predominated and reports of changes in DA metabolism have been less common. Nevertheless, as previously discussed, a significant number of reports have suggested stress-related changes in cerebral DA metabolism. Although many of these have concerned the activation of prefrontal cortex DA terminals, several reports have concerned whole brain[18,19] in which the changes reported cannot have derived solely from this structure that contains only a small proportion of brain DA. For example, Bliss and Ailion found a footshock-induced increased rate of loss of whole brain DA following αMPT treatment, and an increase of homovanillic acid (HVA) in rats following footshock or restraint.[19] Several studies have indicated a reactivity of the nucleus accumbens in stress.[8,10,11,16,20,30,38] Others have noted changes in the hypothalamus.[60] But, still others have noted responses in the striatum.[20,25,29] Most notably, several authors have noted changes of DA release in this structure using *in vivo* voltammetry.[28,30,61,62] Thus these data are generally consistent with our conclusion that there is a global activation of cerebral dopaminergic systems in the brain to parallel the activation of noradrenergic systems during stress. The relative ease with which changes have been observed in the latter may reflect the more tightly coupled feedback mechanisms for the regulation of synthesis in DA relative to NE systems.[2,3,18] This results in the larger changes evident in MHPG, relative to those in DOPAC (see FIGS. 4, 7, and 8) and accounts for the relatively frequent reports of depletions of NE but not DA.[3,18]

We suspect that the reason reports of changes in DOPAC from prefrontal cortex have predominated in the literature is the relatively large magnitude of the stress-related increases in this region, which can approach 100% in the medial division of prefrontal cortex. This is in turn almost certainly due to the relative inactivity of presynaptic autoreceptors in this region. Although it has been suggested that there are no effective presynaptic autoreceptors regulating DA synthesis and release in prefrontal cortex, contrasted with the very effective feedback control in the striatum,[63] more recent studies have indicated the presence of release-inhibiting presynaptic autoreceptors on DA terminals in prefrontal cortex (see reference 64).

We have shown that changes in DA metabolism occur in many brain areas after a variety of different stressors in mice and rats. These changes parallel those observed in NE metabolism, but are the changes truly indicative of stress? The metabolic changes in DA, even in the medial prefrontal cortex, are considerably smaller, and perhaps less sensitive than the changes in plasma corticosterone (see FIGS. 10 and 11). Clearly we need to study other behavioral situations and to manipulate the brain systems to determine which responses are primary and which are secondary, because there is good evidence for complex positive feedback between the catecholaminergic and hypothalamic–pituitary–adrenal (HPA) systems.[5]

It is also clear that we need to revise and refine our concepts of stress. The types of stress that are adequate to initiate activation of cerebral and autonomic catecholaminergic systems and the HPA axis are clearly far less than those required to produce such stress-related phenomena as gastric ulceration, "learned helplessness," and perhaps immunosuppression. Should we then consider the two sets of phenomena causally related? I suggest that the initial response to a novel environmental situation in animals is a coordinated activation of the HPA and catecholaminergic systems, which perhaps we should call arousal rather than stress. If the animal recognizes the situation and considers that it can cope, these activations are turned off, and the potential stress is removed. If not, the activation continues, perhaps fed by positive feedback mechanisms to become more stressful. It is not clear that stress is qualitatively different from the initial arousal, although it may be. However, quantitative factors including the duration of the activation may ultimately account for the qualitatively different behavioral and physiological changes associated with intense or prolonged stress.

## SUMMARY

The changes in dopamine catabolites in various regions of mouse brain have been studied following a variety of behavioral treatments. In confirmation of the results of many others, we find that treatments such as footshock or restraint result in a pronounced activation of dopaminergic systems in the prefrontal cortex, as determined by increases in the content of DOPAC (3,4-dihydroxyphenylacetic acid). However, we also find small but statistically significant increases of DOPAC in the hypothalamus and brain stem even with mild treatments. With restraint and more intense footshock we observe increases of DOPAC in all regions studied, including nucleus accumbens, olfactory tubercle, amygdala, and the striatum. Thus in contrast to previous reports, we find that the DA response in stress is global like that of norepinephrine [as determined by increases of 3-methoxy,4-hydroxyphenylethyleneglycol, (MHPG)], and not specific to the prefrontal cortex. The activation of prefrontal cortex DA metabolism is associated with an activation of the synthetic enzyme tyrosine hydroxylase.

The response pattern of catecholamine metabolites is similar following a variety of stressors, including conditioned footshock, training with one footshock in passive avoidance behavior, performance of passive avoidance behavior, and even following exposure to an apparatus in which mice have been shocked previously. Injection of mice with Newcastle disease virus increases plasma corticosterone, and DOPAC and MHPG in the hypothalamus and brain stem, but not the prefrontal cortex. Thus a virus infection can be considered a stressor. Furthermore, intracerebroventricular (ICV) injection of corticotropin-releasing factor (CRF) produces stresslike increases in DOPAC and MHPG concentrations, suggesting that the release of CRF in the brain during stress may mediate the changes in catecholamine metabolism.

## ACKNOWLEDGMENTS

The skilled technical assistance of Karen Green, Bill Moreshead, and Bunnie Powell is gratefully acknowledged.

## REFERENCES

1.  CANNON, W. B. 1914. The emergency function of the adrenal medulla in pain and the major emotions. Am. J. Physiol. **33:** 356–372.
2.  THIERRY, A.-M., F. JAVOY, J. GLOWINSKI & S. S. KETY. 1968. Effects of stress on the metabolism of norepinephrine, dopamine and serotonin in the central nervous system of the rat. J. Pharmacol. Exp. Ther. **163:** 163–171.
3.  STONE, E. A. 1975. Stress and catecholamines. *In* Catecholamines and Behavior. Vol. 2 Neuropsychopharmacology. A. J. Friedhoff, Ed.: 31–72. Plenum. New York.
4.  ANISMAN, H. 1978. Neurochemical changes elicited by stress. *In* Psychopharmacology of Aversively Motivated Behavior. H. Anisman and G. Bignami, Eds.: 119–172. Plenum. New York.
5.  DUNN, A. J. & N. R. KRAMARCY. 1984. Neurochemical responses in stress: Relationships between the hypothalamic-pituitary-adrenal and catecholamine systems. *In* Handbook of Psychopharmacology, Vol. 18. L. L. Iversen, S. D. Iversen, and S. H. Snyder, Eds.: 455–515. Plenum. New York.
6.  AXELROD, J. & T. D. REISINE. 1984. Stress hormones: Their interaction and regulation. Science **224:** 452–459.
7.  GLAVIN, G. B. 1985. Stress and brain noradrenaline: A review. Neurosci. Biobehav. Rev. **9:** 233–243.
8.  THIERRY, A. M., J. P. TASSIN, G. BLANC & J. GLOWINSKI. 1976. Selective activation of the mesocortical DA system by stress. Nature **263:** 242–244.
9.  LAVIELLE, S., J.-P. TASSIN, A.-M. THIERRY, G. BLANC, D. HERVE, C. BARTHELEMY & J. GLOWINSKI. 1979. Blockade by benzodiazepines of the selective high increase in dopamine turnover induced by stress in mesocortical dopaminergic neurons of the rat. Brain Res. **168:** 585–594.
10. FADDA, F., A. ARGIOLAS, M. R. MELIS, A. H. TISSARI, P. L. ONALI & G. L. GESSA. 1978. Stress-induced increase in 3,4-dihydroxyphenylacetic acid (DOPAC) levels in the cerebral cortex and in n. accumbens: Reversal by diazepam. Life Sci. **23:** 2219–2224.
11. TISSARI, A. H., A. ARGIOLAS, F. FADDA, G. SERRA & G. L. GESSA. 1979. Foot-shock stress accelerates non-striatal dopamine synthesis without activating tyrosine hydroxylase. Naunyn-Schmiedeberg's Arch. Pharmacol. **308:** 155–157.
12. REINHARD, J. F., M. J. BANNON & R. H. ROTH. 1982. Acceleration by stress of dopamine synthesis and metabolism in prefrontal cortex: Antagonism by diazepam. Naunyn-Schmiedeberg's Arch. Pharmacol. **318:** 374–377.
13. BANNON, M. J. & R. H. ROTH. 1983. Pharmacology of mesocortical dopamine neurons. Pharmacol. Rev. **35:** 53–68.
14. KRAMARCY, N. R., R. L. DELANOY & A. J. DUNN. 1984. Footshock treatment activates catecholamine synthesis in slices of mouse brain regions. Brain Res. **290:** 311–319.
15. DUNN, A. J. 1984. Regional responses of biogenic amine catabolites to stressors in the mouse. Trans. Am. Soc. Neurochem. **15:** 203.
16. CLAUSTRE, Y., J. P. RIVY, T. DENNIS & B. SCATTON. 1986. Pharmacological studies on stress-induced increase in frontal cortical dopamine metabolism in the rat. J. Pharmacol. Exp. Ther. **238:** 693–700.
17. DUNN, A. J. 1987. Footshock or restraint stress causes a general activation of cerebral noradrenergic and dopaminergic systems. Psychoneuroendocrinol. In press.
18. BLISS, E. L., J. AILION & J. ZWANZIGER. 1968. Metabolism of norepinephrine, serotonin and dopamine in rat brain with stress. J. Pharmacol. Exp. Ther. **164:** 122–134.
19. BLISS, E. L. & J. AILION. 1971. Relationship of stress and activity to brain dopamine and homovanillic acid. Life Sci. Part I, **10:** 1161–1169.
20. DUNN. A. J. & S. E. FILE. 1983. Cold restraint alters dopamine metabolism in frontal cortex, nucleus accumbens and neostriatum. Physiol. Behav. **31:** 511–513.
21. DUNN, A. J., K. L. ELFVIN & C. W. BERRIDGE. 1986. Changes in plasma corticosterone and cerebral biogenic amines and their catabolites during training and testing of mice in passive avoidance behavior. Behav. Neural Biol. **46:** 410–423.
22. UNDERWOOD. R. H. & G. H. WILLIAMS. 1972. The simultaneous measurement of aldosterone,

cortisol, and corticosterone in human peripheral plasma by displacement analysis. J. Lab. Clin. Med. **79:** 848–862.

23. GWOSDOW-COHEN, A., C. L. CHEN & E. L. BESCH. 1982. Radioimmunoassay (RIA) of serum corticosterone in rats. Proc. Soc. Exp. Biol. Med. **170:** 29–34.

24. WARSH, J. J., D. GODSE, S. W. CHEUNG & P. P. LI. 1981. Rat brain and plasma norepinephrine glycol metabolites determined by gas chromatography-mass fragmentography. J. Neurochem. **36:** 893–901.

25. HUTCHINS, D. A., J. D. M. PEARSON & D. F. SHARMAN. 1975. Striatal metabolism of dopamine in mice made aggressive by isolation. J. Neurochem. **24:** 1151–1154.

26. CURZON, G., P. H. HUTSON & P. J. KNOTT. 1979. Voltammetry in vivo: Effect of stressful manipulations and drugs on the caudate nucleus of the rat. Brit. J. Pharmacol. **66:** 127–128P.

27. KENNEDY, L. T. & M. J. ZIGMOND. 1980. Effects of restraint on dopamine turnover and tyrosine hydroxylase activity in rat frontal cortex. Soc. Neurosci. Abstr. **6:** 44.

28. KELLER, R. W., E. M. STRICKER & M. J. ZIGMOND. 1983. Environmental stimuli but not homeostatic challenges produce apparent increases in dopaminergic activity in the striatum: An analysis by in vivo voltammetry. Brain Res. **279:** 159–170.

29. CULMAN, J., C. C. CHIUEH, M. KOULU & I. J. KOPIN. 1984. Effect of acute restraint stress on dopamine and serotonin turnover in nigrostriatal and mesolimbic dopaminergic systems. Soc. Neurosci. Abstr. **10:** 65.

30. WATANABE, H. 1984. Activation of dopamine synthesis in mesolimbic dopamine neurons by immobilization stress in the rat. Neuropharmacology **23:** 1335–1338.

31. BLANK, C. L., S. SASA, R. ISERNHAGEN, L. R. MEYERSON, D. WASSIL, P. WONG, A. T. MODAK & W. B. STAVINOHA. 1979. Levels of norepinephrine and dopamine in mouse brain regions following microwave inactivation — Rapid post-mortem degradation of striatal dopamine in decapitated animals. J. Neurochem. **33:** 213–219.

32. PONZIO, F., G. ACHILLI & S. ALGERI. 1981. A rapid and simple method for the determination of picogram levels of 3-methoxytyramine in brain tissue using liquid chromatography with electrochemical detection. J. Neurochem. **36:** 1361–1367.

33. ISHIKAWA, K., S. SHIBANOKI, S. SAITO & J. L. MCGAUGH. 1982. Effect of microwave irradiation on monoamine metabolism in dissected rat brain. Brain Res. **240:** 158–161.

34. WESTERINK, B. H. C., F. J. BOSKER & E. WIRIX. 1984. Formation and metabolism of dopamine in nine areas of the rat brain: Modifications by haloperidol. J. Neurochem. **42:** 1321–1327.

35. IKARASHI, Y., T. SASAHARA & Y. MARUYAMA. 1985. Postmortem changes in catecholamines, indoleamines, and their metabolites in rat brain regions: Prevention with 10-kW microwave irradiation. J. Neurochem. **45:** 935–939.

36. MOCHETTI, I., L. DE ANGELIS & G. RACAGNI. 1981. Postmortem changes of normetanephrine determined by a mass-fragmentographic technique in different rat brain areas. J. Neurochem. **37:** 1607–1609.

37. CURZON, G., M. H. JOSEPH & P. J. KNOTT. 1972. Effects of immobilization and food deprivation on rat brain tryptophan metabolism. J. Neurochem. **19:** 1967–1974.

37a. DUNN, A. J. 1988. Changes in plasma and brain tryptophan and brain serotonin and 5-hydroxyindoleacetic acid after footshock stress. Life Sci. **42:** 1847–1853.

38. HERMAN, J. P., D. GUILLONNEAU, R. DANTZER, B. SCATTON, L. SEMERDJIAN-ROUQUIER & M. LE MOAL. 1982. Differential effects of inescapable footshocks and of stimuli previously paired with inescapable footshocks on dopamine turnover in cortical and limbic areas of the rat. Life Sci. **30:** 2207–2214.

39. AKIJA, K., D. P. KALRA, C. P. FAWCETT, L. KRULICH & S. M. MCCANN. 1972. The effect of stress and nembutal on plasma levels of gonadotropins and prolactin in ovariectomized rats. Endocrinology **90:** 707–715.

40. MOORE, K. E. & K. T. DEMAREST. 1982. Tuberoinfundibular and tuberohypophyseal dopaminergic neurons. *In* Frontiers in Neuroendocrinology. Vol. 7. L. Martini and W. F. Ganong, Eds.: 161–190. Raven Press. New York.

41. FUXE, K., K. ANDERSSON, P. ENEROTH, R. A. SIEGEL & L. F. AGNATI. 1983. Immobilization stress-induced changes in discrete hypothalamic catecholamine levels and turnover,

their modulation by nicotine and relationship to neuroendocrine function. Acta Physiol. Scand. **117:** 421–426.

42. DEMAREST, K. T., K. E. MOORE & G. D. RIEGLE. 1985. Acute restraint stress decreases dopamine synthesis and turnover in the median eminence: A model for the study of the inhibitory neuronal influences on tuberoinfundibular dopaminergic neurons. Neuroendocrinology **41:** 437–444.

43. DEMAREST, K. T., K. E. MOORE & G. D. RIEGLE. 1985. Acute restraint stress decreases tuberoinfundibular dopaminergic neuronal activity: Evidence for a differential response in male versus female rats. Neuroendocrinology **41:** 504–510.

44. CASSENS, G., M. ROFFMAN, A. KURUC, P. J. ORSULAK & J. J. SCHILDKRAUT. 1980. Alterations in brain norepinephrine metabolism induced by environmental stimuli previously paired with inescapable shock. Science **209:** 1138–1140.

45. IIMORI, K., M. TANAKA, Y. KOHNO, Y. IDA, R. NAKAGAWA, Y. HOAKI, A. TSUDA & N. NAGASAKI. 1982. Psychological stress enhances noradrenaline turnover in specific brain regions in rats. Pharmacol. Biochem. Behav. **16:** 637–640.

46. TASSIN, J. P., D. HERVE, G. BLANC & J. GLOWINSKI. 1980. Differential effects of a two-minute open-field session on dopamine utilization in the frontal cortices of BALB/c and C57 BL/6 mice. Neurosci. Lett. **17:** 67–71.

47. SMITH, E. M., W. J. MEYER & J. E. BLALOCK. 1982. Virus-induced corticosterone in hypophysectomized mice: A possible lymphoid adrenal axis. Science **218:** 1311.

48. DUNN, A. J., M. L. POWELL, W. V. MORESHEAD, J. M. GASKIN & N. R. HALL. 1987. Effects of Newcastle disease virus to mice on the metabolism of cerebral biogenic amines, plasma corticosterone, and lymphocyte proliferation. Brain, Behav. Immun. **1:** 216–230.

49. DINARELLO, C. A. 1984. Interleukin-1. Rev. Infect. Dis. **6:** 51–95.

50. DUNN A. J. 1988. Stress-related changes in cerebral catecholamine and indoleamine metabolism: Lack of effect of adrenalectomy and corticosterone. J. Neurochem. In press.

51. DUNN, A. J. & C. W. BERRIDGE. 1987. Corticotropin-releasing factor administration elicits a stress-like activation of cerebral catecholaminergic systems. Pharmacol. Biochem. Behav. **27:** 685–691.

52. BROWN, M. R. & L. A. FISHER. 1985. Corticotropin-releasing factor: Effects on the autonomic nervous system and visceral systems. Fed. Proc., Fed. Am. Soc. Exp. Biol. **44:** 243–248.

53. KUROSAWA, M., A. SATO, R. S. SWENSON & Y. TAKAHASHI. 1986. Sympatho-adrenal medullary functions in response to intracerebroventricularly injected corticotropin-releasing factor in anesthetized rats. Brain Res. **367:** 250–257.

54. BRITTON, D. R., G. F. KOOB, J. RIVIER & W. VALE. 1982. Intraventricular corticotropin-releasing factor enhances behavioral effects of novelty. Life Sci. **31:** 363–367.

55. MORLEY, J. E. & A. S. LEVINE. 1982. Corticotrophin releasing factor, grooming and ingestive behavior. Life Sci. **31:** 1459–1464.

56. BERRIDGE, C. W. & A. J. DUNN. 1986. Corticotropin-releasing factor elicits naloxone-sensitive stress-like alterations in exploratory behavior in mice. Regul. Peptides **16:** 83–93.

57. DUNN, A. J. & S. E. FILE. 1987. Corticotropin-releasing factor has an anxiogenic action in the social interaction test. Horm. Behav. **21:** 193–202.

58. IUVONE, P. M. & A. J. DUNN. 1986. Tyrosine hydroxylase activation in mesocortical 3,4-dihydroxyphenylethylamine neurons following footshock. J. Neurochem. **47:** 837–844.

59. IUVONE, P. M., A. L. RAUCH, P. B. MARSHBURN, D. B. GLASS & N. H. NEFF. 1982. Activation of retinal tyrosine hydroxylase in vitro by cyclic AMP-dependent protein kinase: Characterization and comparison to activation in vivo by photic stimulation. J. Neurochem. **39:** 1632–1651.

60. ROTH, K. A., S. L. McINTIRE, R. G. LORENZ & J. D. BARCHAS. 1982. Hypothalamic catecholamine changes under acute stress occur independently of nicotinic stimulation. Neurosci. Lett. **28:** 47–50.

61. IKEDA, M., Y. HIRATA, K. FUJITA, M. SHINZATO, H. TAKAHASHI, S. YAGYU & T. NAGATSU. 1984. Effects of stress on release of dopamine and serotonin in the striatum of spontaneously hypertensive rats: An in vivo voltammetry study. Neurochem. Int. **6:** 509–512.

62. IKEDA, M. & T. NAGATSU. 1985. Effect of short-term swimming stress and diazepam on 3,4-dihydroxyphenylacetic acid (DOPAC) and 5-hydroxyindoleacetic acid (5-HIAA) levels

in the caudate nucleus: An in vivo voltammetric study. Naunyn-Schmiedeberg's Arch. Pharmacol. **331:** 23–26.

63. BANNON, M. J., R. A. MICHAUD & R. H. ROTH. 1981. Mesocortical dopamine neurons: Lack of autoreceptors modulating dopamine synthesis. Mol. Pharmacol. **19:** 270–275.
64. TALMACIU, R. K., I. S. HOFFMANN & L. X. CUBEDDU. 1986. Dopamine autoreceptors modulate dopamine release from the prefrontal cortex. J. Neurochem. **47:** 865–870.

# Mesocorticolimbic Dopamine Systems and Reward

H. C. FIBIGER[a] AND A. G. PHILLIPS[b]

[a]Division of Neurological Sciences
Department of Psychiatry

[b]Department of Psychology
University of British Columbia
Vancouver, B.C., Canada V6T 1W5

## INTRODUCTION

Research during the past decade has generated a substantial body of evidence indicating that mesolimbic dopamine (DA) neurons are an important link in the neural circuitry of reward. Most of this evidence is based on the application of three procedures that are now commonly used to study reward mechanisms: intracranial self-stimulation, intravenous self-administration, and conditioned place preference. Some of the data that have been generated by each approach and that are relevant to the mesolimbic DA hypothesis of reward are reviewed below.

## INTRACRANIAL SELF-STIMULATION

Early indications that DA neurons may be involved in intracranial self-stimulation (ICS) came from studies that indicated that positive electrode sites were located in the region of the substantia nigra and ventral tegmental area (VTA).[1,2] Subsequently, Corbett and Wise[3] used movable stimulating electrodes in conjunction with fluorescence histochemistry to map the midbrain and caudal diencephalon for ICS. These investigators found that positive ICS sites were confined to the layer of DA-containing cell bodies in the mesencephalon, and that ICS current thresholds and response rates were proportional to the density of dopaminergic neurons surrounding the electrode tip. The VTA in particular has been found to be a region from which very high rates of self-stimulation can be obtained.

Pharmacological studies have provided considerable support for the role of DA neurons in brain stimulation reward, despite the fact that interpretation of results has sometimes been difficult. In particular, drugs that block DA receptors (e.g., haloperidol, spiroperidol, pimozide, alpha-flupenthixol) attenuate ICS in a dose-related manner (for reviews see Fibiger,[4] Wise,[5] Fibiger and Phillips[6]). Unfortunately, many of the early pharmacological studies suffered from a failure to distinguish between attenuation of reward processes and the performance deficits that are produced by neuroleptic agents.[4] More recently a considerable amount of research has been devoted to analyzing the mechanisms by which neuroleptics decrease ICS. The majority of this work indicated that although neuroleptic compounds, particularly at higher doses, can decrease self-stimulation rates by producing motoric impairments, these DA receptor antagonists also clearly serve to decrease the reinforcing effects of brain stimulation. Perhaps

206

the strongest support for attenuation of brain stimulation reward by neuroleptics has been generated by studies in which the role of performance variables was minimized by employing rate-free test paradigms. A good example of this approach is the current titration procedure employed by Zarevics and Setler[7] to establish intensity thresholds for reward in drugged and nondrugged animals. Pimozide caused a significant increase in the threshold currents required to maintain ICS responding, thereby indicating that the drug reduced the rewarding value of brain stimulation. Using a similar approach, Esposito et al.[8] found that low doses of haloperidol produced a significant increase in the reward threshold for stimulation of the medial forebrain bundle.

In an attempt to determine the anatomical substrate at which systemic injections of neuroleptics decrease the rewarding impact of brain stimulation, Mogenson et al.[9] found that unilateral injections of the DA receptor antagonist spiroperidol into the nucleus accumbens significantly reduced ICS of the ipsilateral VTA, but did not affect ICS rates obtained from the contralateral VTA. The contrasting effects of the ipsilateral and contralateral nucleus accumbens injections on VTA–ICS indicate that spiroperidol-induced motor deficits could not account for these observations. The specificity of the effect of the ipsilateral nucleus accumbens injections was also demonstrated by the finding that injections of spiroperidol into either the ipsilateral or contralateral prefrontal cortex did not affect VTA–ICS. Therefore, in contrast to the nucleus accumbens, DA receptors in the prefrontal cortex do not appear to be important for mediating the rewarding effects of VTA–ICS. As is discussed below, similar conclusions have been reached with respect to the rewarding properties of intravenously self-administered stimulants such as cocaine and d-amphetamine.

Paralleling the studies on the effects of DA receptor antagonists on ICS are a large number of experiments showing a facilitation of ICS by a variety of indirectly acting agonists that potentiate the function of catecholamine-containing neurons. Reuptake inhibitors such as cocaine enhance ICS.[10] Amphetamine also has potent facilitatory effects on ICS, as revealed by an increased response rate and decreased current threshold.[11] There is considerable evidence that these effects are mediated by dopaminergic mechanisms.[4,5]

Selective lesions of mesolimbic DA neurons also have been used to determine the extent to which stimulation of these neurons mediates some of the rewarding properties of ICS. Employing this strategy, Phillips and Fibiger,[12] found that 6-hydroxy-dopamine (6-OHDA) lesions of the ascending fibers of the mesotelencephalic DA projections resulted in marked decreases in rates of responding for ICS obtained from electrodes in the VTA. ICS obtained from electrodes in the frontal cortex or nucleus accumbens of the same animals was not as severely affected, suggesting that the marked effects on VTA–ICS could not be attributed entirely to lesion-induced motor deficits.

Subsequent work in our laboratories has confirmed and extended these findings.[13] Here again rats were trained to self-stimulate from electrodes in the VTA. In addition, ICS rate–current intensity functions were obtained. These functions determine the rate of responding for ICS at various brain-stimulation current intensities, and provide more detailed information than can be obtained with single-current intensities. After rate intensity functions had been obtained, the animals received 6-OHDA lesions of the mesotelencephalic DA projections at the level of the lateral hypothalamus. These lesions were either ipsilateral or contralateral to the ICS electrode in the VTA. The unilateral 6-OHDA lesions reduced DA concentrations in the nucleus accumbens, olfactory tubercle, and striatum by between 95 and 99% of control concentrations. The 6-OHDA lesions ipsilateral to the ICS electrode produced marked shifts to the right in the rate intensity functions. In contrast, identical lesions contralateral to the electrode failed to produce significant effects on the rate intensity function.

On the basis of ICS rate-stimulus frequency functions, Milliaressis et al.[14] have suggested that changes in the reinforcing efficacy of brain stimulation can be inferred from the shift in the number of rectangular pulses required for the threshold ($\Theta_0$) and half-maximal ($M_{50}$) performance, with the latter measure providing the more accurate index of reward efficacy. Although a sine wave stimulation current was used by Fibiger et al.[13] and current intensity (µamps) rather than pulse frequency was varied, analysis of these data in terms of $M_{50}$ and $\Theta_0$ indicated that the ipsilateral lesions significantly reduced both of these measures of reinforcement efficacy. In contrast, contralateral lesions did not affect either of these measures at any time after the lesions. According to these analyses, therefore, the ipsilateral lesions significantly decreased the reinforcing efficacy of the brain stimulation. In addition to this, however, it is noteworthy that the ipsilateral lesions also resulted in highly significant decreases in the asymptotic rates of responding. Several authors have suggested that decreases in the asymptotic rate of responding indicate that the experimental manipulation in question has interfered with the animal's performance capability.[14,15] According to this formulation, therefore, the ipsilateral lesions also resulted in motoric impairments that interfered with high rates of lever pressing. However, identical contralateral lesions failed to affect the ICS rate–current intensity function, including the asymptotic rate of responding; this dissociation suggests that unilateral lesions of the mesocorticolimbic pathway do not produce motoric impairments. From this pattern of results it may be inferred that changes in asymptotic rates of responding need not reflect changes in performance capacity under all circumstances. Specifically, very extensive lesions of an important reward-related projection may attenuate the value of the rewarding stimulation to such a degree that maximal prelesion rates of responding at electrode sites in this system may never be achieved, regardless of the current intensity employed.

As damage to the contralateral mesotelencephalic DA systems failed to produce significant changes in ICS, the rate intensity data obtained by Fibiger et al.[13] support an important role for DA in mediating the rewarding properties of electrical stimulation of the VTA. As such, these data confirm earlier studies with electrodes in the vicinity of dopaminergic cell bodies in the VTA[12] and axons in the lateral hypothalamus.[16]

Biochemical studies have also generated evidence that DA neurons are an important substrate for ICS obtained from electrodes in the VTA. A number of laboratories have demonstrated that electrical stimulation of the mesotelencephalic DA neurons increases 3,4-dihydroxyphenylacetic acid (DOPAC) and homovanillic acid (HVA) concentrations in the terminal regions of these neurons.[17-19] Because these studies were conducted in anesthetized animals, the relevance of the stimulation parameters to those used in ICS from the VTA is not clear. The first demonstration that DA metabolism, as expressed by the ratio of DOPAC to DA, was increased in the nucleus accumbens and frontal cortex of rats that self-stimulated through electrodes in the VTA was provided by Simon et al.[20] Subsequently, McCowan et al.[21] reported that ICS obtained from electrodes in the lateral hypothalamus did not increase DOPAC concentrations in the striatum, nucleus accumbens, or olfactory tubercles. It is noteworthy, however, that these authors failed to indicate that their DOPAC/DA ratios were increased by nearly 50% in the nucleus accumbens and by more than 100% in the olfactory tubercle of the self-stimulating animals. The ratio effect in the nucleus accumbens was confined to the side ipsilateral to the electrode, while in the olfactory tubercle it was increased bilaterally. Because ratio measures are more sensitive and appropriate indices of DA utilization than are metabolite concentrations, the data of McCowan et al.[21] do in fact support a role for DA neurons in ICS.

To provide additional information concerning the extent to which dopaminergic neurons are activated by ICS obtained from electrodes in the VTA, we recently undertook further experiments to determine the extent to which DA utilization is increased in three DA-rich forebrain regions after a period of self-stimulation.[13] ICS obtained from electrodes in the VTA produced significant increases in the DOPAC/DA and HVA/DA ratios in the striatum, nucleus accumbens, and olfactory tubercles on the side of the brain ipsilateral to the electrode. These increases ranged from a low of 25% in the DOPAC/DA ratio in the olfactory tubercle to a high of 64% in the HVA/DA ratio in the nucleus accumbens. The increases in the metabolite/DA ratios in the ICS group occurred only on the side of the brain ipsilateral to the electrode. Thus, in no instance was there a significant difference between the ratios obtained in the contralateral hemisphere of the ICS animals, and the values obtained in unstimulated controls. This indicates that the increases in DA metabolism observed in the ipsilateral forebrain regions of the ICS group were due to stimulation of the DA neurons, rather than a reflection of the high level of operant responding exhibited by these animals. Further indications that DA metabolism was not affected by the operant behavior *per se* was obtained in an experiment that examined the effects of high rates of lever pressing for food on DA metabolism. In this experiment, animals engaged in this behavior did not display altered rates of DA utilization in the striatum, nucleus accumbens, and olfactory tubercles.[13]

Another biochemical index of the effects of ICS obtained from electrodes in the VTA can be obtained by examining the rates at which 3,4-dihydroxyphenylalanine (DOPA) accumulates in the brain of animals that self-stimulate after inhibition of aromatic amino acid decarboxylase by NSD-1015.[22] This represents an *in vivo* measure of tyrosine hydroxylase activity, the rate-limiting enzyme in the synthesis of DA. Previous research has indicated that *in vivo* tyrosine hydroxylase activity increases in conditions where the physiological activity of dopaminergic neurons is enhanced.[23] In the study by Phillips *et al.*,[22] when compared to implanted unstimulated controls, DOPA concentrations were elevated significantly in the nucleus accumbens, striatum, and olfactory tubercle in the hemisphere ipsilateral to the VTA electrode after 30 minutes of self-stimulation. In agreement with the previously described DA metabolite studies, the concentration of DOPA in contralateral nucleus accumbens and striatum were not significantly different from control levels. In addition, a similar analysis of *in vivo* tyrosine hydroxylase activity in these brain regions following a 30-minute session of lever pressing for food on a fixed ratio (FR-8) schedule did not reveal significant changes relative to control subjects. These, and previous experiments[20] indicate that ICS obtained from electrodes in the VTA increases DA utilization in the major terminal regions of the mesotelencephalic DA systems.

## INTRAVENOUS SELF-ADMINISTRATION

The reinforcing properties of psychoactive drugs have been examined for two decades using the intravenous self-administration procedure developed by Weeks.[24] Alterations in the pattern of drug self-administration produced by specific antagonists or neurotoxins have been used to identify the possible neurochemical and neuroanatomical substrates of drug reinforcement. In the case of psychomotor stimulant drugs such as cocaine and amphetamine, much of this research has suggested that central DA systems play an important role in mediating the rewarding properties of these drugs. For example, Yokel and Wise[25] found that low doses of specific DA receptor antagonists such as pimozide and (+)-butaclamol increased the rate of responding for intravenous injections of d-amphetamine by rats. These results indicated that low doses of the antagonists may have reduced the reinforcing properties of amphetamine by partial blockade of DA receptors, so that higher doses of amphetamine were required to maintain the preferred level of occupancy of postsynaptic DA receptors by DA.

Similar results were observed in animals that self-administer cocaine.[26,27] These pharmacological studies suggested that some of the reinforcing effects of indirectly acting DA receptor agonists such as cocaine and d-amphetamine are due to the ability of these compounds to increase the synaptic concentrations of DA in the brain.

Several studies using 6-OHDA lesions in combination with intravenous self-administration have indicated that the reinforcing properties of stimulants such as cocaine and d-amphetamine are mediated by effects of these compounds on DA release in the nucleus accumbens. In one such study, Roberts et al.[27] trained rats to self-administer cocaine. After stable rates of responding were obtained, the animals received bilateral 6-OHDA lesions of the nucleus accumbens. In animals with extensive losses of DA in the nucleus accumbens there was a substantial decrease in the rate at which these animals lever-pressed for intravenous cocaine. Subsequently, Lyness et al.[28] found that 6-OHDA lesions of the nucleus accumbens produced similar reductions in the rate at which d-amphetamine was self-administered by rats.

Roberts et al.[29] analyzed the pattern of cocaine self-administration after 6-OHDA lesions of the nucleus accumbens. On the first day that cocaine was available after the 6-OHDA lesions, some animals responded rapidly during the early part of the 3-hr test session. The rate of responding then decreased gradually within the first session until there was little or no responding by the end of the 3 hours. Similar patterns were obtained on the following few days; however, the number of responses in the first part of the session was reduced and responding ceased at earlier times in the session. The high rate of responding for intravenous cocaine early in the first postlesion session indicated that the reduction in cocaine self-administration was not due to lesion-induced performance deficits. Perhaps more importantly, the pattern of cocaine self-administration after the 6-OHDA resembled a classic extinction effect, as characterized by high rates of responding when a reinforcer is first removed, followed by a gradual attenuation in responding as the animal learns that the operant response no longer results in the delivery of a reward. The data obtained by Roberts et al.[29] argued strongly that extensive decreases in DA concentrations in the nucleus accumbens produced by 6-OHDA lesions, are accompanied by a reduction or blockade of the reinforcing effects of intravenous cocaine. The data of Lyness et al.[28] also have suggested that DA terminals in the nucleus accumbens are important for the reinforcing effects of d-amphetamine. Further support for this hypothesis came from the demonstration that rats will respond for infusions of amphetamine directly into the nucleus accumbens.[30]

There is also evidence that cocaine may produce some of its reinforcing effects through its actions in the medial prefrontal cortex, a region like the nucleus accumbens, that is innervated by DA terminals originating from cell bodies in the VTA. Goeders and Smith[31] report that rats self-administered cocaine directly into the medial prefrontal cortex, but not into either the nucleus accumbens or VTA. In an attempt to examine the extent to which the reinforcing properties of intravenously administered cocaine are mediated by dopaminergic terminals in the medial prefrontal cortex, Martin-Iverson et al.[32] investigated the effect of destruction of DA-containing terminals in the medial prefrontal cortex on the rate and pattern of intravenous cocaine self-administration. Despite producing substantial depletions of DA in the medial prefrontal cortex, the 6-OHDA lesions did not affect either the rate or pattern of intravenous cocaine self-administration. These data indicate that although rats may respond for cocaine infusions directly into the medial prefrontal cortex, DA terminals in this structure do not contribute significantly to the rewarding action of intravenously administered cocaine.

At present the role of the mesolimbic DA projection in mediating the reinforcing properties of opiates is still uncertain. Bozarth and Wise[33] have demonstrated that rats will self-administer morphine directly into the VTA. In addition, rats will self-administer morphine and D-ala²-methionine enkephalin directly into the nucleus accumbens.[34] Vaccarino et al.[35] have reported that injections of low doses of methyl-naloxone into either the lateral ventricles or directly into the nucleus accumbens significantly increase the rate of intravenous heroin self-administration. Cocaine self-administration was not affected by these manipulations. Although these studies indicate that opiate receptors in the nucleus accumbens are important for mediating some of the reinforcing effects of opiates, there is evidence that these receptors may not be located on dopaminergic terminals. Pettit et al.[36] have observed that destruction of dopaminergic terminals in the nucleus accumbens with 6-OHDA substantially reduces cocaine self-administration, but does not block heroin self-administration in the same animals. This finding suggests that although opiate receptors in the nucleus accumbens may be important for mediating some of the rewarding properties of opiates, this may not be due to an opiate-induced increase in DA release in the nucleus accumbens. Further analysis of the role of the mesotelencephalic DA systems in opiate-induced reward is an important priority for future research.

## PLACE PREFERENCE CONDITIONING

The intracranial self-stimulation and intravenous self-administration procedures have provided valuable information concerning the neural substrates of reinforcement. A limitation of these approaches is that both require animals to perform complex motor responses, often signalled by a tone or light, while under the influence of an agent that may impair sensorimotor processes. An approach that circumvents these potential confounds is place preference conditioning. This technique is based on the fact that neutral environment stimuli paired with drug reinforcement can become conditioned reinforcers for which the animals will respond in the absence of the primary reinforcement produced by the drug. The conditioned place preference paradigm is useful in analyzing the neural mechanisms underlying drug reinforcement because the reward effect is indicated by a preference test conducted after the conditioning sessions and in the absence of the drug. Conditioned place preference is evaluated by the extent to which the undrugged animal approaches and spends time in a distinctive compartment previously paired with the drug. Systemic injections of amphetamine can produce conditioned place preferences.[37,38] The reinforcing properties of d-amphetamine, as assessed by the place preference conditioning procedure, appear to be mediated by the mesolimbic DA system. Spyraki et al.[39] found that amphetamine-induced place preference was blocked by systemic injections of haloperidol and was reduced by 6-OHDA lesions of the nucleus accumbens. The situation appears to be somewhat more complex with respect to nonamphetamine psychomotor stimulants. For example, although cocaine, nomifensine, and methylphenidate all produce conditioned place preferences, haloperidol has no effects on these conditioned preferences, except when very high doses of the neuroleptic are used.[40-42] Furthermore, in contrast to d-amphetamine, cocaine-induced place preferences are not affected by 6-OHDA lesions of the nucleus accumbens. In a study by Mithani et al.[41] haloperidol blocked locomotor activity stimulated by either d-amphetamine or methylphenidate. However, at the same doses the neuroleptic only blocked place preferences induced by d-amphetamine. While these results suggest that the locomotor stimulant properties of methylphenidate and d-amphetamine have common neural substrates, they raise the possibility that the reinforcing properties of these two drugs may be mediated by different mechanisms. The mechanisms by which nonamphetamine stimulants produce their reinforcing effects in the place preference paradigm have yet to be specified.

The extent to which the mesolimbic DA system mediates the reinforcing properties of opiates has also been studied using the conditioned place preference procedure. Schwartz and Marchok[43] first demonstrated that pretreatment with haloperidol blocked place preference conditioning produced by systemic injections of morphine. Subsequently, others reported that heroin-induced place preferences could be attenuated by neuroleptics.[33,44] Spyraki et al.[44] further found that 6-OHDA lesions of the nucleus accumbens reduced heroin-induced place preference conditioning. Additional evidence for a role of the mesolimbic DA system in opiate-induced reinforcement as assessed by place preference conditioning has been obtained in studies where opiates or analogues of enkephalin have been microinjected into discrete brain regions. Phillips and LePiane[45] demonstrated that morphine injections into the VTA could produce place preference conditioning. Place preference conditioning can also be obtained after injections of morphine into the nucleus accumbens.[46] Subsequently, Phillips et al.[47] used the conditioned place preference procedure to demonstrate rewarding properties of unilateral microinjections of (D-ala²)-met⁵-enkephalinamide (D-ALA) into the VTA of the rat. Place preference conditioning produced by this procedure was attenuated in a dose-related manner by systemic injections of haloperidol. In addition, 6-OHDA lesions of the ascending mesotelencephalic DA systems blocked this effect when the lesions were ipsilateral to the injection site in the VTA. Identical lesions in the contralateral hemisphere had no influence on the rewarding effects of intracerebral injections of D-ALA into the VTA. These studies suggest that neurons in the VTA are an important substrate for the rewarding effects of opiates and enkephalin. Furthermore, these data specifically indicate that dopaminergic neurons within the VTA mediate opioid-induced reward, at least when these compounds are directly applied to the VTA. The extent to which systemically administered opiates produce place preference conditioning by acting on systems in addition to the mesolimbic dopaminergic system requires further study.

## CONCLUSIONS

The data just reviewed leave little question that the mesolimbic dopaminergic system mediates some of the rewarding properties of brain-stimulation reward and both stimulant and opiate drugs. Although this general conclusion appears justified, there are many details and discrepancies that require further experimental analysis. For example, the failure of either neuroleptics or 6-OHDA lesions of the nucleus accumbens to block place preferences produced by nonamphetamine stimulants remains to be explained. Additionally, in the absence of potent effects of 6-OHDA lesions of the nucleus accumbens on intravenous self-administration of heroin, it may be concluded that dopaminergic terminals in this region of the forebrain are not involved critically in the reinforcing properties of systemically administered opiates. Nevertheless, several laboratories have demonstrated that activation of dopaminergic neurons in the VTA by opiates is reinforcing. These results indicate that the reinforcing properties of opiates are mediated by at least two distinct mechanisms in the central nervous system: opiate receptors on DA perikarya in the VTA, and opiate receptors on nondopaminergic elements in the nucleus accumbens.

The fact the mesolimbic DA system has reward-related functions raises a number of interesting questions concerning the normal role of this system in behavior. For example, it will be important to delineate the environmental stimuli that normally activate this system. In addition, the extent to which malfunction of this system may contribute to the symptomatology observed in some forms of depression is worthy of detailed investigation. In this regard, it is noteworthy that chronically administered antidepressant drugs appear to enhance the function of this reward-related system via currently unspecified mechanisms.[48] Finally, there is also substantial evidence indicating that the mesolimbic DA system mediates the locomotor stimulant properties of d-amphetamine and other stimulants. The extent to which the reward and motor stimulation functions of this system are related raises many interesting questions concerning the theoretical implications of such an arrangement.[6]

## REFERENCES

1. ROUTTENBERG, A. & C. MALSBURY. 1969. Brainstem pathways of reward. J. Comp. Physiol. Psychol. **68:** 22–30.
2. CROW, T. J. 1972. Catecholamine-containing neurones and electrical self-stimulation. 1. A review of some data. Psychol. Med. **2:** 414–421.
3. CORBETT, D. & R. A. WISE. 1980. Intracranial self-stimulation in relation to the ascending dopaminergic systems of the mid-brain: A moveable electrode mapping study. Brain Res. **185:** 1–15.
4. FIBIGER, H. C. 1978. Drugs and reinforcement: A critical review of the catecholamine theory. Annu. Rev. Pharmacol. Toxicol. **18:** 37–56.
5. WISE, R. A. 1978. Catecholamine theories of reward: A critical review. Brain Res. **152:** 215–247.
6. FIBIGER, H. C. & A. G. PHILLIPS. 1986. Reward, motivation, cognition: Psychobiology of mesotelencephalic dopamine systems. *In* Handbook of Physiology. The Nervous System, Vol. IV. F. E. Bloom and S. R. Geiger, Eds.: 647–675. American Physiological Society. Bethesda, Md.
7. ZAREVICS, P. & P. E. SETLER. 1979. Simultaneous rate-independent and rate-dependent assessment of intracranial self-stimulation: Evidence for the direct involvement of dopamine in brain reinforcement mechanisms. Brain Res. **169:** 499–512.
8. ESPOSITO, R. U., W. FAULKNER & C. KORNETSKY. 1979. Specific modulation of brain stimulation reward by haloperidol. Pharmacol. Biochem. Behav. **10:** 937–940.
9. MOGENSON, G. J., M. TAKIGAWA, A. ROBERTSON & M. WU. 1979. Self-stimulation of the nucleus accumbens and ventral tegmental area of Tsai attenuated by microinjections of spiroperidol into the nucleus accumbens. Brain Res. **171:** 247–259.
10. WAUQUIER, A. 1976. The influence of psychoactive drugs on brain self-stimulation in rats: A review. *In* Brain Stimulation Reward. A. Wauquier and E. T. Rolls, Eds.: 123–170. Elsevier. New York.
11. STEIN, L. 1964. Self-stimulation of the brain and the central stimulant action of amphetamine. Proc. Fed. Am. Soc. Exp. Biol. **23:** 836–841.
12. PHILLIPS, A. G. & H. C. FIBIGER. 1978. The role of dopamine in maintaining intracranial self-stimulation in the ventral tegmentum, nucleus accumbens, and medial prefrontal cortex. Can. J. Physiol. **32:** 58–66.
13. FIBIGER, H. C., F. G. LePIANE, A. JAKUBOVIC & A. G. PHILLIPS. 1987. The role of dopamine in intracranial self-stimulation of the ventral tegmental area. J. Neurosci. **7:** 3888–3896.
14. MILLIARESSIS, E., P.-P. ROMPRE, P. LAVIOLETTE, L. PHILLIPPE & D. COULOMBE. 1986. The curve-shift paradigm in self-stimulation. Physiol. Behav. **37:** 85–91.
15. EDMONDS, D. E. & C. R. GALLISTEL. 1974. Parametric analysis of brain-stimulation reward in the rat. III. Effect of performance variables on the reward summation function. J. Comp. Physiol. Psychol. **87:** 876–883.
16. KOOB, G. F., P. J. FRAY & S. D. IVERSEN. 1978. Self-stimulation at the lateral hypothalamus and locus coeruleus after specific unilateral lesions of the dopamine system. Brain Res. **146:** 123–140.
17. ROTH, R. H., L. C. MURRIN & J. R. WALTERS. 1976. Central dopaminergic neurons: Effects of alterations in impulse flow on the accumulation of dihydroxyphenylacetic acid. Eur. J. Pharmacol. **36:** 163–171.
18. KORF, J., L. GRASDIJK & B. H. C. WESTERINK. 1976. Effects of electrical stimulation of the nigrostriatal pathway of the rat on dopamine metabolism. J. Neurochem. **26:** 579–584.

19.  McCowan, T. J., R. B. Mueller & G. R. Breese. 1983. The effects of anesthetics and electrical stimulation on nigro-striatal dopaminergic neurons. J. Pharmacol. Exp. Ther. 224: 489–493.

20.  Simon, H., L. Stinus, J. P. Tassin, S. Lavielle, G. Blanc, A. M. Thierry, J. Glowinski & M. Le Moal. 1979. Is the dopaminergic mesocorticolimbic system necessary for intracranial self-stimulation? Biochemical and behavioral studies from A10 cell bodies and terminals. Behav. Neural. Biol. 27: 125–145.

21.  McCowan, T. J., T. C. Napier & G. R. Breese. 1986. Effects of chronic electrode implantation in dopaminergic neurons in vivo. Pharmacol. Biochem. Behav. 25: 63–69.

22.  Phillips, A. G., A. Jakubovic & H. C. Fibiger. 1987. Increased in vivo tyrosine hydroxylase activity in rat telencephalon produced by self-stimulation of the ventral tegmental area. Brain. Res. 402: 109–116.

23.  Murrin, L. C. & R. H. Roth. 1976. Dopaminergic neurons: Effects of electrical stimulation on dopamine biosynthesis. Mol. Pharmacol. 12: 463–475.

24.  Weeks, J. R. 1962. Experimental morphine addiction: Method for automatic intravenous injections in unrestrained rats. Science 138: 143–144.

25.  Yokel, R. A. & R. A. Wise. 1976. Attenuation of intravenous amphetamine reinforcement by central dopamine blockade in rats. Psychopharmacology 48: 311–318.

26.  DeWit, H. & R. S. Wise. 1977. Blockade of cocaine reinforcement in rats with the dopamine receptor blocker pimozide, but not with the noradrenergic blockers phentolamine and phenoxybenzamine. Can. J. Psychol. 31: 195–203.

27.  Roberts, D. C. S., M. E. Corcoran & H. C. Fibiger. 1977. On the role of ascending catecholaminergic systems in intravenous self-administration of cocaine. Pharmacol. Biochem. Behav. 6: 615–620.

28.  Lyness, W. H., N. M. Friedle & K. E. Moore. 1979. Destruction of dopaminergic nerve terminals in nucleus accumbens: Effect of d-amphetamine self-administration. Pharmacol. Biochem. Behav. 11: 553–556.

29.  Robert, D. C. S., G. F. Koob, P. Klonoff & H. C. Fibiger. 1980. Extinction and recovery of cocaine self-administration following 6-hydroxydopamine lesions of the nucleus accumbens. Pharmacol. Biochem. Behav. 12: 781–787.

30.  Hoebel, B. G., A. P. Monaco, L. Hernandez, F. F. Aulsi, B. G. Stanley & L. Lenard. 1983. Self-injection of amphetamine directly into the brain. Psychopharmacology 81: 158–163.

31.  Goeders, N. E. & J. E. Smith. 1983. Cortical dopaminergic involvement in cocaine reinforcement. Science 221: 773–775.

32.  Martin-Iverson, M. T., C. Szostak & H. C. Fibiger. 1986. 6-Hydroxydopamine lesions of the medial prefrontal cortex fail to influence intravenous self-administration of cocaine. Psychopharmacology 88: 310–314.

33.  Bozarth, M. A. & R. A. Wise. 1981. Heroin reward is dependent on a dopaminergic substrate. Life Sci. 29: 1881–1886.

34.  Goeders, N. E., J. D. Lane & J. E. Smith. 1984. Self-administration of methionine enkephalin into the nucleus accumbens. Pharmacol. Biochem. Behav. 20: 451–455.

35.  Vaccarino, F. J., F. E. Bloom & G. F. Koob. 1985. Blockade of nucleus accumbens opiate receptors attenuates intravenous heroin reward in the rat. Psychopharmacology 86: 37–42.

36.  Pettit, H. O., A. Ettenberg, F. E. Bloom & G. F. Koob. 1984. Destruction of dopamine in the nucleus accumbens selectively attenuates cocaine but not heroin self-administration in rats. Psychopharmacology 84: 167–173.

37.  Reicher, M. A. & E. W. Holman. 1977. Location preference and flavour aversion reinforced by amphetamine in rats. Anim. Learn. Behav. 5: 343–346.

38.  Sherman, J. E., T. Roberts, S. E. Roskam & E. W. Holman. 1980. Temporal properties of rewarding and aversive effects of amphetamine in rats. Pharmacol. Biochem. Behav. 13: 597–599.

39.  Spyraki, C., H. C. Fibiger & A. G. Phillips. 1982. Dopaminergic substrates of amphetamine-induced place preference conditioning. Brain Res. 253: 185–193.

40.  Martin-Iverson, M. T., R. Ortman & H. C. Fibiger. 1985. Place preference conditioning with methylphenidate and nomifensine. Brain Res. 332: 59–67.

41.  Mithani, S., M. T. Martin-Iverson & A. G. Phillips. 1986. The effects of haloperidol

on amphetamine- and methylphenidate-induced conditioned place preferences and loco-motor activity. Psychopharmacology **90:** 247–252.

42. SPYRAKI, C., H. C. FIBIGER & A. G. PHILLIPS. 1982. Cocaine-induced place preference conditioning: Lack of effects of neuroleptics and 6-hydroxydopamine lesions. Brain Res. **253:** 195–203.

43. SCHWARTZ, A. S. & P. L. MARCHOK. 1974. Depression of morphine-seeking behaviour by dopamine inhibition. Nature **248:** 257–258.

44. SPYRAKI, C., H. C. FIBIGER & A. G. PHILLIPS. 1983. Attenuation of heroin reward in rats by disruption of the mesolimbic dopamine system. Psychopharmacology **79:** 278–283.

45. PHILLIPS, A. G. & F. G. LePIANE. 1980. Reinforcing effects of morphine microinjection into the ventral tegmental area. Pharmacol. Biochem. Behav. **12:** 965–968.

46. VAN DER KOOY, D., R. F. MUCHA, M. O'SHAUGHNESSY & P. BUCKENIEKS. 1982. Reinforcing effects of brain microinjections of morphine revealed by conditioned place preference. Brain Res. **243:** 107–117.

47. PHILLIPS, A. G., F. G. LePIANE & H. C. FIBIGER. 1983. Dopaminergic mediation of reward produced by direct injection of enkephalin into the ventral tegmental area of the rat. Life Sci. **33:** 2505–2511.

48. FIBIGER, H. C. & A. G. PHILLIPS. 1987. Role of catecholamine transmitters in brain reward systems: Implications for the neurobiology of affect. *In* Brain Reward Systems and Abuse. J. Engel, L. Oreland, D. H. Ingvar, B. Pernow, S. Rössner, and L. A. Pellborn, Eds.: 61–74. Raven Press. New York.

# The Functional Output of the Mesolimbic Dopamine System

GEORGE F. KOOB[a] AND

NEAL R. SWERDLOW[b]

[a]Department of Basic and Clinical Research
Scripps Clinic and Research Foundation
La Jolla, California 92037

[b]Department of Psychiatry
University of California
San Diego, California 92093

## INTRODUCTION

The neural substrates for the behavioral expression of mesolimbic or mesocorticolimbic dopamine (DA) activity have been the focus of a substantial amount of interest in recent years for two major reasons. One centers on the repeated observation that direct administration of dopamine or dopamine agonists to the region of the nucleus accumbens (N. Acc.) produces increases in locomotor activity, and destruction of the dopamine projection to this region blocks many stimulant effects.

For example, 6-hydroxydopamine lesions of the region of the nucleus accumbens block the locomotor activation produced by amphetamine[1,2] and cocaine.[3] Such lesions also significantly attenuate the reinforcing properties of cocaine and amphetamine as measured with intravenous self-administration.[4-6] There also appears to be a role in motor activation for the dopamine projection to the nucleus accumbens independent of pharmacological challenges. Six-hydroxydopamine (6-OHDA) lesions of the nucleus accumbens attenuate stress, schedule, and food-deprivation-induced motor activation. Food-deprived rats with nucleus accumbens 6-hydroxydopamine lesions show less locomotor activity in a feeding situation and increases in food intake.[7] Rats with 6-hydroxydopamine lesions to the N. Acc. show decreases in locomotor activity in an open field test.[8,9] Also rats with N. Acc. 6-hydroxydopamine lesions show a decrease in acquisition of schedule-induced polydipsia[10] and the locomotor activation associated with such a schedule.[11]

The second major reason for interest in this brain area centers on neuroanatomical data showing that the nucleus accumbens receives afferent fibers not only from the ventral tegmental area but also from limbic regions such as the amygdala, hippocampus, and cingulate gyrus. This makes the region of the nucleus accumbens a locus for interactions of cortical and midbrain neuroanatomical convergence.

This extensive work describing a functional role for the dopamine projection to the nucleus accumbens has been extended to studies of the neural pathways from the N. Acc. to lower motor circuitry that are involved in modulating locomotor activity.[12,13] In a series of elegant studies, Mogenson and colleagues began to characterize the functional efferent output of the nucleus accumbens. Dopamine injected into the nucleus accumbens produced hyperactivity and this was reversed by injecting gamma-

216

aminobutyric acid (GABA) into the region of the ventral pallidum.[14] Together these results implicated GABA projections from the N. Acc. to the subpallidum in loco-motor activity. In addition, injections of the GABA antagonist, picrotoxin, into the ventral pallidum increased locomotor activity.[15]

## EFFECTS OF DESTRUCTION OF NUCLEUS ACCUMBENS DOPAMINE ON STIMULANT-ENHANCED LOCOMOTION

Another consequence of destruction of presynaptic DA terminals in the N. Acc. is the development of post-synaptic DA receptor supersensitivity that is evidenced bio-chemically by an increase in DA receptor number (B max) in this region,[16] and that is demonstrated behaviorally by a "supersensitive" locomotor response to the direct DA receptor agonist apomorphine.[3]

Animals tested with apomorphine show a clear dose-dependent motor activation that is greatly potentiated in 6-OHDA-injected animals, as indicated by a tenfold in-crease in sensitivity to apomorphine in 6-OHDA-, compared to vehicle-injected animals (FIG. 1). The highest dose of apomorphine (10.0 mg/kg) produced intense gnawing in 6-OHDA-injected animals, with a resultant decrease in locomotor activity.[17]

## EFFECTS OF ELECTROLYTIC- OR IBOTENIC ACID-INDUCED DESTRUCTION OF THE SUBSTANTIA INNOMINATA/LATERAL PREOPTIC AREA ON STIMULANT-ENHANCED LOCOMOTION

In our first attempt to determine the first-order efferent projections from the N. Acc. to the neurons that may eventually activate the spinal "final common pathway," the

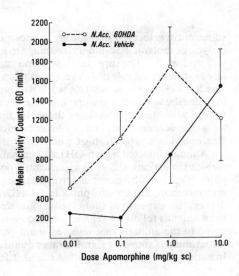

**FIGURE 1.** Locomotor activity elicited by various doses of apomorphine in rats fol-lowing sham and 6-OHDA lesions of the nu-cleus accumbens. Data represents means ($n$ = 4 each dose) ± SEM. (From Van der Kooy, Swerdlow, and Koob.[17] Reproduced by permission.)

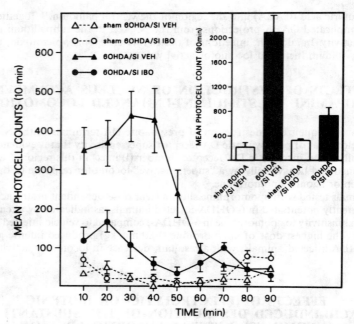

**FIGURE 2.** Locomotor activity following sc injection of 0.1-mg/kg apomorphine. Ordinate refers to mean photocell counts for each 10-min period for the groups represented as follows: △---△, sham 6-OHDA/SI vehicle ($n$ = 6); ○---○, sham 6-OHDA/SI ibotenic acid ($n$ = 6); ▲- - -▲, 6-OHDA/SI vehicle ($n$ = 10); ●---●, 6-OHDA/SI ibotenic acid ($n$ = 9). Statistical analysis was accomplished with a two-way analysis of variance with repeated measures on time, with significance taken at $p < 0.05$. (SI = substantia innominata; IBO = ibotenic acid; for lesion histology) (From Swerdlow, Swanson, and Koob.[25] Reproduced by permission.)

supersensitive locomotor response to apormorphine in rats that received bilateral electrolytic or ibotenic acid-induced damage to a major recipient or N. Acc. efferent fibers was studied.[18,19] The supersensitive locomotor response was chosen so as to functionally exaggerate the role of DA receptors in an easily quantifiable behavioral paradigm. The lesion site chosen for this work was an area ventral to the globus pallidus that includes the substantia innominata/lateral preoptic area (SI/LPO). This region of the ventral pallidum (VP) has been shown by autoradiographic, retrograde transport, anterograde degeneration, immunohistochemical, and electrophysiological techniques to receive a dense projection of fibers from the N. Acc.[12,13,20-22]

Animals injected with 6-OHDA, compared to animals that received N. Acc. sham (vehicle) injections, showed a significantly potentiated locomotor response to apomorphine (FIG. 1). Subsequent electrolytic lesions within the SI/LPO depressed the locomotor response to apomorphine in 6-OHDA-injected animals by 52.7%, but did not depress the response in sham (vehicle) injected animals.[18] FIGURE 2 shows the results from animals following vehicle- and ibotenic-acid injections within the SI/LPO. Compared to the animals that received sham (vehicle) 6-OHDA injections, 6-OHDA injected animals showed a significantly potentiated locomotor response to apomorphine. Injections of ibotenic acid within the SI/LPO significantly diminished (by 65%) the locomotor response to apomorphine in 6-OHDA-injected animals, but not in vehicle-injected animals.

These results indicate that the first-order efferent projection from the N. Acc. onto cells within the ventral pallidum forms a critical output for the behavioral expression of N. Acc. DA receptor stimulation. Thus, locomotor activation produced by stimulation of supersensitive DA receptors within the N. Acc. was significantly decreased by destruction of either cells and fibers within the SI/LPO region — using electrolytic lesions — or by destruction of only cells in this area — using the fiber-sparing neurotoxin ibotenic acid.[23] These results are consistent with those reported by Mogenson and colleagues[14] using different but similar techniques. Apparently, the efferent circuit that translates forebrain DA receptor activation into activation of spinal motorneuron synapses first within this region of the ventral globus pallidus.

Fibers from the N. Acc. containing GABA, enkephalin (ENK), and substance P innervate the SI/LPO.[24] However, ENK-containing fibers do not appear to contribute to the supersensitive locomotor response to apomorphine, since high doses of naloxone do not alter this response.[25] Also, locomotor activation produced by direct application of DA into the N. Acc. is attenuated by infusion of GABA into the SI region.[26] While this DA-stimulated locomotion is distinct from the supersensitive response that follows 6-OHDA-induced denervation, the findings nonetheless suggest that the locomotor-activating properties of DA stimulation within the N. Acc. are opposed by GABAergic transmission within the SI/LPO. One parsimonious explanation for this finding is that DA acts within the N. Acc. to inhibit the release of GABA from terminals within the ventral pallidum, and that this inhibition results in increased locomotor activity.

A series of experiments was conducted to determine whether the locomotor-activating properties of supersensitive DA activity within the N. Acc. results from the interruption of GABAergic transmission within the VP. If such is the case, then stimulation of GABA receptors in the SI with a GABA agonist would be expected to oppose these drug actions.

The effects of injections of the GABA-agonist muscimol into the SI/LPO on apomorphine-stimulated locomotion are seen in FIGURE 3. Injection of low doses of muscimol decreased the locomotor response to apomorphine in 6-OHDA-injected animals in a dose-dependent manner, but had no reliable effect on the locomotor response to apomorphine in vehicle-injected animals (FIG. 3). Higher doses of muscimol (>10 ng) produced an initial blockade of apomorphine-stimulated locomotion, but in both 6-OHDA- and vehicle-injected animals, these higher doses produced a prolonged increase in locomotor activity. However, this increase in motor activity reached its maximum approximately 90 min following muscimol injection, at a point when the supersensitive locomotor response in 6-OHDA-injected rats had subsided.[25]

The locomotor response to amphetamine and heroin is also significantly decreased by muscimol injections into the ventral pallidum; however, the locomotor activation produced by caffeine and corticotropin-releasing factor is not blocked by ventral pallidal injections of muscimol.[27] Thus, injection of the GABA-agonist muscimol into the ventral pallidum differentially blocks the locomotor-activating properties of several stimulants: locomotion stimulated by apomorphine, amphetamine, and heroin is antagonized by these muscimol injections, while locomotion stimulated by caffeine and CRF is not significantly opposed by these injections.

These results are consistent with growing evidence from behavioral investigations that a GABAergic projection from the N. Acc. into the VP provides the first link in the expression of mesolimbic DA stimulation. First, locomotor activation produced by injection of DA into the N. Acc. is disrupted by injection of GABA[26] or ethanola-mine O-sulfate (EOS), an inhibitor of GABA metabolism,[28] into the VP. Second, loco-motor activation resulting from stimulation of supersensitive DA receptors within the

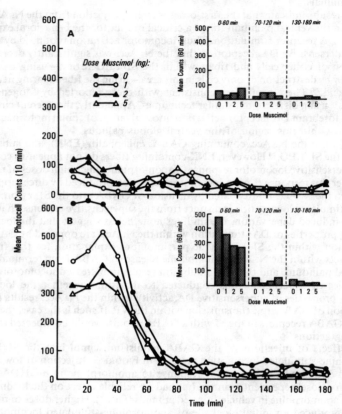

LOCOMOTOR RESPONSE TO 0.1 mg/kg APOMORPHINE (SC)

**FIGURE 3.** Locomotor response to 0.1-mg/kg apomorphine sc in vehicle- (**A**) and 6-OHDA-injected (**B**) rats following intracerebral injection of 0-, 1-, 2-, or 5-μg muscimol into the SI/LPO regions. Insert histogram indicates total locomotor activity collapsed over 60-min intervals. *Significantly different from 0-dose muscimol ($p < 0.05$, Newman–Keuls test following a significant dose × time interaction). (From Swerdlow and Koob.[25] Reproduced by permission.)

N. Acc. is blocked by destruction of cells within the SI/LPO or by injection of the GABA-agonist muscimol into the SI/LPO area.

The effects of muscimol injections into the SI/LPO on amphetamine-, caffeine-, and CRF-induced locomotor activity are strikingly similar to those produced by depletion of DA within the N. Acc., that is, amphetamine-, but neither caffeine- nor CRF-stimulated locomotion is blocked by these injections. In contrast, heroin-induced activation, which is not disrupted by depletion of N. Acc. DA,[40] is clearly opposed by muscimol injections into the SI/LPO. These findings provide evidence for some differentiation in the neural mechanisms of psychostimulant action. Thus, amphetamine activation may depend on two specific sequential neural events: an increase in DA transmission within the N. Acc., and a subsequent inhibition of GABAergic transmission within the ventral pallidum. Heroin activation is known to result from its action on opiate receptors within the N. Acc., since heroin-stimulated activation is opposed by injection of the lipophobic opiate receptor antagonist methylnaloxonium HCL directly into the N. Acc.[29] Furthermore, the present findings suggest that the locomotor-activating properties of heroin, like those of amphetamine and apomorphine, might also depend on the inhibition of GABAergic transmission within the ventral pallidum. In contrast, the activating properties of caffeine and CRF may be mediated by other neural substrates.

## THE EFFECTS OF LESIONS OF SI/LPO EFFERENT FIELDS ON APOMORPHINE-STIMULATED LOCOMOTION

While it appears that the circuitry underlying the stimulant action of at least some psychostimulants involves a GABAergic projection from cells within the N. Acc. onto cells within the SI/LPO, it is still not clear how this circuitry translates drug effects at the level of the ventral pallidum into changes in spinal motorneuron activity. Efferent projections of the SI/LPO region include massive cholinergic projections that traverse rostrally through medial prefrontal cortex (MPC) and then spread caudally to innervate much of the neocortex,[20] as well as fibers that innervate the dorsomedial thalamic nucleus (DMT)[30] and the region of the pedunculopontine nucleus (PPN),[31] which is thought to form a rat homologue to the mesencephalic locomotor region.[32] Indeed using retrograde tracing techniques, injections of the fluorescent tracer Fast Blue and Nuclear Yellow into the PPN or MPC, respectively, resulted in labeling of cells in the ventral pallidum.[33] The majority of the cells labeled from these injections were within the dorsal aspect of the substantia inominata and ventromedial globus pallidus.[33] Particularly heavily labeled were regions immediately ventral to the internal capsule. Significantly, while cells filled from PPN and MPC injection sites occupied many of the same structures within the subpallidal region no cells were identified that labeled *both* Fast Blue and Nuclear Yellow.[33]

The MLR is thought to be involved in triggering rhythmical limb movements via projections to the spinal cord.[34,35] It has been hypothesized that the ventral pallidal projections to the MLR (or by extrapolation PPN) contribute to the locomotor activation associated with natural behavioral responses.[36] In order to examine which of these regions, if any, forms the critical link from the SI/LPO to the lower motor circuitry responsible for translating the effects of forebrain DA receptor stimulation into behavioral activation, the effects of lesions of the MPC, DMT, and PPN on the supersensitive locomotor response to apomorphine were studied using a similar experimental design as for the earlier studies.

Despite massive lesion damage, of the three regions tested, only lesions of the DMT produced a reliable decrease of supersensitive apomorphine-stimulated locomotion (FIG. 4). Especially impressive was the fact that large lesions of the PPN, an area believed to send monosynaptic projections to spinal motoneurons, in fact produced a tendency (nonsignificant) toward increased apomorphine-stimulated locomotion.[37] Furthermore, while extensive damage to the DMT did decrease the supersensitive response, the effect was not one of complete blockade. These results suggest that while some of the SI/LPO efferents critical to the behavioral expression of N. Acc. DA stimulation pass to or through the DMT, other separate critical terminal fields may exist. It is clear from these findings, however, that SI/LPO efferent projections to the areas of MPC and PPN previously described do not serve as a critical substrate for N. Acc. DA-mediated locomotor activation.

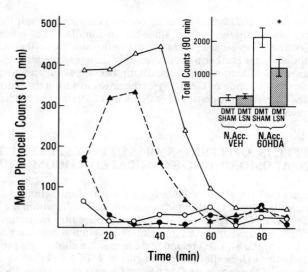

**FIGURE 4.** Locomotor response after sc injection of 0.1-mg/kg apomorphine. Animals had received either vehicle (*circles*) or 6-OHDA (*triangles*) injections into the N. Acc. and either sham (*open figures*) or electrolytic lesions (*solid figures*) of the DMT. *Significantly different from N. Acc. 6-OHDA/DMT sham-lesioned animals, $p < 0.05$, two-way ANOVA with repeated measures on time. (From Swerdlow and Koob.[37] Reproduced by permission.)

In addition picrotoxin, a GABA antagonist, when injected into the ventral pallidum produced a dose-dependent increase in locomotor activity.[37] This picrotoxin-induced locomotor activation was also blocked by lesions of the DMT.[37] These results confirm that the pallido–thalamic connection forms a critical second-order output of the mesolimbic DA system.

## DISCUSSION

A major advantage to the supersensitive locomotor measure used in the present studies is that it permits an anatomical as well as pharmacological analysis of the neural substrates that are important for the behavioral expression of stimulant action. Thus through the use of electrolytic and fiber-sparing lesions, it is possible to demonstrate that the stimulant effects of N. Acc. DA activity are dependent on the integrity of cells within the ventral pallidal region including the SI and LPO. Through the use of local intracerebral injections, it was possible to determine that this critical efferent projection is GABAergic, and thus assign both anatomical and neurochemical identity to this second link in the stimulant "circuit." While the third link in this "output" circuity remains in question, it is apparent from the results presented that fibers projecting to or through the DMT relay at least some of the pallidal information to lower motor circuitry.

One site for a functional DA–opiate interaction might occur presynaptic to mesolimbic DA receptors within the N. Acc.[38] This hypothesis is based on the finding[38] that naloxone antagonizes amphetamine-stimulated locomotion, which depends on presynaptic release of DA onto DA receptors within the N. Acc.; however, naloxone does not antagonize locomotion stimulated by injection of DA into the N. Acc. or by the direct action of apomorphine on postsynaptic DA receptors following denervation of the N. Acc.[39] Furthermore, it is possible that this presynaptic opiate–DA interaction is only one of the central substrates for opiate stimulant properties, since heroin-stimulated locomotion is not antagonized by destruction of the DA-containing fibers innervating the N. Acc.[40]

Another advantage to the locomotor measure is that the index studied is a functional integrated response in a largely intact organism and the response changes can also be interpreted for their functional significance within the animals' behavioral repertoire. For example, the neural substrates for the behaviorally activating properties of amphetamine, apomorphine, and heroin appear to correlate highly within the regions believed to mediate the positively reinforcing properties of these and related agents.[5,6,17,41–45]

The apparent overlap of neural substrates for DA- and opiate-stimulated behavioral activation and those for positive reinforcement leads to the intriguing suggestion that endogenous stimulation of N. Acc. DA and N. Acc. opiate transmission may normally underlie behavioral activation in the rat. It would be unlikely, however, that integrated behavioral displays could be initiated by simple increases and decreases in N. Acc. neurotransmission. It is conceivable, however, that initiation of goal-oriented behavior might follow activation of limbic-cortical glutamate afferents to the N. Acc., which have been shown by Nielsen and Mogenson[46,47] to be a critical substrate for rat exploratory behavior.

The role of limbic–cortical afferent activation of this N. Acc.-ventral pallidal circuitry in locomotor activation in the rat has been addressed by Mogenson and Nielsen.[46] In this work, locomotor activation produced by infusion of carbachol directly into the dentate gyrus of the hippocampus was disrupted by infusion of the glutamate antagonist glutamic acid diethyl ester HCL (GDEE) into the N. Acc., or by infusion of GABA into the ventral pallidum. Interestingly, rat exploratory activation within a novel open-field environment was also inhibited by N. Acc. GDEE infusion or by ventral pallidal GABA infusion.[47] One might speculate that "endogenous" goal-oriented activation may depend on limbic–cortical activation of this N. Acc.-ventral pallidal circuit. Furthermore, these results provide evidence that environment- and psychostimulant-induced behavioral activation in the rat share greatly overlapping neural substrates. Interactions between ascending N. Acc. DA afferent and intrinsic N. Acc. Spiny I circuitry have been proposed to provide a "filter" function that limits the amount or nature of the cortical information that passes beyond the N. Acc. to activate lower motor circuitry.[32] Drugs that alter DA transmission within the N. Acc. may modify these interactions, and thus change the pattern of information that reaches the ventral pallidum.

It is not yet known how ventral pallidal efferents ultimately activate locomotion, although it seems highly unlikely that the complexity of the motor patterns that underlie these behaviors could be supported exclusively at a subcortical level. It is more reasonable to presume that the ultimate "final common pathway" for these behaviors must be the cortico–spinal pathway, which could provide somatotopic organization to the sequences of muscle activation. Activity within pallido–thalamic efferent fibers, and subsequently within thalamo–cortical fibers, might thus serve to direct limbic–cortical information to appropriate effector motor groups through the cortico–spinal pathway (see FIG. 5). According to the findings previously reviewed, stimulation of these substrates can be achieved at many sites proximal to the final common pathway — by carbacol infusions into the hippocampus,[46] glutamate infusions into the N. Acc.,[46] DA-[26] or opiate[29] activation of the N. Acc., or blockade of GABA transmis-

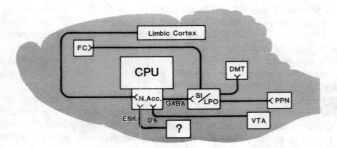

**FIGURE 5.** A model showing the efferent connections of the nucleus accumbens. Results from Mogenson and colleagues and our laboratory concur in describing a functionally significant GABAergic projection from the nucleus accumbens to the ventral pallidum (SI/LPO). The projection from the ventral pallidum to the mesencephalic motor region (PPN in this model) is proposed to be functionally important by Mogenson and colleagues, and a second GABAergic projection from ventral pallidum to the dorsal medial thalamus (DMT) has been proposed to be functionally important by Swerdlow and Koob.

sion within the ventral pallidum.[26] The quantitative and qualitative contribution of each link in this neural circuit to the nature of the resulting behavioral activation is an important issue that awaits further systematic study.

One finding that is evident from recent work is that the stimulant properties of caffeine and centrally administered corticotropin releasing factor (CRF)[48,49] differ markedly from amphetamine, apomorphine, and heroin in their pharmacological and antatomical profiles. Thus, locomotor activity stimulated by caffeine and CRF are not antagonized by selective blockade of receptors for DA or opiates, nor are they antagonized by the destruction of N. Acc. DA terminals or infusion of muscimol into the SI/LPO region.[50] Apparently, these agents exert their stimulant properties through a set of neural elements very distinct from that responsible for the stimulant properties of sympathomimetics and opiates.

The similarity of the pharmacological and behavioral profiles of CRF- and caffeine-activation suggest that hypotheses as to a common mechanism of action should be considered. It is possible that this mechanism might share at least some common elements with the neural substrates of stress-induced behavioral activation, since CRF has been shown to enhance the stress response to novel environments.[48,49] Such a function might employ mechanisms of arousal not involved in the activation produced by the neural circuitry underlying amphetamine-, apomorphine-, and heroin-stimulated locomotion.

## SUMMARY

In summary, the nucleus accumbens, located at the interface of the limbic projections from the amygdala, hippocampus, and cingulate cortex,[20] and receiving extrapyramidal fibers from midbrain DA-containing nuclei,[13] is well situated to form neural circuitry that mediates the behaviorally activating properties of several stimulants. Efferent GABAergic fibers projecting from the nucleus accumbens to the ventral pallidum translate integrated limbic and extrapyramidal information to lower motor circuitry; some of this information appears to be carried by ventral pallidal efferent fibers projecting to the dorsomedial nucleus of the thalamus. It seems very possible that activation of this circuitry by positive reinforcing environmental stimuli, through the release of endogenous DA or opiate compounds, might contribute to motivated behavior. Indeed, environmentally generated locomotor activity can be blocked by disruption of this circuitry following destruction of N. Acc. DA terminals.[10] It is also tempting to speculate that pathological changes in activity within this system might disrupt normal reinforcement contingencies, and contribute to the affective components of both psychiatric and neurologic disease states.

## REFERENCES

1. KELLY, P. H. & S. D. IVERSEN. 1976. Selective 6-OHDA-induced destruction of mesolimbic dopamine neurons: Abolition of psychostimulant induced locomotor activity in rats. Eur. J. Pharmacol. **40:** 45–56.
2. ROBERTS, D. C. S., A. P. ZIS & H. C. FIBIGER. 1975. Ascending catecholamine pathways and amphetamine induced locomotion: Importance of dopamine and apparent non-involvement of norepinephrine. Brain Res. **93:** 441–454.
3. KELLY, P. H., P. SEVIOUR & S. D. IVERSEN. 1975. Amphetamine and apomorphine responses in the rat following 6-OHDA lesions of the nucleus accumbens septi and corpus striatum. Brain Res. **94:** 507–522.
4. ROBERTS, D. C. S., M. E. CORCORAN & H. C. FIBIGER. 1977. On the role of ascending catecholamine systems in intravenous self-administration of cocaine. Pharmacol. Biochem. Behav. **6:** 615–620.
5. ROBERTS, D. C. S., G. F. KOOB, P. KLONOFF & H. C. FIBIGER. 1980. Extinction and recovery of cocaine self-administration following 6-hydroxydopamine lesions of the nucleus accumbens. Pharmacol. Biochem. Behav. **12:** 781–787.
6. LYNESS, W. H., N. M. FRIEDLE & K. E. MOORE. 1979. Destruction of dopaminergic nerve terminals in the nucleus accumbens: Effect on d-amphetamine self-administration. Pharmacol. Biochem. Behav. **11:** 553–556.
7. KOOB, G. F., S. J. RILEY, S. C. SMITH & J. W. ROBBINS. 1975. Effects of 6-hydroxydopamine lesions of the nucleus accumbens septi and olfactory tuberele on feeding locomotor activity and amphetamine anorexia in the rat. J. Comp. Physiol. Psychol. **92:** 917–927.
8. JOYCE, E. M., L. STINUS & S. D. IVERSEN. 1983. Effect of injection of 6-OHDA into either nucleus accumbens septi or frontal cortex on spontaneous and drug-induced activity. Neuropharmacology. **22:** 1141–1145.
9. TAGHZOUTI, K., H. SIMON, A. LOUILOT, J. P. HERMAN & M. LE MOAL. 1985. Behavioral study after local injection of 6-hydroxydopamine into the nucleus accumbens in the rat. Brain Res. **344:** 9–20.
10. ROBBINS, T. W. & G. F. KOOB. 1980. Selective disruption of displacement behaviour by lesions of the mesolimbic dopamine system. Nature. **285:** 409–412.
11. ROBBINS, T. W., D. C. S. ROBERTS & G. F. KOOB. 1983. The effects of amphetamine and apomorphine upon operant behavior and schedule-induced licking in rats with 6-hydroxydopamine-induced lesions of the nucleus accumbens. J. Pharmacol. Exp. Ther. **224:** 662–673.
12. NAUTA, W. J. H., G. P. SMITH, V. B. DOMESICK & R. L. M. FAULL. 1978. Efferent connections and nigral afferents of the nucleus accumbens septi in the rat. Neuroscience. **3:** 385–401.
13. MOGENSON, G. J., L. W. SWANSON & M. WU. 1983. Neural projections from the nucleus accumbens to globus pallidus, substantia innominata, and lateral preoptic-lateral hypothalmic area: An anatomical and electrophysiological investigation in the rat. J. Neurosci. Res. **3:** 189–202.
14. JONES, D. L. & G. J. MOGENSON. 1980. Nucleus accumbens to globus pallidus GABA projection subserving ambulatory activity. Am. J. Physiol. **238:** R63–R69.
15. MOGENSON, G. J., M. WU & D. L. JONES. 1980. Locomotor activity elicited by injections

of picrotoxin into the ventral tegmental area is attenuated by injections of GABA into the globus pallidus. Brain Res. **191:** 569.

16.  STAUNTON, D. A., P. J. MAGISTRETTI, G. F. KOOB, W. J. SHOEMAKER & F. E. BLOOM. 1982. Dopaminergic supersensitivity induced by denervation and chronic receptor blockade is additive. Nature. **299:** 72–74.

17.  VAN DER KOOY, D., N. R. SWERDLOW & G. F. KOOB. 1983. Paradoxical reinforcing properties of apomorphine: Effects of nucleus accumbens and area postrema lesions. Brain Res. **259:** 111–118.

18.  SWERDLOW, N. R., L. W. SWANSON & G. F. KOOB. 1983. Electrolytic lesions of the substantia inominata and lateral preoptic area attenuate the "supersensitive" locomotor response to apomorphine resulting from denervation of the nucleus accumbens. Brain Res. **306:** 141–148.

19.  SWERDLOW, N. R., L. W. SWANSON & G. F. KOOB. 1984. Substantia innominata: Critical link in the behavioral expression of mesolimbic dopamine stimulation in the rat. Neurosci. Lett. **50:** 19–24.

20.  HEIMER, L. & R. D. WILSON. 1975. The subcortical projections of the allocortex: Similarities in the neural associations of the hippocampus, the piriform cortex, and the neocortex. *In* Golgi Centennial Symposium Proceedings. M. Santini, Ed.: 177–193. Raven Press. New York.

21.  SWANSON, L. W. & W. M. COWAN. 1975. A note on the connections and development of the nucleus accumbens. Brain Res. **92:** 324–330.

22.  WILLIAMS, D. J., A. R. CROSSMAN & P. SLATER. 1977. The efferent projections of the nucleus accumbens in the rat. Brain Res. **130:** 217–227.

23.  SCHWARCZ, R., T. HOKFELT, K. FUXE, G. JONSSON, M. GOLDSTEIN & L. TERENIUS. 1979. Ibotenic acid-induced neuronal degeneration: A morphological and neurochemical study. Exp. Brain Res. **37:** 199–216.

24.  ZABORSKY, L., G. F. ALHEID, V. E. ALONES, W. H. OERTEL, D. E. SCHMECHEL & L. HEIMER. 1982. Afferents of the ventral pallidum studied with a combined immunohistochemical-anterograde degeneration method. Soc. Neurosci. Abstr. **8:** 218.

25.  SWERDLOW, N. R. & G. F. KOOB. 1984. Neural substrates of apomorphine-stimulated locomotor activity following denervation of the nucleus accumbens. Life Sci. **35:** 2537–2544.

26.  MOGENSON, G. J. & M. A. NIELSON. 1983. Evidence that an accumbens to subpallidal GABAergic projection contributes to locomotor activity. Brain Res. Res. Bull. **11:** 309–314.

27.  SWERDLOW, N. R. & G. F. KOOB. 1985. Separate neural substrates of the locomotor-activity properties of amphetamine, heroin, caffeine, and corticotropin releasing factor (CRF) in the rat. Pharmacol. Biochem. Behav. **23:** 303–307.

28.  PYCOCK, C. & R. HORTON. 1976. Evidence for an accumbens-pallidal pathway in the rat and its possible gabaminergic control. Brain Res. **110:** 629–634.

29.  AMALRIC, M. & G. KOOB. 1985. Methylnaloxonium in the nucleus accumbens blocks heroin locomotion in the rat. Pharmacol. Biochem. Behav. **23:** 411–415.

30.  ZAHM, D. S., L. ZABORSKY, W. H. OERTEL, D. E. SCHMECHEL & L. HEIMER. 1984. The ventral pallido-thalamic projection. Soc. Neurosci. Abstr. **10:** 10.

31.  SWANSON, L. W., G. J. MOGENSON, C. R. GERFEN & P. ROBINSON. 1984. Evidence for a projection from the lateral preoptic area and substantia innominata to the 'mesencephalic locomotor region' in the rat. Brain Res. **295:** 161–178.

32.  GROVES, P. M. 1983. A theory of the functional organization of the neostriatum and the neostriatal control of voluntary movement. Brain Res. Rev. **5:** 109–132.

33.  SWERDLOW, N. R. 1986. Ventral striato-pallidal circuitry and the neural substrates of dopamine-stimulated locomotor activity in the rat. Ph.D. Dissertation, University of California.

34.  SKINNER, R. D. & E. GARCIA-RILL. 1984. The mesencephalic locomotor region (MLR) in the rat. Brain Res. **323:** 385–389.

35.  STEEVES, J. D. & L. M. JORDAN. 1980. Localization of a descending pathway in the spinal cord which is necessary for controlled treadmill locomotion. Neurosci. Lett. **20:** 283–288.

36.  MOGENSON, G. J. 1984. Limbic-motor integration with emphasis on initiation of exploratory and goal depicted locomotion. *In* Modulation of Sensorimotor Activity During Alterations in Behavioral States. R. Bandler, Ed.: 121–137. Alan Liss. New York.

37.  SWERDLOW, N. R. & G. F. KOOB. 1987. Lesions of the dorsomedial nucleus of the thal-
     amus, medial prefrontal cortex and pedunculo pontine nucleus: Effects on locomotor
     activity mediated by nucleus accumbens-ventral pallidal circuitry. Brain Res. **412:** 233–243.
38.  SWERDLOW, N. R., F. J. VACCARINO & G. F. KOOB. 1985. Effects of naloxone on heroin-
     amphetamine-, and caffeine-stimulated locomotor activity in the rat. Pharmacol. Bio-
     chem. Behav. **23:** 499–501.
39.  BATLLE, F. J. & M. F. LOPEZ. 1979. Interrelationships between complement and coagula-
     tion systems in human DIC. II. Role of complement. Sangre. **24:** 513–518.
40.  VACCARINO, F. J., M. AMALRIC, N. R. SWERDLOW & G. F. KOOB. 1986. Blockade of am-
     phetamine but not opiate-induced locomotion following antagonism of dopamine func-
     tion in the rat. Pharmacol. Biochem. Behav. **24:** 61–65.
41.  ETTENBERG, A., H. O. PETTIT, F. E. BLOOM & G. F. KOOB. 1982. Heroin and cocaine self-
     administration in rats: Mediation by separate neural systems. Psychopharmacology.
     **78:** 204–209.
42.  MUCHA, R. F., D. VAN DER KOOY, M. O'SHAUGHNESSY & P. BUCENIEKS. 1982. Drug rein-
     forcement studied by the use of place conditioning in rat. Brain Res. **243:** 91–105.
43.  PETTIT, H. O., A. ETTENBERG, F. E. BLOOM & G. F. KOOB. 1984. Destruction of dopamine
     in the nucleus accumbens selectively attenuates cocaine but not heroin self-administration
     in rats. Psychopharmacology. **24:** 167–173.
44.  SPYRAKI, C., H. C. FIBIGER & A. G. PHILLIPS. 1982. Dopaminergic substrates of amphetamine-
     induced place preference conditioning. Brain Res. **253:** 185–193.
45.  VACCARINO, F. J., F. E. BLOOM & G. F. KOOB. 1985. Blockade of nucleus accumbens opiate
     receptors attenuates intravenous heroin reward in the rat. Psychopharmacology. **85:** 37–42.
46.  MOGENSON, G. J. & M. NIELSON. 1984. A study of the contribution of hippocampal-
     accumbens-subpallidal projections to locomotor activity. Behav. Neural. Biol. **42:** 38–51.
47.  MOGENSON, G. J. & M. NIELSON. 1984. Neuropharmacological evidence to suggest that
     the nucleus accumbens and subpallidal regions contribute to exploratory locomotion.
     Behav. Neural. Biol. **42:** 52–60.
48.  BRITTON, D. R., G. F. KOOB, J. RIVIER & W. VALE. 1982. Intraventricular corticotropin-
     releasing factor enhances behavioral effects of novelty. Life Sci. **31:** 363–367.
49.  SUTTON, R. E., G. F. KOOB, M. LE MOAL, J. RIVIER & W. VALE. 1982. Corticotropin releasing
     factor (CRF) produces behavioral activation in rats. Nature. **297:** 331–333.
50.  KOOB, G. F., N. SWERDLOW, M. SEELIGSON, M. EAVES, R. SUTTON, J. RIVIER & W. VALE.
     1984. CRF-induced locomotor activation is antagonized by alpha-flupenthixol but not
     by naloxone. Neuroendocrinology. **39:** 459–464.

# Psychomotor Stimulant Properties of Addictive Drugs

ROY A. WISE

*Center for Studies in Behavioral Neurobiology*
*Department of Psychology*
*Concordia University*
*Montreal, P.Q., Canada H3G 1M8*

Electrical stimulation of the medial forebrain bundle produces two powerful motivational effects: drive and reinforcement. The thesis offered here (and elsewhere[1,2,3]) is that these two effects are manifestations of a single biological mechanism and process — psychomotor activation — and that all rewarding events, including injections of the variety of habit-forming drugs, activate that mechanism and contribute to that process.

First, consider the case of brain-stimulation effects. The appearance of two distinct effects — drive effects and reinforcement effects — is a consequence of the two different paradigms in which the consequences of the stimulation are assessed. When we focus our attention on the behavior of the animal just prior to the delivery of the stimulation, and when we make delivery of the stimulation contingent upon some particular feature of that behavior, we notice an increase in the frequency or probability of the act in question. This effect is termed the rewarding effect in everyday language and termed the "reinforcing" effect by Skinner,[4] who developed what is known as the "operant" paradigm (the "Skinner box" is the best known example) for studying the importance of this phenomenon in the establishment of the habits that Skinner and his followers have taken to be the basic units of behavior. The reinforcing effects of brain stimulation have been extensively studied in the operant paradigm since their discovery in 1954 by Olds and Milner.[5]

Another great tradition in psychology was inspired by the work of Pavlov, who ignored the behavior of his animals — or waited for it to cease — before administering the stimuli of interest in his very different but equally important paradigm. It was Pavlov,[6] not Skinner, who first coined the term "reinforcer"; he used the term to designate the unconditioned stimulus in his conditioning paradigm, termed the "respondent" paradigm by Skinner.[4] If we take medial forebrain bundle stimulation as our reinforcer and study it in the paradigm of Pavlov, we wait for the animal to be still, and then we apply the stimulation and note the unconditioned response. It is when medial forebrain bundle stimulation is studied in this way that it is seen to have *drive*-like effects; the unconditioned consequence of the stimulation is an increase in exploration of and interaction with the biologically significant stimuli (food, water, nesting material, sex partner, etc.) in the environment.[2] These drivelike effects of medial forebrain bundle stimulation have also been intensively studied, largely, but not exclusively, by different workers than those who have studied brain stimulation as operant reinforcement. Hess won the Nobel Prize for such work in the second quarter of this century,[7] and Miller and his students established it in the English literature in the third.[8]

When the study of the drivelike effects of medial forebrain bundle stimulation came to the attention of the students of the rewardlike effects, and vice versa, there was considerable interest in the "drive–reward paradox": Why should an animal work for stimulation that induces a drivelike state resembling, in most important ways,[9] natural hunger, thirst, sexual activation, and the like? One resolution of the paradox involved rejection of the notion — then losing favor for other reasons — that drive states are aversive and that their reduction is a necessary condition for reinforcement. Another resolution involved the assumption that different, but adjacent or interwoven, hypothalamic elements mediated the drivelike effects and the rewardlike effects. In support of this view was the fact that there were persistent differences in the intensity thresholds for stimulation-induced feeding and for stimulation-induced reinforcement; reward thresholds were generally much higher than feeding thresholds.[10] The reason for this may have to do with response requirements, however; when animals poke their nose in a hole[11] or rear[12] for stimulation, their reward thresholds are much lower.

Against the view that different hypothalamic elements mediate the drivelike and rewardlike effects of stimulation were reports of several manipulations that altered the two effects in parallel. Physiological and pharmacological manipulations that increase or decrease the threshold for brain stimulation reward almost always similarly increase or decrease the threshold for stimulation-induced feeding.[13] More recently we have found much stronger data to suggest that common medial forebrain bundle fibers contribute to the rewardlike effects and the drivelike effects of medial forebrain bundle stimulation. The refractory periods for the directly activated fibers of stimulation-induced eating[14] reflect the same two subpopulations as are implicated in self-stimulation.[15] The conduction velocities are also similar, as are the anterior–posterior alignments of the relevant fibers as they pass, without synaptic interruption, between the lateral hypothalamus and the ventral tegmental area.[4] These findings suggest that the motivational fibers of the medial forebrain bundle should be considered neither "reward fibers" nor "drive fibers," but rather should be seen as fibers serving a function that is common to both reward and drive. Such a function is psychomotor activation.

Psychomotor activation is the unconditioned response to reinforcing electrical stimulation of the medial forebrain bundle.[2] Psychomotor activation takes several forms; the two reflections that are of particular interest for the present are increased tendencies to locomote and to eat. These two effects[16,17] and the rewarding effects[18] of medial forebrain bundle stimulation appear to depend on the transsynaptic activation[19] of the mesocorticolimbic and perhaps the nigrostriatal[20] dopamine system. We have recently proposed that activation of this system or its efferents may be common to all major classes of addictive drugs.[21,22]

The evidence for this suggestion is strong for two classes of drug: the nominal psychomotor stimulants and the opiates. The evidence is suggestive for the following additional cases: alcohol, nicotine, caffeine, cannabis, phencyclidine, barbiturates, and benzodiazepines. These cases will be taken up in turn.

The nominal psychomotor stimulants are amphetamine, cocaine, and related compounds. The qualifier "psychomotor" is used to distinguish these drugs from convulsants such as picrotoxin, pentylene tetrazol, and strychnine, and calls attention to their effects on human performance on a variety of vigilance and coordination tasks.[23] In animals psychomotor stimulants cause obvious locomotor responses and variously cause stereotyped head and eye movements or orofacial movements, depending on the species and the situation. The view that is advanced here is that the mechanism of psychomotor stimulant effects is the same as the mechanism of the psychomotor activation caused by medial forebrain bundle electrical stimulation: the mesocorticolimbic dopamine system, the nigrostriatal dopamine system, and their efferents. The psychomotor stimulant effect on locomotion involves, primarily, the mesocorticolimbic system[24] and the stereotypy effect involves, primarily, the nigrostriatal system.[25] The same systems mediate the direct rewarding effects[26,27] of amphetamine. That a common final path — through the dopamine synapse — accounts for both the locomotor stimulant effects and the direct rewarding effects of amphetamine on the one hand and of medial forebrain bundle brain stimulation on the other hand fits well with the fact that amphetamine enhances the rewarding effects of such brain stimulation by actions in the same two sites.[28,29]

A fact that has seemed to go against the view that the rewarding and the drivelike effects of hypothalamic stimulation reflect activation of a common mechanism — and one that is shared with that of the behavioral effects of amphetamine — is that amphetamine is generally thought to facilitate brain stimulation reward,[30] while it is generally thought to inhibit both natural and stimulation-induced feeding.[31] Our recent work — and that of others[32] — reopens this question. We have found that low doses of systemic amphetamine facilitate both deprivation-induced and stimulation-induced feeding, and they do so when the drug is microinjected directly into its reward and reward-enhancing site in the nucleus accumbens.[33] High doses, on the other hand, have mixed effects. They increase the probability that the animal will fail to feed on a given trial, but they accelerate feeding on those trials where it does occur. Only minimal effects are seen with injections of the dextroisomer into the caudate nucleus or into the accumbens contralateral to the stimulation site; the levoisomer is effective only when injected into the ipsilateral accumbens, and even then it is only minimally effective.

By traditional classifications, the opiates are not psychomotor stimulants. When injected into the region of the ventral tegmental dopamine-containing cell bodies, however, opiates have psychomotor stimulant effects. These injections activate mesocorticolimbic and substantia nigra dopamine neurons[34] and stimulate locomotor activity.[35] When administered unilaterally, they normally[36] cause contraversive circling.[37] Such injections are rewarding in their own right,[38,39] and they facilitate brain-stimulation reward.[40,41] They also facilitate stimulation-induced feeding.[42] The rewarding effects of ventral tegmental morphine as revealed by place preference conditioning using low (200–250-ng) doses are restricted to the region of dopaminergic cells; injections rostral, caudal, or ventral[43] or dorsal[39] to the dopamine cell layer fail to cause conditioned place preference or psychomotor activation.[37] Conditioned place preference has been reported after 10-μm injections into the periaqueductal gray, lateral hypothalamus, and nucleus accumbens, but ventricular injections at this dose are also effective and require less powerful statistics to demonstrate.[44] Just as low doses of morphine are effective in the ventral tegmental area, but ineffective in the accumbens in place preference tests, so are they effective in the ventral tegmental area, but ineffective in the accumbens in intracranial self-administration tests in our hands.[38]

While ventral tegmental morphine is effective in locomotion tests, feeding tests, self-stimulation tests, and direct reinforcement tests, there is some indication of multiple contributions to the mechanisms of these behaviors, and it appears that they are not completely overlapping. While the selective delta agonist D-Pen2,D-Pen5 enkephalin and the selective kappa agonist U-50,488H are as effective as morphine in facilitating feeding,[45] only the delta agonist and morphine are effective in the self-stimulation[46] and locomotion tests.[47] Dynorphin, a kappa agonist, though not a particularly selective one, is even more effective in feeding tests; picomole doses of ventral tegmental dynorphin can induce feeding in sated rats.[48]

A second site at which opioids can have psychomotor stimulant[49] and reinforcing[50,51] effects is the nucleus accumbens. As mentioned, low doses are not as effective as reinforcers when injected here;[38,44] similarly, they are not as effective as locomotor stimulants.[49] Indeed, nucleus accumbens opiates seem rather weak as locomotor stimulants unless the dopamine system has been depleted or blocked.[52,53] Thus nucleus accumbens seems a less preferred site at which opiates have secondary access to the circuitry of psychomotor activation.

The low-dose reinforcing effects of ventral tegmental morphine are *positive* reinforcing effects. Morphine injections in this area do not alleviate pain[54] and they do not appear likely to alleviate withdrawal symptoms (see below). Dopamine antagonists block the positive reinforcing[18] but not the negative reinforcing[55] effects of brain stimulation. Thus ventral tegmental morphine injections activate a mesocorticolimbic system that participates in positive reinforcement (reinforcement involving induction of a positive state) rather than negative reinforcement (reinforcement involving alleviation of a negative state). The negative state most often associated with natural reinforcers like food and water is a drive state, but no drive state is needed for medial forebrain bundle stimulation[56] or ventral tegmental opiate injections to be reinforcing.[38] The negative state most often associated with drugs of addiction is a state of withdrawal distress, but there is no evidence for such a state in animals working for, or receiving passively, ventral tegmental morphine.[57]

The negative reinforcing effects of morphine would appear to be mediated primarily by mechanisms of quite a separate part of the brain: the periaqueductal gray matter. Morphine microinjection into this area alleviates pain[58] and, if chronic, causes physical dependence.[57] There is some evidence to suggest that opioid systems of the periaqueductal gray are also involved in the distress symptoms caused by social isolation;[59] this may be related to relief of loneliness or lovesickness by opiates.[60]

Two findings provide strong support for the notion that ventral tegmental opiates and nucleus accumbens amphetamines act at different synaptic links of the same locomotor and positive reinforcement circuitry. First, the locomotor-stimulating effects of systemic amphetamine[61] and ventral tegmental morphine[62] each undergo sensitization or "reverse tolerance." Moreover, there is cross-sensitization; that is, repeated exposure to amphetamine sensitizes animals to the locomotor stimulant effects of ventral tegmental morphine.[63] Just as cross-tolerance suggests a common mechanism of drug action, so does cross-sensitization or "cross-reverse-tolerance."

Second, there is cross-substitution of ventral tegmental morphine with intravenous cocaine in an animal model of addiction relapse. In this paradigm, animals are trained to respond for intravenous injections of cocaine[64] or heroin.[65] During testing the injection lines are disconnected, and the response habit is "extinguished." Various stimuli are then tested for their ability to trigger response reinitiation, even though the animals are still under conditions of extinction (they can no longer *earn* drug injections). In this paradigm, the most effective stimulus to relapse is an intravenous injection of the training drug. Other drugs reinitiate responding in proportion to their similarity to the training drug. Ventral tegmental morphine injections reinstate responding in animals trained with either intravenous heroin or intravenous cocaine;[66] in a sense, the animals fail to respond as if they distinguish ventral tegmental morphine from intravenous heroin or cocaine. The stimulus dimension on which morphine and cocaine are similar is the dimension of euphoria.[67]

Thus the narcotic analgesic, morphine, has in common with the psychomotor stimulant, amphetamine, the ability to activate a feeding, locomotor, and reinforcement system involving mesocorticolimbic dopamine projections and their efferents. That is, while not a nominal psychomotor stimulant, morphine has psychomotor stimulant properties. These properties are subtle compared to the sedation that is triggered by slightly higher systemic doses than the doses producing locomotor stimulation. The psychomotor stimulant effects involve actions in the ventral tegmental area and nucleus accumbens; the sedative effects involve actions in the mesencephalic reticular formation.[68] The fact that morphine can be a narcotic analgesic and yet have psychomotor stimulant properties that are reinforcing raises the possibility that other sedative drugs might also have reinforcing psychomotor stimulant actions.

Evidence in support of this notion is scattered but suggestive. While neither barbiturates nor benzodiazepines appear to stimulate dopamine turnover,[69] each may act in GABAergic efferents thought to participate in locomotion[70] and stereotypy.[71] Barbiturates and benzodiazepines have each been reported to facilitate brain stimulation reward,[19] to facilitate feeding,[72,73] and to enhance locomotion;[74,75] the threshold dose for these effects is only slightly lower than the anesthetic or sedative doses, and thus the locomotor effects are seen only for a brief period as the animal recovers from intoxication. Ethanol is more frankly a psychomotor stimulant; this fact is almost completely obscured in behavioral tests in the rat because sedative effects are seen at the same doses.[76] However, even in rats, ethanol stimulates dopamine turnover[77] and cell firing,[78] stimulates locomotion,[79] and enhances brain-stimulation reward.[80] It can also facilitate feeding.[81] Cannabis also facilitates feeding and locomotion at low doses,[82] and it stimulates dopamine turnover.[83]

Nicotine, caffeine, and phencyclidine qualify more obviously as psychomotor stimulants, though they are not traditionally classified as such. Nicotine stimulates dopamine cell firing[84,85] and dopamine turnover;[86,87] caffeine stimulates dopamine turnover.[88] Phencyclidine either causes dopamine release[89] or blocks dopamine reuptake.[90] All three stimulate locomotion,[91,92,93] and nicotine facilitates brain stimulation reward[94] and causes conditioned place preference.[95]

These data suggest psychomotor activation as a common denominator of a wide range of addictive drugs. While it is clear that the negative reinforcing effects (relief of dysphoria) of different drugs are mediated by a variety of dependence mechanisms, it would appear that the positive reinforcing effects (induction of euphoria) result from actions in a shared or common mechanism. This shared mechanism is activated by drive states as well as reinforcing conditions, and is best characterized as a mechanism of psychomotor activation. This view fits well with theory in experimental psychology, in which increased activity is associated with deprivation conditions, positive reinforcement, and exposure to incentive stimuli, and in which withdrawal, inactivity, or freezing is associated with satiety, negative reinforcement, or aversive stimuli.

This view suggests that difficulty in developing a unified theory of addiction has been caused, in part, by the dominance of sedative "side-effects" of the most obviously dependence-producing drugs—the opiates, ethanol, barbiturates, and benzodiazepines. These sedative effects have obscured the psychomotor stimulant effects that offer a common denominator for all positive reinforcers and, in our view, an unappreciated key to the addictive process.[21,22]

## REFERENCES

1. SCHNEIRLA, T. C. 1959. *In* Proc. Nebraska Symposium on Motivation. M. R. Jones, Ed.: 1–42. Univ. Nebraska Press. Lincoln.
2. GLICKMAN, S. E. & B. B. SCHIFF. 1967. Psychol. Rev. **74:** 81–109.
3. BINDRA, D. 1974. Psychol. Rev. **81:** 199–213.
4. SKINNER, B. F. 1937. J. Gen. Psychol. **16:** 272–279.
5. OLDS, J. & P. M. MILNER. 1954. J. Comp. Physiol. Psychol. **47:** 419–427.
6. PAVLOV, I. 1927. Conditioned Reflexes. Oxford University Press. Oxford.
7. HESS, W. R. 1957. The Functional Organization of the Diencephalon. J. R. Hughes, Ed. Grune & Stratton. New York.
8. MILLER, N. E. 1960. Fed. Proc., Fed. Am. Soc. Exp. Biol. **19:** 846–854.
9. WISE, R. A. 1974. Brain Res. **67:** 187–209.
10. HUSTON, J. P. 1971. Physiol. Behav. **6:** 711–716.
11. ETTENBERG, A., G. F. KOOB & F. E. BLOOM. 1981. Science **213:** 357–359.

12. WISE, R. A. 1985. Behav. Brain Sci. **8:** 178–186.
13. HOEBEL, B. G. 1969. Proc. N.Y. Acad. Sci. **157:** 758–778.
14. GRATTON, A. & R. A. WISE. 1985. Soc. Neurosci. Abstr. **11:** 1176.
15. GRATTON, A. & R. A. WISE. 1985. Science **227:** 545–548.
16. GALLISTEL, C. R., M. BOYTIM, Y. GOMITA & L. KLEBANOFF. 1982. Pharmacol. Biochem. Behav. **17:** 769–781.
17. JENCK, F., A. GRATTON & R. A. WISE. 1986. Brain Res. **375:** 329–337.
18. FOURIEZOS, G. & R. A. WISE. 1976. Brain Res. **103:** 377–380.
19. WISE, R. A. 1980. Pharmacol. Biochem. Behav. (Suppl. 1) **13:** 213–223.
20. CORBETT, D. & R. A. WISE. 1980. Brain Res. **185:** 1–15.
21. WISE, R. A. 1987. Pharmaco. Therap. **35:** 227–263.
22. WISE, R. A. & M. A. BOZARTH. 1987. Psychol. Rev. **94:** 469–492.
23. HINDMARCH, I. 1980. Br. J. Clin. Pharmacol. **10:** 189–209.
24. KELLY, P. H., P. W. SEVIOUR & S. D. IVERSEN. 1975. Brain Res. **94:** 507–522.
25. CREESE, I. & S. D. IVERSEN. 1974. Psychopharmacologia **39:** 345–357.
26. PHILLIPS, A. G., F. MORA & E. T. ROLLS. 1981. Neurosci. Lett. **24:** 81–86.
27. HOEBEL, B. G., A. MONACO, L. HERNANDES, E. AULISI, B. G. STANLEY & L. LENARD. 1983. Psychopharmacologia **81:** 158–163.
28. BROEKKAMP, C. L. E., A. J. J. PIJNENBURG, A. R. COOLS & J. M. VAN ROSSUM. 1975. Psychopharmacologia **42:** 179–183.
29. GALLISTEL, C. R. & D. KARRAS. 1984. Pharmacol. Biochem. Behav. **20:** 73–77.
30. COLLE, L. & R. A. WISE. 1986. Soc. Neurosci. Abstr. **12:** 930.
31. STARK, P. & C. W. TOTTY. 1967. J. Pharmacol. Exp. Ther. **158:** 272–278.
32. BLUNDELL, J. E. & C. J. LATHAM. 1980. Pharmacol. Biochem. Behav. **12:** 717–722.
33. COLLE, L. & R. A. WISE. 1988. Facilitory and inhibitory effects of nucleus accumbens amphetamine on feeding. This volume.
34. MATTHEWS, R. T. & D. C. GERMAN. 1984. Neuroscience **11:** 617–626.
35. JOYCE, E. M. & S. D. IVERSEN. 1979. Neurosci. Lett. **14:** 207–212.
36. WISE, R. A. & L. J. HOLMES. 1986. Brain Res. Bull. **16:** 267–269.
37. HOLMES, L. J. & R. A. WISE. 1985. Brain Res. **326:** 19–26.
38. BOZARTH, M. A. & R. A. WISE. 1981. Life Sci. **28:** 551–555.
39. PHILLIPS, A. G. & F. G. LEPIANE. 1980. Pharmacol. Biochem. Behav. **12:** 965–968.
40. BROEKKAMP, C. L. E., J. H. VAN DEN BOGAARD, H. J. HEIJNEN, R. H. ROPS, A. R. COOLS & J. M. VAN ROSSUM. 1976. Eur. J. Pharmacol. **36:** 443–446.
41. JENCK, F., A. GRATTON & R. A. WISE. 1987. Brain Res. **423:** 34–38.
42. JENCK, F., A. GRATTON & R. A. WISE. 1986. Brain Res. **399:** 24–32.
43. BOZARTH, M. A. 1987. Brain Res. **414:** 77–84.
44. VAN DER KOOY, D., R. F. MUCHA, M. O'SHAUGHNESSY & P. BUCENIEKS. 1982. Brain. Res. **243:** 107–117.
45. JENCK, F., R. QUIRION & R. A. WISE. 1987. Brain Res. **423:** 39–44.
46. JENCK, F., A. GRATTON & R. A. WISE. 1987. Brain Res. **423:** 34–38.
47. JENCK, F., M. A. BOZARTH & R. A. WISE. 1988. Brain Res. In press.
48. HAMILTON, M. E. & M. A. BOZARTH. 1986. Soc. Neurosci. Abstr. **12:** 412.
49. KALIVAS, P. W., E. WIDERLOV, D. STANLEY, G. BREESE & A. J. PRANGE. 1983. J. Pharmacol. Exp. Ther. **227:** 229–237.
50. GOEDERS, N. E., J. D. LANE & J. E. SMITH. 1984. Pharmacol. Biochem. Behav. **20:** 451–455.
51. OLDS, M. E. 1982. Brain Res. **237:** 429–440.
52. STINUS, L., M. WINNOCK & A. E. KELLEY. 1985. Psychopharmacology **85:** 323–328.
53. STINUS, L., D. NADAUD, J. JAUREGUI & A. E. KELLEY. 1986. Biol. Psychiat. **21:** 34–48.
54. MOREAU, J-L., P. SCHMITT & P. KARLI. 1985. Pharmacol. Biochem. Behav. **23:** 931–936.
55. WASSERMAN, E., Y. GOMITA & C. R. GALLISTEL. 1982. Pharmacol. Biochem. Behav. **17:** 783–787.
56. FRUTIGER, S. A. 1986. Behav. Neurosci. **100:** 221–229.
57. BOZARTH, M. A. & R. A. WISE. 1984. Science **224:** 516–517.
58. YAKSH, T. L. & T. A. RUDY. 1978. Pain **4:** 299–359.
59. HERMAN, B. H. & J. PANKSEPP. 1981. Science **211:** 1060–1062.
60. PANKSEPP, J., B. H. HERMAN, R. CONNER, P. BISHOP & J. P. SCOTT. 1978. Biol. Psychiat. **13:** 607–618.

61. TILSON, H. A. & R. H. RECH. 1973. Pharmacol. Biochem. Behav. **1:** 149–153.
62. VEZINA, P. & J. STEWART. 1984. Pharmacol. Biochem. Behav. **20:** 925–934.
63. STEWART, J. & P. VEZINA. 1987. Psychobiology **15:** 144–153.
64. DE WIT, H. & J. STEWART. 1981. Psychopharmacologia **75:** 134–143.
65. DE WIT, H. & J. STEWART. 1983. Psychopharmacologia **79:** 29–31.
66. STEWART, J. 1984. Pharmacol. Biochem. Behav. **20:** 917–923.
67. HAERTZEN, C. A. 1966. Psychol. Rep. **18:** 163–194.
68. BROEKKAMP, C. L. E., M. LEPICHON & K. G. LLOYD. 1984. Neurosci. Lett. **50:** 313–318.
69. WOOD, P. L. 1982. J. Pharmacol. Exp. Ther. **222:** 674–679.
70. GARCIA-RILL, E. 1986. Brain Res. Rev. **11:** 47–63.
71. REDGRAVE, P., P. DEAN, T. P. DONOHOE & S. G. POPE. 1980. Brain Res. **196:** 541–546.
72. SOPER, W. Y. & R. A. WISE. 1971. J. Life Sci. **1:** 79–84.
73. JACOBS, B. L. & P. B. FAREL. 1971. Physiol. Behav. **6:** 473–476.
74. WINTERS, W. D., K. MORI, C. E. SPENCER & R. O. BAUER. 1967. Anesthesiology **28:** 65–80.
75. MARGULES, D. L. & L. STEIN. 1968. Psychopharmacologia **13:** 74–80.
76. FRYE, G. D. & G. R. BREESE. 1981. Psychopharmacologia **75:** 372–379.
77. CARLSSON, A. & M. LINDQVIST. 1973. J. Pharm. Pharmacol. **25:** 437–440.
78. GESSA, G. L., F. MUNTONI, M. COLLU, L. VARGIU & G. MEREU. 1985. Brain Res. **348:** 201–204.
79. CARLSSON, A., J. ENGEL & T. H. SVENSSON. 1972. Psychopharmacologia **26:** 307–312.
80. DE WITTE, P. & M. F. BADA. 1983. Exp. Neurol. **82:** 675–682.
81. BRITTON, D. R. & K. T. BRITTON. 1981. Pharmacol. Biochem. Behav. **15:** 577–582.
82. GLICK, S. D. & S. MILLOY. 1972. Psychonom. Sci. **29:** 6.
83. HARRIS, L. S., W. L. DEWEY & R. K. RAZDAN. 1986. *In* Handbook of Experimental Pharmacology. W. R. Martin, Ed.: 372–429. Springer-Verlag. New York.
84. SVENSSON, T. H., J. GRENHOFF & G. ASTON-JONES. 1986. Soc. Neurosci. Abstr. **12:** 1154.
85. YOON, K-W. P., G. L. GESSA, V. BOI, L. NAES, G. MEREU & T. C. WESTFALL. 1986. Soc. Neurosci. Abstr. **12:** 1515.
86. LICHTENSTEIGER, W., D. FELIX, R. LIENHART & F. HEFTI. 1976. Brain Res. **117:** 85–103.
87. ARQUIEROS, L., D. NAQUIRA & E. ZUNINO. 1978. Biochem. Pharmacol. **27:** 2667–2674.
88. GOVONI, S., V. V. PETKOV, O. MONTEFUSCO, C. MISSALE, F. BATTAINI, P. F. SPANO & M. TRABUCCHI. 1984. J. Pharm. Pharmacol. **36:** 458–460.
89. JOHNSON, K. M. 1978. *In* Phencyclidine (PCP) Abuse: An Appraisal. R. C. Petersen & R. C. Stillman, Eds.: 44–52. National Institute of Drug Abuse. Rockville, Md.
90. GERHARDT, G. & G. ROSE. 1985. Soc. Neurosci. Abstr. **11:** 1205.
91. IWAMOTO, E. T. 1984. Psychopharmacology **84:** 374–382.
92. WALDECK, B. 1973. J. Neural Trans. **34:** 61–72.
93. CASTELLANI, S. & P. M. ADAMS. 1981. Neuropharmacology **20:** 371–374.
94. CLARKE, P. B. S. & R. KUMAR. 1984. Psychopharmacologia **84:** 109–114.
95. FUDALA, P. J., K. W. TEOH & E. T. IWAMOTO. 1985. Pharmacol. Biochem. Behav. **222:** 237–241.

# Mesencephalic Dopaminergic Neurons:
# Role in the General Economy of the Brain

HERVÉ SIMON AND MICHEL LE MOAL

*Laboratoire de Psychobiologie des Comportements Adaptatifs*
*INSERM U.259, Université Bordeaux II*
*Domaine de Carreire*
*Rue Camille Saint-Saëns*
*33077 Bordeaux Cedex, France*

## INTRODUCTION

The mesolimbic–mesocortical dopamine (DA) network can be considered as the Cinderella of the catecholamine family, at least by comparison with the nigrostriatal and the tuberoinfundibular pathways that are better characterized functionally. In fact, functional studies on these neurons face three main difficulties: first, no disease or clinical syndrome with anatomical or biochemical abnormalities directly attributable to these structures has yet been demonstrated; second, the neuronal systems to which they project are functionally more complex and less well understood than structures such as the striatum; and third, the effects of selective interventions (lesions, stimulation, etc.) on a specific transmission system are target-dependent, since cell bodies, fibers of passage, and terminal fields are intimately intertwined. Some of the results presented in this review are based on a working hypothesis formulated in 1984.[1] This hypothesis has received considerable support from the results of experiments published in the last few years, whose conclusions can be summarized briefly as follows: (1) DA neurons do not have specific functions; (2) they regulate and enable functions in the neuronal systems on which they project; (3) lesion of their terminals induces neuropsychological deficits that are characteristic of the functions of the neuronal systems they regulate; and (4) the deficits observed depend on the situations or the tasks that are used to explore the functional role of the particular neuronal system.

A further viewpoint is represented by a consideration of the DA neuronal network within a wider framework.

## LESION OF A DOPAMINERGIC TERMINAL FIELD INDUCES DEFICITS THAT REFLECT THE DISTURBANCE OF THE FUNCTION INTEGRATED BY THE WHOLE STRUCTURE OF PROJECTION

In the first part of this review we examine some of the consequences of manipulations of the DA projections within their terminal fields. Our first approach can be schema-

235

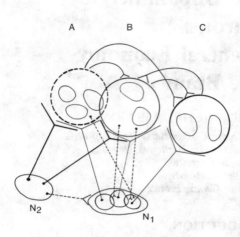

**FIGURE 1.** Symbolic representation of the DA network. N1 represents the DA cell bodies within the ventral tegmental area, with subsets of cell groups sending axons to a given terminal field, in a given forebrain cortical, limbic, or striatal region or system: A, B, or C. These regions are interconnected directly or indirectly via the DA cell bodies; a given region may control its own DA innervation or the innervation of another area; N2 represents another transmitter cell group (e.g., noradrenergic, serotinergic, etc.) and provides a biochemically heterogeneous regulation of the DA network. This intermingled and intraregulated DA network can be studied at various levels of complexity: (1) the role of a given projection after lesion, blockade, or stimulation; (2) the nature of regulation of one terminal field on the functioning of the others, after lesion, stimulation, blockade, and by various behavioral and biochemical techniques; (3) the role of other neuroregulatory systems on the DA network; (4) the network within the general economy of the brain, particularly with respect to the kind of information it receives or translates, or from the meaning, functionally speaking, of the regulatory system.

tized as follows (cf. FIG. 1). It can be seen as a linear point-to-point conception of the DA network, that is, one group of cells projecting to one terminal field. Lesion of the terminals within this region should therefore provide information about the role of DA transmission, particularly the function integrated in this region, or at least about the functioning of the region when deprived of the regulating influence of the DA neurons. This phenomenological approach does tell us something important, albeit somewhat trivial: namely, that the effects of the DA lesions do not stem directly from the 6-hydroxydopamine (6-OHDA) lesion *per se*, but are characteristic of the terminal field, that is of the function integrated in this executive neuronal system. The postsynaptic cells of the terminal region are themselves connected (considering only the direct efferents and afferents) to other nuclei or structures. The integrated function results, to some extent, from the coordination of all these monosynaptically connected structures that could thus be referred to as a neuronal system.[1] Two examples can be considered: the effects of lesions of the DA terminals in the frontal cortex, or in the lateral septum. Other examples, such as the nucleus accumbens projection, have been described in recent publications.[2-4] These studies were essentially designed to evaluate the functions modulated by the DA neurons.

## Dopaminergic Transmission in the Prefrontal Neuronal System Is Involved in Cognitive Functions

**(1) The so-called prefrontal system.** As initially proposed,[5] the prefrontal neuronal system mainly includes the prefrontal cortex and the anteromedial part of the striatum. The prefrontal cortex in the rat is defined anatomically as the region of projection of efferent fibers from the mediodorsal thalamic nucleus.[6-9] This particular site receives DA projections from the ventral tegmental area (VTA).[10-15]

The caudate nucleus is classically a DA innervated structure receiving its major DA innervation from the substantia nigra. However, in the anteromedial part of the caudate nucleus, there is a further set of DA projections with cell bodies in the VTA-A10 area.[13-17] Interestingly, this anteromedial part of the caudate nucleus receives afferents not only from the mediodorsal thalamic nucleus[18] but also from the prefrontal cortex.

(2) **A functional definition of the prefrontal system.** Delayed response tasks are widely considered to be particularly sensitive to cognitive deficits after lesions of the prefrontal system in all species of mammal. In rodents, these deficits are usually tested in a T-maze. In general, they are more pronounced after lesion of the striatum than after ablation of the prefrontal cortex.[19] Indeed, the striatum tends to assume cortical functions either when the prefrontal cortex is poorly developed, as in the lower mammals, or when immature, as in the early life of primates.[20,21] Moreover it has been shown that the prefrontal region that receives projections from the mediodorsal thalamic nucleus, and which sends axons to the anterior striatum and thalamus,[7,22] is especially involved in delayed alternation.

These findings suggest to us that DA modulation of this region might be involved in cognitive processes, especially those required for the performance of delayed alternation tasks. The cognitive and attentional disorders in schizophrenic patients, generally attributed to a dysfunction of both the prefrontal cortex and the striatum, encouraged us to find out whether the dopaminergic neurons projecting to these regions are involved in the functions reflected by accomplishment of delayed alternation. We tested the effects of (1) an electrolytic lesion of the DA cell bodies in the VTA (results not reported here); (2) a 6-OHDA lesion in the same area; and (3) a 6-OHDA lesion of the terminals in the prefrontal cortex or the anterior and medial parts of the striatum.[23-25]

(3) **Experiments and results.** In the delayed alternation task, deprived rats are food-reinforced to enter alternatively each arm of a T-maze. Between each trial, the rat is placed for 20 sec in its own cage. The 6-OHDA lesions of the cell bodies in the VTA were made after the animals had learned the task. After 10 days of postoperative recovery, the animals were tested again for retention of the delayed alternation under the same conditions as those used for the learning sessions. Training was continued until the preinjection criterion was reached. Considering the number of errors in the last 60 preoperative and in the first 60 postoperative trials, the control rats showed no deterioration in performance. Moreover, the number of trials for retention was only slightly higher than the number of trials imposed to reach the learning criterion (TABLE 1). In contrast, the lesioned rats performed badly, not only compared to the controls but also to their own preoperative performance. Observation of the behavior of the animals during the preoperative learning period showed that they exhibited collateral behaviors such as rearing, stopping, and returning before entering the chosen arm of the T-maze. These collateral behaviors were frequently observed at the beginning of acquisition, disappearing progressively as the numbers of errors decreased. After the lesion, all the experimental rats displayed more collateral behaviors than the controls (FIG. 2).

Interestingly, the disturbance observed in the delayed alternation task was not the result of a more general learning disability. This was demonstrated by testing food-deprived animals in a Y-maze using a visual discrimination task. Food reward signaled by light was randomly placed in the right or left arm of the maze. After the acquisition of the task, control rats received a saline injection, while the experimental rats received

**TABLE 1.** Learning and Retention Scores of Delayed Alternation Response (Mean ± SEM)

| Experiment and Groups (n) | Errors in the First 60 Postoperative Trials | Number of Trials to Reach Criterion | |
|---|---|---|---|
| | | Preoperative | Postoperative |
| VTA | | | |
| 6-OHDA lesions | | | |
| Control (6) | 5.2 ± 0.7 | 146.6 ± 12.3 | 70.0 ± 4.5 |
| 6-OHDA (9) | 19.6 ± 1.3*• | 148.9 ± 10.1 | 313.3 ± 33.9*• |
| Terminals | | | |
| 6-OHDA lesions | | | |
| Control (6) | 6.9 ± 1.0 | 190.0 ± 8.4 | 86.7 ± 11.4 |
| Antero median caudate (6) | 18.2 ± 3.0• | 183.3 ± 16.7 | 213.3 ± 46.4§ |
| Frontal cortex (6) | 17.3 ± 2.7• | 193.3 ± 16.1 | 153.3 ± 27.7§ |

Comparison between controls and lesioned rats: Student's $t$-test: •$p < 0.001$; § $p < 0.001$.
Comparison between pre- and postoperative scores in the same rats: paired $t$-test *$p < 0.001$.

a 6-OHDA injection in the VTA region, under identical conditions to those employed in the delayed alternation experiments. After postoperative recovery the rats were tested for retention of the visual discrimination. As indicated in TABLE 2, the number of trials to reach the criterion and the mean of errors in the first 60 postoperative trials were similar for the two groups of rats.

The previously described delayed alternation experiment was also carried out following lesions made in two DA terminal regions included in the frontal system: the prefrontal cortex and the anteromedial striatum. The results obtained are presented in TABLE 1. The performance of the rats bearing the lesions was markedly impaired compared to the control group. After the operation, they made many more errors, and they needed many more trials to reach the same learning criteria. These results are in agreement with those of Brozoski et al.,[26] who demonstrated an impairment in delayed alternation in the monkey after lesion of the prefrontal cortex with 6-OHDA.

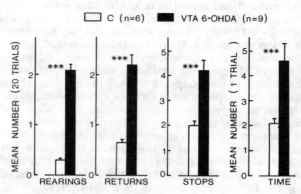

**FIGURE 2.** Collateral behaviors displayed in the T-maze and time spent to reach the goal box during the postoperative retention of the delayed alternation task. These data were collected during the third postoperative session. *Open column*: control groups; *shaded column*: 6-OHDA lesion at the level of the VTA-A-10 cell bodies. (Modified from Simon.[25])

**TABLE 2.** Learning and Retention Score of Visual Discrimination (Mean ± SEM)

| Groups (n) | Errors in the First 60 Postoperative Trials | Number of Trials to Reach Criterion | |
| --- | --- | --- | --- |
| | | Preoperative | Postoperative |
| Control (5) | 6.6 ± 0.5 | 116 ± 4 | 72 ± 5 |
| VTA-A10 (7) | 6.3 ± 0.4 | 111.4 ± 6 | 71.4 ± 4 |

NOTE: No statistical difference was observed between control and 6-OHDA-A10-lesioned rats. The number of trials for all rats in retention was only slightly greater than the 60 trails imposed to reach the criterion.

In conclusion, these results suggest that lesion of DA neurons, and more specifically of the DA terminals in the frontal system, induced deficits corresponding to the function integrated in these regions. In some respects, the impairment was similar to that seen after a large lesion of the innervated structure (in this case, the frontal cortex). However, the nature of the impaired function is more difficult to explain. Since the 6-OHDA–VTA rats exhibited more collateral or "irrelevant" behaviors, it could be suggested that they had an attentional deficit resulting from an enhanced distractibility or responsiveness to environmental stimuli. The animals are thus unable to select the relevant information for correct performance of the task. In this respect, it is interesting that the frontal syndrome has also been interpreted in terms of an impairment in attention.[27] These deficits are revealed in the delayed alternation task.[28,29]

### Dopaminergic Transmission in the Lateral Septum Is Involved in the Frustration Effect and in Spatial Memory

**(1) The so-called septal system and its functional characterization.** Electrolytic lesions of the septal nuclei lead to a complex behavioral syndrome[30-32] characterized by (1) hyperreactivity and hyperemotionality associated with increased intraspecies aggressiveness, (2) exaggerated relativity to unexpected omission of reward, and various behavioral responses interpreted in terms of a frustration effect, (3) disruption of alternation and reversal responses, and (4) learning deficits in spatial tasks. It is generally acknowledged that these disturbances are the result of large lesions with damage in both the medial and lateral septum, including cell bodies and fibers of passage. Little is currently known about the role of the septal dopaminergic innervation arising in the VTA. In a series of experiments[33-36] we showed that the lesion of DA terminals in the septum induced the same type of disturbances as those observed after total lesion of this structure. In other words, we showed that destruction of the DA innervation induced a behavioral syndrome characterized by a global dysfunction of the septal system rather than a specific or circumscribed deficit.

**(2) Experiments and results.**

*Behavioral activation produced by an enhanced frustration effect.* The animals were tested in a situation made aversive by the complete or partial withdrawal of a food reward. Three types of behavior were studied: (1) development of a displacement activity (polydipsia); (2) locomotor activity in a straight double runway; and (3) lever presses during the extinction of a food-reinforced operant conditioning task.

• *Polydipsia.*[36] Displacement activities are generally observed in a conflict situation. If food-deprived animals are submitted to an intermittent schedule of food

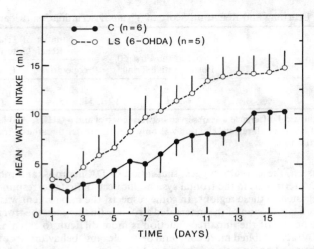

**FIGURE 3.** Mean water intake in schedule-induced polydipsia experiment, following 6-OHDA lesions of the lateral septum. Each session lasted 30 min. The rats, maintained at 80% of their body weight were supplied automatically with 1 pellet/min. Water was freely available throughout the experimental session. (Modified from Taghzouti et al.[36])

delivery, they drink excessively when they have free access to a water spout.[37] Lesion of septal DA innervation reduced the latency to drink, and led to an increase in water intake (FIG. 3). Further experiments with these animals showed that this DA lesion had no effect on (1) spontaneous drinking; water intake after 24 hr food or water deprivation, or after an hypertonic challenge; (2) eating behavior with or without food deprivation; or (3) spontaneous locomotor activity. These results argue in favor of an enhanced frustrative effect. They are comparable to those obtained after large electrolytic lesions of the septum.[38-40] In contrast, lesions of the mesolimbic DA system in the nucleus accumbens induced an opposite effect, that is, a disruption of the acquisition of polydipsia.[41,42]

• *Locomotor responses in the double runway.*[34] The experimental situation of the double runway has a certain similarity to the polydipsia situation in that the animals are exposed to a schedule of partial reinforcement. In the two situations, the omission of an expected reward leads to energizing effects on behavior. In the double runway experiment, when the animal is not rewarded in the goal box of the first runway, it runs faster in the second runway.[43] The experiment was designed to test for the generalization of the effects of nonreward after lesion of dopaminergic transmission in the septum. The animals were submitted to three phases of testing with different degrees of reinforcement: (a) an acquisition phase, in which the reinforcement was continuously delivered in both goal boxes; (b) a partial reinforcement phase, in which animals received 50% partial reinforcement in the first alley, and continuous reinforcement in the second alley; and (c) an extinction phase carried out in one alley with no reinforcement. Animals with DA lesions ran faster for food than controls in the partial reinforcement or extinction situation. However, there was no difference between the two groups in the acquisition phase of the continuous schedule of reinforcement, or in the 50% reinforced trials of the partial reinforcement phase. The two groups also behaved similarly after the first six trials in the extinction phase.

- *Food-reinforced conditioning*.[34] Omission of reward has opposite effects on behavior. The immediate effect is a potentiation of the previously rewarded responses (running speed, or number of lever presses), or an increased probability of displacement activities; this phase is one of behavioral activation. In the longer term, responding is suppressed, corresponding to the phenomenon of extinction *per se*. Here we shall only examine effects of lesions of the DA innervation of the septum on the first phase of this behavior. Animals with lesions and controls learned this task equally well, both with respect to the number of lever presses, and the time to obtain a fixed number of food pellets. However, in the first 5 min following the omission of reward, the experimental animals made more lever presses than the controls. This difference disappeared in the later stages of the test. These results showing an increased responsiveness appearing in the first few minutes or in trials following omission of reinforcement are indicative of a frustration effect. These results also support the idea that the loss of septal DA innervation leads to similar behavioral effects to those obtained after total destruction of the same region by electrocoagulation.

- *Spatial memory*.[33] A final and important characteristic of the septal syndrome is the disruption of spatially guided behaviors and memory processes. These have been explored after lesions of the septum or of the septohippocampal pathway in a variety of different tasks.[44-49] The results have been generally attributed to lesion of the cholinergic cell bodies located in the medial septum,[50-52] although mesoseptal DA innervation is usually destroyed as well. In contrast to studies on cholinergic transmission, little has been published on the role of DA neurons in the memory deficits seen after septohippocampal lesions.[33] Nevertheless, a few studies have been devoted to catecholaminergic systems, essentially the noradrenergic pathways.[50,53]

We investigated the effect of bilateral lesion of the mesoseptal DA projection in two tests of spatial memory: a radial 8-arm maze and a T-maze. The lesions were shown to have selectively depleted dopamine concentrations in the septum without damaging noradrenergic terminals or cholinergic cell bodies. Moreover, it has been reported by Harrell *et al.*[54] that lesion of noradrenergic terminals by 6-OHDA injected into the medial septum (as opposed to the lateral septum, as in our experiments) led to different and even opposite results to ours. Three different experiments were conducted in the radial maze. In experiment I, rats learned the task with food reinforcement in all arms of the maze. In experiment II, retention of the spatial information (working memory) learned in experiment I was tested by interposing various time intervals between choices 4 and 5 of each trial. In experiment III, reference and working memory were simultaneously assessed by only reinforcing four choices in the radial maze. Performance was compared between spaced and massed trials. In the T-maze, the rats were first tested on a spatial discrimination between the two arms of the maze, and subsequently for reversal of the previously learned response. The results showed that the rats with lesions were impaired in all experimental situations. The impairment was particularly marked in (1) the search for the last four pellets in experiment I; (2) the first presentations of various intervals interposed between choices 4 and 5 in experiment II; and (3) the search for food in the baited arms of the previously learned spatial discrimination in the T-maze. These behavioral deficits observed in the rats with septal DA lesions were interpreted as an increased susceptibility to interference.

Experiment III is of particular interest. Here only four nonadjacent arms of the maze (1,2,5,6) were reinforced, and the location of the reinforced arms was unchanged throughout the testing period. The rats were tested over a 7-day period. They were

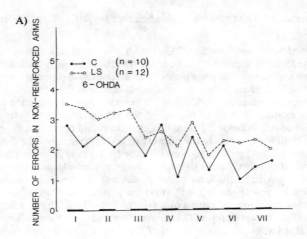

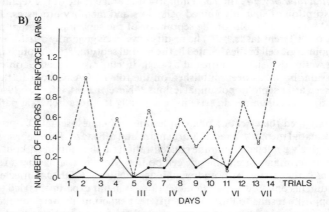

**FIGURE 4.** Effects of 6-OHDA injections in the lateral septum on the performance of rats in the radial maze when only 4 arms were baited. Two consecutive trials were performed each day during 7 days. (**A**) Representation of the mean number of errors in the nonbaited arm (index of reference memory). (**B**) Representation of the mean number of errors in the baited arms (index of working memory). (Modified from Simon *et al.*[33])

replaced in the central platform for 10 sec (time required for placing pellets in the four arms). The numbers of errors or reentries in the reinforced and nonreinforced arms were recorded. It was found that the number of errors in the nonreinforced arms (index of reference memory) for control rats varied in a "sawtooth" pattern (Fig. 4A): on each day, the mean number of errors was always lower in the second trial, which took place immediately after the first trial. In addition, more errors were made in the first trial than in the preceding trial performed 24 hr earlier (ANOVA: $F\ 1.120\ =\ 11.3$ ; $p < 0.003$, trials effect). This follows the classical learning curve with an improvement in performance with repeated stimulus–response associations over a short period of time. A similar time-course in the performance of rats with lesions was observed, although it was much less pronounced. Overall, the two groups of rats improved their performance with a reduction in the number of errors over subsequent trials. However, the performance in the baited reinforced arms (index of working memory) of the animals with lesions displayed an opposite effect (FIG. 4B): the number of errors increased in the second daily trial. The sawtooth pattern was more pronounced in the group of rats with lesions ($F(1/20) = 36.4$; $p < 0.001$, group effect; $F\ 1/20 = 29.4$; $p < 0.001$, group × trials). These results can be explained by the influence of interfering factors left over from the preceding trial on the response made in the second trial. This interpretation is consistent with the characteristics of working memory that is thought to be particularly sensitive to proactive interference.[47] The lesion is thought to lead to enhanced sensitivity to interference, resulting in a more pronounced second trial effect.

The difference in the results of massed and spaced trials provide additional evidence in favor of a dissociation between reference and working memory. In conclusion, these data show that DA innervation plays an important role in memory by interfering with the functioning of the septohippocampal system.

# RECOVERY OF FUNCTIONS LOST AFTER LESION OF DOPAMINERGIC CELL BODIES OR TERMINAL FIELDS

The idea that DA neurons do not have a specific behavioral role, but seem to facilitate processes in the region they innervate, has an important consequence. Since the neurons involved in specific functions are not damaged, some functional recovery should be possible even in the absence of the dopaminergic innervation. This functional recovery was demonstrated by restoration of different behaviors in animals with lesions in DA cell bodies or in various DA terminal fields. A number of different experimental procedures have produced essentially similar results.

## Pharmacological Treatment (L-DOPA)

Lesion of dopaminergic neurons in the nucleus accumbens abolishes or markedly reduces hoarding behavior in rats.[55] These lesioned rats, after optimization of the dose, received an individual dose of L-DOPA (50 to 200 mg/kg) in a small ball of moist crushed food, 1 hr before the hoarding tests. The results (FIG. 5) showed that treatment with L-DOPA restored hoarding scores to control levels.

## Dopaminergic Neuronal Grafting

The effects of DA neuronal grafting were tested on the deficit of hoarding behavior induced by dopaminergic lesion in the nucleus accumbens.[56] The grafting of embryonic DA cell bodies in the nucleus accumbens was performed four weeks after the initial lesion. The technique used was basically that described by Björklund et al.[57] Three groups were used: a nonlesioned, nongrafted group (control group); a lesioned, nongrafted group (lesion group; and a lesioned, grafted group (grafted group). Twelve weeks after the grafting procedure, hoarding behavior was tested in two different sessions separated by a 2-day interval: either after treatment with saline or 10 min after an injection of d-amphetamine (0.2 mg/kg). The results (cf. FIG. 6) demonstrated a marked deficit in hoarding behavior following the lesion (FIG. 6A) as found in the previous

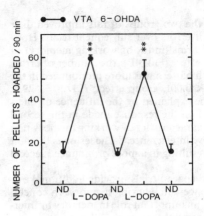

**FIGURE 5.** Effect of 6-OHDA lesion of VTA on hoarding behavior with or without treatment (ND: no drug) with L-DOPA. Bars represent standard errors of the mean. Statistical significance: ** $p < 0.001$. (Modified from Kelley and Stinus.[55])

studies.[55] This deficit in the lesioned group was not affected by pretreatment with *d*-amphetamine. However, hoarding in the grafted group was significantly improved by the *d*-amphetamine. In fact, the scores of almost all of the grafted rats were improved by pretreatment with *d*-amphetamine (FIG. 6B).

### *Changes in Internal State*

The effects of lesion of DA terminals in the lateral septum on spontaneous alternation behavior in a Y-maze, and on spatially oriented behavior in an 8-arm radial maze were also investigated.[35] Exploratory behaviors were tested without any food reward in both mazes. The performance of the animals under two different physiological states, either food-satiated or food-deprived, was assessed. Selective depletion of septal DA led to an impaired performance in both the Y- (FIG. 7) and the radial mazes. However, the deficits disappeared when the animals with lesions were deprived of food (FIG. 7). This phenomenon is robust, as it has been repeatedly demonstrated in both behavioral paradigms (Y- and radial mazes). However, we can only provide a rather speculative interpretation of these results. Food deprivation could conceivably activate the DA septal terminals spared by the lesions, or act on other cerebral structures leading to increased behavioral arousal.

### *Lesion of Noradrenergic Neurons*

As previously mentioned, lesion of DA terminals in the lateral septum induces a disturbance of spontaneous alternation behavior in food-satiated rats tested for free exploration in a Y-maze. This "model" was chosen to test the effect of a further lesion, this time of noradrenergic (NA) fibers originating in the locus coeruleus. Three groups of rats were used: a control group received only vehicle solution, a group with DA lesions (in this group the noradrenergic terminals in the lateral septum were protected from 6-OHDA lesion by pretreatment with desmethylimipramine), and a group with a combined DA + NA lesion (in this group, the 6-OHDA was injected in the lateral septum without prior injection of desmethylimipramine). The results presented in FIGURE

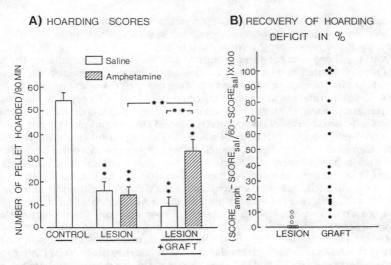

**FIGURE 6.** Hoarding behavior after 6-OHDA lesion of the nucleus accumbens. Effect of d-amphetamine (0.2 mg/kg sc) 12 weeks after transplantation of embryonic VTA cells in the nucleus accumbens. Statistical significance: ** $p < 0.001$. (From Herman *et al.*[56] Reproduced by permission.)

8 show that lesion of DA innervation alone in the lateral septum led to the expected disturbance of spontaneous alternation. However, the combined lesion of DA + NA innervation did not affect performance. Three weeks later, the three groups of rats were retested for spontaneous alternation under the same conditions, except that rats

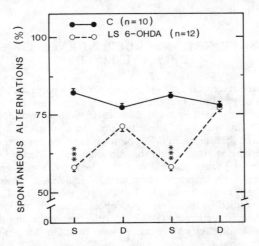

**FIGURE 7.** Spontaneous alternation (mean percentage + SEM) in a Y-maze after lesion of the dopaminergic innervation of the lateral septum. Effect of internal state: satiated (S) or deprived (D). Notice that 50% alternation represents the chance level. Statistical significance. ** $p < 0.001$. (Modified from Taghzouti *et al.*[35])

with selective lesion of the septal DA innervation were reoperated on, receiving a 6-OHDA injection in the pedunculus cerebellaris superior (PCS) in order to destroy the ascending dorsal noradrenergic pathway.

FIGURE 8 shows that the three groups of rats displayed approximately the same percentage of alternation. This was a clear demonstration that the lesion of NA neurons made at the same time as, or some days after, the lesion of DA neurons could compensate for the impairment in alternation resulting from lesion of septal DA innervation.

It is interesting that this type of interaction between dopaminergic and noradrenergic neurons was also observed following destruction of DA neurons by electrolytic lesions of the cell bodies in the ventral tegmental area. Two important characteristics of the ventral tegmental area syndrome, that is, locomotor hyperactivity and disruption of alternation behavior[1] were not observed after an additional lesion of noradrenergic neurons.[58] Interactions between NA and DA neurons in the central nervous system are well documented, but our data emphasize the view that behavioral disturbances result from an imbalance between the normal activities of these neuronal systems rather than from a dysfunction of either one *per se*. The interactions were demonstrated in the lateral septum, but they could have involved any of the structures innervated by the relevant DA neurons. Although the mechanisms involved are unknown, we have shown that NA fibers in the prefrontal cortex modulate the sensitivity of DA receptors via adenylate cyclase.[59,60] The DA1 supersensitivity induced by electrolytic lesion of DA cell bodies in the VTA was abolished after a combined lesion of the dorsal noradrenergic pathway in the PCS.

In conclusion, these various findings support the idea that lesion of DA neurons does not suppress any specific function. Such lesions lead to behavioral deficits that can be corrected either by supplying substantial amounts of dopamine (exogenously by treatment with L-DOPA, or endogenously by grafting embryonic DA neurons) or by interventions on other neural systems (as yet unidentified in the experiments on food deprivation, or identified in the case of lesion of NA neurons). These data may have relevance for the treatment of neurological or mental disorders involving DA neurons.

## FUNCTIONAL INTERDEPENDENCE OF DA TERMINAL FIELDS

In the conclusion of a review on the functional role of DA neurons, published in 1984,[1] we wrote ". . . one can imagine that the dopaminergic neurons act on the integrating systems (frontal, limbic, striato-limbic and extrapyramidal system) not only in insuring an optimal level of functioning of these systems but also in tuning their respective activity." This implies that the various DA pathways act in a coordinated manner, and consequently that there are interregulations between them. This hypothesis has been the subject of recent experimental verification. The activity of a given DA pathway was manipulated by direct injection of dopaminergic agonists or antagonists, or by destruction of DA terminals with the specific neurotoxin 6-OHDA. The effect on other DA pathways was studied by measuring the concentration of one of the metabolites of DA, dihydroxyphenylacetic acid (DOPAC) either *in vivo* using differential pulse voltammetry, or postmortem by biochemical assay of brain tissue samples from anatomically defined regions.

We initially investigated the functional interdependence between the dopaminergic projection of the nucleus accumbens and the amygdala by pharmacological manipulation of DA transmission in the amygdala.[61] The results of *in vivo* voltammetry showed (FIG. 9) that local injection of *d*-amphetamine into the basolateral nucleus of the amyg-

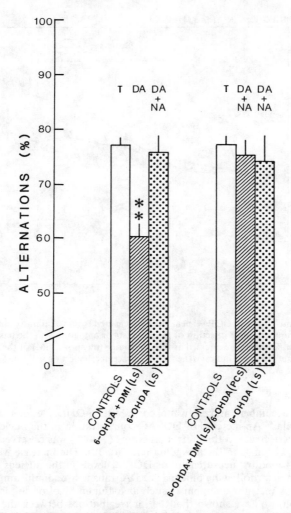

**FIGURE 8.** Effect of the type of catecholaminergic lesion on spontaneous alternation behavior. The lesion type is indicated in the upper part of the figure. DA: lesion of dopaminergic innervation; DA + NA: combined lesion of dopaminergic and noradrenergic innervations. Drug treatments are indicated at the bottom of the figure. Performance of animals is represented on the left panel for the first test, and on the right panel for the second test. Between two behavioral tests, the 6-OHDA + DMI group (*hatched column*) was reoperated and injected with 6-OHDA at the level of the dorsal noradrenergic bundle in the PCS. Statistical significance: ** $p < 0.01$ in comparison to the performance of controls (C) and double-lesioned rats (DA + NA).

dala induced a reduction in the DOPAC peak height recorded in the nucleus accumbens. Conversely, DA receptor blockade in the amygdala by local injection of sulpiride or α-flupenthixol raised DOPAC levels in the nucleus accumbens. These acute findings were subsequently confirmed by postmortem neurochemical assays of DA and DOPAC

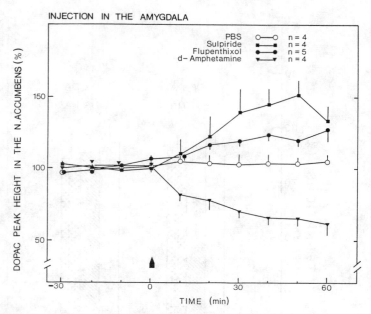

**FIGURE 9.** Time-course of DOPAC peak height measured from voltammograms recorded from the nucleus accumbens after injection of DA agonists or antagonists in the basolateral nucleus of the amygdala. Results are expressed as the percentage (mean + SEM) of the respective mean preinjection value. The arrow indicates the time of intracerebral injection in the amygdala. (Modified from Louilot et al.[61])

in the nucleus accumbens and prefrontal cortex after 6-OHDA lesions of DA terminals in the amygdala.[62] An increase of DOPAC concentration in the nucleus accumbens (+35%) and a decrease in the prefrontal cortex (−40%) was observed 5 weeks after lesion of DA terminals in the amygdala (cf. FIG. 10). The increase was in the same range as that found by measurement of DOPAC levels in the nucleus accumbens by *in vivo* voltammetry following blockade of DA transmission in the amygdala by local infusion of DA receptor antagonists such as α-flupenthixol or sulpiride.[61]

In addition, we have shown that the interregulations between the DA pathways in the amygdala, nucleus accumbens, and prefrontal cortex have behavioral consequences. Lesion of DA innervation in the amygdala does not affect spontaneous locomotor activity of rats, but it does enhance the locomotor response after an intraperitoneal injection of *d*-amphetamine. This is consistent with an increase in DOPAC in the nucleus accumbens. Many studies[63-65] have shown that spontaneous locomotor activity and the locomotor response to *d*-amphetamine are controlled by the activity of DA neurons in the nucleus accumbens. Furthermore, we showed in previous studies that manipulations that have opposite effects on DA activity in the nucleus accumbens (increase) and prefrontal cortex (reduction) lead to locomotor hyperactivity.[66-68] It must also be emphasized that the behavioral effects of disruption of DA activity in the amygdala are not restricted to alterations in locomotor activity. For example, we have shown that DA lesions in the amygdala enhance the acquisition of intravenous self-administration of *d*-amphetamine.[69] A relationship between DA function in amygdala and

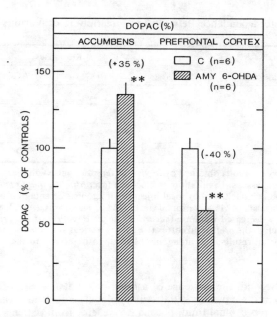

**FIGURE 10.** DOPAC concentrations measured postmortem in the nucleus accumbens and prefrontal cortex five weeks after lesion of the dopaminergic innervation in the amygdala. Results are expressed as the percentage of control values. Statistical significance: ** $p < 0.01$.

nucleus accumbens may account for the interesting findings of pathological studies that have detected alterations of DA in the amygdala[70] and nucleus accumbens[71] of schizophrenic patients.

Interregulations between DA activity in amygdala and nucleus accumbens have been extended to other DA forebrain terminal fields using the technique of *in vivo* voltammetry. These data are summarized in the TABLE 3. Blockade of DA transmission in the prefrontal cortex of the rat (the anteromedial part as well as the suprarhinal region) by α-flupenthixol resulted in an increase in DOPAC peak height in the nucleus accumbens. This is in agreement with the results of postmortem neurochemical assays of the nucleus accumbens following lesion of DA innervation in the anteromedial part of the prefrontal cortex.[72] In addition, we have found that facilitation of DA transmission in the nucleus accumbens and in the lateral septum by local injection of *d*-amphetamine leads to increases in DOPAC peak height in striatum and nucleus accumbens, respectively.[73]

These results provide some glimpses into brain function. First, the interregulations between the different DA pathways do appear to be coordinated and are not coincidental. There also appears to be a functional hierarchy between the pathways. The prefrontal region is a good candidate for major organizer of the activation of other DA pathways. This idea is consistent with the results presented in TABLE 3. For example, alteration of DA activity in the amygdala could indirectly affect DA activity in the nucleus accumbens by interference with DA pathways in the prefrontal cortex. Thus, an increase in DOPAC levels in the nucleus accumbens was found[73] after local injection of DA antagonists into the cortex, mimicking the effect of DA lesions in

**TABLE 3.** Interdependence Between the Functioning of Various DA Forebrain Projections

| Facilitation or Blockade | Responses | | | |
|---|---|---|---|---|
| | AMY | PFC | ACC | STR |
| AMY ↘ | | ↙ | ↗ | |
| PFC ↘ | | | ↗ | |
| ACC ↗↗ | | | | ↗ |
| LS ↗↗ | | | ↗ | |

NOTE: Summary of results obtained by *in vivo* differential pulse voltammetry and postmortem radioenzymatic assays. Facilitation or blockade (*according to the direction of the arrow*) of DA transmission was achieved by local injection of agonists or antagonists in the following DA structures: amygdala (AMY), prefrontal cortex (PFC), accumbens, (ACC), and lateral septum (LS). Increased or decreased response (*according to the direction of the arrow*) in the other DA pathways, such as the prefrontal cortex (PFC), the nucleus accumbens, and striatum (STR) are indicated. For all results, DA antagonists had opposite effects to those of the agonists.

the amygdala. Second, the existence of a functional balance between DA pathways could explain some discrepancies in the result of global neurochemical assays performed on samples of cerebrospinal fluid, plasma, urine, etc., from patients with neuropsychiatric disorders. Disappointing results could be, at least in part, attributed to the counterbalancing effects of reciprocal alterations in DA activity in the different cerebral regions.

## CONCLUSIONS

From this overview of selected results of our investigation of the role of the mesencephalic DA neurons obtained over the last few years, three main points emerge: first, the behavioral disturbances following DA lesions are characteristic of a dysfunction in the structures innervated rather than of a specific effect of the loss of the DA neurons themselves. This argues in favor of a permissive nonspecific role for DA neurons in the VTA. A similar conclusion has been reached by Stricker and Zigmond[74,75] for the DA neurons in the nigro-striatal pathway. Overall, these data underline the danger of relating behavior or cerebral function to one particular class of neuron, neglecting the dynamic aspects of cerebral function.

Second, recovery of function can be obtained in DA-depleted rats. This was demonstrated in various situations, such as food deprivation, after pharmacological treatment, or following transplantation of DA embryonic cells. Recovery of function has also been observed following lesions in a second neuronal system (e.g., noradrenergic). The effect of food deprivation can be viewed in the light of the results showing that rats with 6-OHDA lesions in the lateral hypothalamus will not eat dry laboratory chow but are able to consume more palatable foods.[76,77] Also, rats made akinetic by lesion of DA neurons in the substantia-nigra can show periods of normal activity when placed in a group cage with other rats, and can swim normally when placed in a tank of water.[78,79] Recovery of function after DA lesions in both the VTA and substantia nigra by means of endocrinelike interventions, such as treatment with dopamine agonists or neuronal grafting, is already well documented, but recovery of function after lesion in NA pathways is somewhat unexpected. It may represent a new method for investigation of DA–NA interactions, and it suggests new, less direct, therapeutic approaches to the treatment of clinical syndromes involving alterations in brain DA activity.

Third, the interregulation in DA activity in forebrain structures is an important feature of the functioning of these neurons. Changes in a defined DA pathway can therefore only be understood by taking account of the activity of other DA efferents. Moreover, the largely negative results of attempts to find a direct anatomical substrate of various psychiatric disorders, as opposed to those of a more neurological nature like Parkinson's disease, may be attributed to the disruption of such subtle interplays as those we have found between the various DA pathways. By analogy with the disconnection syndrome of Geschwind,[80] disorganization in DA neuronal interdependence can be thought to lead to "a dysregulation syndrome," that is, dysregulation of integrative brain regions modulated by DA efferents. Further studies will no doubt shed more light on these ideas. Certainly, more detailed information is required on the functional aspects of regulatory neurons in general. The DA pathways would seem to represent a particularly important example, as well as a system accessible to current techniques of investigation.

## REFERENCES

1. SIMON, H. & M. LE MOAL. 1984. *In* Catecholamines: Neuropharmacology and Central Nervous System. Vol. 86. E. Usdin, A. Carlsson, A. Dahlstrom, and J. Engel, Eds.: 293–307.
2. TAGHZOUTI, K., A. M. GARRIGUES, J. LABOUESSE, M. LE MOAL & H. SIMON. 1987. Life Sci. **40:** 127–137.
3. TAGHZOUTI, K., A. LOUILOT, J. P. HERMAN, M. LE MOAL & H. SIMON. 1985. Behav. Neural Biol. **44:** 354–363.
4. TAGHZOUTI, K., A. LOUILOT, J. P. HERMAN, M. LE MOAL & H. SIMON. 1985. Brain Res. **344:** 9–20.
5. ROSVOLD, H. E. & M. K. SZWARCBART. 1984. *In* The Frontal Granular Cortex and Behavior. J. M. Warren and K. Akert, Eds.: 1–15. McGraw-Hill. New York.
6. AKERT, K. 1964. *In* The Frontal Granular Cortex and Behavior. J. M. Warren and K. Akert, Eds.: 372–396. McGraw-Hill. New York.
7. LEONARD, C. M. 1969. Brain Res. **12:** 321–343.
8. LEONARD. C. M. 1972. Brain Behav. Evol. **6:** 524–541.
9. KRETTEK, J. E. & J. L. PRICE. 1977. J. Comp. Neurol. **17:** 157–192.
10. BERGER, B., A. M. THIERRY, J. P. TASSIN & M. A. MOYNE. 1976. Brain Res. **106:** 133–145.
11. LINDVALL, O., A. BJÖRKLUND, R. Y. MOORE & U. STENEVI. 1974. Brain Res. **81:** 321–331.
12. LINDVALL, O., A. BJÖRKLUND & J. DIVAC. 1977. Acta Physiol. Scand. **Suppl. 452:** 35–38.
13. SIMON, H., M. LE MOAL, D. GALEY & B. CARDO. 1976. Brain Res. **115:** 215–232.
14. SIMON, H., M. LE MOAL & A. CALAS. 1979. Brain Res. **178:** 17–40.
15. THIERRY, A-M., G. BLANC, A. SOBEL, L. STINUS & J. GLOWINSKI. 1973. Science **182:** 499–501.
16. BJÖRKLUND, A. & O. LINDVALL. 1984. *In* Handbook of Chemical Neuroanatomy. 2: Classical Transmitter in the CNS, Part I: A. Björklund and T. Hökfelt, Eds.: 55–122. Elsevier. Amsterdam.
17. SWANSON, L. V. 1982. Brain Res. Bull. **9:** 321–353.
18. TOBIAS, T. J. & F. F. EBNER. 1973. Brain Res. **52:** 79–96.
19. WIKMARK, R. G. E., I. DIVAC & R. WEISS. 1973. Brain. Behav. Evol. **8:** 329–339.
20. GOLDMAN, P. S. 1971. Exp. Neurol. **32:** 366–387.
21. OBERG, R. G. & I. DIVAC. 1975. Acta Neurobiol. Exp. **35:** 429–432.
22. LARSEN, J. K. & I. DIVAC. 1978. Physiol. Psychol. **6:** 15–17.
23. SIMON, H., B. SCATTON & M. LE MOAL. 1979. Neurosci. Lett. **15:** 319–324.
24. SIMON, H., B. SCATTON & M. LE MOAL. 1980. Nature **286:** 150–151.
25. SIMON, H. 1981. J. Physiol., Paris **77:** 81–95.

26. Brozoski, T. J., R. M. Brown, M. E. Rosvold & P. S. Goldman. 1979. Science **205:** 929–931.
27. Nauta, W. J. H. 1971. J. Psychiat. Res. **8:** 167–187.
28. Finan, J. L. 1942. Am. J. Psychol. **55:** 202–214.
29. Malmö, R. B. 1942. J. Neurophysiol. **5:** 295–308.
30. Caplan, M. 1973. Behav. Neural Biol. **9:** 129–167.
31. Dickinson, A. 1974. Physiol. Psychol. **2:** 444–456.
32. Gray, J. A. & N. McNaughton. 1983. Neurosci. Biobehav. Rev. **7:** 119–188.
33. Simon, H., K. Taghzouti & M. Le Moal. 1986. Behav. Brain Res. **19:** 7–16.
34. Taghzouti, K., M. Le Moal & H. Simon. 1985. Behav. Neurosci. **99:** 1066–1073.
35. Taghzouti, K., H. Simon & M. Le Moal. 1986. Behav. Neural Biol. **45:** 48–56.
36. Taghzouti, K., H. Simon, A. Tazi, R. Dantzer & M. Le Moal. 1985. Behav. Brain Res. **15:** 1–8.
37. Falk, J. L. 1971. Physiol. Behav. **6:** 577–588.
38. Albert, D. J. & G. L. Chew. 1980. Behav. Neural Biol. **30:** 357–388.
39. Poplawsky, A. & S. L. Cohen. 1977. Physiol. Behav. **18:** 983–985.
40. Wayner, J. M. & I. Greenberg. 1972. Physiol. Behav. **9:** 663–669.
41. Robbins, T. W. & G. F. Koob. 1980. Nature **285:** 409–412.
42. Wallace, M., G. Singer, J. Finlay & S. Gibson. 1983. Pharmacol. Biochem. Behav. **18:** 129–136.
43. Amsel, A. & J. Roussel. 1952. J. Exp. Psychol. **43:** 363–368.
44. Beatty, W. W. & C. P. Carbone. 1980. Physiol. Behav. **24:** 675–679.
45. Brito, G. N. O. & C. J. Thomas. 1981. Behav. Brain Res. **3:** 319–340.
46. O'Keefe, J. & L. Nadel. 1979. Behav. Brain Sci. **2:** 487–533.
47. Olton, D. S. & B. C. Pappas. 1979. Neuropsychologia **17:** 669–682.
48. Olton, D. S., J. A. Walker & F. Gage. 1978. Brain Res. **139:** 295–308.
49. Thomas, G. J. & P. S. Spafford. 1984. Behav. Neurosci. **98:** 394–404.
50. Brito, G. N. O., B. J. Davis, C. L. Stopp & M. E. Stanton. 1983. Psychopharmacology **81:** 315–320.
51. Low, W. C., P. R. Lavis, S. T. Bunch, S. B. Dunnett, S. R. Thomas, S. D. Iversen, A. S. Björklund & U. Stenevi. 1982. Nature **300:** 260–262.
52. Mitchell, S. J., J. A. Rawlins, O. Steward & D. S. Olton. 1982. J. Neurosci. **2:** 292–302.
53. Beatty, W. W., R. A. Bierle & J. Boyd. 1984. Behav. Neural Biol. **42:** 169–176.
54. Harrell, L. E., T. S. Barlow, M. Miller, J. H. Haring & J. N. Davis. 1984. Exp. Neurol. **85:** 69–77.
55. Kelley, A. E. & L. Stinus. 1985. Behav. Neurosci. **99:** 531–545.
56. Herman, J. P., S. Nadaud, K. Choulli, K. Taghzouti, H. Simon & M. Le Moal. 1985. In Neural Grafting in the Mammalian CNS. A. Bjorklund and U. Stenevi, Eds.: 519–527. Elsevier. Amsterdam.
57. Björklund, A., R. H. Schmidt & U. Stenevi. 1980. Cell. Tiss. Res. **212:** 39–45.
58. Taghzouti, K., H. Simon, D. Herve, G. Blanc, J. M. Studler, J. Glowinski, M. Le Moal & J. P. Tassin. 1988. Brain Res. **440:** 172–176.
59. Glowinski, J., D. Hervé & J. P. Tassin. 1988. Heterologous regulation of receptors on target cells of dopamine neurons in the prefrontal cortex, nucleus accumbens, and striatum. This volume.
60. Tassin, J. P., J. M. Studler, D. Herve, G. Blanc & J. Glowinski. 1986. J. Neurochem. **46:** 243–248.
61. Louilot, A., H. Simon, K. Taghzouti & M. Le Moal. 1985. Brain Res. **346:** 141–145.
62. Simon, H., K. Taghzouti, H. Gozlan, J. M. Studler, A. Louilot, D. Herve, J. Glowinski, J. P. Tassin & M. Le Moal. 1988. Brain Res. **447:** 335–340.
63. Costall, B. & R. J. Naylor. 1975. Eur. J. Pharmacol. **32:** 87–92.
64. Iversen, S. D. & G. F. Koob. 1977. In Nonstriatal Dopamine Neurons. Advancement in Biochemical Psychopharmacology, Vol. 16. E. Costa and G. L. Gessa, Eds.: 589–595. Raven Press. New York.
65. Kelly, P. H., P. W. Seviour & S. D. Iversen. 1975. Brain Res. **94:** 507–522.
66. Blanc, G., D. Herve, H. Simon, A. Lisoprawski, J. Glowinski & J. P. Tassin. 1980. Nature **284:** 265–267.

67. HERVE, D., H. SIMON, G. BLANC, M. LE MOAL, J. GLOWINSKI & J. P. TASSIN. 1981. Brain Res. **216:** 422–428.
68. TASSIN, J. P., H. SIMON, J. GLOWINSKI & J. BOCKAERT. 1982. *In* Brain Peptides and Hormones. R. Collu, J. R. Ducharme, A. Barbeau, and M. D. Tolis, Eds.: 17–30. Raven Press. New York.
69. DEMINIERE, J. M., K. TAGHZOUTI, J. P. TASSIN, M. LE MOAL & H. SIMON. 1988. Psychopharmacology **94:** 232–236.
70. REYNOLD, G. P. 1983. Nature **305:** 527–529.
71. CROWN, T. J., A. J. CROSS, J. A. JOHNSON, E. C. JOHNSTONE, M. H. JOSEPH, F. OWEN, D. G. C. OWENS & M. POULTER. 1984. *In* Catecholamines: Neuropharmacology and Central Nervous System, Vol. 8C. Therapeutic Aspects. E. Usdin, A. Carlsson, A. Dahlstrom, and J. Engel, Eds.: 259–269. Alan Liss. New York.
72. PYCOCK, C. J., C. J. CARTER & R. W. KERWIN. 1980. J. Neurochem. **34:** 91–99.
73. LOUILOT, A., K. TAGHZOUTI, H. SIMON & M. LE MOAL. 1987. Brain Behav. Evol. In press.
74. STRICKER, E. M. & M. J. ZIGMOND. 1976. *In* Progress in Psychobiology and Physiological Psychology. J. M. Sprague and A. N. Epstein, Eds.: 121–189. Academic. New York.
75. STRICKER, E. M. & M. J. ZIGMOND. 1984. *In* Catecholamines: Neuropharmacology and Central Nervous System, Vol. 8B. E. Usdin, A. Carlsson, A. Dahlstrom, and J. Engel, Eds.: 259–269. Alan Liss. New York.
76. TEITELBAUM, P. & E. STELLAR. 1954. Science **120:** 894–895.
77. ZIGMOND, M. J. & E. M. STRICKER. 1973. Science **182:** 717–720.
78. LEAVITT, D. R. & P. TEITELBAUM. 1975. Proc. Nat. Sci. U.S.A. **72:** 2819–2823.
79. MARSHALL, J. F., D. LEVITAN & E. M. STRICKER. 1976. J. Comp. Physiol. Psychol. **90:** 536–546.
80. GESCHWIND, N. 1965. Brain **88:** 237–294.

# Relationships between Mesolimbic Dopamine Function and Eating Behavior[a]

GERARD P. SMITH AND LINDA H. SCHNEIDER

*Department of Psychiatry*
*Cornell University Medical College*
*and*
*Edward W. Bourne Behavioral Research Laboratory*
*The Eating Disorders Institute*
*The New York Hospital–Cornell Medical Center*
*Westchester Division*
*White Plains, New York 10605*

## INTRODUCTION

That central dopamine (DA) neurons have an important role in the control of eating behavior was first demonstrated by Ungerstedt in 1971 when he reported that 6-hydroxydopamine (6-OHDA) lesions of the nigro-striatal tract produced aphagia and adipsia.[1] While these lesions also destroyed some mesolimbicocortical dopaminergic neurons, this aspect of the neuropathology was not emphasized. Further analysis indicated that the nigro-striatal system was especially critical for sensory-motor aspects of eating behavior.[2-4] The potential role of the mesolimbicocortical system in sensory-hedonic aspects of ingestion was largely neglected, although eating decreased for about a week after bilateral 6-OHDA injections into the anterolateral hypothalamus that spared most of the nigro-striatal dopaminergic terminals.[5]

The involvement of nonstriatal DA neurons in the motivational components of eating behavior was suggested by the report that the dopamine receptor antagonist pimozide apparently reduced the reinforcing effect of food.[6] Wise argued that the effect of pimozide on eating was comprehensible within his more general hypothesis of the role of the mesolimbicocortical DA system in the reinforcement produced by natural and experimental stimuli.[7] (It is beyond the scope of this paper to evaluate the considerable literature that bears on Wise's interpretation of the effect of pimozide on eating or on his more general hypothesis.)

Neurochemical evidence to support the proposed role of central dopamine in the positive reinforcing effect of food was sought. Although Biggio *et al.*[8] reported an increase in central DA metabolism correlated with food intake after a period of food deprivation, the first clear correlation between the mesolimbic DA system and eating came from Seiden's laboratory.[9] They demonstrated that when food-deprived rats ate, the dihydroxyphenylacetic acid to dopamine ratio (DOPAC/DA) increased in the

[a] The preparation of the manuscript and the work from the Edward W. Bourne Behavioral Research Laboratory that is cited were supported in part by Grants MH15455 and MH00149 (to G. P. S.) and in part by Grants MH09400 and NS24781 (to L. H. S.).

254

hypothalamus, accumbens, and amygdala. Neither food deprivation nor *ad lib.* feeding produced these increases in dopamine metabolism. Although the dopaminergic response in the amygdala appeared to be a postingestive effect because it could be produced by gastric intubation of food, the responses in the hypothalamus and accumbens were not. In a subsequent experiment, however, Heffner *et al.*[10] could not correlate these increases in dopamine metabolism of the hypothalamus or accumbens with any specific aspect of eating, such as the beginning of a meal, meal duration, or amount of food ingested or the onset of satiation.

Our laboratory attempted to replicate the results of Heffner *et al.*[9] We found that the ingestion of sweet milk following 20 hours of food deprivation increased DOPAC/DA in the hypothalamus, but not in the accumbens, striatum, frontal cortex, olfactory tubercle, or the amygdala–piriform cortex.[11] Furthermore, we observed that hypothalamic DOPAC/DA also increased significantly in rats that did not receive the sweet milk diet, but were exposed to the stimuli of other rats eating during the usual test hour.[11] Blackburn *et al.*[12] also observed an increase in accumbens DOPAC/DA in rats scheduled to eat food, but not actually given food. More recently, Blackburn *et al.*[13] reported that an increase in DOPAC/DA was found in the accumbens and the striatum when animals ingested a liquid food, but not when they ingested solid food or a saccharin solution.

These results may be summarized by saying that the anticipation of eating and the ingestion of liquid or solid foods can produce an increase in dopamine metabolism within mesolimbic terminal fields, but the relationship(s) between the dopaminergic changes and the specific food-related stimulus is not clear. To facilitate the analysis of the relationship(s), we attempted to get better stimulus control of eating by analyzing the effect of the ingestion of sucrose on mesolimbic dopaminergic metabolism. Sucrose has several advantages for this purpose: first, its reinforcing effect is concentration-dependent;[14] second, sucrose elicits intake and manifestations of pleasurable affective displays in the newborn human[15] and in the 3-day-old rat pup;[16] third, central dopaminergic damage decreases the intake of sucrose by rats without abolishing their discrimination of sucrose from water;[17,18] fourth, a dopaminergic antagonist, such as pimozide, decreases the intake of sucrose.[19,20]

The inhibitory effect of dopaminergic antagonists[19,20] had been observed in intake tests in which both the orosensory and the postingestive effects of sucrose occurred. In order to maximize the relationship of the orosensory, reinforcing the effect of sucrose to any central dopaminergic changes, we studied the *sham* feeding of sucrose using the chronic gastric fistula rat (FIG. 1). Since sham feeding minimizes or removes the postingestive effects of sucrose, it eliminates the usual decrease in intake that is observed with concentrations of sucrose above 10%.[22-24] Thus, when rats sham feed sucrose, there is a sigmoid-shaped relationship between sucrose concentration and 30-minute intake.[25]

## PHARMACOLOGY OF SUCROSE SHAM FEEDING

Using this technique, Geary and Smith[26] showed that pimozide (0.25 mg/kg⁻¹, ip) decreased the intake of sucrose solutions during sham feeding (FIG. 2). Note that the pimozide-treated rats ingested 20% sucrose at the same rate throughout the test as they ingested 5% sucrose when they were not pretreated with pimozide. Thus, pimozide decreased the sham intake of sucrose in a manner that was functionally equivalent to decreasing sucrose concentration. This suggested that dopaminergic synaptic mechanisms antagonized by pimozide were necessary for the normal sensory and/or hedonic

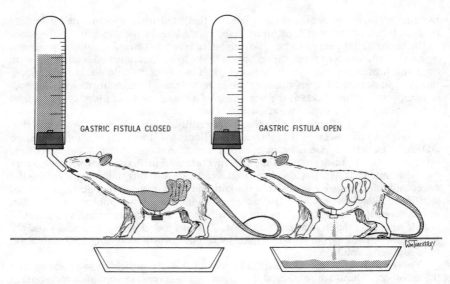

**FIGURE 1.** When the gastric cannula is closed (*left*), the sucrose solution is tasted and swallowed. Since it accumulates in the stomach and enters the small intestine, postingestive effects occur. When the gastric cannula is open (*right*), the sucrose solution is tasted and swallowed, but it does not accumulate in the stomach and does not enter the small intestine. Thus, its postingestive effects are minimized. (From Smith *et al.*[21] Reproduced by permission.)

processing of the oral stimulus provided by sucrose and that the decrease of intake was not the result of a simple motor deficit that was insensitive to the strength of the stimulus.

Subsequently, we conducted a series of experiments that sought to define the dopaminergic receptor mechanisms that were important for this inhibitory effect of pimozide on sucrose sham feeding. Two subtypes of DA receptors are now well characterized: the $D_1$ type stimulates a DA-sensitive adenylate cyclase and the $D_2$ type does not.[27] Since pimozide is a potent, preferential, but not purely selective, $D_2$ receptor antagonist, we tested three selective $D_2$ receptor antagonists, sulpiride, sultopride, and raclopride,[28] and the selective $D_1$ receptor antagonist, SCH 23390,[29,30] and compared their effects on sham feeding of sucrose with those produced by the preferential $D_2$ receptor antagonists, pimozide and haloperidol. We found that all of these antagonists decreased the sham intake of sucrose.[31,32] In the case of sulpiride, we demonstrated stereospecificity of the inhibitory effect because (−)-sulpiride produced a significant inhibition of sham intake of sucrose, but an equivalent dose of (+)-sulpiride did not.[31] We concluded that central dopaminergic (DA) activity at both $D_1$ and $D_2$ receptors was necessary for the normal sham feeding response to sucrose.

Analysis of the cumulative intake curves during 30 min of sham feeding by the method of Davis *et al.*[33] revealed that at least one dose of each antagonist that decreased 30-min intake of 10% sucrose also decreased the initial rate of intake without affecting the rate of decay of intake that occurred over the 30-min test.[34] The decrease in the initial rate of intake is consistent with an action of the $D_1$ and $D_2$ antagonists on the palatability of sucrose, that is, its sensory and/or hedonic effects. The failure of the antagonists to affect the rate of decay of intake suggests that the antagonists

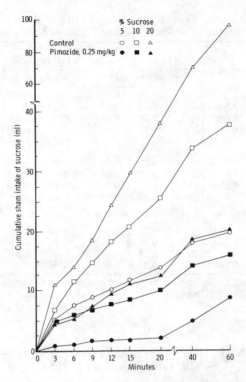

**FIGURE 2.** The effects of sucrose concentration and pimozide injections on sham intake of sucrose. Data are mean cumulative sham intakes for 60 min after presentation of 3 different concentrations of sucrose 4 hr after injection of 0.25 mg/kg[-1] pimozide (*closed symbols*) or injection of the vehicle control (*open symbols*). (From Geary and Smith.[26] Reproduced by permission.)

did not decrease intake by producing a deficit in the ingestive movements made during sham feeding, such as opening the mouth, licking, and swallowing.

To obtain further evidence regarding a possible motor deficit produced by these antagonists, we tested pimozide, haloperidol, (−)-raclopride, and SCH 23390 on the sham feeding of 10% sucrose after 4.75 hr of food deprivation and on the sham drinking of water after 17–18 hr of water deprivation. The longer deprivation for the water test was required to produce water intake equivalent to sucrose intake. Our rationale was that equivalent intakes required equivalent ingestive movements. Thus, if the antagonists decreased intake by producing a deficit in ingestive movements, then the threshold dose of the antagonists for decreasing sucrose and water intake should be identical. But the results were not what the motor deficit hypothesis predicted—all four antagonists decreased sucrose intake at a lower dose than they decreased water intake.[31,35] The preferential effect of the antagonists on sucrose intake compared to water intake strongly suggests that the antagonists were not merely interfering with the ingestive movements, but were interfering with the sensory and/or reinforcing effects of the orosensory stimulation by sucrose during sham feeding.

**TABLE 1.** Hypothalamic Concentrations of DOPAC and DA, and Ratios of DOPAC/DA after 9 Minutes of Sham Feeding Different Concentrations of Sucrose

| Group | $n$ | Intake (ml) | DOPAC (ng/mg$^{-1}$ tissue) | DA (ng/mg$^{-1}$ tissue) | DOPAC/DA |
|---|---|---|---|---|---|
| | | | Experiment 1 | | |
| Control | 12 | 0 | $0.16 \pm 0.02$ | $0.60 \pm 0.04$ | $0.28 \pm 0.02$ |
| 1–1.25% | 9 | $9.6 \pm 20.4$ | $0.23 \pm 0.02$ | $0.83 \pm 0.08$ | $0.30 \pm 0.04$ |
| 10% | 26 | $16.0 \pm 10.1*$ | $0.20 \pm 0.01$ | $0.58 \pm 0.03$ | $0.35 \pm 0.02$ |
| 40% | 16 | $18.2 \pm 10.2*$ | $0.23 \pm 0.01$ | $0.47 \pm 0.03**$ | $0.50 \pm 0.03**$ |
| | | | Experiment 2 | | |
| Control | 5 | 0 | $0.20 \pm 0.06$ | $0.72 \pm 0.07$ | $0.27 \pm 0.05$ |
| 2.5% | 6 | $7.8 \pm 2.2$ | $0.12 \pm 0.02$ | $0.54 \pm 0.05*$ | $0.22 \pm 0.02$ |
| 10% | 6 | $19.2 \pm 2.0*$ | $0.17 \pm 0.01$ | $0.53 \pm 0.01*$ | $0.32 \pm 0.02$ |
| 40% | 6 | $22.8 \pm 2.2*$ | $0.33 \pm 0.02*$ | $0.68 \pm 0.04$ | $0.48 \pm 0.02**$ |
| | | | Experiment 3 | | |
| Control | 6 | 0 | $0.15 \pm 0.01$ | $0.64 \pm 0.04$ | $0.23 \pm 0.04$ |
| 2.5% | 6 | $4.3 \pm 0.8$ | $0.19 \pm 0.02$ | $0.60 \pm 0.01$ | $0.28 \pm 0.01$ |
| 10% | 6 | $9.8 \pm 2.2*$ | $0.23 \pm 0.03*$ | $0.74 \pm 0.04$ | $0.30 \pm 0.02*$ |
| 40% | 6 | $16.8 \pm 2.3*$ | $0.23 \pm 0.01*$ | $0.66 \pm 0.06$ | $0.36 \pm 0.02**$ |

NOTE: Data are mean ± SE. **$p < 0.01$, *$p < 0.05$ compared to Control by Tukey's HSD test after a significant treatment effect by one-way ANOVA. (From Smith *et al.*[36] Reprinted by permission.)

## CENTRAL DOPAMINE METABOLISM DURING SUCROSE SHAM FEEDING

The pharmacological results suggested that sucrose stimulated DA neuronal activity during sham feeding. To investigate this inference, we studied the effect of sham feeding different concentrations of sucrose on dopamine metabolism in hypothalamus, olfactory tubercle, accumbens, striatum, frontal cortex, and amygdala-piriform cortex. We found that 10% and 40% sucrose produced a significant increase in DOPAC/DA in the hypothalamus after 9 min of sham feeding[36] (TABLE 1). No concentration of sucrose increased DOPAC/DA metabolism in any of the other regions samples. But failure to see similar increases in sites such as the accumbens or the amygdala may be accounted for by the insensitivity of the postmortem technique, the use of regional dissection rather than punch dissection, and/or other factors having to do with the accumulation of DOPAC in these regions under our experimental conditions. Thus, we emphasize the positive results in the hypothalamus, aware of the dictum that absence of proof is not proof of absence.

## SUMMARY

These experiments are the first to correlate a specific stimulus of eating—the orosensory stimulation by sucrose—to mesolimbic dopaminergic activity. The pharmacological results and the increase in hypothalamic DOPAC/DA are convergent evidence for this relationship.

The meaning of the relationship is not clear. The possibility that the decreased intake after dopaminergic receptor antagonist treatment and the increase in hypothalamic DOPAC/DA is related to the ingestive movements necessary for sham feeding seems unlikely for the following reasons: first, at least one dose of the antagonist had a preferential inhibition on sucrose intake compared to water intake;[31,35] second, the $D_1$ and $D_2$ selective receptor antagonists decreased the initial rate of sucrose intake, but did not affect the rate of decay of sucrose intake over a 30-min test;[34] third, in the second neurochemical experiment (TABLE 1), the volume ingested during 9 min of sham feeding 10% sucrose was not significantly different from the volume ingested from sham feeding 40% sucrose, but there was a significantly larger increase in the hypothalamic DOPAC/DA after 40% sucrose.[36] Of course, a finer measurement of movements, such as lick rate, may reveal a significant difference that would correlate with the metabolic change. Fourth, striatal DOPAC/DA did not change during sham feeding of sucrose.[36] Fifth, Bailey et al.[20] demonstrated that a response-frequency summation analysis of the inhibitory effect of pimozide on sucrose intake did not reveal a motoric deficit.

Thus, we interpret the increase of hypothalamic DOPAC/DA during the sham feeding of sucrose as evidence that activation of mesolimbic dopaminergic terminals in the hypothalamus is necessary for the normal processing of the central sensory and/or positive-reinforcing information produced by oral sucrose stimulation. Experiments are in progress to test this hypothesis and to attempt to distinguish between the sensory and positive-reinforcing effects of sucrose during sham feeding.

In addition to generating this specific hypothesis concerning sucrose and hypothalamic DA activity, the results of these experiments suggest that the sham feeding preparation will be useful for the analysis of the important problem of the natural reinforcing properties of sweet taste.[37] And finally, since sham feeding of sucrose is a form of oral self-stimulation,[36] it provides a new experimental tool for comparing the role of central DA mechanisms in the positive-reinforcing effects of food, psychostimulant self-administration, and intracranial electrical self-stimulation.[7,38]

## ACKNOWLEDGMENTS

We thank Mrs. Marion Jacobson and Mrs. Jane Magnetti for processing this manuscript for publication.

### REFERENCES

1. UNGERSTEDT, U. 1971. Adipsia and aphagia after 6-hydroxydopamine induced degeneration of the nigro-striatal dopamine system. Acta Physiol. Scand., Suppl. **367:** 95–122.
2. STRICKER, E. M. & M. J. ZIGMOND. 1976. Recovery of function after damage to central catecholamine-containing neurons: A neurochemical model for the lateral hypothalamic syndrome. In Progress in Psychobiology and Physiological Psychology, Vol. 6. J. M. Sprague and A. N. Epstein, Eds.: 121–188. Academic Press. New York.
3. ZIS, A. P. & H. C. FIBIGER. 1975. Neuroleptic-induced deficits in food and water regulation: Similarities to the lateral hypothalamic syndrome. Psychopharmacologia **43:** 63–68.
4. MARSHALL, J. F., J. S. RICHARDSON & P. TEITLEBAUM. 1974. Nigrostriatal bundle damage and the lateral hypothalamic syndrome. J. Comp. Physiol. Psychol. **86:** 375–395.
5. SMITH, G. P., A. J. STROHMAYER & D. J. REIS. 1972. Effect of lateral hypothalamic injections of 6-hydroxydopamine on food and water intake in rats. Nature New Biol. **235:** 27–29.
6. WISE, R. A., J. SPINDLER, H. DEWIT & G. J. GERGER. 1978. Neuroleptic-induced "anhedonia" in rats: Pimozide blocks the reward quality of food. Science **201:** 262–264.
7. WISE, R. A. 1982. Common neural basis for brain stimulation reward, drug reward, and

food reward. *In* The Neural Basis of Feeding and Reward. B. G. Hoebel and D. Novin, Eds.: 445–454. Haer Institute for Electrophysiological Research. Brunswick, Maine.

8. BIGGIO, G., M. L. PORCEDDU, W. FRATTA & G. L. GESSA. 1977. Changes in dopamine metabolism associated with fasting and satiation. *In* Advances in Biochemical Psychopharmacology, Vol. 16. E. Costa & G. L. Gessa, Eds.: 377–380. Raven Press. New York.

9. HEFFNER, T. G., J. A. HARTMAN & L. S. SEIDEN. 1980. Feeding increases dopamine metabolism in the rat brain. Science **208:** 1168–1170.

10. HEFFNER, T. G., G. VOSMER & L. S. SEIDEN. 1984. Time-dependent changes in hypothalamic dopamine metabolism during feeding in the rat. Pharmacol. Biochem. Behav. **20:** 947–949.

11. SIMANSKY, K. J., K. A. BOURBONAIS & G. P. SMITH. 1985. Food-related stimuli increase the DOPAC/DA ratio in rat hypothalamus. Pharmacol. Biochem. Behav. **23:** 253–258.

12. BLACKBURN, J. R., A. G. PHILLIPS, A. JAKUBOVIC & H. C. FIBIGER. 1986. Dopamine turnover increases in anticipation of a meal. Appetite **7:** 243.

13. BLACKBURN, J. R., A. G. PHILLIPS, A. JAKUBOVIC & H. C. FIBEGER. 1986. Increased dopamine metabolism in the nucleus accumbens and striatum following consumption of a nutritive meal but not a palatable non-nutritive saccharin solution. Pharmacol. Biochem. Behav. **25:** 1095–1100.

14. PFAFFMANN, C. 1982. Taste: A model of incentive motivation. *In* The Physiological Mechanisms of Motivation, D. W. Pfaff, Ed.: 61–97. Springer-Verlag. New York.

15. STEINER, J. E. 1977. Facial expressions of the neonate infant indicating the hedonics of food-related chemical stimuli. *In* Taste and Development: The Genesis of Sweet Preference. J. M. Weiffenbach, Ed.: 173–187. DHEW Publication (NIH) 77–1068. Bethesda, Md.

16. HALL, W. G. & T. E. BRYAN. 1981. The ontogeny of feeding in rats: IV. Taste development as measured by intake and behavioral responses to oral infusions of sucrose and quinine. J. Comp. Physiol. Psychol. **95:** 240–251.

17. SORENSON, C. A., G. D. ELLISON & D. MASUOKA. 1972. Changes in fluid intake suggesting depressed appetites in rats with central catecholaminergic lesions. Nature New Biol. **237:** 279–281.

18. BREESE, G. R., R. C. SMITH, B. R. COOPER & L. D. GRANT. 1973. Alterations in consummatory behavior following intracisternal injection of 6-hydroxydopamine. Pharmacol. Biochem. Behav. **1:** 319–328.

19. SANDBERG, D., M. VAILLANCOURT, R. WISE & J. STEWART. 1982. Effects of pimozide on saccharin and sucrose consumption. Soc. Neurosci. Abstr. **8:** 603.

20. BAILEY, C. S., S. HSIAO & J. E. KING. 1986. Hedonic reactivity to sucrose in rats: Modification by pimozide. Physiol. Behav. **38:** 447–452.

21. SMITH, G. P., J. GIBBS & R. C. YOUNG. 1974. Cholecystokinin and intestinal satiety in the rat. Fed. Proc. Fed. Am. Soc. Exp. Biol. **33:** 1146–1149.

22. MOOK, D. G. 1963. Oral and postingestional determinants of the intake of various solutions in rats with esophageal fistulas. J. Comp. Physiol. Psychol. **56:** 645–659.

23. SCLAFANI, A. & J. W. NISSENBAUM. 1985. On the roles of the mouth and gut in the control of saccharin and sugar intake: A reexamination of the sham-feeding preparation. Brain Res. Bull. **14:** 569–576.

24. WEINGARTEN, H. P. & S. D. WATSON. 1982. Sham feeding as a procedure for assessing the influence of diet palatability on food intake. Physiol. Behav. **28:** 401–407.

25. BERNZ, J. A., G. P. SMITH & J. GIBBS. 1983. A comparison of the effectiveness of intraperitoneal injections of bombesin (BBS) and cholecystokinin (CCK-8) to reduce sham feeding of different sucrose solutions. *In* Proceedings of the Eastern Psychological Association, p. 94.

26. GEARY, N. & G. P. SMITH. 1985. Pimozide decreases the positive reinforcing effect of sham fed sucrose in the rat. Pharmacol. Biochem. Behav. **22:** 787–790.

27. KEBABIAN, J. W. & D. B. CALNE. 1979. Multiple receptors for dopamine. Nature (London), **277:** 93–96.

28. KOHLER, C., H. HALL, S. O. OGREN & L. GAWELL. 1985. Specific in vitro and in vivo binding of tritiated raclopride: A potent substituted benzamide drug with high affinity for dopamine $D_2$ receptors in the rat brain. Biochem. Pharmacol. **34:** 2251–2259.

29. IORIO, L. C., A. BARNETT, F. H. LEITZ, V. P. HOUSER & C. A. KORDUBA. 1983. SCH 23390,

a potential benzazepine antipsychotic with unique interactions on dopaminergic systems. J. Pharmacol. Exp. The. **226:** 462–468.

30.  HYTTEL, J. 1983. SCH 23390 – The first selective dopamine $D_1$ antagonist. Eur. J. Pharmacol. **91:** 153–154.

31.  SCHNEIDER, L. H., J. GIBBS & G. P. SMITH. 1986. $D_2$ selective receptor antagonists suppress sucrose sham feeding in the rat. Brain Res. Bull. **17:** 605–611.

32.  L. H. SCHNEIDER, J. GIBBS & G. P. SMITH. 1986. Selective $D_1$ or $D_2$ receptor antagonists inhibit sucrose sham feeding in rats. Appetite **7:** 294–295.

33.  DAVIS, J. D., B. J. COLLINS & M. W. LEVINE. 1978. The interaction between gustatory stimulation and gut feedback in the control of the ingestion of liquid diets. *In* Hunger Models. D. A. Booth, Ed.: 109–142. Academic Press. New York.

34.  DAVIS, J. D., L. H. SCHNEIDER, J. GIBBS & G. P. SMITH. 1986. $D_1$ and $D_2$ receptor antagonists reduce initial rate of intake in sham feeding rats. Soc. Neurosci. Abstr. **12:** 1557.

35.  SCHNEIDER, L. H., D. GREENBERG & G. P. SMITH. 1988. Comparison of the effects of selective $D_1$ and $D_2$ receptor antagonists on sucrose sham feeding and water sham drinking. This volume.

36.  SMITH, G. P., K. BOURBONAIS, C. JEROME & K. J. SIMANSKY. 1987. Sham feeding of sucrose increases the ratio of 3,4-dihydroxyphenylacetic acid to dopamine in the hypothalamus. Pharmacol. Biochem. Behav. **26:** 585–591.

37.  NORGREN, R. E. 1977. Gustatory pathways and their relations to catecholamine pathways. *In* Neuronal and Neurochemical Substrates of Reinforcement. Neuroscience Research Program Bulletin, Vol. 15. 169–172.

38.  HOEBEL, G. G., L. HERNANDEZ, S. MCLEAN, B. G. STANLEY, E. F. AULISSI, P. GLIMCHER & D. MARGOLIN. 1982. Catecholamines, enkephalin and neurotensin in feeding and reward. *In* The Neural Basis of Feeding and Reward. B. G. Hoebel and D. Novin, Eds.: 465–478. Haer Institute for Electrophysiological Research. Brunswick, Maine.

# Stress and Enhanced Dopamine Utilization in the Frontal Cortex: The Myth and the Reality[a]

SEYMOUR M. ANTELMAN,[b] STEVEN KNOPF,[b]
ANTHONY R. CAGGIULA,[c] DONNA KOCAN,[b]
DONALD T. LYSLE,[b] AND DAVID J. EDWARDS[d]

[b] Department of Psychiatry
School of Medicine
University of Pittsburgh
Pittsburgh, Pennsylvania 15213

[c] Departments of Psychology and Behavioral Neuroscience
University of Pittsburgh
Pittsburgh, Pennsylvania 15213

[d] Department of Physiology/Pharmacology
School of Dental Medicine
University of Pittsburgh
Pittsburgh, Pennsylvania 15213

Fashions are seen in science as they are in other arenas of society. Some findings, as certain areas of research, are "in" and others are not. Unfortunately, those results that fit in with the zeitgeist are often subject to less scrutiny than they might otherwise be and perhaps than they ought to be. One such example relates to the currently fashionable and widespread belief that mild stress causes a "selective activation of the mesocortical dopaminergic system."[1] There is no question that there have been a number of reports suggesting an increase in dopamine (DA) utilization in the frontal cortical terminal region of the mescortical DA pathway following several different stressors.[1-10] However, questions can and should be raised regarding the issues of (1) whether this is true of all stressors, (2) whether the stressors employed to induce this effect can truly be considered "mild," and (3) whether the effects of stressors are selective for the mesocortical DA system. Interest in some of these issues began as a result of experiments designed to determine whether prior exposure to a benzodiazepine (BZD) could sensitize the response to a subsequent encounter with the same agent. Our initial finding was that the ability of diazepam (0.5 mg/kg, ip) to antagonize convulsions induced by pentylenetetrazole (PTZ) was significantly enhanced when the same dose of this BZD had been administered once, weeks earlier.[11] We next inquired whether the demonstrated antistress effects of diazepam on DA metabolism in the nucleus accumbens[3] and frontal and cortex[1,6] would show similar evidence of sensitization over time.[12] Since PTZ produces stresslike effects, including anxiogenic actions in rats[13]

[a] This work was supported in part by Grants MH24114 and Research Career Development Award MH00238 (to S. M. A.) and in part by Clinical Research Center Grant MH30915.

and humans[14] and pronounced elevation of plasma corticosterone[12] and norepinephrine metabolism (unpublished observations), it was the stressor used in this experiment. Male rats received one injection of diazepam (0.5 mg/kg, ip), or two such treatments 28 days apart, with a convulsant dose of PTZ (40 mg/kg, ip) administered one
hour following the last injection. Sacrifice occurred 10 min after PTZ administration,
by which time all seizure activity was complete. Frontal cortices (FC) and accumbens
nuclei (Acc.) were immediately dissected according to the procedure of Heffner *et al.*[15]
and stored at $-50°C$ until assay. Tissue concentrations of DA and dihydroxyphenylacetic acid (DOPAC), one of its principal metabolites, were determined by high-
performance liquid chromatography with electrochemical detection according to an
adaptation of the procedures of Reinhard and Roth.[16]

The results can be seen in TABLE 1. PTZ induced a marked and significant increase
in DA levels both in the Acc. (+42%) and in the FC (+123%). Since there were no
changes in DOPAC, the DOPAC/DA ratios decreased, although due to high variability
this was significant only in the Acc. Diazepam, administered one hour before, prevented
completely the influence of PTZ on DA levels in both regions and antagonized the
decreased DOPAC/DA ratio in the accumbens. Interestingly, the effect of diazepam,
like that of PTZ, was also much greater in the FC (where DA went from 223 to 94%
of control) than in the Acc. (where it dropped from 142 to 79% of control). *Remarkably, this preventive effect of diazepam on the PTZ-induced elevation of DA in both
the FC and Acc. was itself significantly antagonized in animals receiving a single in-
jection of isotonic saline 28 days earlier (saline $\xrightarrow{28 \text{ days}}$ diazepam $\xrightarrow{1 \text{ hr}}$ PTZ)*, but was
reinstated in the Acc. but not the FC when another diazepam treatment was substituted
for saline (diazepam $\xrightarrow{28 \text{ days}}$ diazepam $\xrightarrow{1 \text{ hour}}$ PTZ). This experiment was repeated
in the FC, substituting a 2-hour period of immobilization in lieu of the saline injection
28 days prior to diazepam. The results were the same. PTZ significantly increased DA
from $32.7 \pm 3.7$ ng/g to $76.0 \pm 7.5$, an increase of 132%. Diazepam, one hour earlier,
lowered this significantly to $45.9 \pm 3.1$ and, in turn, the effect of diazepam was completely antagonized to $79.6 \pm 12.7$ in animals subjected to the stress of immobilization
one month earlier. There were no significant effects on DOPAC, and DOPAC/DA
ratios were significantly depressed to 55–64% of control values by all manipulations.

These findings are important to the literature on the effects of stress on mesocortical and mesolimbic DA systems in several ways. First, in contrast to the well-established
view that stressors increase DA utilization in the FC[1-10] and the less accepted view that
they also do so in the Acc.,[3,7] and that these effects can be antagonized by diazepam,[1,3,6]
our findings very clearly indicate that PTZ (which at the dose used elevates plasma
corticosterone, an index of degree of stress, to 12 times control values)[12] decreases DA
utilization in both areas, while diazepam reverses this effect. In other words, diazepam's
actions on DA utilization were opposite to those it exerts when stressors enhance DA
activity and indicate that under circumstances where DA utilization is depressed, BZDs
can actually activate DA neurons in the Acc. and FC. Interestingly, this occurred at
a dose one-quarter to one-tenth that used to inhibit DA utilization following its increase by stressors.[1,3,6] Another major point that emerged from these studies was that
even a single exposure to a brief stressful event — in this case, a saline injection or a
period of immobilization — can have an extremely long-lasting, sensitizing influence
on DA utilization in the FC and Acc. In the present case, this influence served to reinstate the decrease in DA utilization induced by PTZ after its inhibition by diazepam.
It is presumed that by sensitizing the animal to the stress of PTZ, the saline injection
and immobilization obviated the static effect of the unvarying dose of diazepam. Since
diazepam itself was able to overcome the effect of the injection stressor and bring back
the antagonistic effect of diazepam administered one hour before PTZ, it may have
exerted a preferential sensitizing influence on the second BZD injection.

**TABLE 1.** The Effects of Spaced Diazepam (0.5-mg/kg) Treatments on PTZ (40-mg/kg)-Induced Changes in Dopamine and DOPAC

| Group | Nucleus Accumbens % of Control | | | Frontal Cortex % of Control | | |
|---|---|---|---|---|---|---|
| | DA | DOPAC | DOPAC/DA | DA | DOPAC | DOPAC/DA |
| No treatment | 100 ± 4 | 100 ± 5 | 1.01 ± 0.09 | 100 ± 18 | 100 ± 20 | 1.00 ± 0.22 |
| PTZ | 142 ± 8* | 100 ± 11 | 0.71 ± 0.07¶ | 223 ± 57¶ | 122 ± 12 | 0.55 ± 0.15 |
| Diazepam $\xrightarrow{1\,hr}$ PTZ | 79 ± 10† | 100 ± 10 | 1.25 ± 0.08† | 94 ± 7† | 68 ± 10 | 0.72 ± 0.14 |
| Saline $\xrightarrow{28\,days}$ diazepam $\xrightarrow{1\,hr}$ PTZ | 129 ± 5** | 100 ± 3 | 0.78 ± 0.04*** | 169 ± 25*** | 94 ± 14 | 0.56 ± 0.07 |
| Diazepam $\xrightarrow{28\,days}$ PTZ | 123 ± 11 | 100 ± 10 | 0.83 ± 0.09 | 144 ± 17 | 100 ± 10 | 0.68 ± 0.12 |
| Diazepam $\xrightarrow{28\,days}$ diazepam $\xrightarrow{1\,hr}$ PTZ | 88 ± 9‡ | 100 ± 7 | 1.19 ± 0.09‡ | 127 ± 12 | 95 ± 12 | 0.75 ± 0.09 |

NOTE: *$p < 0.05$ relative to no treatment; ¶$p < 0.01$ relative to no treatment; †$p < 0.01$ relative to PTZ; **$p < 0.05$ relative to diazepam $\xrightarrow{1\,hr}$ PTZ; ***$p < 0.01$ relative to diazepam $\xrightarrow{1\,hr}$ PTZ; ‡$p < 0.01$ relative to saline 28 days before diazepam $\xrightarrow{1\,hr}$ PTZ; Newman-Keuls test, $n = 5$–$9$.

**TABLE 2.** Effect of a Subconvulsant Dose of Pentylenetetrazole (PTZ: 25 mg/kg) on DA and DOPAC in the Nucleus Accumbens and Frontal Cortex

| | Nucleus Accumbens (μg/g) | | | Frontal Cortex (ng/g) | | |
|---|---|---|---|---|---|---|
| | DA | DOPAC | DOPAC/DA | DA | DOPAC | DOPAC/DA |
| Control | 5.37 ± 0.59 | 1.70 ± 0.13 | 0.331 ± 0.027 | 32.50 ± 2.02 | 17.99 ± 0.80 | 0.561 ± 0.023 |
| PTZ (25 mg/kg) | 4.94 ± 0.71 | 1.46 ± 0.10 | 0.329 ± 0.041 | 42.20 ± 3.90 | 23.70 ± 1.90* | 0.567 ± 0.026 |
| Diaz. (0.5 mg/kg) $\xrightarrow{1\,hr}$ PTZ | 5.88 ± 0.54 | 1.55 ± 0.07 | 0.270 ± 0.013 | 40.03 ± 2.98 | 22.82 ± 1.05* | 0.579 ± 0.028 |

NOTE: Diaz. = diazepam; *$p < 0.05$ relative to control; Newman-Keuls test, $n = 6$–$8$.

A stimulus severe enough to cause the type of paroxysmal firing of neurons associated with convulsions would also have the potential to send cells into depolarization blockade. If this had occurred in the experiments described, it could explain our results. Cells in depolarization blockade should not be able to release significant amounts of transmitter and therefore no change in DOPAC would be expected, although DA synthesis might continue and/or that already synthesized would not be discharged. Moreover, if diazepam were acting through presynaptic gamma-aminobutyric acid (GABA) receptors, it might be expected to repolarize FC and Acc. DA neurons and reverse the effects of depolarization blockade. Cessation of neuronal firing would also be consistent with the immobility that followed PTZ convulsions. This theoretical scenario does occur in large part in the midbrain DA cell body regions following long-term neuroleptic treatment,[17-19] although supposedly it is not seen in mesocortical cells after such treatment.[18]

If the decreased DA utilization we obtained were indeed due to cessation of neuronal firing stemming from depolarization blockade, it should be possible to actually obtain evidence of increased DA utilization by administering PTZ in a subconvulsant dose. This was done and plasma corticosterone was also measured in the same animals in order to obtain an index of whether at the lowered dose, PTZ could still be considered a stressor. The results are seen in TABLES 2 and 3. At the subconvulsant dose of 25 mg/kg, PTZ induced a modest, though significant 31% elevation of DOPAC in the FC ($F = 6.69$, $df = 2.18$, $p < 0.01$; Newman–Keuls $p < 0.05$, PTZ vs. control). No change was seen in DA or the DOPAC/DA ratio in the FC, and there were no significant changes of any kind in the Acc. Also, in contrast to the marked action of diazepam in reversing the decrease in FC DA utilization after 40 mg/kg of PTZ, it failed to modify the increased DOPAC in the present experiment. PTZ elevated corticosterone values more than eightfold (TABLE 3), and this was not modified by diazepam.

Although our data are apparently consistent with the belief that stress can cause increased activation of DA activity in the FC,[1-10] they are also somewhat troublesome for that view. For instance, considered relative to the more than eightfold change in corticosterone after PTZ, the increase in FC DOPAC pales by comparison and begins to raise thoughts about whether very severe, rather than so-called "mild" stressors,[1,6,8] are actually necessary to induce substantial increases in DA utilization. Thus, one cannot help but wonder whether stressors that induce much less marked changes in corticosterone would have any effect at all on FC DA utilization. The failure to find any increase in the DOPAC/DA ratio is equally disturbing, since this has been proposed as a sensitive measure of changes in DA activity.[1] This experiment does help to clarify the interpretation of the results seen after 40 mg/kg of PTZ (TABLE 1) by suggesting that they may, in fact, have been due to a stressor severe enough to cause cessation of neuronal firing.

We next investigated the effect of a 45-min period of restraint on DA and DOPAC in FC and Acc. Plasma corticosterone was again sampled as an independent measure

**TABLE 3.** Effect of a Subconvulsant Dose of Pentylenetetrazole (PTZ: 25 mg/kg) on Plasma Corticosterone

| Treatment | Corticosterone (μg/dl) |
|---|---|
| Control | $6.61 \pm 2.1$ |
| PTZ | $53.60 \pm 7.6*$ |
| Diazepam/PTZ | $62.60 \pm 8.2*$ |

NOTE: $F = 22.3$ (2,20) $p < 0.001$; $*p < 0.01$ relative to control; Newman–Keuls test, $n = 6$–8.

**TABLE 4.** Effects of a 45-min Immobilization Period on Dopamine and DOPAC in the Nucleus Accumbens and Frontal Cortex

| | Nucleus Accumbens (µg/g) | | | Frontal Cortex (ng/g) | | |
|---|---|---|---|---|---|---|
| | DA | DOPAC | DOPAC/DA | DA | DOPAC | DOPAC/DA |
| No treatment | 4.17 ± 0.49 | 2.18 ± 0.14 | 0.559 ± 0.041 | 32.70 ± 2.80 | 23.16 ± 1.29 | 0.741 ± 0.065 |
| Immobilization | 4.08 ± 0.49 | 2.18 ± 0.18 | 0.583 ± 0.083 | 35.99 ± 2.07 | 29.36 ± 1.60* | 0.835 ± 0.067 |
| Diazepam (0.5 mg/kg) $\xrightarrow{30 \text{ min}}$ immobilization | 3.64 ± 0.25 | 2.27 ± 0.15 | 0.655 ± 0.071 | 36.99 ± 2.25 | 29.61 ± 1.28* | 0.824 ± 0.052 |

NOTE: *$p < 0.01$ relative to no treatment, Newman-Keuls test, $n = 9$-11.

of the stressfulness of the procedure. Most reports of the effect of stressors on DA metabolism in these regions have used footshock.[1-3,6,8] Dunn and File[7] reported a large increase in FC DOPAC after a 2-hour period of restraint; however, this was complicated by the fact that it was done in a cold room at 4°C. On the other hand, an abstract by Kennedy and Zigmond[20] reported only a modest, 30% increase in DOPAC following 15 min of restraint.

Our results (TABLE 4), which are essentially the same as those of Kennedy and Zigmond,[20] indicate only a 27% increase in FC DOPAC ($F = 6.66$, $df = 2,26$, $p < 0.005$), no change in DA or the DOPAC/DA ratio, and no modification of any kind in the Acc. Also, diazepam (0.5 mg/kg), administered 30 min prior to the start of the immobilization period, failed to alter the increase in FC DOPAC. In sharp contrast to its relatively puny effect on FC DOPAC, the immobilization induced a greater than ninefold increase in corticosterone in the same animals (TABLE 5).

The nature and pattern of these results are virtually identical to those obtained after the subconvulsant dose of PTZ and once again indicate that even very severe stressors have surprisingly little impact on a region supposedly sensitive to "mild" stressors.[1,6,8]

Out last series of experiments examined the effects of signaled footshock (1.6 mA; 5 sec of shock every 4 min on a variable schedule for 64 min or a total of 16 shocks) and intense sound (120-dB white noise, given according to a regimen identical to that used for shock) on DA and DOPAC in FC and Acc. and also on plasma corticosterone and the *in vitro* mitogenic response of splenic lymphocytes to phytohemagglutinin A (PHA) and concanavalin A (CONA). As expected, shock resulted in large increases in both FC DOPAC (+124%) and the DOPAC/DA ratio (+56%). DOPAC was also significantly increased in the Acc. (+31%) (TABLE 6). Plasma corticosterone showed almost a fourfold elevation (TABLE 7) and there is reason to believe that even this large increase may considerably underestimate the true effect, since the animals in this experiment had a much higher baseline than those in TABLES 3 and 5 as a result of being housed in a different, more stressful, animal room. A large decrease was also observed in the mitogenic responses of splenic lymphocytes to both CONA and PHA (TABLE 8). The corticosterone and immune measures indicate that the shock was extremely stressful even though investigators have characterized 45–1350 times the number of shocks given here [1,3,6] at the same or even 25% greater amperage and over a shorter time, as "mild footshock stress".[1,6,8]

Astonishingly, the sound stressor — which, incidentally, is particularly relevant to humans — failed to produce any effect whatever on either our brain or blood measurements even though it also occurred in a novel environment. At present, this result is not understood, although several findings in the literature suggest that as sound intensity is increased, it may paradoxically inhibit the responses to other stressors.

The data presented in this manuscript coupled with that available in the literature suggest the following conclusions.

**TABLE 5.** Plasma Corticosterone in Rats Exposed to 45 min of Immobilization

| Treatment | Corticosterone (μg/dl) |
|---|---|
| Control | 4.4 ± 1.8 |
| Immobilization | 41.0 ± 3.5* |
| Diazepam (0.5 mg/kg) $\xrightarrow{30 \text{ min}}$ immobilization | 41.0 ± 3.5* |

NOTE: $F = 45.9$ (2,25) $p < 0.00001$; *$p < 0.01$ relative to controls; Newman–Keuls test, $n = 9$–10.

**TABLE 6.** Effects of Footshock (1.6 mA) or Intense Sound (120-dB White Noise for 1 hr) on DA and DOPAC in Rat Nucleus Accumbens and Frontal Cortex

| | Nucleus Accumbens (µg/g) | | | Frontal Cortex (ng/g) | | |
|---|---|---|---|---|---|---|
| | DA | DOPAC | DOPAC/DA | DA | DOPAC | DOPAC/DA |
| Controls | 5.47 ± 0.67 | 1.82 ± 0.10 | 0.344 ± 0.033 | 48.02 ± 1.44 | 25.48 ± 1.26 | 0.534 ± 0.039 |
| Sound | 6.48 ± 0.29 | 1.89 ± 0.10 | 0.291 ± 0.009 | 45.90 ± 2.00 | 25.40 ± 0.20 | 0.557 ± 0.029 |
| Shock | 6.36 ± 0.35 | 2.39 ± 0.18* | 0.382 ± 0.046 | 71.02 ± 12.03 | 57.07 ± 4.59** | 0.833 ± 0.060** |

NOTE: *$p < 0.05$, **$p < 0.01$ relative to no treatment; Newman–Keuls test, $n = 3$–4.

**TABLE 7.** Plasma Corticosterone in Rats Exposed to Footshock or Intense Sound

| Treatment | Corticosterone ($\mu$g/dl) |
|-----------|---------------------------|
| Control | 20.0 ± 8.5 |
| Sound | 22.6 ± 6.8 |
| Shock | 73.9 ± 6.3* |

NOTE: $F = 19.1\ (2,8)\ p < 0.001$; $*p < 0.01$ relative to controls; Newman–Keuls test, $n = 3-4$.

(1) *Not all stressors increase DA utilization in the FC.* Some stressors can decrease DA utilization, while others have no apparent effect. The type of stressful stimulus represented by a convulsant dose of PTZ decreased DA activity both in this region and the Acc. (TABLE 1). Similarly, long-term isolation — which is usually thought of as a stressor — also significantly decreased measures of FC DA activity,[5] although, for some unexplained reason, no reference was made to its stressful properties. Still other recognized stressors at times have no effect on FC DA neurons. Here we have reported no apparent change after a sound stimulus so intense that it rattled the animal's cage and also evoked a startle response. Also, in a paper frequently cited in support of stressor-induced increases in FC and Acc. DA metabolism,[3] the following statement was noted in the Methods section: "We found that by placing rats in the boxes for electric shocks, but without delivering electric current caused no changes in DA metabolism in any of the brain areas examined." Although Fadda *et al.*[3] said no more about this, it very clearly indicates that exposure to a novel environment had no effect on FC DA activity, even though, according to Hennessy and Levine,[21] novelty "invariably results in an increase in adrenocortical activity" and is a potent stressor. Finally, a study of Hadfield[22] is relevant although it dealt with prefrontal cortical uptake rather than metabolism. This report observed significant increases in $K_m$ and $V_{max}$ in mesocortical synaptosomes of isolated fighting mice but not in fighting-observation or simulated-fighting controls, even though these groups preserved the affective/anticipatory and physical stress components of fighting.

(2) *Severe, not "mild stress" appears necessary to increase DA metabolism in the FC.* Perhaps the strongest of the conclusions that can be drawn from our data is that even some severely stressful stimuli induce only very modest increases in FC DA utilization. Since the implications of this are completely antithetical to the claims that the mesocortical DA system is responsive to "mild stress,"[1,2,6,8] the latter needs to be examined more closely. Our attention will be focused on footshock, since this is the stressor most frequently employed.[1-3,6,8] Although "only 16 shocks" were used over a 64-min period in our own experiments, they were sufficient to induce not only a fourfold increase in plasma corticosterone (TABLE 7) but also an 80–97% decrease in mitogenic stimulation of splenic lymphocytes (TABLE 8). Moreover, other experiments by some of us have shown that the identical shock regimen produced a suppression of mitogenic response in whole blood that persisted for between 48 and 96 h.[23] That research also indicated a significant decrease in blood lymphocytic response with as few as four shocks.

In light of such findings, it is difficult to understand how 720[1]-2400[3,6] shocks in 20 min, or an astounding 21,600 shocks in 3 h[3] at the same or greater[3,6] intensity as that used here, could conceivably be fairly characterized as "mild footshock stress"[6,8] or "mild electric foot shock."[1] Moreover, the dependence of any change in rat FC DOPAC on such severe conditions is clearly brought home by the failure of Lavielle *et al.*[1] to observe any change whatever in this measure during 10 min of shock, although 360 1.6-mA shocks were delivered during this period. The authors did observe a signifi-

**TABLE 8.** Effects of Electric Shock (1.6 mA) and Intense Sound (120 dB) on Mitogenic Stimulation of Splenic Lymphocytes

| | 0 | 5.0 µg/mL CONA | 10 µg/mL CONA | 5.0 µg/mL PHA | 10 µg/mL PHA |
|---|---|---|---|---|---|
| Home cage control | 5,333 ± 1,138* | 184,945 ± 14,445 | 202,755 ± 5,947 | 78,292 ± 7,425 | 166,663 ± 19,641 |
| Sound stress | 7,946 ± 1,280 | 192,281 ± 10,201 | 204,646 ± 11,800 | 83,659 ± 5,304 | 194,467 ± 5,931 |
| Shock stress | 5,812 ± 2,109 | 19,282 ± 4,537** | 40,339 ± 9,280** | 10,703 ± 3,593** | 5,781 ± 1,608** |

NOTE: * Scintillation counts/min after incubation with mitogen for 48 hr and $^3$H-thymidine for last 5 hr. ** $p < 0.01$ relative to home cage control; Newman–Keuls test following significant ANOVAs.

cant decrease in DA at that time, and this resulted in an increase in the DOPAC/DA ratio, which was interpreted as indicating increased utilization. However, we find it of questionable validity to emphasize changes in the DOPAC/DA ratio based exclusively on decreased DA levels. Therefore, the point previously made still stands: 360 shocks failed to alter DA metabolism.

The findings reported and discussed here make it amply clear that an independent measure of stressfulness such as corticosterone levels or an index of immune competence is required before a stimulus can be categorized as "mildly stressful," and that arbitrary assignment to such a category may turn out to be completely misleading. Only when increases in FC DA metabolism are accompanied by significant though minimal changes in an independent measure such as corticosterone will it be accurate to depict the stimuli producing such changes as "mildly stressful." Our own opinion is that if the mesocortical DA system is truly responsive to mild stress, changes should be seen after stimuli such as a single shock or one jab with a needle. Although we have focused only on footshock, our comments apply equally well to the other stressors used to date.

(3) *The effect of stressors on DA is not selective for the mesocortical system.* This point, which is reinforced by the present findings (TABLES 1 and 6), should already be abundantly clear from the literature.[3,24,25] Although, it is equally clear that the FC is more sensitive than, for example, the Acc.

## REFERENCES

1. LAVIELLE, S., J. TASSIN, A. THIERRY, G. BLANC, D. HERVE, C. BARTHELMY & J. GLOWINSKI. 1978. Brain Res. **168:** 585–594.
2. THIERRY, A. M., J. P. TASSIN, G. BLANC & J. GLOWINSKI. 1976. Nature (London) **263:** 242–244.
3. FADDA, F. A., ARGIOLAS, M. R. MELIS, A. H. TISSARI, P. L. ONALI & G. L. GESSA. 1978. Life Sci. **23:** 2219–2224.
4. HERVE, D., J. P. TASSIN, C. BARTHELEMY, G. BLANC, S. LAVIELLE & J. GLOWINSKI. 1979. Life Sci. **25:** 1659–1664.
5. BLANC, G., D. HERVE, H. SIMON, A. LISOPRAWSKI, J. GLOWINSKI & J. P. TASSIN. 1980. Nature **284:** 265–267.
6. REINHARD, J. F., M. J. BANNON & R. H. ROTH. 1982. Arch. Pharmacol. **318:** 374–377.
7. DUNN, A. J. & S. E. FILE. 1983. Physiol. Behav. **31:** 511–513.
8. DEUTCH, A. Y., S. Y. TAM & R. H. ROTH. 1985. Brain Res. **333:** 143–146.
9. TAM, S. Y. & R. H. ROTH. 1985. Biochem. Pharmacol. **34:** 1595–1598.
10. CLAUSTRE, Y., J. P. RIVY, T. DENNIS & B. SCATTON. 1986. J. Pharmacol. Exp. Ther. **238:** 693–700.
11. ANTELMAN, S. M., D. KOCAN, D. J. EDWARDS & S. KNOPF. 1987. Psychopharm. Bull. **23:** 430–434.
12. ANTELMAN, S. M., S. KNOPF, D. KOCAN, D. J. EDWARDS, C. B. NEMEROFF & J. C. RITCHIE. 1988. Brain Res. **445:** 380–385.
13. LAL, H. & M. W. EMMETT-OGLESBY. 1983. Neuropharmacology **22:** 1423–1441.
14. RODIN, E. 1958. Electroencephalogr. Clin. Neurophysiol. **10:** 433–446.
15. HEFFNER, T. G., J. A. HARTMANN & L. S. SEIDEN. 1980. Pharmac. Biochem. Behav. **13:** 453–456.
16. REINHARD, J. E., JR. & R. H. ROTH. 1981. J. Pharmacol. Exp. Ther. **321:** 541–546.
17. BUNNEY, B. S. & A. A. GRACE. 1978. Life Sci. **23:** 1715–1728.
18. CHIODO, L. A. & B. S. BUNNEY. 1983. J. Neurosci. **3:** 1607–1619.
19. WHITE, F. J. & R. Y. WANG. 1983. Science **221:** 1054–1057.
20. KENNEDY, L. T. & M. J. ZIGMOND. 1980. Soc. Neurosci. Abstr. **6:** 44.

21. HENNESSY, J. W. & S. LEVINE. 1979. Prog. Psychobiol. Physiol. Psychol. **8:** 133–178.
22. HADFIELD, M. G. 1983. Behav. Brain Res. **7:** 269–281.
23. LYSLE, D. T., M. LYTE, H. FOWLER & B. S. RABIN. 1987. Life Sci. **41:** 1805–1814.
24. ANTELMAN, S. M. & L. A. CHIODO. 1984. *In* Handbook of Psychopharmacology. L. L. Iversen, S. D. Iversen, and S. H. Snyder, Eds.: 279–341. Plenum. New York.
25. ROBINSON, T. E., J. B. BECKER, E. A. YOUNG, H. AKIL & E. CASTANEDA. 1987. Neuropharmacology **26:** 679–691.

# Neuropeptides, Dopamine, and Schizophrenia[a]

CHARLES B. NEMEROFF AND GARTH BISSETTE

*Departments of Psychiatry and Pharmacology*
*Duke University Medical Center*
*Durham, North Carolina 27710*

## INTRODUCTION

Any conference on dopamine (DA), especially mesolimbic and mesolimbic DA systems, must include a discussion of schizophrenia. With the exception of the destruction of nigro-neostriatal DA neurons in Parkinson's disease, pathological involvement of DA neurons in neuropsychiatry has been most often postulated to occur in schizophrenia. Much of the pertinent data have been reviewed in this volume in papers by Weinberger and by Pickar. In this paper we review the data concerning neuropeptide–dopamine interactions and their relevance to the pathogenesis of schizophrenia.

Elucidation of the physiological and pathological roles and effects of an increasingly large number of peptides in the central nervous system (CNS) is a major focus of neuroscience research. More than 50 peptides have been isolated and sequenced from the mammalian brain. They range in size from dipeptides (two amino acids joined by a single peptide bond such as carnosine) to large molecules such as growth hormone-releasing factor (GRF), which contains 40 amino acids. Detailed and comprehensive reviews by our group and others [1-3] of the neuroanatomical distribution and neurochemical, neurophysiological, neuropharmacological, and behavioral effects of a variety of neuropeptides have appeared recently. This paper reviews some of the evidence that neuropeptides are involved in the pathophysiology of schizophrenia. We have focused on peptides known to interact with DA neurons.

With a few exceptions, peptide discovery has occurred as follows: first, a crude extract of brain (or some other tissue) is found to possess a specific biological activity. This activity is then found to be due to the presence of a peptide, and the peptide is eventually purified and sequenced.

For many years, the greatest impetus for research in neuropeptide neurobiology was the discovery that the various endocrine axes are organized in hierarchical fashion, with the CNS at the summit. The chemical regulators of adenohypophysical hormone secretion, the release and release-inhibiting factors, are known to be neuropeptides. The chemotransmitter-portal-vessel hypothesis, posited by Harris and his colleagues,[4] postulated the presence of neurohormones that are released from nerve endings in the median eminence region of the hypothalamus and are transported from the primary capillary plexus to the anterior pituitary gland by the hypothalamo–hypophyseal portal system. Once in the anterior pituitary, these peptides bind to specific membrane receptors, which results in the release (or inhibition of release) of one (or more) pitu-

[a] This work was supported in part by MERIT award MH-39415 from the National Institute of Mental Health and in part by a grant from the Schizophrenia Research Foundation.

273

itary trophic hormones. Millions of sheep and pig hypothalami were extracted to eventually yield a few precious milligrams of the first hypothalamic releasing hormones to be discovered.[5] These included thyrotropin-releasing hormone (TRH), gonadotropin-releasing hormone (GnRH or LHRH), and somatostatin (SRIF).

These findings have resulted in major diagnostic and treatment breakthroughs in endocrinology and have had considerable impact in psychiatry as well. The major reason for this chapter's review of the possible role of neuropeptides in schizophrenia rests on several distinct, but related, discoveries that have led to one inexorable conclusion — that neuropeptides are important neuroregulators in the CNS. They function in the CNS as neurotransmitters and neuromodulators and, consequently, they also modulate behavior. Moreover, some evidence is concordant with the view that alterations of specific neuropeptide-containing neurons occur in certain neuropsychiatric diseases, including schizophrenia.

Neuropeptides are heterogeneously distributed in the CNS. The pattern of distribution of each peptide is relatively unique. Thus, in man and other mammals, neurotensin (NT) is found in high concentrations in the hypothalamus, amygdala, nucleus accumbens, and septum.[6,7] In contrast, vasoactive intestinal peptide (VIP) and cholecystokin in (CCK) are present in high concentrations in the cerebral cortex, as well as in the hippocampus.[8,9]

Unlike the monoamines, neuropeptides, once released into the synaptic cleft, are inactivated primarily by enzymatic degradation. Current knowledge about the transduction of the signal that occurs after neuropeptides bind to their membrane receptor(s) is also quite limited. However, changes in neuronal firing rates have repeatedly been observed after microiontophoretic application of neuropeptides such as NT.[10] Finally, behavioral changes and modifications in responses to centrally acting pharmacological agents have been observed after intracerebroventricular or direct CNS administration of neuropeptides.[11] These latter findings suggest that changes in the extracellular fluid concentration of neuropeptides can produce marked physiological and pharmacobehavioral alterations.

An exciting observation by Hokfelt and colleagues[12] and others[13] is the convincing demonstration of co-localization of neuropeptides and monoamines. The co-localization of sub P and serotonin (5HT) in descending spinal pathways has been the most closely scrutinized example of co-localization. Compelling evidence for co-localization of CCK and dopamine (DA) and neurotensin and DA has appeared.[14]

Thus, a large number of neuropeptides are now known to be present in the mammalian CNS. Their unique anatomical localization and the concatenation of behavioral, electrophysiological, and pharmacological properties attributed to them make neuropeptides prime candidates for one of the classes of endogenous substances that modulate normal and abnormal physiology and behavior.

In this paper, three types of evidence for the possible role of neuropeptides in the pathophysiology of schizophrenia are considered. First, studies in postmortem brain tissues and cerebrospinal fluid (CSF) have been conducted to determine whether the integrity or activity of neuropeptide-containing systems and their receptors is altered in schizophrenia. Second, studies in which peptides have been administered to schizophrenic patients to evaluate their potential therapeutic use are reviewed. Finally, the effects of peptide receptor antagonists on the symptoms of schizophrenic patients are reviewed.

There are, of course, problems with each of these approaches. The postmortem tissue and CSF studies have recently been reviewed by Edwardson and McDermott[15] and Rossor,[16] and by Post and co-workers,[17] respectively. In both types of studies, several potentially confounding variables must be carefully evaluated; these include patient age and sex, and drug effects. Such considerations increase the likelihood that alterations in peptide concentration (or receptor number) are related to schizophrenia and are not artifactual. In postmortem tissue studies, stability of the peptide to be measured must be taken into consideration, as well as agonal state, postmortem delay, and cause of death. In CSF and postmortem studies, the time of day (and year) the sample is obtained may be important because of possible circadian (and circannual) rhythms in the concentrations of certain neurotransmitters and their metabolites.[18] In general, neuropeptides have been found to be remarkably stable in postmortem brain tissue and CSF. However, the complexity of neuropeptide neurobiology is demonstrated by the multiple forms of certain neuropeptides that have been found in the brain and CSF.[19]

The studies in which peptides have been administered to schizophrenic patients as potential treatments are also problematical. It is unclear at this time whether neuropeptides penetrate the blood–brain barrier in appreciable quantities after systemic injection; therefore, any observed effects may not be due to direct peptide actions on the CNS. Studies of peptides as putative pharmacotherapeutic agents must be evaluated with the same rigor as any other drug trial. Ideally, these should be randomized, placebo-controlled, double-blind studies with large numbers per group and conducted by clinically experienced investigators. The peptide antagonist studies, largely limited at this time to naloxone and naltrexone, the opiate receptor antagonists, also have problems. The duration of action of the antagonists is relatively brief, and at higher doses, they may have effects on nonopioid systems.[20]

The neuropeptides given the most attention in this chapter are CCK, NT, and the opioids. For all these peptides, interactions with CNS DA systems, in general, and mesolimbicocortical DA circuits, in particular, have been demonstrated.

## STUDIES OF NEUROPEPTIDE CONCENTRATIONS IN SCHIZOPHRENIA

### Endorphin Concentrations in Schizophrenia

Terenius et al.[21] first reported alterations in endogenous opioid peptide concentrations in CSF of schizophrenic patients. Their radioreceptor assay utilized $^3$H-dihydromorphine as the ligand and measured total opioid activity without discrimination as to which particular opioid was present. In this original report, the CSF opioid activity of four chronic schizophrenic patients (ill for at least ten years, but drug-free for four weeks) was compared before, and two and four weeks after, clozapine treatment. The CSF was filtered and chromatographed on Sephadex G-10; two fractions with opiate receptor activity were isolated (Fraction I and II). Methionine–enkephalin (Met–ENK) co-eluted with Fraction II, but only the concentration of Fraction I was changed after neuroleptic treatment. Two of the four schizophrenic patients had elevated CSF Fraction I opioid concentrations after four weeks of neuroleptic treatment, but no statistical test was performed on this small sample.

In a later study by the same group of Swedish investigators, Lindstrom et al.[22] reported that when CSF opioid activity, as defined with the same radioreceptor assay, was measured in nine chronic schizophrenic patients after a drug-free period of 12 months, six of the patients had higher Fraction I opioid concentrations than the mean Fraction I concentration of 19 normal volunteers. In addition, when retested after treatment with antipsychotic drugs for 12 days and 2 months, the schizophrenic patients with higher pretreatment CSF Fraction I levels exhibited values close to the mean of the normal controls. In another study[23] using the same methods, CSF Fraction I opioid activity was measured in 18 drug-free acute schizophrenic patients (11 had never received neuroleptics; seven had stopped neuroleptic treatment four to eight weeks before this study) and in 24 chronic schizophrenic patients who had been neuroleptic-free for at least two weeks. The schizophrenic patients fulfilled Feighner's criteria[24] for definite schizophrenia, and only the chronic patients whose symptoms worsened during the two-week drug holiday were studied (9 of 12). Two of the nine chronic schizophrenic patients, four of the six relapsed patients, and six of the nine acute schizophrenic patients had elevated CSF Fraction I opioid concentrations when compared to mean values for normal controls from the Lindstrom et al.[22] study.

Dupont et al.,[25] using a radioreceptor assay employing $^3$H-naloxone as the radio-active ligand, found decreased CSF concentrations of opioid activity in 19 chronic schizophrenic patients when compared to nine controls. The diagnostic criteria used were not specified, and all of the schizophrenic patients were receiving neuroleptics.

In a preliminary report, Domschke et al.[26] presented data on the CSF concentrations of β-endorphin in five acute and seven chronic (>10 years) schizophrenic patients compared to seven normal controls and ten patients with herniated vertebral discs. No diagnostic criteria for schizophrenia were provided and all psychiatric patients were receiving neuroleptic drug therapy. The CSF was extracted in silicic acid and acetone, and β-endorphin was estimated by radioimmunoassay (RIA). Inappropriately using Student's t-test to analyze the data, this group claimed that the acute schizophrenic patients had increased, and the chronic schizophrenic patients had decreased, CSF β-endorphin concentrations, when compared to the controls.

Burbach et al.[27] compared CSF concentrations of β-endorphin and Met-ENK in nine neurologically diseased controls and nine schizophrenic patients. No diagnostic criteria were reported for the schizophrenic patients, and all were treated with neuroleptics. Both peptides were measured by RIA. No significant group-related differences in CSF β-endorphin or Met-ENK concentrations were observed.

Naber et al.[28,29] and Naber and Pickar,[30] using a radioreceptor assay for opioid activity and an RIA for β-endorphin, studied CSF from psychiatric patients with a variety of diagnoses, including schizophrenia ($n = 27$), schizoaffective disorder ($n = 17$), depression ($n = 35$), and mania ($n = 13$), as well as for normal controls. Schizophrenic patients were diagnosed by research diagnostic criteria (RDC)[24] and were medication-free for two weeks prior to the study. The radioreceptor assay used a Met-ENK analog, $^3$H-D-Ala-L-Leu-enkephalinamide (D-ALA), and the RIA used $^{125}$I-β-endorphin as the tracer. Opiate receptor activity was significantly reduced in the schizophrenic males only ($p < 0.005$, Student's t-test, two-tailed).

Emrich et al.[31,32] and Hollt et al.[33] measured the concentration of β-endorphinlike immunoreactivity by RIA in CSF and plasma of eight controls compared to fifteen schizophrenic patients and a variety of other neurological patients. Schizophrenic patients were diagnosed by the International Classification of Disease (ICD) nomenclature[24] and were medication-free for four weeks. Plasma, but not CSF, β-endorphin was extracted with a silicic acid/acetone mixture. No significant differences between controls and schizophrenic patients were detected.

Van Kammen et al.[34] measured both β-endorphin concentration and opioid activity in CSF from 30 schizophrenic patients and 52 normal controls; in addition, vasopressin and angiotensin I and II concentrations were assayed. Schizophrenic patients fulfulled RDC criteria[24] and were drug-free for an average of 33 days before treatment. Concentrations of β-endorphin, vasopressin and angiotensin I and II were measured by RIA using $^{125}$I-labeled peptides and opioid activity was assessed by radioreceptor assay with $^3$H-D-ALA as the radioligand. The concentration of vasopressin was found to be reduced by approximately 40% ($p < 0.01$) in the CSF of male schizophrenic patients. No differences were found in the concentrations of the other peptides.

Recently, Wen et al.[35] measured CSF Met-ENK levels in chronic schizophrenic patients ($n = 18$; duration of illness greater than ten years) and neurological controls ($n = 18$; eight stroke, ten headache). The patients were rated before CSF withdrawal with the Brief Psychiatric Rating Scale (BPRS); no mention was made of medication status. The RIA employed recognized Met-O-enkephalin, and therefore [125]I-Met-O-enkephalin was used as the radioactive trace. All CSF samples were passed through Sep-Pak filters and oxidized with hydrogen peroxide to form Met-O-enkephalin. Recovery was estimated at 70%, and schizophrenic patients were reported to have significantly less Met-ENK present in CSF than controls ($p < 0.02$, Students' t-test). No significant correlation was seen between BPRS score and Met-ENK concentration. This group used identical biochemical methodology in a second study[36] while investigating the purported antipsychotic effects of naloxone in schizophrenic patients. They found a significant correlation between the increase in CSF Met-ENK concentrations and the naloxone-induced decrease in psychotic symptoms in seven schizophrenic patients.

Thus, at the present time, the data provided by measuring opioid peptides in CSF is contradictory and confusing and provides no compelling evidence for a significant role of endorphins in schizophrenia. Much of the controversy in this field arises from assay differences. Recently the complexity of opioid peptide neurobiology and its relevance to CSF measurements of opioid activity is becoming clear. Nyberg et al.[37] have recently discovered the presence of a whole family of peptides from the two proenkephalin genes in human CSF. Similar results have been obtained by Bach et al.[38]

Wagemaker and Cade[39] reported a little more than a decade ago, in an open and uncontrolled trial, that weekly hemodialysis in schizophrenic subjects produced improvement in their schizophrenic symptoms. Simultaneously, they and their collaborators, Palmour et al.[40] reported the existence of a previously unknown peptide, a leucine-5-β-endorphin. This group further argued that the effectiveness of the hemodialysis in schizophrenia depended on the removal of leucine-5-β-endorphin from the plasma. Thus, several issues were brought together in a very complex package: the issue of the clinical efficacy of hemodialysis in schizophrenia, and the issue of whether removal of that compound by dialysis was an effective means of treating schizophrenia. To address the first issue, several studies using hemodialysis or peritoneal dialysis were carried out in medical centers across the country. To date, these studies have failed to confirm the clinical utility or efficacy of hemodialysis as a treatment for schizophrenia.[41] Moreover, Lewis et al.[42] studied the hemofiltrate from dialyzed schizophrenics and could dectect no methionine-5- or leucine-5-β-endorphin in the hemofiltrate.

There have been several reports in which nonopioid peptides have been measured in the CSF of schizophrenic patients. Based on a myriad of preclinical data that have unequivocally demonstrated NT–DA interactions (see Bissette and Nemeroff, this volume), we have measured the concentration of NT in CSF of patients with schizophrenia. Led by Widerlov, we assayed CSF NT concentrations by RIA in 21 schizophrenic patients diagnosed by RDC[24] and 12 age- and sex-matched healthy volunteers. The schizophrenic patients were drug-free for at least two weeks, and psychiatric symptoms were assessed with the Comprehensive Psychopathological Rating Scale (CPRS).[43] Group mean CSF concentrations of NT-like immunoreactivity were not significantly different, but the schizophrenic group was shown to consist of two subgroups; one of these had very low CSF concentrations of NT-like immunoreactivity. After neuroleptic treatment, this latter subgroup exhibited normalization of CSF NT concentrations. Only one of 16 items in the CPRS was significantly correlated with the concentration of NT in CSF from the schizophrenic group: slowness of movement ($p <$

0.01). In this regard, it is of interest that all of the catatonic patients were in the low NT subgroup.

Recently, we have confirmed the decrease of NT-like immunoreactivity in the CSF of schizophrenic patients, but changes in NT concentration after neuroleptic treatment were not found.[44] No such CSF NT reductions were observed in patients with major depression, anorexia–bulimia, or premenstrual syndrome.[45]

The involvement of SRIF, the endogenous tetradecapeptide, has also been investigated in schizophrenia by our group and others. In our study,[46] the CSF concentration of SRIF was measured in ten healthy volunteers, 29 demented patients, 23 patients with major depression, and ten schizophrenic patients (DSM-III criteria).[24] All three psychiatric diagnostic groups had significantly reduced CSF concentrations of SRIF when compared to controls. Thus, decreases in CSF SRIF appear not to be specific to a particular disease state, but may reflect cognitive impairment. Gattaz et al.[47] measured the concentration of CSF SRIF in 14 schizophrenic patients before and after three weeks of haloperidol treatment. Although baseline levels of SRIF in CSF were negatively correlated with BPRS items related to psychosis, the increase in CSF SRIF after haloperidol treatment did not correlate with psychopathological improvement.

Gerner and Yamada[48] assayed CSF concentrations of immunoreactive CCK, SRIF, and bombesin (BOM) in normal healthy volunteers ($n = 29$) and patients with anorexia nervosa ($n = 23$), mania ($n = 10$), primary depression ($n = 28$), and chronic schizophrenia ($n = 13$), all ill for more than six months. Diagnoses were made using RDC criteria,[24] and schizophrenic patients were neuroleptic-free for 14 days prior to CSF sampling. No diagnostic group-related statistically significant differences in CSF concentrations of any neuropeptide were found.

In a second study, Gerner[49] measured BOM, SRIF, and CCK by RIA in CSF obtained from 31 normal controls, 19 schizophrenic patients from California hospitals, and 53 schizophrenic patients from the National Institute of Mental Health (NIMH). All schizophrenic patients fulfilled RDC criteria[24] and were neuroleptic-free for at least 14 days. Only the schizophrenic patients from the NIMH exhibited significant elevations in CCK and SRIF concentrations and decreases in BOM, when compared to controls. Rubinow et al.[50,51] who were the first to demonstrate reductions in CSF SRIF in depressed patients, found no alterations in CSF SRIF concentrations in drug-free schizophrenic patients.

As noted in the introduction, the discovery of co-localization of CCK with DA in certain midbrain neurons, particularly those of the ventral tegmental area,[14] has provided an impetus for study of potential interactions of these two neurotransmitter substances in normal and abnormal behavioral states. This subject is discussed in detail in this volume in papers by Crawley and by Wang.

Verbank et al.[52] measured CSF CCK concentrations in control subjects and in patients with Parkinson's disease ($n = 13$), depression ($n = 30$), and schizophrenia ($n = 15$). Schizophrenic patients were diagnosed using Feighner's criteria.[24] Nine patients were drug-free for six weeks, and six received haloperidol prior to CSF withdrawal. The antiserum used to measure CCK also recognized gastrin and caerulein, and $^{125}$I-gastrin was used as the radioligand in the CCK assay. The concentration of CCK in CSF was reported to be significantly decreased in the drug-free schizophrenic patients when compared to the normal controls. Tamminga and her colleagues[53] could not confirm these findings. In fact, drug-free schizophrenic patients had elevated concentrations of CCK when compared to controls. These findings are described in further detail in this volume in the paper by Tamminga.

Rimon et al.[54] recently measured the concentration of sub P in CSF from 15 controls (X-ray or urology patients), 12 depressed patients, and 12 schizophrenic patients.

Schizophrenic patients fulfilled Feighner's criteria[24] and were drug-free for two weeks. Samples of CSF were filtered on Sep-Pak cartridges and sub P was measured by RIA. The schizophrenic patients had significantly increased CSF concentrations of this undecapeptide. Gel electrophoresis of the sub P immunoreactivity in CSF revealed that less than 10% of the observed immunoreactivity was due to the presence of the intact sub P molecule; fragments co-eluting with sub $P_{5-11}$ and sub $P_{3-11}$ represented the bulk of the immunoreactivity.

Lindstrom et al.[55] measured the CSF concentrations of immunoreactive delta sleep-inducing peptide (DSIP) in healthy volunteers ($n = 20$), schizophrenic patients ($n = 22$), and depressed patients ($n = 10$). Schizophrenic patients fulfilled RDC criteria[24] and were drug-free for two weeks before the first CSF sample was obtained. Schizophrenic patients had significantly lower CSF DSIP concentrations than controls, both in the drug-free state and after four weeks of neuroleptic treatment.

### Neuropeptide Concentrations in Postmortem Brain in Schizophrenia

In addition to neuropeptide measurement in CSF, investigators have also examined postmortem brain tissue from schizophrenic patients.

Recently, Crow and his colleagues have measured the concentrations of several centrally active neuropeptides in brain regions from 12 controls and 14 schizophrenic patients.[56-58] All schizophrenic patients fulfilled Feighner's criteria[24] and were further subclassified into Type I ($n = 7$) and Type II ($n = 7$) based on the presence or absence of "positive" and "negative" symptoms, as described by Crow.[58] Five neuropeptides (NT, sub P, CCK, SRIF, and VIP) were assayed by RIA in temporal, frontal, parietal, and cingulate cortices and several subcortical regions, including the hippocampus, amygdala, globus pallidus, putamen, dorsomedial thalamus, and lateral thalamus. Significant alterations were observed for CCK (reduced in temporal cortex) and sub P (increased in hippocampus) in the total group of schizophrenic patients compared to controls. Type II schizophrenic patients had significantly decreased concentrations of CCK in the amygdala and significantly decreased SRIF and CCK concentrations in the hippocampus; Type I schizophrenic patients had elevated levels of VIP in the amygdala. No significant correlation was seen for any regional neuropeptide concentration with age, postmortem delay, or presence of neuroleptic medication. This same group has reported reduced numbers of CCK receptors in the frontal cortex of schizophrenic patients.[59]

Nemeroff et al.[60,61] measured the regional postmortem brain concentrations of NT, SRIF, and TRH in controls (free of neurological or psychiatric disease, $n = 50$), patients with Huntington's chorea ($n = 24$), and schizophrenic patients ($n = 46$). Schizophrenic patients were diagnosed by RDC criteria[24] and were on various neuroleptic regimens before and, in some cases, up to the time of death. No significant differences in NT, SRIF, or TRH concentrations were seen between controls and schizophrenic patients in the caudate nucleus, nucleus accumbens, amygdala, or hypothalamus. A significant decrease in SRIF ($p < 0.05$) and TRH ($p < 0.004$) concentrations in Brodmann's area 12 (frontal cortex) and a significant decrease ($p < 0.05$) in TRH concentration in Brodmann's area 32 (frontal cortex) were observed in the schizophrenic patients when compared to the controls; in contrast, NT content was significantly elevated ($p < 0.006$) in Brodmann's area 32 (frontal cortex) in the schizophrenic group (FIG. 1).

Kleinman et al.[62] measured the concentration of four neuropeptides (Met–ENK, sub P, NT, and CCK) by RIA in postmortem brain regions from normal control sub-

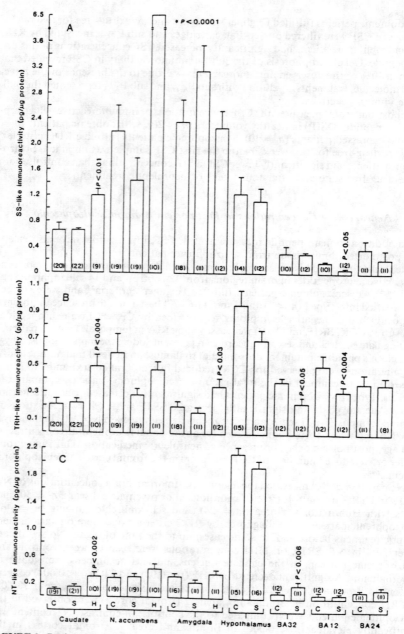

**FIGURE 1.** Regional brain concentrations of (**A**) somatostatin (SS)-like, (**B**) TRH-like, and (**C**) NT-like immunoreactivity in normal controls (C), schizophrenics (S), and Huntington's chorea patients (H). Values are means ± standard errors; numbers in parentheses refer to the number of samples per group. Huntington's chorea patients had significantly higher concentrations of ▶

jects ($n$ = 18), alcoholic patients ($n$ = 7), opiate users ($n$ = 12), suicide victims ($n$ = 19), and psychotic patients ($n$ = 40). The psychotic group was subdivided by RDC criteria[24] into chronic paranoid schizophrenic patients ($n$ = 11), chronic undifferentiated schizophrenic patients ($n$ = 6), and patients with "other" psychotic disorders (unspecified functional psychoses and affective psychoses). No significant differences between normals and psychotic patients were found in Met–ENK concentrations in nucleus accumbens, hypothalamus, globus pallidus, or putamen. Similarly, no significant group-related differences in NT concentrations in nucleus accumbens, globus pallidus, or hypothalamus were observed. Moreover, no significant differences were seen between control and psychotic patients in CCK concentrations in amygdala, nucleus accumbens, caudate nucleus, frontal cortex, substantia-nigra, hippocampus, or temporal cortex. Met–ENK concentrations were reported to be significantly ($p$ < 0.05) decreased in the caudate nucleus of chronic paranoid schizophrenics compared to other diagnostic groups or controls; sub P levels were significantly increased in the caudate nucleus of patients with psychoses when compared to diagnoses other than schizophrenia.

Biggins et al.[63] have recently measured amygdaloid concentrations of NT and TRH by RIA in normals ($n$ = 7) and patients with senile dementia of Alzheimer's type ($n$ = 7), depressive illness ($n$ = 7), or schizophrenia ($n$ = 7). No criteria were given for the diagnosis of schizophrenia, and no mention was made of medication status. No significant difference was seen in amygdaloid concentrations of TRH or NT between the four diagnostic groups. No correlation was seen between patient age and peptide concentration.

Recently, Zech et al,[64] using immunohistochemical methods, have examined the localization of four neuropeptides, Met–ENK, NT, neuropeptide Y, and vasoactive intestinal polypeptide (VIP) in the amygdala of controls ($n$ = 7) and schizophrenic patients ($n$ = 5). The distribution and staining intensity of the first three neuropeptides were unchanged in the amygdala, but VIP staining was reportedly increased in the central amygdaloid nucleus of the schizophrenic patients. Recently Kleinman[65] has comprehensively reviewed postmortem neurochemical studies in schizophrenia.

# STUDIES USING NEUROPEPTIDES AS TREATMENTS FOR SCHIZOPHRENIA

## β-Endorphin in Schizophrenia

Kline et al.[66] administered 1.5-mg β-endorphin iv to three schizophrenic patients and reported a rapid worsening of their cognitive difficulties. Less than two weeks later, a second trial was conducted with higher doses of β-endorphin. One schizophrenic patient who had not responded to the previous 1-mg dose responded to 4-mg of β-endorphin iv by looking more energetic, smiling frequently, and speaking rapidly. He spoke of plans for the future and a new lack of fear of others. However, after 7-mg of β-endorphin iv, he again looked fatigued and spoke in a halting manner. Two other schizophrenic patients who received 3-mg β-endorphin iv showed no behavioral changes.

---

SS, TRH, and NT in the caudate nucleus, SS in nucleus accumbens, and TRH in the amygdala. The schizophrenics had significantly lower concentrations of SS and TRH in one frontal cortical region (BA12) and reduced levels of TRH in another frontal cortical region (BA32) as well. In the latter region the concentration of NT was elevated. $p$ values were derived from analysis of variance. (From Nemeroff et al.[60] Reprinted by permission.)

The Stanford group[67] reported on a double-blind, crossover investigation in ten male, drug-free veterans with the diagnosis of chronic schizophrenia who were given a single injection of 20-mg β-endorphin iv or placebo on three consecutive Mondays. Two investigators rated the patients' symptoms using the BPRS and the CGI.[68,69] Frequent ratings were performed on the day of the infusion and daily ratings were continued until the following Monday. Prolactin concentrations were elevated by β-endorphin, suggesting that the β-endorphin was pharmacologically active. The CGI scores were consistent with the impressions of both staff and patients that neither could distinguish the response to β-endorphin from the response to saline. However, when the BPRS scores were analyzed, there was a statistically significant, but not clinically obvious, improvement following β-endorphin injection compared to placebo injection.

Gerner et al.[70] administered β-endorphin to eight schizophrenic patients in a double-blind, placebo-controlled crossover design. Subjects in this investigation were rated by self-rating scales. As a group, the schizophrenic subjects were not significantly different after β-endorphin administration than after placebo on overall ratings. However, as a general observation, the condition of six of the eight subjects worsened after β-endorphin, while only one subject worsened after placebo.

Pickar et al.[71] administered 4- to 15-mg β-endorphin iv to six schizophrenic patients in a double-blind, placebo-controlled investigation. Individual physician raters recorded pertinent clinical observations and completed the BPRS at baseline and at regular intervals. Comparison of the BPRS change scores for placebo and β-endorphin indicated that β-endorphin did not cause significant behavioral changes in the six schizophrenic subjects.

Petho et al.[72] gave human β-endorphin to six acute schizophrenic patients using a double-blind, parallel-groups design. Six patients were given 4-mg β-endorphin iv, while three patients were given the same volume of physiological saline solution. Each of the six schizophrenic patients given β-endorphin demonstrated some change following the β-endorphin infusion. The changes were reported as an improvement in the areas of mood and activity. However, there was no improvement in specific psychotic symptoms or in the cognitive disorders of schizophrenia. The investigators concluded that there was very little evidence that β-endorphin had any influence whatsoever in relieving psychosis.

## Enkephalin Analogs in Schizophrenia

The effects of a potent and stable Met–ENK analog, FK-33-824, have been studied in schizophrenia. The studies by Nedopil, Jungkunz, and co-workers have been summarized by Klein et al.[73] In an open study of nine paranoid schizophrenic patients, treatment with FK-33-824 (0.5 mg iv on day 1, 1.0 mg on day 2), resulted in three patients dropping out of the study because of a dramatic worsening of symptoms. However, five of the remaining six patients were improved, as evidenced by a significant decrease in BPRS scores. In contrast, in a later double-blind two-day study,[11] the effects of FK-33-824 (3 mg im per day) in 16 schizophrenic patients were evaluated and no clinical improvement was observed.

## DTγE and DEγE in Schizophrenia

In a series of reports, De Wied, van Ree, Verhoeven, and their associates from Utrecht in the Netherlands have postulated that schizophrenia is a disorder of endorphin metabolism — an overproduction of α-type endorphins, which purportedly have am-phetaminelike properties, and/or an underproduction of the γ-type endorphins, which purportedly possess neuroleptic properties. Such theoretical considerations and the preclinical data concordant with these hypotheses have led to clinical trials of des-tyrosine-γ-endorphin (DTγE) and related peptides in schizophrenic patients. DTγE is γ-endorphin with the tyrosine removed; it has no opioid activity. In addition, Burbach and De Wied found evidence of naturally occurring DTγE in rat pituitary, rat brain, and human CSF. They also report that incubation of β-endorphin with homogenates of rat forebrain yield DTγE, suggesting that DTγE may be an endogenously formed compound.[74,75] These theoretical issues and early clinical trials have been described in a series of reviews.[76-79]

The preclinical studies with γ-endorphin fragments by the Utrecht group have been criticized on the grounds that the tests used to detect "neuroleptic activity" are atyp-ical (e.g., the pole-jumping test, and the paw-grip test[80]) when compared to standardly used tests, such as effects on the extinction of conditioned avoidance responding or blockade of the actions of DA agonists. Such criticisms are only partially warranted, because use of standard neuroleptic screening tests may only reveal activity of com-pounds with DA receptor blocking action, and these drugs may possess unwanted side effects, such as extrapyramidal symptoms, and may eventually produce tardive dys-kinesia. Using atypical or novel screening tests for neuroleptics may eventually pro-duce medications useful for schizophrenia without the usual neuroleptic side effects.

γ-Endorphin derivatives with purported antipsychotic activity have been tested for antipsychotic efficacy in schizophrenic patients by the Utrecht group. In the first study,[81] six schizophrenic patients were withdrawn from neuroleptic drugs one week prior to the clinical trial. The patients then received daily treatments with 0.5–1.0-mg DTγE im for ten days. All six patients were reported to show dramatic improvement, though three patients rapidly relapsed during treatment with the peptide.

In a second study by the same group,[79,81] schizophrenic patients were maintained on neuroleptics during treatment with DTγE. In this double-blind, crossover-designed study, 16 patients received DTγE (1 mg im daily for 16 days) or placebo. The authors reported a significant improvement after combining neuroleptic and DTγE treatment when compared to the combined neuroleptic and placebo treatment. The patients be-came progressively less psychotic, and hallucinations and delusions were significantly reduced.

In contrast to these findings, Emrich and his colleagues,[82] in a double-blind trial using daily injections of 2-mg DTγE im, found no significant antipsychotic effects of the peptide in 13 patients maintained on neuroleptics in an attempt to replicate the conditions used by Verhoeven et al.[81] Other largely negative studies have been pub-lished, including those of Fink et al.,[83] Manchandra and Hirsch,[84] Tamminga et al.,[85] and Meltzer et al.[86] In these studies and in the recent study by Volavka et al.,[87] the antipsychotic effects of DTγE, when evident at all, were short-lived, barely attained statistical significance, and were not clinically robust.

Recently, the Utrecht group has studied the clinical effects of des-enkephalin-γ-endorphin (DEγE), the shortest fragment of γ-endorphin with neurolepticlike activity in preclinical studies. Similar to DTγE, DEγE has no opioid activity. Both single- and double-blind studies have been conducted.[88,89] In a single-blind study of four patients (one neuroleptic-free), two patients received 1-mg DEγE im and two received 10-mg DEγE im. All four patients were reported to show a marked amelioration of psychotic symptomatology, and two of these were discharged from the hospital. In the double-blind study, 19 patients were studied and received 3-mg DEγE im. A significant reduc-tion in BPRS scores was associated with the peptide treatment. Two patients showed no response, four a slight to moderate response, four a moderate to marked response, and three a very marked response.

In a recent review, van Ree and De Wied,[78] adding together results from several of their studies, reported that of 43 schizophrenic patients treated with DTγE and 21 treated with DEγE (total of 64 patients), 13 showed no response (<20% improvement), 19 showed a slight response (20–50% improvement), 16 showed a moderate response (50–80% improvement), and 16 showed a marked response (>80% improvement).

## Clinical Trials of Nonendorphin Peptides in Schizophrenia

Two other neuropeptides have been tested clinically for antipsychotic effects: CCK and TRH. As noted earlier, based on compelling evidence of the coexistence of CCK and DA in the mesolimbic system,[14] the effects of treatment with CCK or a related homologous decapeptide, ceruletide, on the symptoms of schizophrenia have been studied. Moroji et al.[90–92] treated 20 chronic schizophrenic patients maintained on antipsychotic drugs with a single injection of ceruletide (0.3 or 0.6 µg/kg iv) and used the BPRS to rate symptoms in this open study. After the low dose, five of the 12 patients showed improvement in mood, and one patient reported a reduction in auditory hallucinations. After the high dose of the peptide, improved mood was noted in 16 patients, and reduction in auditory hallucinations was observed in three patients. These improvements persisted for three weeks postinjection.

The effects of CCK-33 (0.3 µg/kg iv) in chronic schizophrenia were studied by another group.[93,94] Six chronic paranoid schizophrenic patients maintained on neuroleptic drugs were studied in the first trial. In this open, uncontrolled study, CCK-33 produced a significant reduction in the BPRS score that was maintained for six weeks. In a second study, a single dose of CCK-8 (0.04 µg/kg iv) was administered to eight chronic schizophrenic patients maintained on neuroleptic drugs. A rapid improvement in psychopathology was reported. Peak improvement was observed six days post-CCK injection. Nair et al.[95] have reviewed these early studies in detail. More recently Verhoeven et al.[96] treated schizophrenic patients maintained on antipsychotic drugs with ceruletide with remarkably beneficial effects. Stimulated by these preliminary findings, several research groups have evaluated the effects of ceruletide in schizophrenia using a double-blind, placebo-controlled protocol. The results have been quite disappointing.

Hommer et al.[97] treated eight neuroleptic-treated schizophrenic patients with ceruletide with increasing im doses beginning at 0.3 µg/kg twice per day to reach a final dose of 0.6 µg/kg. The peptide produced no amelioration in schizophrenic symptoms as assessed by several rating scales, including the BPRS. Albus et al.[98] have conducted both an open study (six patients) and a double-blind study (20 patients) with ceruletide. No antipsychotic effects of the peptide were observed. Mattes et al.[99] in a double-blind study of 17 chronic, neuroleptic-treated schizophrenic patients, administered two injections of either ceruletide (0.6 µg/kg im) or placebo one week apart. The evaluation included ratings of 29 variables related to prognosis in schizophrenia, as well as BPRS and SCL-90 scales. No beneficial effects of the peptide were observed. Recently, Tamminga and her colleagues [reference 53, and this volume] used both fixed and rising-dose schedules in drug-free schizophrenic patients and administered a fixed dose of caerulein to neuroleptic-treated schizophrenic patients. No beneficial effects were observed. Peselow et al.[100] treated 14 chronic schizophrenic patients receiving neuroleptic drugs with CCK-8 using a double-blind crossover design. No beneficial effects of the peptide were noted.

The effects of TRH have been most widely studied in affective disorders; a few studies with schizophrenic patients have been conducted. This literature has been comprehensively reviewed most recently by Loosen and Prange.[101] In general, the results of TRH trials in schizophrenia are disappointing. In a single-blind study, TRH was administered orally (4 mg/day) to 62 chronic, neuroleptic-treated schizophrenic patients. A beneficial effect was reported within two weeks in 75% of the patients.[101] A double-blind study of 143 chronic schizophrenic patients by the same Japanese group confirmed the initial findings.[101] Motivation and social contact were reportedly the most improved. The studies in which TRH was administered intravenously to schizophrenic patients have been disappointing. Moreover, several investigators have reported that TRH apparently worsens the symptoms of paranoid schizophrenic patients.[102] Recently, however, Mizuki et al.[103] treated six schizophrenic patients maintained on antipsychotic drugs with the potent TRH analog, DN-1417, for 2 weeks. Both BPRS scores and scores on hallucinatory behavior and unusual thought content were significantly decreased. Moreover, Brambilla et al.[104] recently treated chronic schizophrenic patients with a preponderance of negative symptoms with iv TRH every other day for 30 days. In this open study, TRH improved negative symptoms.

## TREATMENT OF SCHIZOPHRENIA WITH OPIOID ANTAGONISTS

The only neuropeptide receptor antagonists that have been evaluated as putative antipsychotic agents are the opiate/opioid receptor blockers naloxone and naltrexone. We have recently comprehensively reviewed these data,[11] and the interested reader can refer to the reviews of Mueser and Dysken[105] and McNichols and Martin[106] as well. These studies are, of course, based on the hypothesis that schizophrenia is associated with excess CNS opioid activity, and therefore the opioid receptor blockade should ameliorate the symptoms of schizophrenia. In the space below we briefly review this literature.

The first attempt to reverse schizophrenia symptoms with naloxone was carried out by Gunne et al.[107] This initial study was a single-blind study in which a low dose of naloxone (0.4 mg) was given to six schizophrenic patients. Four of the six patients reported significantly decreased auditory hallucinations for up to four hours following naloxone, but not following saline.

This original report led to several attempted replications using a double-blind crossover design that produced basically negative results. Volavka et al.[108] used 0.4-mg naloxone iv in seven patients and reported that naloxone had no effects. Janowsky et al.[109] used 1.2-mg naloxone administered over one hour in a study of a heterogeneous group of patients. This group also failed to find an effect of naloxone in their eight subjects. Kurlan et al.[110] administered between 0.4 and 1.2 mg naloxone and also found no effect on their eight patients. Lipinski et al.,[111] using a double-blind crossover design, gave 1.6-mg naloxone to schizophrenic patients and reported no effects. Naber et al.[112] performed a double-blind crossover study with 10 mg per day naloxone in acute and chronic schizophrenics for five days. No beneficial effects were observed. Another investigation using multiple doses of naloxone performed by Verhoeven et al.[113] also failed to demonstrate positive effects of this opiate antagonist. Thus, in these investigations there is no evidence that naloxone had an effect on schizophrenic symptoms.

There are, however, a series of investigations that seem to support the original finding of Gunne et al.[107] suggesting that naloxone decreases schizophrenic auditory hallucinations. Davis et al.,[114] in a double-blind crossover design, using low doses (0.4 mg and in a few instances 10 mg) of naloxone, studied 14 schizophrenic patients and found a change in the "unusual thought content" item on the BPRS.

In a study conducted at Stanford,[115] a large number of schizophrenic subjects (1800) were prescreened in order to identify 18 patients who met RDC and DSM-III criteria for schizophrenia and who exhibited constant auditory hallucinations. They were chronic undifferentiated or paranoid schizophrenics, were stable on their medication, and had at least a twice-per-hour pattern of hallucinations. In this double-blind crossover design, 10 mg of naloxone was used and the patients were followed for up to two days after the infusion. Naloxone was found to produce a statistically significant reduction of hallucinations as rated by the BPRS at one and one-half to two hours after naloxone administration. The decrease was observed in patients receiving neuroleptics, as well as in patients who were drug-free.

Emrich et al.[116,117] reported two studies in which they evaluated the effects of naloxone in schizophrenia. Their general impression in the first study was that naloxone was effective in reducing schizophrenic hallucinations between two and seven hours after administering 1.2 to 4 mg naloxone. In the second study, using much larger doses of naloxone (24.8 mg), there was a reduction in both psychotic symptoms and hallucinations. Davis et al.,[118] in another double-blind study using 15 mg of naloxone, found that there was a significant reduction in unusual thought content in their schizophrenic patients.

In a large, multicentered investigation organized and coordinated by the World Helath Organization (WHO), six groups participated in a study on the effects of naloxone on schizophrenic symptoms. The WHO collaborative study found significant reductions in hallucinations in 32 schizophrenic subjects who received 0.3 mg/kg naloxone subcutaneously.[119] The reduction in schizophrenic hallucinations in the WHO study occurred in the neuroleptic-treated patients ($n = 19$), but not in the drug-free patients ($n = 13$). Another group of investigators led by Kleinman also reported positive effects of naloxone on schizophrenic symptoms in patients currently being treated with neuroleptics, but not in patients who were drug-free.[120]

Thus, the investigations using naloxone to treat schizophrenic symptoms have produced inconsistent results. However, when one examines high-dose, double-blind crossover naloxone studies, which use between 4 and 25 mg naloxone in schizophrenic patients, the majority of studies report positive, if somewhat variable, results.

The opiate antagonist naltrexone would appear to have several advantages over naloxone in the study of the effects of opiate antagonists in schizophrenia. It can be given in large doses, in an oral form, and has a very long period of action. There have been a few attempts to study naltrexone in schizophrenia. Mueser and Dysken[105] have reviewed these studies and summarized the current literature; of 42 schizophrenics treated with naltrexone (50–800 mg orally for 2 to 6 weeks), only seven improved.

## DISCUSSION

We have attempted to provide an overview of neuropeptides in schizophrenia, with an emphasis on neuropeptides that interact with CNS DA neurons. Much of our ignorance concerning the possible role of neuropeptides in the pathogenesis of schizophrenia resides with the lack of tools necessary to assess the functional activity of neuropeptide-containing systems in the CNS.

We still cannot measure neuropeptide turnover, and peptide biosynthesis using rates of mRNA synthesis is only now being routinely measured. Structural analogs of neuropeptides are now available that, when radiolabeled, result in radioligands suitable to detect high-affinity binding sites for these substances in brain membranes. Simply stated, when neuropeptide concentrations are found to be altered in postmortem brain tissue or CSF in a disease such as schizophrenia, the meaning of this finding remains difficult to interpret. Whether CSF or tissue concentrations of neuropeptides accurately reflect extracellular fluid concentrations at relevant synaptic receptor sites in the CNS also remains to be determined.

To draw conclusions from the present literature is difficult. Although the CSF opioid peptide studies in schizophrenia have not been fruitful, the NT and DSIP studies in similar patient populations showed differences worthy of additional study.

As treatments for schizophrenia, neuropeptides have certainly not yet been shown to be effective. β-Endorphin is clearly not a practical treatment for schizophrenia, and the use of DTγE in schizophrenia remains quite controversial. As noted in this chapter, the Utrecht group has consistently observed antipsychotic effects of DTγE in schizophrenic patients. In open studies, CCK seemed to possess antipsychotic effects, but this has not been confirmed in double-blind studies. One must conclude that the neuropeptide treatment strategy for schizophrenia is in its infancy, and considerable work in drug design and clinical neuropsychopharmacology must take place.

The peptide antagonist studies are of considerable interest. It seems clear that naloxone reduces hallucinations and unusual thought content in a subset of schizophrenic patients. Unfortunately, these effects are fleeting, difficult to measure, and variable from investigator to investigator. It is not clear whether the naloxone effect is due to opiate receptor blockade or is the result of secondary or tertiary effects resulting from that blockade.

If we regard the last 25 years of research as preliminary findings, then the next decade shall almost certainly witness a veritable explosion in neuropeptide research, with an emphasis on molecular biology. The impact of this research in psychiatry, especially in the area of the pathophysiology of schizophrenia, may be extremely important. Thus, the wisest course will be to withhold conclusions on the possible role of neuropeptides in schizophrenia until more extensive basic science information is available to clarify the various clinical controversies and yield new data.

# ACKNOWLEDGMENTS

We are grateful to Sheila Walker for manuscript preparation.

## REFERENCES

1. NEMEROFF, C. B., Ed. 1988. Neuropeptides in Psychiatric and Neurological Disorders. Johns Hopkins Univ. Press. Baltimore, Md.
2. NEMEROFF, C. B. & P. T. LOOSEN, Eds. 1987. Handbook of Clinical Psychoneuroendocrinology. Guilford Press. New York.
3. IVERSEN, L. L., S. D. IVERSEN & S. H. SNYDER, Eds. 1983. Handbook of Psychopharmacology, Vol. 16. Plenum Press. New York.
4. HARRIS, G. W. 1972. J. Endocrinol. **53**: ii–xxiii.
5. VALE, W. & C. RIVIER. 1975. *In* Handbook of Psychopharmacology, Vol. V. L. L. Iversen, S. D. Iversen, and S. H. Snyder, Eds.: 195–237. Plenum Press. New York.
6. JENNES, L., W. E. STUMPF & P. W. KALIVAS. 1982. J. Comp. Neurol. **210**: 211–224.
7. MANBERG, P. J., W. W. YOUNGBLOOD, C. B. NEMEROFF, M. N. ROSSOR, L. L. IVERSEN, A. J. PRANGE, JR. & J. S. KIZER. 1982. J. Neurochem. **38**: 1777–1780.
8. LAMERS, C. B., J. E. MORLEY, P. POITRAS, B. SHARP, H. E. CARLSON, J. E. HERSHMAN & J. H. WALSH. 1980. Am. J. Physiol. **239**: E232–E235.
9. MUTT, V. 1983. *In* Brain Peptides. D. T. Krieger, M. J. Brownstein, and J. B. Martin, Eds.: 871–902. Wiley-Interscience. New York.

10. HENRY, J. L. 1982. Ann. N.Y. Acad. Sci. **400:** 216–227.
11. JUNGKUNZ, G., N. NEDOPIL & E. RUTHER. 1984. Pharmacopsychiatra **17:** 76–78.
12. HOKFELT, T., B. J. EVERITT, E. THEODORSSON-NORHEIM & M. GOLDSTEIN. 1984. J. Comp. Neurol. **222:** 543–559.
13. IBATA, Y., F. H. OKAMURA, T. KAWAKAMI, M. TANAKA, H. L. OBATA, O. T. TSUTO, H. TEROBAYASHI, C. YANAIHARA & N. YANAIHARA. 1983. Brain Res. **269:** 177–179.
14. HOKFELT, T., J. F. REHFELD, L. SKIRBOLL, B. IVEMARK, M. GOLDSTEIN & K. MARKEY. 1980. Nature **285:** 476–478.
15. EDWARDSON, J. A. & J. R. McDERMOTT. 1982. Brit. Med. Bull. **38:** 259–264.
16. ROSSOR, M. 1984. J. Psychiat. Res. **18:** 457–465.
17. POST, R. M., P. W. GOLD, D. R. RUBINOW, W. E. BUNNEY, JR., J. C. BALLENGER & F. K. GOODWIN. 1983. *In* Neurobiology of Cerebrospinal Fluid. J. H. Wood, Ed.: 107–141. Plenum Press. New York.
18. VON KNORRING, L., B. G. L. ALMAY, F. JOHANSSON, J. TERENIUS & A. WAHLSTROM. 1982. Pain **12:** 265–272.
19. TERENIUS, L. & F. NYBERG. 1983. *In* Biochemical and Clinical Aspects of Neuropeptides: Synthesis, Processing and Gene Function. G. Kock and D. Richter, Eds.: 99–112. Academic Press. New York.
20. SAWYNOK, J., C. PINSKEY & F. S. LaBELLA. 1979. Life Sci. **9:** 213–225.
21. TERENIUS, L., A. WAHLSTROM, L. H. LINDSTROM & E. WIDERLOV. 1976. Neurosci. Lett. **3:** 157–162.
22. LINDSTROM, L. H., E. WIDERLOV, L. M. GUNNE, A. WAHLSTROM & L. TERENIUS. 1978. Acta Psychiat. Scand. **57:** 153–169.
23. RIMON, R., P. LeGREVES, F. NYBERG, L. HEIKKILA, L. SALMELA & L. TERENIUS. 1984. Biol. Psychiatry **19:** 509–516.
24. BERNER, P., G. GABRIEL, H. KATSCHNIG, W. KIEFFER, G. LENZ & C. SIMHANDL. Diagnostic Criteria for Schizophrenia and Affective Disorders. World Psychiatric Association, American Psychiatric Press. Washington, D.C.
25. DUPONT, A., A. VILLENEUVE, J. P. BOUCHARD, R. BOUCHARD, Y. MERAND, D. ROULEAU & F. LABRIE. 1978. Lancet ii: 1107.
26. DOMSCHKE, W., A. DICKSCHAS & P. MITZNEGG. 1979. Lancet i: 1024.
27. BURBACH, J. P. H., J. G. LOEBER, J. VERHOEF, E. R. DE KLOET, J. M. VAN REE & D. DE WIED. 1979. Lancet ii: 480–481.
28. NABER, D., D. PICKAR, R. M. POST, D. P. VAN KAMMEN, J. BALLENGER, D. RUBINOW, R. N. WATERS & W. E. BUNNEY, JR. 1981. *In* Biological Psychiatry. C. Perris, G. Struwe, and B. Jansson, Eds.: 372–375. Elsevier. Amsterdam/New York.
29. NABER, D., D. PICKAR, R. M. POST, D. P. VAN KAMMEN, R. N. WATERS, J. C. BALLENGER, F. K. GOODWIN & W. E. BUNNEY, JR. 1981. Am. J. Psychiatry. **138:** 1457–1462.
30. NABER, D. & D. PICKAR. 1983. Psychiatric Clinics of North America **6:** 443–456.
31. EMRICH, H. M., V. HOLLT, W. KISSLING, M. FISCHLER, H. HEINEMANN, D. VAN ZERSSEN & A. HERZ. 1979. *In* Modulators, Mediators and Specifiers in Brain Function. Y. H. Erlich, J. Volavka, L. G. Davis, and E. G. Brunngraber, Eds.: 307–317. Plenum Press. New York.
32. EMRICH, H. M., V. HOLLT, W. KISSLING, M. FISCHLER, H. LASPE, H. HEINEMANN, D. VON ZERSSEN & A. HERZ. 1979. Pharmakopsychiatria **12:** 269–276.
33. HOLLT, V., H. M. EMRICH, M. BERGMANN, N. NEDOPIL, D. DIETERIE, H. J. GURLAND, L. NUSSETT, D. VON ZERSSEN & A. HERZ. 1982. *In* Endorphins and Opiate Antagonists in Psychiatry. N. S. Shah and A. G. Donald, Eds.: 231–243. Plenum Press. New York.
34. VAN KAMMEN, D. P., R. N. WATERS, P. GOLD, D. STERNBERG, G. ROBERTSON, D. GANTEN, D. PICKAR, D. NABER, J. C. BALLENGER, W. H. KAYE, R. M. POST & W. E. BUNNEY, JR. 1981. *In* Biological Psychiatry. C. Perris, G. Struwe, and B. Jansson, Eds.: 339–344. Elsevier. Amsterdam/New York.
35. WEN, H. L., C. W. LO & W. K. HO. 1983. Clin. Chim. Acta **128:** 367–371.
36. LO, C. W., H. L. WEN & W. K. K. HO. 1983. Eur. J. Pharmacol. **92:** 77–81.
37. NYBERG, F., I. NYLANDER & L. TERENIUS. 1986. Brain Res. **371:** 278–286.
38. BACH, F. W., R. EKMAN & F. M. JENSEN. 1986. Regul. Pept. **16:** 189–198.
39. WAGEMAKER, H. & R. CADE. 1977. Am. J. Psychiatry **134:** 684–685.

40. PALMOUR, R. M., F. R. ERVIN, H. WAGEMAKER & R. CADE. 1977. Soc. Neurosci. Abstr. **4:** 320.
41. EMRICH, H. M., W. KISSLING, M. FISCHLER, D. F. ZERSSEN, H. RIEDHAMMER & H. H. EDEL. 1979. Am. J. Psychiatry **136:** 1095.
42. LEWIS, R. V., L. D. GERBER, S. STEIN, R. L. STEPHEN, B. I. BROSSER, S. F. VELICK & S. UDENFRIEND. 1979. Arch. Gen. Psychiatry **36:** 237–239.
43. WIDERLOV, E., L. H. LINDSTROM, G. BESEV, P. J. MANBERG, C. B. NEMEROFF, G. R. BREESE, J. S. KIZER & A. J. PRANGE, JR. 1982. Amer. J. Psychiatry **139:** 1122–1126.
44. LINDSTROM, L. H., E. WIDERLOV, G. BISSETTE & C. B. NEMEROFF. 1988. Schizophrenia Res. In press.
45. MANBERG, P. J., C. B. NEMEROFF, G. BISSETTE, A. J. PRANGE, JR. & R. H. GERNER. 1983. Soc. Neurosci. Abstr. **9:** 1034.
46. BISSETTE, G., E. WIDERLOV, H. WALLEUS, I. KARLSSON, K. EKLUND, A. FORSMAN & C. B. NEMEROFF. 1986. Arch. Gen. Psychiatry **43:** 1148–1154.
47. GATTAZ, W. F., K. RISSLER, D. GATTAZ & H. CRAMER. 1986. Psychiatr. Res. **17:** 1–6.
48. GERNER, R. H. & T. YAMADA. 1982. Brain Res. **238:** 298–302.
49. GERNER, R. H. 1984. *In* Neurobiology of Mood Disorders. R. M. Post and J. C. Ballenger, Eds.: 388–392. William & Wilkins. Baltimore, Md.
50. RUBINOW, D. R., P. W. GOLD, R. M. POST, J. C. BALLENGER, R. COWDRY, J. BOLLINGER & S. REICHLIN. 1983. Arch. Gen. Psychiatry **40:** 409–413.
51. RUBINOW, D. R. 1986. Biol. Psychiatry **21:** 341–365.
52. VERBANCK, P. M. P., F. LOTSTRA, C. GILLES, P. LINKOWSKI, J. MENDLEWICZ & J. J. VANDERHAEGHEN. 1983. Life Sci. **34:** 67–72.
53. TAMMINGA, C. A., R. L. LITTMAN, L. D. ALPHS, T. N. CHASE, G. K. THAKER & A. M. WAGMAN. 1986. Psychopharmacology **88:** 387–391.
54. RIMON, R., P. LEGREVES, F. NYBERG, L. HEIKKILA, L. SALMELA & L. TERENIUS. 1984. Biol. Psychiatry **19:** 509–516.
55. LINDSTROM, L. H., R. EKMAN, H. WALLEUS & E. WIDERLOV. 1985. Progr. Neuro-Psychopharmacol. Biol. Psychiatry **9:** 83–90.
56. FERRIER, I. N., T. J. CROW, G. W. ROBERTS, E. C. JOHNSTONE, D. G. C. OWENS, Y. LEE, A. BARACESE-HAMILTON, G. MCGREGOR, D. O'SHAUGHNESSY, J. M. POLAK & S. R. BLOOM. 1984. *In* Psychopharmacology of the Limbic System. M. R. Trimble and E. Zaritan, Eds.: 244–254. Oxford Univ. Press. London/New York.
57. FERRIER, I. N., G. W. ROBERTS, T. J. CROW, E. C. JOHNSTONE, D. G. C. OWENS, Y. C. LEE, D. O'SHAUGHNESSY, T. E. ADRIAN, J. M. POLAK & S. R. BLOOM. 1983. Life Sci. **33:** 475–482.
58. CROW, T. J., Ed. 1982. Disorders of Neurohumoural Transmission. 287–340. Academic Press. New York.
59. FARMERY, S. M., F. OWEN, M. POULTER & T. J. CROW. 1985. Life Sci. **36:** 472–476.
60. NEMEROFF, C. B., W. W. YOUNGBLOOD, P. J. MANBERG, A. J. PRANGE, JR. & J. S. KIZER. 1983. Science **221:** 972–975.
61. NEMEROFF, C. B. & G. BISSETTE. 1987. *In* Handbook of Schizophrenia, Vol. 2. F. A. Henn and L. E. Delisi, Eds.: 297–317. Elsevier. Amsterdam/New York.
62. KLEINMAN, J. E., M. IADAROLA, S. GOVONI, J. HONG, J. C. GILLIN & R. J. WYATT. 1983. Psychopharmacol. Bull. **19:** 375–377.
63. BIGGINS, J., E. K. PERRY, J. R. MCDERMOTT, I. A. SMITH, R. H. PERRY & J. A. EDWARDSON. 1983. J. Neurol. Sci. **58:** 117–122.
64. ZECH, M., G. W. ROBERTS, B. BOGERTS, T. J. CROW & J. M. POLAK. 1986. Acta Neuropathol. **71:** 259–266.
65. KLEINMAN, J. E. 1986. *In* Handbook of Schizophrenia, Vol. 1. H. A. Nasrallah and D. R. Weinberger, Eds.: 349–360. Elsevier. Amsterdam/New York.
66. KLINE, N. S. & H. E. LEHMANN. 1979. *In* Endorphins in Mental Health Research. E. Usdin, W. E. Bunney, Jr., and N. S. Kline, Eds.: 500–517. Macmillan. London.
67. BERGER, P. A., S. J. WATSON, H. AKIL, G. R. ELLIOT, R. T. RUBIN, A. PFEFFERBAUM, K. L. DAVIS, J. D. BARCHAS & C. H. LI. 1980. Arch. Gen. Psychiatry **37:** 635–640.
68. BERGER, P. A., S. J. WATSON, H. AKIL & J. D. BARCHAS. 1985. *In* Neuropeptides: Implications for Neurologic and Psychiatric Diseases. J. Martin and J. Barchas, Eds.: 309–334. Raven Press. New York.

69. THE CLINICAL GLOBAL IMPRESSIONS SCALE (CGI). 1967. Psychopharmacological Research Branch of the National Institute of Mental Health, March.
70. GERNER, R. H., D. H. CATLIN, D. A. GORELICK, K. K. HUI & C. H. LI. 1980. Arch. Gen. Psychiatry 37: 642–647.
71. PICKAR, D., G. D. DAVIS, S. C. SCHULZ & W. E. BUNNEY, JR. 1981. Am. J. Psychiatry 138: 160–166.
72. PETHO, B., G. LASZLO, I. KARCZAG, J. BORVENDEG, I. BITTER, I. BARNA, H. ILONA, J. TOLNA & K. BARACZKA. 1983. In Proceedings of the Conference on Opioids in Mental Illness, Vol. 398. K. Verebey, Ed.: 460–469. Ann. N.Y. Acad. Sci. New York.
73. KLEIN, H., G. JUNGKUNZ, N. NEDOPIL, E. RUTHER & R. SPIEGEL. 1981. In Biological Psychiatry. C. Perris, G. Struwe, and B. Jansson, Eds.: 390–393. Elsevier. Amsterdam/New York.
74. BURBACH, P. & D. DE WIED. 1980. In Enzymes and Neurotransmitters in Mental Diseases. E. Usdin, T. S. Sourkes, and M. B. H. Youdim, Eds.: 103–114. Wiley. New York.
75. DORSA, D. M., J. M. VAN REE & D. DE WIED. 1979. Pharmacol. Biochem. Behav. 10: 899–905.
76. DE WIED, D. 1982. In Brain Peptides and Hormones. R. Collu, Ed.: 137–147. Raven Press. New York.
77. VAN PRAAG, H. M. & W. M. A. VERHOEVEN. 1981. In Handbook of Biological Psychiatry, Part IV, Brain Mechanisms and Abnormal Behavior-Chemistry. H. M. van Praag, M. H. Lader. O. J. Rafaelson, and E. J. Sachar, Eds.: 511–545. Dekker. New York.
78. VAN REE, J. M. & D. DE WIED. 1984. In Central and Peripheral Endorphins: Basic and Clinical Aspects. E. E. Muiler and R. Genazzani, Eds.: 325–332. Raven Press. New York.
79. VAN REE, J. M., W. M. A. VERHOEVEN, H. M. VAN PRAAG & D. DE WIED. 1978. In Characteristics and Functions of Opioids. J. M. van Ree and L. Terenius, Eds.: 181–184. Elsevier/North Holland. Amsterdam.
80. DE WIED, D., B. BOHUS, J. M. VAN REE, G. L. KOVACS & H. M. GREVEN. 1978. Lancet i: 1046.
81. VERHOEVEN, V. M. A., H. M. VAN PRAAG, P. A. BOTTER, A. SUNIER, J. M. VAN REE & D. DE WIED. 1978. Lancet i: 1046–1047.
82. EMRICH, H. M., M. ZAUDIG, W. KISSLING, G. DIRLICH, D. VON ZERSSEN & A. HERZ. 1980. Pharmakopsychiatria 13: 290–298.
83. FINK, M., Y. PAPAKOSTAS, J. LEE & L. JOHNSON. 1981. In Biological Psychiatry. C. Perris, G. Struwe, and B. Jansson, Eds.: 398–401. Elsevier. Amsterdam/New York.
84. MANCHANDRA, R. & S. R. HIRSCH. 1981. Psychol. Med. 11: 401–403.
85. TAMMINGA, C. A., P. J. TIGHE, T. N. CHASE, G. DE FRATTES & M. H. SCHAEFFER. 1981. Arch. Gen. Psychiatry 38: 167.
86. MELTZER, H. Y., D. A. BUSCH, B. J. TRICON & A. ROBERTSON. 1982. Psychiatry Res. 6: 313–326.
87. VOLAVKA, J., K.-S. HUI, B. ANDERSON, Z. NEMES, J. O'DONNELL & A. LAYTHA. 1983. Psychiatry Res. 10: 243–252.
88. VERHOEVEN, W. M. A., H. M. VAN PRAAG, J. M. VAN REE & D. DE WIED. 1979. Arch. Gen. Psychiatry 36: 294–298.
89. VERHOEVEN, W. M. A., J. M. VAN REE, A. HEEZIUS-VAN BENTUM, D. DE WIED & H. M. VAN PRAAG. 1982. Arch. Gen. Psychiatry 39: 648–654.
90. MOROJI, T., N. WATANABE, N. AOKI & S. ITOH. 1982. Int. Pharmacopsychiatry 17: 255–273.
91. MOROJI, T., N. WATANABE, N. AOKI & S. ITOH. 1982. Arch. Gen. Psychiatry 39: 485–486.
92. MOROJI, T., N. WATANABE & S. ITOH. 1982. Proc. World Psychiatr. Ass.: 165–169.
93. BLOOM, D. M., N. P. V. NAIR & G. SCHWARTZ. 1983. Psychopharmacology 69: 133–136.
94. NAIR, N. P. V., D. M. BLOOM & J. D. NESTOROS. 1982. Prog. Neuropsychopharmacol. Biol. Psychiatry 6: 509–512.
95. NAIR, N. P. V., S. LAL & D. M. BLOOM. 1985. Prog. Neuropsychopharmacol. Biol. Psychiatry 9: 515–524.
96. VERHOEVEN, W. M. A., H. G. M. WESTERBERG & J. M. VAN REE. 1986. Acta Psychiatry Scand. 13: 372–382.
97. HOMMER, D. W., D. PICKAR, A. ROY, P. NINAN, J. BORONOW & S. M. PAUL. 1984. Arch. Gen. Psychiatry 41: 617–619.

98. ALBUS, M., M. ACKENHEIL, U. MUNCH & D. NABER. 1984. Arch. Gen. Psychiatry **41**: 528.
99. MATTES, J. A., W. HUM, J. M. ROCHFORD & M. ORLOSKY. 1985. Biol. Psychiatry **20**: 533–538.
100. PESELOW, E., B. ANGRIST, A. SUDILOVSKY, J. CORWIN, J. SIEKIERSKI, F. TRENT & J. ROTROSEN. 1987. Psychopharmacology **91**: 80–84.
101. LOOSEN, P. T. & A. J. PRANGE, JR. 1984. *In* Peptides, Hormones and Behavior. C. B. Nemeroff and A. J. Dunn, Eds.: 533–577. Spectrum Publishers. New York.
102. DAVIS, K. L., L. E. HOLLISTER & P. A. BERGER. 1975. Am. J. Psychiatry **132**: 9.
103. MIZUKI, Y., S. NISHIKORI, N. KAJIMURA, J. IMAIZIMI, M. YAMADA & K. INANAAGA. 1985. Biol. Psychiatry **20**: 1030–1035.
104. BRAMBILLA, F., E. AGUGULIA, R. MASSIRORI, M. MAGGIONI, W. GRILLO, R. CASTIGLIORI, M. CATALENO & F. DRAGO. 1986. Neuropsychobiology **15**: 114–121.
105. MUESER, K. T. & M. W. DYSKEN. 1983. Schizophrenia Bull. **9**: 213–225.
106. MCNICHOLS, L. F. & W. R. MARTIN. 1984. Drugs **27**: 81–93.
107. GUNNE, L. M., L. LINDSTROM & L. TERENIUS. 1977. J. Neural. Trans. **40**: 13–19.
108. VOLAVKA, J., A. MALLYA, S. BAIG & J. PEREZ-CRUET. 1977. Naloxone in chronic schizophrenia. Science **196**: 1227–1228.
109. JANOWSKY, D. S., D. S. SEGAL, F. BLOOM, A. ABRAMS & R. GUILLEMIN. 1977. Am. J. Psychiatry **134**: 926–927.
110. KURLAND, A. A., O. L. MCCABLE, T. E. HANLON & D. SULLIVAN. 1977. Am. J. Psychiatry **134**: 1408–1410.
111. LIPINSKI, J., R. MEYER, C. KORNETSKY & B. M. COHEN. 1979. Lancet **i**: 1292–1293.
112. NABER, D., U. MUNCH, J. WISSMANN, R. GROSSE, R. RITT & R. WELTER. 1983. Acta Psychiatry Scand. **67**: 265–271.
113. VERHOEVEN, W. M. A., H. M. VAN PRAAG & J. M. VAN REE. 1984. Psychiatry Res. **12**: 297.
114. DAVIS, G. C., W. E. BUNNEY, E. G. DE FRAITES, J. E. KLEINMAN, D. P. VAN KAMMEN, R. M. POST & R. J. WYATT. 1977. Science **197**: 74–77.
115. WATSON, S. J., P. A. BERGER, H. AKIL, M. J. MILLS & J. D. BARCHAS. 1978. Science **201**: 73–76.
116. EMRICH, H. M., C. CORDING, S. PIREE, D. KOLLING, D. UZERSSEN & A. HERZ. 1977. Pharmakopsychiatria **10**: 265–270.
117. EMRICH, H. M., H. J. MOLLER, H. LASPE, I. MEISEL-KOSIK, H. DWINGER, R. OECHSNER, W. KISSLING & D. VON ZERSSEN. 1979. *In* Biological Psychiatry Today. J. Obiols, C. Ballus, E. Gonzalez Monclus, and J. Pujol, Eds.: 798–805. Elsevier/North Holland. Amsterdam.
118. DAVIS, G. C., W. E. BUNNEY, E. G. DE FRAITES, I. EXTEIN, F. K. GOODWIN, W. HAMILTON, J. KLEINMAN, W. MENDELSON, R. POST, V. RECES, D. SHILING, D. VAN KAMMEN, D. WEINBERGER, R. J. WYATT & C. H. LI. 1978. Human studies of opioid antagonists and endorphins. Presented at the Annual Meeting of the American College of Neuropsychopharmacology, Maui, Hawaii, December.
119. PICKAR, D., F. VARTANIAN & W. E. BUNNEY. 1982. Arch. Gen. Psychiatry **39**: 313.
120. KLEINMAN, J. E., D. R. WEINBERGER, A. ROGOL, D. J. SHILING, W. B. MENDELSON, G. C. DAVIS, W. E. BUNNEY, JR. & R. J. WYATT. 1982. Psychiatry Res. **7**: 1.

# Cocaine-Induced Behavioral Sensitization and Kindling: Implications for the Emergence of Psychopathology and Seizures

ROBERT M. POST,[a] SUSAN R. B. WEISS, AND AGU PERT

*Biological Psychiatry Branch*
*National Institute of Mental Health*
*Bethesda, Maryland 20892*

## INTRODUCTION

With the increasing recognition of the behavioral and physiological toxicities of the chronic use of cocaine in man, elucidation of potential anatomical, biochemical, and physiological substrates underlying these effects in animals is of considerable importance. In this manuscript, we focus on two interesting characteristics of repeated cocaine administration—that of increased behavioral responsivity to the same low to moderate dose over time (behavioral sensitization) and increased electrophysiological and convulsive responsivity to repeated administration of the same high dose over time (pharmacological kindling). Investigations of the biochemical and anatomical basis of these effects in animals may enlarge our understanding of mechanisms involved in the progressive development of the psychiatric and physiologic toxicities (lethal convulsions) in human cocaine users.

The phenomenon of behavioral sensitization is pertinent to this conference on mesolimbic and mesocortical dopamine systems, since stimulant-induced hyperactivity is thought to be mediated in part through mesolimbic dopamine systems, particularly in the nucleus accumbens.[1] In addition, the limbic system is implicated in the pharmacological kindling effect of local anesthetics such as lidocaine,[2] as well as the mixed psychomotor stimulant–local anesthetic cocaine.[3-5] Additionally, a considerable body of data reviewed elsewhere suggests that mesolimbic and mesocortical substrates may be directly involved in the rewarding effects of psychomotor stimulants such as amphetamine and cocaine as assessed by either intravenous self-administration or paradigms involving direct intracerebral self-administration of drugs into these areas[6,7] (see also Wise, this conference). Thus, limbic mechanisms may not only be involved in the behavioral sensitization and pharmacological kindling effects of cocaine in animals, but may also be relevant to related effects in man.

[a] Address for correspondence: Robert M. Post, M.D., Chief, Biological Psychiatry Branch, NIMH, Bldg. 10, Room 3N212, 9000 Rockville Pike, Bethesda, Maryland 20892.

# THE ROLE OF CONDITIONING IN BEHAVIORAL SENSITIZATION TO COCAINE

The increased response to repeated cocaine treatment appears to be related to initial dose, number of repetitions, genetic strain, gender (females > males), and an intact vasopressinergic substrate (see review by Post and Contel[8]). Environmental context and conditioning variables are also critical to the emergence of some types of cocaine-induced behavioral sensitization.[9,10] That is, animals repeatedly given cocaine in the test environment showed greater hyperactivity upon rechallenge (with cocaine or saline) in this environment compared to animals that had been given the same dose of cocaine in a different environment.[9] These data suggest that powerful conditioning of cocaine-induced behavioral sensitization is occurring over the course of repeated daily administration of this low dose of cocaine (10 mg/kg ip).

## *Amphetamine Injections into Accumbens and Caudate in Chronic Cocaine-Sensitized Rats*

We attempted to elucidate possible neural substrates of this effect by pretreating animals with cocaine and challenging them with the psychomotor stimulant amphetamine injected directly into the nucleus accumbens or into the caudate nucleus. In this study, 7–10 days following the implantation of cannulae into the nucleus accumbens, rats were treated with two daily injections (10 mg/kg ip) for ten days. One injection was given just prior to the animal's being placed in the test chamber in which activity was being measured, and a second injection was given when animals were returned to their home cage. The first group received cocaine (10 mg/kg ip) repeatedly in the test environment and saline upon return to the home cage. The second group received saline repeatedly in the test environment and cocaine upon return to the home cage. The third group received repeated saline injections in both environments. Following this chronic ten-day pretreatment regimen, animals were challenged acutely with amphetamine (10 µg in 1 µl) injected directly into the nucleus accumbens bilaterally (i.e., 10 µg in each side).

As illustrated in FIGURE 1, animals with repeated experience of cocaine in the context of the test cage were significantly more active upon amphetamine challenge in the nucleus accumbens compared with the other two groups ($F = 3.19$, $p < 0.09$; two-tailed ANOVA with repeated measures; $p < 0.05$, one-tailed). It is of interest that animals receiving cocaine in the context of the home cage were no more active than the saline controls that had never received cocaine in either environment.

This differential responsivity was also apparent when saline was injected into the nucleus accumbens, as illustrated in FIGURE 2. Again, rats having repeated pretreatment experience with cocaine in the context of the test cage environment were significantly more active than animals receiving cocaine in the home cage, or the saline controls ($F = 7.79$, $p < 0.02$: ANOVA with repeated measures). These data taken together with the amphetamine-challenge data in FIGURE 1, suggest an environmental-context and/or conditioning effect of the cocaine pretreatment in the test environment rather than a differential sensitivity to amphetamine based on prior cocaine experience.

In contrast to the injections of amphetamine or saline into the nucleus accumbens, amphetamine administered into the caudate nucleus revealed no evidence of differential sensitization on the basis of prior cocaine-induced hyperactivity and stereotypy in the test cage. In this study, 7–10 days following caudate nucleus cannula implantation, groups of rats received twice-daily injections of cocaine or saline for a total of

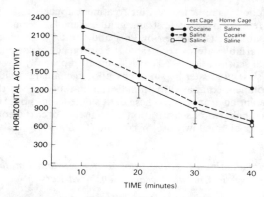

**FIGURE 1.** Three groups of rats received two daily ip injections of cocaine (10 mg/kg) or saline for 10 days. One group received cocaine in the test environment and saline in the home cage; a second group received saline in the test environment and cocaine in the home cage; and the third group received two saline injections. Following this chronic regimen, an acute challenge with amphetamine (10 μg) injected directly into the nucleus accumbens bilaterally revealed a significant difference in the locomotor activity exhibited by the rats that previously received cocaine in the test chamber and those that had never received cocaine. No difference between the rats that received cocaine in the home cage and those that had never received cocaine was seen.

17 days in order to ensure the adequate development of substantial amounts of stereotypic behavior. During the first ten days, cocaine was administered at a dose of 10 mg/kg, ip, and, in order to induce more intense stereotypes, the dose was raised to 20 mg/kg, ip, for an additional seven days. Animals received saline upon return to the home cage. A second group of animals received saline in the test cage and the same doses (as in group one) of cocaine in the home cage over the 17 days. The third group of animals received saline (1 ml/kg—an equivalent volume to that of cocaine) in the test and home cages. Stereotypic ratings were performed using a modification of the Creese and Iversen scale[11] at 10-minute intervals beginning 5 minutes after the injection and extending for 55 minutes postinjection.

Acute administration of amphetamine (10 μg bilaterally in the caudate) produced significant degrees of stereotypy, but there were no differences among groups (FIG. 3). Thus, amphetamine-induced stereotypic behavior appeared to be, if anything, less robust in animals previously exhibiting cocaine-induced stereotypic behaviors either in the test-cage or the home-cage environments.

Taken together, the data from intracerebral injections of amphetamine into the nucleus accumbens and caudate nucleus in cocaine-pretreated animals suggests a possible role for the nucleus accumbens in the conditioned component of cocaine-induced locomotor hyperactivity, but a lack of effect of the caudate in cocaine-induced sensitization to stereotypic behavior. It is pertinent to note that in other paradigms designed to induce stereotypic behavior to cocaine (40 mg/kg ip for 3 days) that both a conditioned and unconditioned component of stereotypic behavior can be revealed (see FIG. 4) following rechallenge with a low dose of cocaine (10 mg/kg ip) on day 4. These and other data suggest that cocaine-induced stereotypic behavior does display a sen-

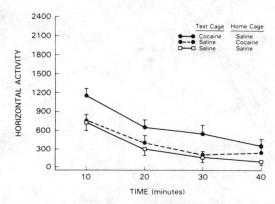

**FIGURE 2.** Rats received daily ip injections of cocaine (10 mg/kg) in the test or home cage (as described in FIG. 1). Following this chronic regimen and five days after the amphetamine challenge, an acute challenge with saline injected directly into the nucleus accumbens revealed a significant increase in the locomotor activity exhibited by the rats that previously received cocaine in the test chamber compared to those that had never received cocaine. No difference between the rats that received cocaine in the home cage and those that had never received cocaine was seen.

sitization phenomenon following rechallenge with systemic administration of cocaine, and a lack of sensitization to stereotypic effects is not the reason that no effect was observed upon administration of amphetamine into the caudate. Rather, it suggests that the caudate is not the substrate subserving context-dependent or context-independent cocaine-induced sensitization of stereotypic behavior. Further examination of mesolimbic dopaminergic substrates, such as those residing in the nucleus accumbens or amygdala, would appear to deserve exploration as potential mediators of sensitization to cocaine's stereotypic effects.

### Conditioned Cocaine-Induced Behavioral Sensitization Revealed by a Single High-Dose Pretreatment

As illustrated in FIGURE 4, an interaction of cocaine dose and number of repetitions appears to be involved in inducing the type and duration of behavioral sensitization. Injection of a single high-dose of cocaine (40 mg/kg) reveals substantial sensitization to a rechallenge dose (10 mg/kg) the next day, where a single administration of a low dose of cocaine (10 mg/kg) is unable to induce the sensitization effect. Yet, if this same low dose of cocaine (10 mg/kg ip) is repeated enough times, it also can induce a robust degree of sensitization that is long-lasting. If high doses of cocaine (40 mg/kg ip) are repeated for three days, the type of behavior shifts from predominantly locomotor activity to stereotypic responses, and the sensitization shifts from one that is entirely environmental-context-dependent (following a single cocaine pretreatment) to a sensitization demonstrating both context-independent and context-dependent properties. Thus, with increasing doses and numbers of repetitions of cocaine adminis-

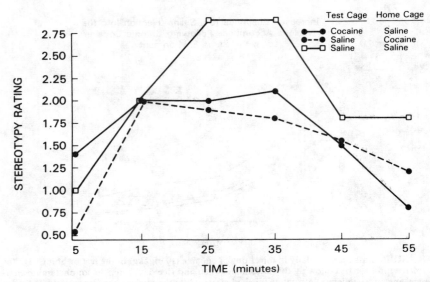

**FIGURE 3.** Lack of effect of prior cocaine treatment on amphetamine-induced stereotypy following caudate injection. Three groups of rats received 2 daily ip injections of cocaine or saline for a total of 17 days. Stereotypy ratings were made using a modified version of the Creese and Iverson scale (1974) at 10-min intervals beginning 5 min after the injection and lasting for 55 min postinjection. The group mean ratings are plotted on the ordinate and time is plotted on the abscissa. One injection was given to the rats just prior to being placed in the test cage in which stereotypy was rated and a second injection occurred when the rats were returned to the home cage. One group received cocaine in the test environment and saline in the home cage; a second group received saline in the test environment and cocaine in the home cage; and the third group received two saline injections. Following this chronic regimen, an acute challenge with amphetamine injected directly into the caudate revealed no significant differences among the three groups, although the cocaine pretreated groups (regardless of location or injection) showed slightly less stereotypic behavior.

tration, there is a shift from a locomotor hyperactivity pattern and sensitization that is environmental-context-dependent to behavior that involves more predominant stereotypes where sensitization does not depend entirely on conditioning.

### Stimulus Generalization: Similarity of Environmental Context

Consistent with the conditioned effect achieved with a single cocaine dose, we have observed that the degree of environmental similarity in which the animals receive the pretreatment dose and the subsequent cocaine challenge is related to the degree of behavioral sensitization obtained.[12] If the pretreatment and test environments are highly similar, robust behavioral sensitization is induced; if the environments are highly dissimilar, no sensitization occurs. Thus, principles derived from learning theory, such as stimulus generalization, appear to be relevant to cocaine-induced sensitization. Convergent with these data are our observations that blockade of the initial day of cocaine-induced hyperactivity is sufficient to block the development of sensitization to a

| COCAINE | | EFFECT | | | | | | | | | |
|---|---|---|---|---|---|---|---|---|---|---|---|
| Number of Injections | Dose mg/kg i.p. | Behavioral Sensitization | Duration | Activity Context Dep. | Indep. | Stereotypy Context Dep. | Indep. | Saline Conditioning | Sensitization Neuroleptic Independent | Seizure Kindling | Death |
| ↑↑↑ | COC$_{65}$ | | | | | | | | | ++ | ++ |
| x 10 days | COC$_{160}$ subcut. (K. Gale) | ++ | | | ++ | | ++ | | ++ | | |
| ++++++++++ | COC$_{10}$ | ++ | months | ++ | 0 | | | ++ | | | |
| ↑↑↑ | COC$_{40}$ | + | | 0 | ++ | ++ | ++ | ± | | | |
| ↑ | COC$_{40}$ | ++ | days | ++ | 0 | 0 | 0 | 0 | 0 | | |
| ↑↑↑ | COC$_{20}$ | 0 | 0 | 0 | 0 | 0 | + | | | | |
| ↑↑↑ | COC$_{10}$ | 0 | 0 | 0 | 0 | 0 | 0 | | | | |
| ↑ | COC$_{10}$ | 0 | 0 | | | | | | | | |

**FIGURE 4.** A schematic representation of the increasing behavioral effects of cocaine following repeated administration and increasing doses. At the lower doses, or with few repetitions, cocaine produced a sensitization of locomotor activity and stereotypy that was context-dependent and moderately long-lasting. At higher doses, or with greater repetitions, the behavior became more pathologic (intense stereotypes and/or seizures), less dependent on context and conditioning principles, and changes were longer lasting.

rechallenge on the next day. This blockade can be achieved with either direct dopamine receptor antagonists, for example, haloperidol (0.2 or 0.5 mg/kg), or with sedating doses of diazepam (5 mg/kg). These data imply that the behavior must be manifest in order for conditioning or sensitization effects to be observed.

*Neuroleptics Block Development but not Expression of Sensitization*

A remarkable dissociation in the ability of neuroleptics to block the development vs. the expression of cocaine-induced behavioral sensitization is illustrated in FIGURE 5. That is, doses of haloperidol administered prior to the initial cocaine injection on day 1, are sufficient to block the development of cocaine-induced behavioral sensitization, as revealed by a test dose of cocaine (10 mg/kg ip) on day 2. In contrast, the same doses of neuroleptics (either 0.20 or 0.50 mg/kg) are not able to block the effects

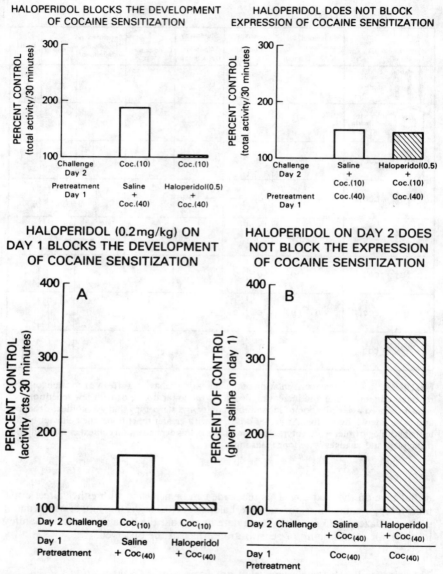

**FIGURE 5.** The total horizontal activity (30 min) in the experimental groups is expressed as the percentage of activity in the control groups. *Left side*: the control groups were pretreated with saline alone for the cocaine plus saline group and haloperidol alone for the cocaine plus haloperidol group. Only the group of rats that received cocaine without haloperidol showed sensitization to cocaine on the following day. *Right side*: Haloperidol was administered to one-half of the cocaine- and saline-pretreated rats during the cocaine challenge day. On the challenge day, rats that received haloperidol and cocaine, but had been pretreated with saline, served as the controls for those that were pretreated with cocaine. Rats that received saline and cocaine, but had been pretreated with saline, served as the controls for those that were pretreated with cocaine. Neuroleptics blocked the development of cocaine sensitization, but once established, neuroleptic blockade did not prevent its expression.

of prior cocaine if the neuroleptic is administered only prior to the cocaine challenge on day 2. These data replicate and extend those of Beninger and Hahn,[13] Beninger and Herz,[14] and Tadokoro and Kuribara,[15] who also found that doses of neuroleptics that were capable of blocking stimulant-induced behavioral sensitization or conditioning (to cocaine, amphetamine, or methamphetamine) were not cabable of blocking the expression of these behaviors when the neuroleptics were administered prior to the challenge only.

These data suggest that dopaminergic or other neuroleptic blockable mechanisms are critical to the developing phase of psychomotor stimulant-induced behavioral sensitization, but once this sensitizing effect has been induced, even high sedating doses of neuroleptics are no longer able to block the expression of this effect; that is, it has become independent of dopamine mechanisms. Further exploration of the neurotransmitter systems involved in this conditioned component of cocaine-induced behavioral sensitization and expression would appear warranted.

## Effect of Nucleus Accumbens and Amygdala Lesions on Cocaine Sensitization

Given the robust and highly replicable nature of the conditioned component, that is, environmental context dependency of cocaine-induced behavioral sensitization, we attempted to further explore possible neuroanatomical substrates of this conditioned component. In a series of studies (Weiss and Pert, unpublished data), preliminary data suggested that electrolytic lesions of the amygdala and selective dopaminergic lesions of the nucleus accumbens (with 6-hydroxydopamine and desmethylimipramine [DMI] blockade) blocked the expression of cocaine-induced behavioral sensitization compared with sham-lesioned controls or electrolytic lesions of the dorsal hippocampus (FIG. 6b). The nucleus accumbens lesions produced approximately 60% dopamine depletion, but left the day-1 cocaine-induced hyperactivity intact (FIG. 6a). In a second study, electrolytic lesions of the ventral hippocampus did not appear to impair the expression of cocaine-induced behavioral sensitization and neither did large cerebellar lesions of midline nuclear structures, in spite of the fact that they left the animals generally ataxic with impaired locomotor capabilities. A third study replicated the effects of amygdala lesions on cocaine-induced behavioral sensitization and also demonstrated that these effects were more robust with selective depletions of dopamine in the amygdala than with electrolytic lesions. While these studies remain to be further analyzed following histological confirmation of the lesions, these preliminary data suggest the possibility that dopamine substrates in the nucleus accumbens and in the amygdala may be critically involved in the expression of the conditioned component of cocaine-induced behavioral sensitization.

Several caveats are in order regarding these preliminary conclusions. Nucleus accumbens lesions did not significantly reduce locomotor activity induced following cocaine (40 mg/kg ip) on day 1. These data are at variance with those of Kelly and Iversen,[1] who reported that lesions of the nucleus accumbens reduced activity following cocaine (20 mg/kg). However, in their study, greater depletions of dopamine were produced in the nucleus accumbens, which may account for this difference. In our study, despite the fact that robust cocaine-induced hyperactivity was achieved following cocaine challenge on day 1, the accumbens-lesioned animals still showed a response on day 2 to cocaine (10 mg/kg) that was no greater than in animals that had been pretreated with saline on day 1. These data suggest that the partial depletion, while insufficient to prevent cocaine-induced hyperactivity, was nevertheless able to block the cocaine sensitization or conditioning and that this aspect of cocaine's effects may be more sensitive to dopamine depletion than just the motor activating effect of cocaine.

NO EFFECT OF LESIONS OF THE AMYGDALA,
NUCLEUS ACCUMBENS OR DORSAL HIPPOCAMPUS
ON COCAINE-INDUCED HYPERACTIVITY

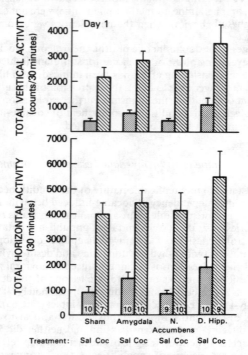

**FIGURE 6a.** The mean and standard error of the total horizontal and vertical (rearing) loco-motor activity for 30 min is illustrated for groups of rats that received lesions in one of the fol-lowing areas: sham (surgical control); amygdala; nucleus accumbens (6-OHDA); or dorsal hip-pocampus. The number of subjects in each group is illustrated in the bars in the lower half of the figure. Rats from each of these groups that received cocaine (40 mg/kg) exhibited a marked hyperactivity compared to saline-treated controls.

**FIGURE 6b.** Horizontal and vertical locomotor activity in response to a cocaine challenge ▶
(10 mg/kg) is illustrated for the same animals shown in FIG. 6a. These rats were pretreated with either cocaine (40 mg/kg) or saline, and also had sham lesions or lesions of the amygdala, nu-cleus accumbens, or dorsal hippocampus. The number of subjects in each group is illustrated in the bars on the lower half of the figure. Rats with sham lesions or lesions of the dorsal hip-pocampus that were pretreated with cocaine showed an enhanced response to cocaine compared to saline-pretreated controls. Rats with lesions of the amygdala or nucleus accumbens failed to show a differential response to the cocaine despite the difference in pretreatments.

# INHIBITION OF COCAINE SENSITIZATION
# BY AMYGDALA AND
# NUCLEUS ACCUMBENS LESIONS

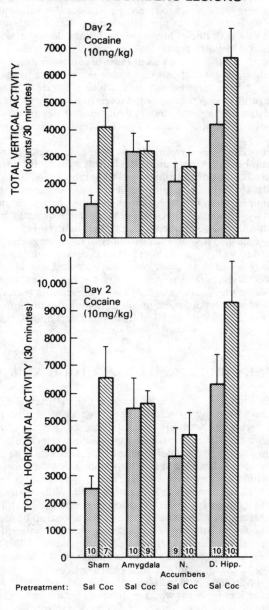

A second caveat to consider in evaluating our data is that the lack of sensitization to prior cocaine in both the amygdala- and nucleus-accumbens-lesioned animals was, in part, attributable to the increases in activity in the saline-pretreated lesioned animals that were challenged with cocaine on day 2. This raises the possibility that the lesioned control animals were more prone to stress sensitization[16-18] following saline administration than are rats with no lesions or sham-lesions. Against this interpretation is the finding that the rats with dorsal hippocampal lesions demonstrated sensitization to prior cocaine despite elevated activity in both saline- and cocaine-pretreated animals.

A last caveat is that the nucleus accumbens lesions were able to block the expression of the conditioned components of cocaine sensitization on day 2, while leaving the day 1 unconditioned component intact, which is contrary to what would be expected from the results using the dopamine receptor antagonists previously presented. This may be related to the partial (60%) depletions of dopamine achieved, but also suggests that the neuroleptic blockade of systems other than dopamine should be further investigated.

Gold and associates[19] have reported that more extensive dopaminergic lesions of the nucleus accumbens (91% dopamine depletion) were sufficient to block both the unconditioned and conditioned components of amphetamine-induced locomotor activity. These data, in conjunction with our lesions of the nucleus accumbens, as well as the direct administration of amphetamine into the nucleus accumbens in cocaine-pretreated animals, all suggest that the nucleus accumbens may be importantly involved in the conditioned component of stimulant-induced behavioral sensitization. Our preliminary data also suggest the possibility that the amygdala may play a critical role in this regard as well. These data are of considerable interest in light of the role of the amygdala in a variety of other conditioning paradigms including conditioned startle,[20] conditioned emotional responses, and a variety of other conditioned autonomic effects. Moreover, Squillace et al.[21] also observed that lesions of the amygdala blocked the progressive development of lidocaine-induced omniphagic behavior, another endpoint that appears to show sensitization effects upon repetition of the same dose of drug.

## COCAINE-INDUCED PHARMACOLOGICAL KINDLING

As illustrated in Figure 7, if doses of cocaine are sufficiently high at the outset, repetition of administration may lead to the emergence of seizures to a dose that was previously subconvulsant. A variety of data discussed in detail elsewhere[7,22] suggest that this may represent a true pharmacological kindling effect rather than one related to pharmacokinetics, tissue accumulation, or other artifacts. The phenomenon may closely resemble that of electrophysiological kindling first described by Goddard and associates,[23] in which repeated stimulation of the amygdala evokes seizures to stimulus characteristics that had previously been subthreshold. While many areas of the brain can be electrically kindled (with the exception of the cerebellum), the amygdala and related limbic system sites such as the hippocampus appear to be most easily kindled, as revealed by the fewest number of stimulations prior to onset of the first seizure. Moreover, 2-deoxyglucose and electrophysiological studies of local anesthetics suggest that lidocaine-induced seizures may importantly involve limbic system substrates such as the amygdala, hippocampus, and perirhinal cortex.[2]

In contrast to lidocaine-induced seizures, which are relatively well tolerated even with repeated inductions for many weeks or months, cocaine-induced seizures are highly lethal, with most animals dying after the first or second seizure (FIG. 7a). This suggests that the properties of cocaine that confer its psychomotor stimulant attributes (possibly its ability to potentiate catecholamines) may be involved in the increased lethality of cocaine-induced seizures compared with a similar dose of the equipotent local anesthetic lidocaine. It is of interest that chronic, but not acute, treatment with the anticonvulsant carbamazepine is capable of blocking the development of lidocaine-induced and cocaine-induced pharmacologically kindled seizures (FIG. 7b). Carbamazepine exerts complex effects on dopaminergic mechanisms as well as a multiplicity of other neurotransmitter–neuromodulator substances, as reviewed elsewhere,[24] and it is not at all clear which effect may relate to the ability of this anticonvulsant to inhibit local anesthetic-induced kindling. Nonetheless, carbamazepine is among the most potent of the anticonvulsants in inhibiting amygdala-kindled compared with cortical-kindled seizures.[25]

## CLINICAL IMPLICATIONS OF COCAINE-INDUCED BEHAVIORAL SENSITIZATION AND PHARMACOLOGICAL KINDLING

Along with a growing recognition of cocaine's exquisitely psychologically addicting properties is its capacity to induce a variety of dysfunctional mood and cognitive states. Cocaine-induced dysphoria is increasingly apparent with high-dose administration associated with either peak dose effects or with the wearing off and withdrawal phases. Recent laboratory studies of this effect under controlled circumstances by Sherer and associates[26] indicate that dysphoric elements do emerge, even with maintenance of high cocaine levels with a continuous intravenous infusion. Therefore, cocaine-induced dysphoria cannot be attributable solely to cocaine withdrawal effects. This has long been recognized by street users of cocaine who administer cocaine with heroin and other drugs in an attempt to decrease the dysphoric and anxiogenic components of cocaine. In the studies of Sherer *et al.* emerging evidence of paranoia was also observed with maintenance of cocaine levels, supporting the less controlled self-reports of a high incidence of cocaine-induced paranoia in callers to the Cocaine Hotline.

In addition to these well-described effects, which have also been reported and observed with the related psychomotor stimulant amphetamine, a unique syndrome has been reported — that of cocaine-induced panic attacks. As described in detail elsewhere,[7] Uhde and associates have observed that a number of patients presenting to their clinic for the study and treatment of panic anxiety disorders, reported the onset of their panic attacks following cocaine administration. In particular, it appears that repeated cocaine use for many months or years is not associated with the induction of panic attacks initially, but, with more chronic administration, may be a more consistent concomitant of the use of cocaine. With sufficient repetition, these cocaine-induced panic attacks may become spontaneous, perhaps akin to the phenomenon of spontaneity in electrophysiological kindling where repeated seizures induced by electrical stimulation eventually leaves the animal susceptible to the appearance of spontaneous seizures without further exogenous electrophysiological stimulation.

While cocaine-induced seizures are not evident in patients experiencing cocaine-related panic attacks, it is also apparent that seizures are an increasingly recognized concomitant of cocaine deaths in emergency room statistics, (e.g., Len Bias clearly had a seizure prior to his terminal events). While it is unclear what the prior history of cocaine use is in many clinical situations, extrapolations from the data on pharmacological kindling observed in rats, cats, dogs, and rhesus monkeys (see review of Post and Contel[8]) suggest the possibility that seizures might also develop in man to a dose similar to one that had previously been tolerated.

Conditioned components of the clinical syndromes of cocaine use in man are also

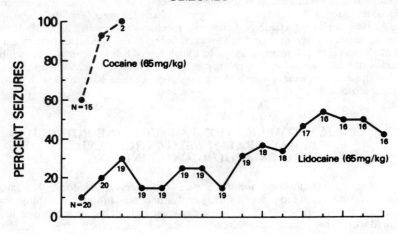

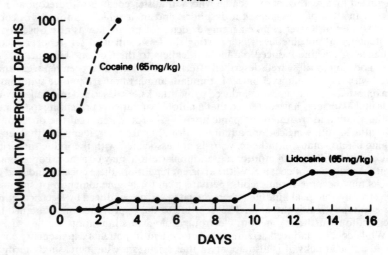

**FIGURE 7a.** The percentage of rats experiencing lidocaine- or cocaine-induced seizures and deaths is shown over days. Rats received a single ip injection (65 mg/kg) each day. The study began with 20 subjects per group, and the number remaining each day is shown in the top half of the figure. Despite the equal potency of these drugs as local anesthetics, cocaine is much more toxic than lidocaine.

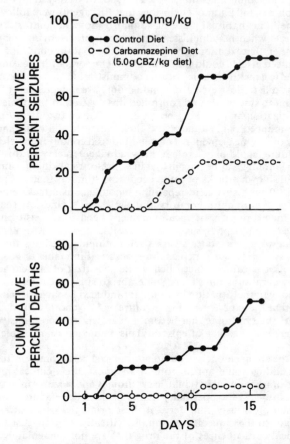

CHRONIC CARBAMAZEPINE PREVENTS THE
DEVELOPMENT OF COCAINE KINDLED SEIZURES
AND MORTALITY

**FIGURE 7b.** The percentage of rats experiencing cocaine-induced seizures and deaths is shown over days with or without carbamazepine cotreatment (N = 20/group). Rats treated with carbamazepine were fed a diet containing the drug beginning 4 days before the first cocaine injection and were continued on this diet throughout the experiment. Note that a lower dose of cocaine (40 mg/kg) was used in this experiment compared with the study illustrated in FIG. 7a. Carbamazepine markedly suppressed the development of the cocaine-induced seizures and deaths.

increasingly being recognized. Gawin and Kleber[27] reported many clinical vignettes of the powerful effects of cocaine-conditioned cues for inducing "highs," craving, and relapse phenomena. In more systematic studies, Childress *et al.*[28] have reported that viewing slides of cocaine-related paraphernalia induces high levels of craving in cocaine users who were abstinent for many weeks, similar to what has previously been reported for opiate users. These investigators are now attempting to decondition cocaine users to these powerful conditioning mechanisms. A context-dependent induction of cocaine-induced dysphoria and paranoia has also been reported by a high-dose user (D.L., personal communication, Nov. 27, 1986) who consistently noted increased degrees of dysphoria and paranoid delusions that FBI agents were following him when he used cocaine in his habitual place of administration. In contrast, he experienced more mild effects when he administered cocaine in other environmental contexts.

Taken together, these data suggest the possibility that the conditioned component of cocaine-induced effects could play a role in the reports of increasingly prominent psychological effects with chronic cocaine administration. Of course, many of these effects could be due to dose escalation and chronic use independent of sensitization, requiring that more systematic and controlled observation of the clinical phenomena related to sensitization and kindling be conducted. Given the interesting time course of the cocaine-induced panic attacks and their emergence into the spontaneous variety, it is likely that some elements of cocaine-induced conditioned behavioral sensitization and kindling could play a role in the gradual emergence of this phenomenon. The analogy to kindling is appealing in that in both electrical kindling and panic-attack evolution (1) full-blown attacks begin to occur to a stimulus that was previously subthreshold, and (2) with sufficient repetition, spontaneous attacks emerge.

A series of studies in our laboratory and elsewhere[13-15] indicate that the development, but not the expression, of cocaine-induced behavioral sensitization is responsive to blockade by neuroleptics, suggesting a possible model for neuroleptic nonresponsiveness in some psychotic states such as schizophrenia. Perhaps the experience of activated and psychotic states, such as those observed in mania or schizophreniform psychosis may, like cocaine-induced behavioral sensitization, be capable of making the underlying neural substrates more vulnerable to subsequent reactivation. If there is a direct analogy to the situation in stimulant-induced behavioral sensitization, one would predict that the experience of these untreated psychotic episodes could lead to a component of the syndrome that becomes neuroleptic nonresponsive upon subsequent reexperience of this type of episode. This prediction is amenable to direct clinical testing.

Obviously, the animal models of stimulant-induced behavioral sensitization or pharmacological kindling would appear to have the most direct clinical relevance to the induction of cocaine-induced psychiatric syndromes and seizures in man. The current series of studies suggest the possibility that cocaine may be a more insidiously dangerous drug than previously considered if these principles of sensitization and kindling are relevant to the clinical situation. Specifically, they suggest that behavioral and physiological consequences of the drug that are not immediately apparent at a given dose may, with sufficient repetition, emerge and induce increasingly pathological behaviors and, possibly, pharmacologically kindled seizures.

Preliminary data from our laboratory and that from Gold and associates[19] suggest the possibility that mesolimbic dopamine substrates in the nucleus accumbens and amygdala may be involved in some aspects of the conditioned component of stimulant-induced behavioral effects. Further work is required to elucidate the critical anatomical and neurotransmitter pathways involved in this component of cocaine-induced sensitization and also to elucidate the possible clinical correlates of this conditioned phenomenon in man. Similarly, controlled clinical trials are required in order to assess the potential clinical efficacy of blockade of cocaine-induced kindled seizure phenomena utilizing the anticonvulsant carbamazepine. Considerable caution would be required in the potential clinical application of this drug, as we have observed increased cocaine-induced convulsive toxicity and lethality following acute, rather than chronic, pretreatment with carbamazepine.

Nonetheless, we would suggest that the preclinical studies of behavioral sensitization and pharmacological kindling give an important new orientation and focus to the longitudinal and potentially progressive toxicities of repeated use of cocaine. The sensitization studies raise the possibility that powerful conditioned components of the drug may be occurring in man as have already been preliminarily documented. They further suggest the possibility that pharmacological interventions (for example, with neuroleptics) may differ in their efficacy as a function of development vs. expression of behavioral sensitization. Conversely, under some circumstances, lesions of the amygdala and nucleus accumbens may be capable of blocking the expression of cocaine-induced sensitization, while leaving unaltered the ability of cocaine to induce hyperactivity on day 1. Similar principles are also apparent for pharmacological interventions in kindling that differ as a function of stage of development.[29] Further elucidation of the role of mesolimbic and mesocortical dopamine systems in the conditioned component of psychomotor stimulant-induced behavioral sensitization may provide new clues to the mechanisms underlying these phenomena and new methods to intervene in its induction.

## REFERENCES

1. KELLY, P. H. & S. D. IVERSEN. 1976. Selective 6-OHDA-induced destruction of mesolimbic dopamine neurons: Abolition of psychostimulant-induced locomotor activity in rats. Eur. J. Pharmacol. **40:** 45–56.
2. POST, R. M., C. KENNEDY, M. SHINOHARA, K. SQUILLACE, M. MIYAOKA, S. SUDA, D. H. INGVAR & L. SOKOLOFF. 1984. Metabolic and behavioral consequences of lidocaine-kindled seizures. Brain Res. **324:** 295–304.
3. POST, R. M. & R. T. KOPANDA. 1976. Cocaine, kindling, and psychosis. Am. J. Psychiatry **133:** 627–634.
4. ELLINWOOD, E. H., M. M. KILBEY, S. CASTELLANI & C. KHOURY. 1977. Amygdala hyperspindling and seizures induced by cocaine. *In* Cocaine and Other Stimulants, Advances in Behavioral Biology, Vol. 21. E. H. Ellinwood and M. M. Kilbey, Eds.: 303–326. Plenum Press. New York.
5. STRIPLING, J. S. 1982. Origin of cocaine-induced and lidocaine-induced spindle activity within the olfactory forebrain of the rat. Electroencephalogr. Clin. Neurophysiol. **53:** 208–219.
6. WISE, R. A. 1984. Neural mechanisms of the reinforcing action of cocaine. *In* Cocaine: Pharmacology, Effects, and Treatment of Abuse. J. Grabowski, Ed. NIDA Monograph Series 50: 15–33. U.S. Government Printing Office, Washington, D.C.
7. POST, R. M., S. R. B. WEISS, A. PERT & T. W. UHDE. 1987. Chronic cocaine administration: Sensitization and kindling effects. *In* Cocaine: Clinical and Biobehavioral Aspects. S. Fisher, A. Raskin, and E. H. Uhlenhuth, Eds.: 109–173. Oxford Univ. Press. London/New York.
8. POST, R. M. & N. R. CONTEL. 1983. Human and animal studies of cocaine: Implications for development of behavioral pathology. *In* Stimulants: Neurochemical, Behavioral, and Clinical Perspective. I. Creese, Ed.: 169–203. Raven Press. New York.
9. POST, R. M., A. LOCKFELD, K. M. SQUILLACE & N. R. CONTEL. 1981. Drug-environment interaction: Context dependency of cocaine-induced behavioral sensitization. Life Sci. **28:** 755–760.
10. HINSON, R. E. & C. X. POULOS. 1981. Sensitization to the behavioral effects of cocaine: Modulation by pavlovian conditioning. Pharmacol. Biochem. Behav. **15:** 559–562.
11. CREESE, I. & S. D. IVERSEN. 1974. The role of forebrain dopamine systems in amphetamine-induced sterotypy in the adult rat following neonatal treatment with 6-hydroxydopamine. Psychopharmacologia **39:** 345–357.
12. WEISS, S. R. B., D. MURMAN, R. M. POST & A. PERT. 1986. Conditioning in cocaine-induced behavioral sensitization. Abstracts, Society for Neuroscience, 16th Annual Meeting, Washington, D.C., Nov. 9–14: 914.

13. BENINGER, R. J. & B. L. HAHN. 1983. Pimozide blocks establishment but not expression of amphetamine-produced environment-specific conditioning. Science 220: 1304.

14. BENINGER, R. J. & R. S. HERZ. 1986. Pimozide blocks establishment but not expression of cocaine-produced environment-specific conditioning. Life Sci. 38: 1425–1431.

15. TADOKORO, S. & H. KURIBARA. 1986. Reverse tolerance to the ambulation-increasing effect of the methamphetamine in mice as an animal model of amphetamine-psychosis. Psychopharmacol. Bull. 22: 757–762.

16. ANTELMAN, S. M., A. J. EICHLER, C. A. BLACK & D. KOCAN. 1980. Interchangeability of stress and amphetamine in sensitization. Science 207: 329–331.

17. ANTELMAN, S. M. & L. A. CHIODO. 1984. Stress: Its effect on interactions among biogenic amines and role in the induction and treatment of disease. In Handbook of Psychopharmacology, Vol. 18. L. L. Iversen, S. D. Iversen, and S. H. Snyder, Eds.: 279–341. Plenum Press. New York.

18. KALIVAS, P. W. & P. DUFFY. 1988. Similar effects of daily cocaine and daily stress on mesocorticolimbic dopamine neural transmission. Unpublished manuscript.

19. GOLD, L. H., N. R. SWERDOW & G. F. KOOB. 1988. The role of mesolimbic dopamine in conditioned locomotion produced by amphetamine. Behav. Neurosci. In press.

20. HITCHCOCK, J. & M. DAVIS. 1986. Lesions of the amygdala, but not of the cerebullum or red nucleus, block conditioned fear as measured with the potentiated startle paradigm. Behav. Neurosci. 100: 11–22.

21. SQUILLACE, K. M., R. M. POST & A. PERT. 1982. Effect of lidocaine pretreatment of cocaine-induced behavior in normal and amygdala-lesioned rats. Neuropsychology 8: 113–122.

22. POST, R. M., R. T. KOPANDA & K. E. BLACK. 1976. Progressive effects of cocaine on behavior and central amine metabolism in rhesus monkeys: Relationship to kindling and psychosis. Biol. Psychiatry 11: 403–419.

23. GODDARD, G. V., D. C. MCINTYRE & C. K. LEECH. 1969. A permanent change in brain function resulting from daily electrical stimulation. Exp. Neurol. 25: 295–330.

24. POST, R. M. 1987. Mechanisms of action of carbamazepine and related anticonvulsants in affective illness. In Psychopharmacology: A Third Generation of Progress. H. Meltzer, Ed.: 567–576. Raven Press. New York.

25. ALBRIGHT, P. S. & W. M. BURNHAM. 1980. Development of a new pharmacological seizure model: Effects of anticonvulsants on cortical- and amygdala-kindled seizures in the rat. Epilepsia 21: 681–689.

26. SHERER, M. A., K. M. KUMAR & J. H. JAFFE. 1986. Infusions of cocaine: A model for cocaine induced psychosis? Abstracts, American Psychiatric Association, 139th Annual Meeting, Washington, D.C., May 10–16: 54.

27. GAWIN, F. H. & H. KLEBER. 1987. Issues in cocaine abuse treatment research. In Cocaine: Clinical and Biobehavioral Aspects. S. Fisher, A. Raskin and E. H. Uhlenhuth, Eds.: 174–192. Oxford Univ. Press. London/New York.

28. CHILDRESS, A. R., A. T. MCLELLAN, R. N. EHRMAN & C. P. O'BRIEN. 1987. Extinction of conditioned responses in abstinent cocaine or opioid users. In NIDA monograph, Problems of Drug Dependence. U.S. Government Printing Office. Washington. D.C. In press.

29. POST, R. M., D. R. RUBINOW & J. C. BALLENGER. 1986. Conditioning and sensitization in the longitudinal course of affective illness. Br. J. Psychiatry 149: 191.

# A Critical Appraisal of CSF Monoamine Metabolite Studies in Schizophrenia

ERIK WIDERLÖV

*Department of Psychiatry and Neurochemistry*
*University of Lund*
*220 06 Lund, Sweden*

## INTRODUCTION

During the late 1950s and the following decades increasing evidence for a connection between central dopamine (DA) functions and schizophrenia emerged. The DA hypothesis of schizophrenia was based primarily on indirect pharmacological evidences, for example, the antipsychotic action of neuroleptic drugs correlated with their propensity to reduce DA function (phenothiazines, reserpine); neuroleptic drugs bind to dopamine receptors with affinities that are proportional to their antipsychotic potencies; high doses of amphetamine or other DA agonists can induce psychotic states resembling schizophrenia or exacerbate schizophrenic symptoms in patients with schizophrenia. Several extensive reviews of this field have previously been presented.[1-5]

More recent support for the hypothesis are findings of increased numbers of DA-$D_2$ (but not DA-$D_1$ receptors) in postmortem brains of schizophrenic patients unrelated to previous neuroleptic treatment.[6-8] Interestingly, Wong and collaborators[9] have recently found increased DA-$D_2$ receptor densities *in vivo* in the caudate nucleus of drug-naive schizophrenic patients using positron emission tomography.

Several different approaches have been used to test the DA hypothesis of schizophrenia, for example, measurements of DA and its major metabolites homovanillic acid (HVA), or 3,4-dihydroxyphenylacetic acid (DOPAC) in postmortem brains, or cerebrospinal fluid (CSF) from schizophrenic patients and controls; measurements of enzyme activities involved in DA synthesis or degradation; assessments of central DA receptor sensitivity; and evaluation of clinical effects of drugs that alter DA function (for an extensive review, see reference 5).

In the present paper, the focus is on findings in CSF monoamine and monoamine metabolite studies in schizophrenia. Emphasis is on the DA system, but also noradrenaline and serotonin and their principal metabolites, 3-methoxy-4-hydroxyphenyl glycol (MHPG) and 5-hydroxyindoleacetic acid (5-HIAA), are briefly discussed.

## CSF MONOAMINE METABOLITE STUDIES IN SCHIZOPHRENIA

The first indication of altered neurotransmitter function related to psychiatric illness by assessment of a CSF monoamine metabolite concentration was reported by Ashcroft and Sharman in 1960,[10] when they showed a reduced 5-HIAA concentration in depressed patients. Since then a large number of CSF studies have been presented, the majority related to manic-depressive illness, but also a number of papers related to other neuropsychiatric illnesses like schizophrenia, different types of dementias, and Huntington's chorea.

Bowers[11] concluded in an overview of the field that clinical studies so far have failed to define specific monoamine changes in nosologically defined neuropsychiatric syndromes.

In the earliest reports fluorometric methods were the only analytic methods available for the monoamine metabolites. In the early 1970s mass fragmentographic methods with much higher sensitivity and specificity[12] were introduced. Later also high-performance liquid chromatography (HPLC) methods have increasingly been used.

In TABLE 1 a number of CSF monoamine metabolite studies in schizophrenia have been summarized.[13-41] The table is by no means complete; in particular, many of the earliest studies have been excluded and so have many studies related to clinical trials of drugs.

The majority of the studies have not shown any consistent differences in CSF monoamine metabolite concentrations between schizophrenic patients and control subjects.

A major methodological problem is the influence of antipsychotic drugs on the CSF metabolite concentrations.

The rapid increase in DA release and elevation of DA metabolite concentrations following acute neuroleptic administration to animals was first demonstrated by Carlsson and Lindquist[42] and Andén and co-workers.[43] Later it was demonstrated that a region-specific tolerance developed to the increase in DA turnover following chronic neuroleptic administration to animals.[44-46]

Several clinical papers have also demonstrated elevated DA metabolite concentrations in CSF during the initial phase of antipsychotic medication (e.g., references 25, 38, 47, 48).

Results from human CSF studies are conflicting with regard to the tolerance development after chronic treatment. Post and Goodwin[38] found a time-dependent reduction of HVA in CSF after an initial increase of the metabolite. Sedvall's group in Stockholm[25,47,48] found the same HVA elevation in CSF at two and four weeks of neuroleptic treatment, while others have found mixed patterns.[49,50] Bowers[19] reported that in a group of 24 patients receiving neuroleptics, the 11 patients whose HVA levels in CSF showed no tolerance to neuroleptics at one month had significantly more residual symptoms, extrapyramidal side effects, and family history of psychiatric illness. The occurrence of CSF HVA tolerance may thus be an indicator of responsiveness to neuroleptics that may be predicted by the family history.

A reduction of DA as well as its metabolites DOPAC and HVA in CSF of poorly responding schizophrenics following withdrawal of long-term neuroleptic treatment has been reported.[13,14] The reductions correlated inversely with the plasma concentrations of the total neurolepticlike activity in plasma assessed with a radioreceptor assay. The authors conclude that even if an eventual reduction of DA turnover is observed following withdrawal of neuroleptics, more than a two-week washout period is required to reach pretreatment steady-state conditions. They also suggested that the lack of tolerance noted in these patients may play a role in the poor clinical response.

The same group[20] also demonstrated that the decrease in CSF DA and DOPAC following withdrawal of long-term neuroleptic medication was correlated with positive symptoms of postwithdrawal deterioration, and a low prewithdrawal CSF DOPAC level predicted severe relapse.

In an early report by Chase et al.[51] high levels of HVA in CSF after a year or more of neuroleptic treatment were associated with an absence of extrapyramidal side effects, whereas Bowers and Heninger[50] have suggested that tolerance, or decrease in

CSF HVA levels, is associated with fewer Parkinsonian side effects and greater clinical improvement.

Particularly many of the early clinical studies used quite short washout periods between the drug withdrawal and the lumbar puncture. In more recent studies a drug-free period of two weeks or more is commonly used. However, no study has been found using exclusively drug-naive patients. Central pharmacodynamic effects of antipsychotic agents can remain even at very low plasma concentrations of the compound,[52] and it is questioned whether a two- week washout period is sufficient for a return to baseline conditions of the central DA functions.

Central monoamine turnover is at least partly regulated by the availability of the precursor amino acids tyrosine, phenylalanine, or tryptophan. The brain levels of these amino acids are dependent on active transport mechanisms across the blood–brain barrier by the neutral L-amino acid transport system,[53] thereby competing with other amino acids for their access to the brain. Interestingly, Bjerkenstedt and co-workers[17] found negative correlations between the CSF concentrations of HVA and 5-HIAA and the plasma levels of those amino acids that are competing with tyrosine and tryptophan for transport across the blood–brain barrier.

Gattaz and co-workers[22] found no differences in CSF levels of DA or noradrenaline in schizophrenic patients without neuroleptic treatment when compared to healthy controls. Patients treated with neuroleptics, however, showed significantly higher concentrations of both amines in the CSF. Further, Kemali et al.[29] reported elevated CSF noradrenaline levels in drug-free schizophrenic patients compared to healthy subjects, whereas no difference was observed in the CSF DA concentrations.

Several groups have recently studied the relationship between CSF monoamine metabolite concentrations and computerized tomography (CT) measures of brain atrophy in schizophrenics.[26-28,34,35,39] All studies demonstrated an inverse relationship between brain atrophy (ventricle–brain ratio, third or lateral ventricle size, cortical atrophy) and measures of central monoamine function. The reduced CSF monoamine metabolite concentrations were considered not to be a simple dilution effect because of the increased CSF space, but rather to reflect reduced central monoaminergic functions. For instance, Losonczy et al.[34] found a significant negative correlation between CSF HVA levels following probenecid and the ventricle–brain ratios (VBR) in a group of drug-free chronic schizophrenic males. Houston et al.[26] found a strong negative correlation between CSF HVA concentrations and third ventricle widths or severity rating of schizophrenics using the Global Assessment Scale (in GAS a low score corresponds to severe illness). Jennings and co-workers[27] came to similar conclusions when they found negative correlations between CSF HVA and VBRs in psychotic teenagers. Reduced CSF concentrations of HVA and DOPAC as well as indexes of both intracellular and extracellular DA metabolism were also found by van Kammen et al.[28] in drug-free schizophrenic patients with cortical atrophy.

Bjerkenstedt et al.[17] and Lindström[30] have found lower CSF HVA concentrations in drug-free schizophrenic patients when compared to matched healthy controls. In the study by Lindström[30] low CSF HVA levels were associated with negative schizophrenic symptoms like lassitude, psychomotor retardation, and social withdrawal.

Rimon and co-workers[40] and Bartfai et al.[15] found elevated CSF HVA concentrations in paranoid psychotic patients.

## METHODOLOGICAL ASPECTS

A number of factors are known to influence CSF monoamine metabolite concentrations. Post and co-workers[54] have demonstrated that increased motor activity before

**TABLE 1.** Cerebrospinal Fluid Dopamine and Monoamine Metabolite Concentrations in Schizophrenia

| Authors | Patient Characteristics | Number of Patients | DA | DOPAC | HVA | 5-HIAA | MHPG | Comments |
|---|---|---|---|---|---|---|---|---|
| Bagdy & Perényi 1984[13] and Bagdy et al. 1985[14] | Chronic S-NL (RDC) | 15 | ↗ | ↗ | ↗ | | | NL-treatment ≥ 3 years with poor response. Reduced levels 2 weeks after NL withdrawal. The lack of tolerance may play a role in the poor clinical response. |
| Bartfai et al. 1984[15] | S-DF Paranoid psychosis-DF (RDC) | 13 / 5 | | | ↑↗ | ↑↗ | ↓↑ | Unmedicated recently admitted patients compared to sex- and age-matched controls. |
| Berger et al. 1980[16] | S-DF (Feighner) | 7 | | ↑ | ↑ | ↑ | ↑ | No differences in baseline concentrations before or after probenecid administration in normal subjects (n = 14) and patients with S. |
| Bjerkenstedt et al. 1985[17] | S-DF (RDC) | 37 | | | ↗ | ↑ | ↗ | Unmedicated patients compared to healthy volunteers (n = 65). In the patients a negative correlation between HVA and 5-HIAA vs. the plasma levels of those amino acids that compete with tyrosine and tryptophan for transport across the blood-brain barrier. |
| Bowers 1974[18] | S | 17 | | | ↗ | | | Accumulation of HVA following probenecid was substantially lower in patients with poor prognosis than in patients with good prognosis. |

| Study | Diagnosis | n | | | | | Comments |
|---|---|---|---|---|---|---|---|
| Bowers 1984[19] | S-NL (DSM-III) | 24 | | ↗ | | | In the 24 patients on NL, the 11 patients whose HVA showed no tolerance to NL had significantly more residual symptoms, more EPS and a family history of psychiatric hospitalization. |
| Frecska et al. 1985[20] | Chronic S-NL (RDC) | 14 | | ↗ | ↗ | ↗ | NL-treatment ≥ 5 years. Significant reductions 2 weeks after NL withdrawal. The decrease in DA and DOPAC correlated with positive symptoms of postwithdrawal deterioration. Low prewithdrawal DOPAC predicted severe relapse. |
| Gattaz et al. 1982[21] | Paranoid S (RDC) | 28 | ↑ | ↗ | ↑ | | Reduced 5-HIAA when compared to neurological controls ($n = 16$). 5-HIAA correlated positively with symptoms of grandiosity and hallucinatory behavior. |
| Gattaz et al. 1983[22] | S-NL<br>S-DF (RDC) | | ↖ ↑ | | | | Higher DA (and NA) in the NL-treated group. S-DF was equal to controls for DA (and NA). |
| Gerner et al. 1984[23] | Chronic S-DF (RDC) | 20 | | ↑ | ↖ | | Patients had been NL-free for at least 2 weeks (mean = 64 days). $p = 0.086$ for the 5-HIAA increase. |
| Gomes et al. 1980[24] | Acute S-(NL)<br>Chronic S-NL (WHO) | 10<br>11 | | ↑↑ | ↑↑ | | No difference vs. nonpsychiatric controls. The NL-treated chronic S patients had higher CSF noradrenaline levels. |

**TABLE 1.** (*Continued*) Cerebrospinal Fluid Dopamine and Monoamine Metabolite Concentrations in Schizophrenia

| Authors | Patient Characteristics | Number of Patients | DA | DOPAC | HVA | 5-HIAA | MHPG | Comments |
|---|---|---|---|---|---|---|---|---|
| Härnryd et al. 1984[25] | S-NL (RDC) | 25 + 25 | | | ↗ | ↑ | ↗ | Pretreatment levels identical to historical control values. HVA reached peak levels after 1 (cpz) or 2 (sulp) weeks of treatment and subsequently declined almost to the pretreatment values at 8 weeks. |
| Houston et al. 1986[26] | Chronic S (RDC) | 16 | | | ↗ | | | HVA correlated negatively with CT measures of brain third ventricle size (CT) and with the overall level of functioning (GAS). |
| Jennings et al. 1985[27] | Psychotics-DF Nonpsychotics-DF (Various DSM-III diagnoses) | 21 18 | | | ↑ | ↑ | | Psychotic and nonpsychotic adolescents had similar levels of HVA and 5-HIAA. The psychotic group displayed negative correlations between VBR (CT) and HVA and between VBR and 5-HIAA. |
| van Kammen et al. 1986[28] | S-DF (RDC + DSM-III) | 53 | | ↗ | ↗ | | | Patients had been DF for at least 2 weeks (mean = 32 days). HVA and DOPAC reduced in patients with cortical atrophy (CT). Substantially reduced indexes of DA turnover in S patients with cortical atrophy. |
| Kemali et al. 1982[29] | S-DF (ICD-9) | 8 | ↑ | | | | | DA (and adrenaline) was unchanged when compared to controls (n = 10), whereas noradrenaline was higher in CSF and plasma of S. |

| Reference | Diagnosis | n | | Comments |
|---|---|---|---|---|
| Lindström 1985[30] | S-DF (RDC) | 40 | ↑ ↗ | Significantly reduced HVA levels in S-DF compared to controls (n = 21). Low HVA levels were associated with negative symptoms like lassitude, psychomotor retardation, and social withdrawal. |
| Lindström et al. 1986[31] | S-DF (RDC) | 44 | ↗ | Increased levels of Fraction I opioid radioreceptor activity were associated with low HVA levels. |
| Linnoila et al. 1983[32] | S-DF (RDC) | 28 | Intraindividual variation | Considerable intraindividual variability of HVA, 5-HIAA, and MHPG in serial samples. |
| Losonczy et al. 1984[33] | S-DF (F or RDC) | 24 | Seasonal variation | Samples taken Oct.-Mar. had significantly higher levels of HVA and 5-HIAA, but not MHPG, than samples from Apr. to Sept. |
| Losonczy et al. 1986[36] | Chronic S-DF (F or RDC) | 28 | ↗ | Significant negative correlation between HVA and VBR (CT) following probenecid. |
| Nybäck et al. 1983[35] | S-DF (RDC) | 26 | ↑ ↑ ↗ | No difference compared to healthy volunteers (n = 43). A significant negative correlation was obtained between the size of the lateral ventricles and the levels of HVA and 5-HIAA in patients, but not in controls. |

**TABLE 1.** (*Continued*) Cerebrospinal Fluid Dopamine and Monoamine Metabolite Concentrations in Schizophrenia

| Authors | Patient Characteristics | Number of Patients | DA | DOPAC | HVA | 5-HIAA | MHPG | Comments |
|---|---|---|---|---|---|---|---|---|
| Persson & Roos 1969[36] | S-(NL) | 40 | | | ↑ | ↑ | | NL treatment stopped 4 days before lumbar puncture. No significant difference vs. healthy volunteers ($n = 34$). Patients with previously high NL doses had significantly higher HVA levels. |
| Post et al. 1975[37] | Acute S-DF (DSM-II) (F) | 20 | | | ↑ (↗) | ↑ | ↑ | Baseline levels were not significantly different from those in normal ($n = 10$) and neurological ($n = 19$) controls. After patients had recovered from their acute S illness, HVA accumulations following probenecid were significantly reduced, suggesting an underlying deficit in DA function in patients predisposed to S. |
| Post & Goodwin 1975[38] | S-NL Manic-NL | | | | ↑ transient | | | The probenecid-induced HVA accumulation increased during short-term (15–19 days), but normalized after extended (25–77 days) phenothiazine treatment. |

| Study | Diagnosis | n | Findings |
|---|---|---|---|
| Potkin et al. 1983[39] | Chronic-S (RDC) | 24 | No overall difference between S patients and control patients with neurological disorders. However, ventricular size (CT) correlated inversely with 5-HIAA, and the 5-HIAA concentrations were significantly reduced in patients with enlarged ventricles. |
| Rimon et al. 1971[40] | S-DF | 30 | No difference between S-DF and non-S control patients. Patients with paranoid symptoms had higher HVA levels. |
| Sedvall & Wode-Helgodt 1980[41] | S-DF (RDC) | 36 | Patients with a family history of S ($n = 11$) had higher HVA and 5-HIAA concentrations, whereas those S without a family history ($n = 25$) had similar concentrations as healthy controls ($n = 32$). |

ABBREVIATIONS: cpz = chlorpromazine; DF = drug-free; DSM-III;[65] F = Feighner criteria;[65] ICD-9 = International Classification of Diseases, 9 ed.; NL = neuroleptic; RDC = Research Diagnostic Criteria;[64] S = schizophrenia, schizophrenic; WHO = unspecified WHO criteria.

the lumbar puncture caused elevated metabolite levels in lumbar CSF. Further, inpatients have higher HVA and 5-HIAA concentrations in CSF than outpatients.[55] A rostrocaudal gradient, more pronounced for HVA and 5-HIAA than for MHPG, with higher concentrations in ventricular than in lumbar CSF, is well established.[56,57] However, these gradients are not affected by body position.[58] Also the site of lumbar puncture influences these levels.[59]

The CSF monoamine metabolite concentrations fluctuate considerably over time in schizophrenic patients.[32] Diurnal[60] and seasonal variations[33] of CSF and postmortem brain concentrations[61] of monoamine metabolites have also been demonstrated. The influences of age, sex, and height of the subjects must be considered[32,48,62,63] as additional sources for this variability.

The large number of possible factors that can influence the CSF monoamine metabolite concentrations emphasize the importance of a strict standardization of the lumbar puncture procedure. It is also of great importance that CSF from patients and controls are collected using the same standardized technique. The necessity of a careful selection of the patient sample must also be emphasized. Many studies, particularly many of the earlier ones, used heterogenous, poorly defined patient samples. However, the more recent studies generally use commonly accepted diagnostic criteria like research diagnostic criteria (RDC)[64] or DSM-III criteria[65] together with internationally accepted psychiatric rating scales, like the Brief Psychiatric Rating Scale (BPRS)[66] or items from the Comprehensive Psychopathological Rating Scale (CPRS).[67] A fruitful approach has been the introduction of the concept "positive" vs. "negative" symptoms of schizophrenia[68] or the "Type I" vs. "Type II" syndromes.[69] Those patients with negative symptoms or Type II syndrome also seem to have reduced CSF levels of HVA[30] or impaired DA function concomitantly with signs of brain atrophy (see the preceding).

The control groups often consist of unspecified neurological patients. At best, age- and sex-matched healthy control subjects have been used. Considering the large number of factors that can influence the CSF monoamine metabolite concentrations, the importance of a careful selection and matching of the contrast subjects must also be emphasized. Ideally, not only age and sex, but also height, dietary habits, drug treatment (other than neuroleptics, which should be excluded) and seasonal variation, should be taken into consideration in this matching procedure.

## FUTURE PERSPECTIVES

For a long time the concept "one neuron–one transmitter" was generally accepted. This is referred to as "Dale's principle," a popular version of which states that one neuron produces and releases only one transmitter (for a discussion of the principle, see reference 70).

During recent years a number of neuronal coexistences between classical neurotransmitters, like DA, noradrenaline, and serotonin, together with one or more neuropeptides have been demonstrated using sensitive immunohistofluorescence techinques.[71] Also, numerous recent reports have demonstrated biochemical and behavioral interactions between classical neurotransmitter functions and various neuropeptides within the central nervous system. For instance, endorphins, neurotensin, cholecystokinin, and somatostatin have been demonstrated to interact with several central dopaminergic functions.[72-75]

These novel findings will predictively have great impact on our future concepts of biochemical mechanisms in the etiology and pathogenesis of psychiatric disorders. The DA hypothesis of schizophrenia and the monoamine hypotheses of affective disorders presumably have to be expanded to also involve this novel knowledge. Instead of measuring only the CSF monoamine metabolite concentrations, determinations of some CSF neuropeptide concentrations must also be considered. In fact, several studies have demonstrated altered CSF neuropeptide concentrations in schizophrenia, for example, elevated endorphins,[76] as well as reduced delta sleep-inducing peptide,[77] neurotensin,[78] and somatostatin,[79] which are all peptides known to be involved in central DA functions.

## CONCLUSION

The hypothesis of schizophrenia postulates an overactivity of central DA-dependent functions. It is supported by a quantity of evidence that drugs that increase DA activity may induce or aggravate psychotic symptoms. A large number of scientific reports have tried to test the hypothesis by measuring concentrations of DA and its principal metabolites in CSF of patients with schizophrenia compared to healthy controls. The vast majority of the reports did not verify a DA hyperactivity in schizophrenia. However, some reports demonstrated positive correlations between DA hyperactivity and productive paranoid symptoms. More recent studies lend support for a decrease in DA function, particularly in association with negative symptoms and brain atrophy revealed by computerized tomography. Recent discoveries that DA coexists with neuropeptides (e.g., neurotensin, cholecystokinin, endorphins) in some DA-rich mesolimbic regions suggest that other transmitters than DA itself also may be involved in schizophrenia. It is therefore proposed that the DA hypothesis of schizophrenia should be expanded to also include one or more neuropeptides.

### REFERENCES

1. MATTHYSSE, S. 1974. Dopamine and the pharmacology of schizophrenia: The state of the evidence. J. Psychiatr. Res. **11:** 107–113.
2. SNYDER, S. H., S. P. BANERJEE, H. I. YAMAMURA & D. GREENBERG. 1974. Drugs, neurotransmitters, and schizophrenia. Science **184:** 1243–1253.
3. CARLSSON, A. 1978. Antipsychotic drugs, neurotransmitters, and schizophrenia. Am. J. Psychiatry **135:** 164–173.
4. HORNYKIEWICZ, O. 1978. Psychopharmacological implications of dopamine and dopamine antagonists: A critical evaluation of current evidence. Neuroscience **3:** 773–783.
5. HARACZ, J. L. 1982. The dopamine hypothesis: An overview of studies with schizophrenic patients. Schizophrenia Bull. **8:** 438–469.
6. LEE, T. & P. SEEMAN. 1980. Elevation of brain neuroleptic/dopamine receptors in schizophrenia. Am. J. Psychiatry **137:** 191–197.
7. MACKAY, A. V. P., L. L. IVERSEN, M. ROSSOR, E. SPOKES, E. BIRD, A. ARREGUI, I. CREESE & S. H. SNYDER. 1982. Increased brain dopamine receptors in schizophrenia. Arch. Gen. Psychiatry **39:** 991–997.
8. OWEN, F., A. J. CROSS, T. CROW, A. LONGDEN, M. POULTER & G. J. RILEY. 1978. Increased dopamine-receptor sensitivity in schizophrenia. Lancet **ii:** 223–226.
9. WONG, D. F., H. N. WAGNER, JR., L. E. TUNE, R. F. DANNALS, G. D. PEARLSON, J. M. LINKS, C. A. TAMMINGA, E. P. BROUSSOLLE, H. T. RAVERT, A. A. WILSON, J. K. T. TOUNG, J. MALAT, J. A. WILLIAMS, L. A. O'TUAMA, S. H. SNYDER, M. J. KUHAR & A. GJEDDE. 1986. Positron emission tomography reveals elevated $D_2$ dopamine receptors in drug-naive schizophrenics. Science **234:** 1558–1563.
10. ASHCROFT, G. W. & D. F. SHARMAN. 1960. 5-Hydroxyindoles in human cerebrospinal fluids. Nature **186:** 1050–1051.

11. Bowers, M. B. 1984. Sixteen years of CSF research. American College of Neuropsychopharmacology, Annual meeting, Dec. 1984: 13.

12. Sjöquist, B. & B. Johansson. 1978. A comparison between fluorometric and mass fragmentographic determinations of homovanillic acid and 5-hydroxyindoleacetic acid in human cerebrospinal fluid. J. Neurochem. 31: 621–625.

13. Bagdy, G. & A. Perènyi. 1984. Decrease of CSF dopamine, its metabolites, and noradrenalin after withdrawal of chronic neuroleptic treatment in schizophrenic patients. Psychiatry Res. 12: 177–178.

14. Bagdy, G., A. Perènyi, E. Frecska, K. Rèvai, Z. Papp, M. I. K. Fekete & M. Arató. 1985. Decrease in dopamine, its metabolites and noradrenaline in cerebrospinal fluid of schizophrenic patients after withdrawal of long-term neuroleptic treatment. Psychopharmacology 85: 62–64.

15. Bartfai, A., G. Edman, S. E. Levander, D. Schalling & G. Sedvall. 1984. Bilateral skin conductance activity, clinical symptoms and CSF monoamine metabolite levels in unmedicated schizophrenics, differing in rate of habituation. Biol. Psychol. 18: 201–218.

16. Berger, P. A., K. F. Faull, J. Kilkowski, P. J. Anderson, H. Kraemer, K. L. Davis & J. D. Barchas. 1980. CSF monoamine metabolites in depression and schizophrenia. Am. J. Psychiatry 137: 174–180.

17. Bjerkenstedt, L., G. Edman, L. Hagenfeldt, G. Sedvall & F.-A. Wiesel. 1985. Plasma amino acids in relation to cerebrospinal fluid monoamine metabolites in schizophrenic patients and healthy controls. Brit. J. Psychiatry 147: 276–282.

18. Bowers, M. B. 1974. Central dopamine turnover in schizophrenic syndromes. Arch. Gen. Psychiatry 31: 50–54.

19. Bowers, M. B. 1984. Family history and CSF homovanillic acid pattern during neuroleptic treatment. Am. J. Psychiatry 141: 296–298.

20. Frecska, E., A. Perènyi, G. Bagdy & K. Rèvai. 1985. CSF dopamine turnover and positive schizophrenic symptoms after withdrawal of long-term neuroleptic treatment. Psychiatry Res. 16: 221–226.

21. Gattaz, W. F., P. Waldmeier & H. Beckmann. 1982. CSF monoamine metabolites in schizophrenic patients. Acta Psychiatry Scand. 66: 350–360.

22. Gattaz, W. F., P. Riederer, G. P. Reynolds, D. Gattaz & H. Beckmann. 1983. Dopamine and noradrenalin in the cerebrospinal fluid of schizophrenic patients. Psychiatry Res. 8: 243–250.

23. Gerner, R. H., L. Fairbanks, G. M. Anderson, J. G. Young, M. Scheinin, M. Linnoila, T. A. Hare, B. A. Shaywitz & D. J. Cohen. 1984. CSF neurochemistry in depressed, manic, and schizophrenic patients compared with that of normal controls. Am. J. Psychiatry 141: 1533–1540.

24. Gomes, U. C. R., B. C. Shanley, L. Potgieter & J. T. Roux. 1980. Noradrenergic overactivity in chronic schizophrenia: Evidence based on cerebrospinal fluid noradrenaline and cyclic nucleotide concentrations. Brit. J. Psychiatry 137: 346–351.

25. Härnryd, C., L. Bjerkenstedt, B. Gullberg, G. Oxenstierna, G. Sedvall & F.-A. Wiesel. 1984. Time course for effects of sulpiride and chlorpromazine on monoamine metabolite and prolactin levels in cerebrospinal fluid from schizophrenic patients. Acta Psychiatry Scand., Suppl. 311: 75–91.

26. Houston, J. P., J. W. Maas, C. L. Bowden, S. A. Contreras, K. L. McIntyre & M. A. Javors. 1986. Cerebrospinal fluid HVA, central brain atrophy, and clinical state in schizophrenia. Psychiatry Res. 19: 207–214.

27. Jennings, W. S., Jr., S. C. Schulz, N. Narasimhachari, R. M. Hamer & R. O. Friedel. 1985. Brain ventricular size and CSF monoamine metabolites in an adolescent inpatient population. Psychiatry. Res. 16: 87–94.

28. Van Kammen, D. P., W. B. van Kammen, L. S. Mann, T. Seppala & M. Linnoila. 1986. Dopamine metabolism in the cerebrospinal fluid of drug-free schizophrenic patients with and without cortical atrophy. Arch. Gen. Psychiatry 43: 978–983.

29. Kemali, D., M. Del Vecchio & M. Maj. 1982. Increased noradrenaline levels in CSF and plasma of schizophrenic patients. Biol. Psychiatry 17: 711–717.

30. Lindström, L. H. 1985. Low HVA and normal 5HIAA CSF levels in drug-free schizophrenic patients compared to healthy volunteers: Correlations to symptomatology and family history. Psychiatry Res. 14: 265–273.

31. LINDSTRÖM, L. H., G. BESEV, L. M. GUNNE & L. TERENIUS. 1986. CSF levels of receptor-active endorphins in schizophrenic patients: Correlations with symptomatology and mono-amine metabolites. Psychiatry Res. **19:** 93–100.
32. LINNOILA, M., P. T. NINAN, M. SCHEININ, R. N. WATERS, W.-H. CHANG, J. BARTKO & D. P. VAN KAMMEN. 1983. Reliability of norepinephrine and major monoamine metabolite measurements in CSF of schizophrenic patients. Arch. Gen. Psychiatry **40:** 1290–1294.
33. LOSONCZY, M. F., R. C. MOHS & K. L. DAVIS. 1984. Seasonal variations of human lumbar CSF neurotransmitter metabolite concentrations. Psychiatry Res. **12:** 79–87.
34. LOSONCZY, M. F., I. S. SONG, R. C. MOHS, A. A. MATHÉ, M. DAVIDSON, B. M. DAVIS & K. L. DAVIS. 1986. Correlates of lateral ventricular size in chronic schizophrenia, II: Biological measures. Am. J. Psychiatry **143:** 1113–1118.
35. NYBÄCK, H., B.-M. BERGGREN, T. HINDMARSH, G. SEDVALL & F.-A. WIESEL. 1983. Cerebroventricular size and cerebrospinal fluid monoamine metabolites in schizophrenic patients and healthy volunteers. Psychiatry Res. **9:** 301–308.
36. PERSSON, T. & B.-E. ROOS. 1969. Acid metabolites from monoamines in cerebrospinal fluid of chronic schizophrenics. Brit. J. Psychiatry **115:** 95–98.
37. POST, R. M., E. FINK, W. T. CARPENTER, JR. & F. K. GOODWIN. 1975. Cerebrospinal fluid amine metabolites in acute schizophrenia. Arch. Gen. Psychiatry **32:** 1063–1069.
38. POST, R. M. & F. K. GOODWIN. 1975. Time-dependent effects of phenothiazines on dopa-mine turnover in psychiatric patients. Science **190:** 488–489.
39. POTKIN, S. G., D. R. WEINBERGER, M. LINNOILA & R. J. WYATT. 1983. Low CSF 5-hydroxyindoleacetic acid in schizophrenic patients with enlarged cerebral ventricles. Am. J. Psychiatry **140:** 21–25.
40. RIMÒN, R., B.-E. ROOS, V. RÄKKÖLÄINEN & Y. ALANEN. 1971. The content of 5-hydroxyindoleacetic acid and homovanillic acid in the cerebrospinal fluid of patients with acute schizophrenia. J. Psychosomat. Res. **15:** 375–378.
41. SEDVALL, G. C. & B. WODE-HELGODT. 1980. Aberrant monoamine metabolite levels in CSF and family history of schizophrenia. Arch. Gen. Psychiatry **37:** 1113–1116.
42. CARLSSON, A. & M. LINDQUIST. 1983. Effect of chlorpromazine or haloperidol on forma-tion of 3-methoxytyramine and normetanephrine in mouse brain. Acta Pharmacol. Tox-icol. **20:** 140–144.
43. ANDÉN, N. E., B.-E. ROOS & B. WERDINIUS. 1964. Effect of chlorpromazine, haloperidol, and reserpine on the levels of phenolic acids in rabbit corpus striatum. Life Sci. **3:** 149–158.
44. BOWERS, M. B. & A. ROZITIS. 1974. Regional differences in homovanillic acid concentra-tion after acute and chronic administration of antipsychotic drugs. J. Pharm. Pharmacol. **26:** 743–745.
45. SCATTON, B. 1977. Differential regional development of tolerance to increase in dopamine turnover upon repeated neuroleptic administration. Eur. J. Pharmacol. **46:** 363–369.
46. BACAPOULOS, N. G., D. E. REDMOND, J. BAULU & R. H. ROTH. 1980. Chronic haloperidol or fluphenazine: Effects on dopamine metabolism in brain, cerebrospinal fluid and plasma of cercopithecus aethiops (vervet monkey). J. Pharmacol. Exp. Ther. **212:** 1–5.
47. SEDVALL, G. 1980. Concentrations of monoamine metabolites and chlorpromazine in cerebrospinal fluid for prediction of therapeutic response in psychotic patients treated with neuroleptic drugs. Prog. Biochem. Pharmacol. **16:** 133–140.
48. WODE-HELGODT, B., B. FYRÖ, B. GULLBERG & G. SEDVALL. 1977. Effect of chlorproma-zine treatment on monoamine metabolite levels in CSF of psychotic patients. Acta Psy-chiatry Scand. **56:** 129–142.
49. GERLACH, J., K. THORSEN & R. FOG. 1975. Extrapyramidal reactions and amine metabo-lites in CSF during haloperidol and clozapine treatment of schizophrenic patients. Psy-chopharmacology **40:** 341–350.
50. BOWERS, M. B. & G. R. HENINGER. 1981. Cerebrospinal fluid homovanillic acid patterns during neuroleptic treatment. Psychiatry Res. **4:** 285–290.
51. CHASE, T. N., J. A. SCHNUR & E. K. GORDON. 1970. Cerebrospinal fluid monoamine catabo-lites in drug-induced extrapyramidal disorders. Neuropharmacology **9:** 265–268.
52. SEDVALL, G., L. FARDE, A. PERSSON & F.-A. WIESEL. 1986. Imaging of neurotransmitter receptors in the living human brain.
53. FERNSTROM, J. D. & R. J. WURTMAN. 1978. Neutral amino acids in the brain: Changes in response to food ingestion. J. Neurochem. **30:** 1531–1538.

54. POST, R. M., J. C. BALLINGER & F. K. GOODWIN. 1980. Cerebrospinal fluid studies of neu-
    rotransmitter function in manic and depressive illness. *In* Neurobiology of Cerebrospinal
    Fluid. J. H. Wood, Ed.: 685–717. Plenum Press. New York.
55. GUTHRIE, S. K., W. BERETTINI, D. R. RUBINOW, J. I. NURNBERGER, J. J. BARTKO & M.
    LINNOILA. 1986. Different neurotransmitter metabolite concentrations in CSF samples
    from inpatient and outpatient normal volunteers. Acta Psychiatry Scand. **73:** 315–321.
56. SIEVER, L., H. KRAEMER, R. SACK, P. ANGWIN, P. BERGER, V. ZARCONE, J. BARCHAS
    & H. K. BRODIE. 1975. Gradients of biogenic amine metabolites in cerebrospinal fluid.
    Dis. Nerv. Syst. **36:** 13–16.
57. ZIEGLER, M. G., J. H. WOOD, C. R. LAKE & I. J. KOPIN. 1977. Norepinephrine and 3-
    methoxy-4-hydroxyphenyl glycol gradients in human cerebrospinal fluid. Am. J. Psy-
    chiatry **134:** 565–568.
58. GATELESS, D., M. STANLEY, L. TRÄSKMAN-BENDZ & J. GILROY. 1984. The influence of the
    lying and sitting positions on the gradients of 5-HIAA and HVA in lumbar cerebrospinal
    fluid. Biol. Psychiatry **19:** 1585–1589.
59. NORDIN, C., B. SIWERS & L. BERTILSSON. 1982. Site of lumbar puncture influences levels
    of monoamine metabolites. Arch. Gen. Psychiatry **39:** 1445.
60. NICOLETTI, F., R. RAFFAELE, A. FALSAPERLA & R. PACI. 1981. Circadian variation in 5-
    hydroxyindoleacetic acid levels in human cerebrospinal fluid. Eur. Neurol. **20:** 9–12.
61. CARLSSON, A., L. SVENNERHOLM & B. WINBLAD. 1980. Seasonal and circadian monoamine
    variations in human brains examined post mortem. Acta Psychiatry Scand., **Suppl.**
    **280:** 75–85.
62. GOTTFRIES, C. G., I. GOTTFRIES, B. JOHANSSON, R. OLSSON, T. PERSSON, B.-E. ROOS &
    R. SJÖSTRÖM. 1971. Acid monoamine metabolites in human cerebrospinal fluid and their
    relations to age and sex. Neuropharmacology **10:** 665–672.
63. WODE-HELGODT, B. & G. SEDVALL. 1978. Correlations between height of subject and con-
    centrations of monoamine metabolites in cerebrospinal fluid from psychotic men and
    women. Commun. Psychopharmacol. **2:** 177–183.
64. SPITZER, R. L., J. ENDICOTT & E. ROBINS. 1977. Research diagnostic criteria (RDC) for
    a selected group of functional disorders, 3rd. ed. New York State Psychiatric Institute,
    Biometrics Research. New York.
65. AMERICAN PSYCHIATRIC ASSOCIATION. 1980. DSM-III: Diagnostic and Statistical Manual
    of Mental Disorders, 3rd ed. American Psychiatric Association. Washington, D.C.
66. OVERALL, J. E. & D. R. GORHAM. 1962. The brief psychiatric rating scale. Psychol. Rep.
    **10:** 799–812.
67. ÅSBERG, M., S. MONTGOMERY, C. PERRIS, D. SCHALLING & G. SEDVALL. 1978. CPRS—
    The comprehensive psychopathological rating scale. Acta Psychiatry Scand., **Suppl. 271.**
68. ANDREASEN, N. C. 1981. Scale for the Assessment of Negative Symptoms (SANS). Univ.
    of Iowa. Iowa City.
69. CROW, T. J. 1982. Two syndromes in schizophrenia? Trends Neurosci. **5:** 351–354.
70. POTTER, D. D., E. J. FURSHPLAN & S. G. LANDIS. 1981. Multiple transmitter status and
    "Dale's principle." Neurosci. Comment. **1:** 1–9.
71. HÖKFELT, T., O. JOHANSSON & M. GOLDSTEIN. 1984. Chemical anatomy of the brain. Science
    **225:** 1326–1334.
72. WIDERLÖV, E., C. D. KILTS, R. B. MAILMAN, C. B. NEMEROFF, T. J. MCCOWN, A. J. PRANGE,
    JR. & G. R. BREESE. 1982. Increase in dopaminergic metabolites in rat brain by neu-
    rotensin. J. Pharmacol. Exp. Ther. **222:** 1–6.
73. KALIVAS, P. V., E. WIDERLÖV, D. STANLEY, G. R. BREESE & A. J. PRANGE, JR. 1983. En-
    kephalin action on the mesolimbic system: A dopamine-dependent and a dopamine-
    independent increase in locomotor activity. J. Pharmacol. Exp. Ther. **227:** 229–237.
74. MEYER, D. K. & J. KRAUSS. 1983. Dopamine modulates cholecystokinin release in neostri-
    atum. Nature **301:** 338–340.
75. NEMEROFF, C. B., D. LUTTINGER, D. E. HERNANDEZ, R. B. MAILMAN, G. A. MASON, S. D.
    DAVIS, E. WIDERLÖV, G. D. FRYE, C. D. KILTS, K. BEAUMONT, G. R. BREESE & A. J.
    PRANGE, JR. 1983. Interactions of neurotensin with brain dopamine systems: Biochem-
    ical and behavioural studies. J. Pharmacol. Exp. Ther. **225:** 337–345.
76. LINDSTRÖM, L. H., E. WIDERLÖV, L. M. GUNNE, A. WAHLSTRÖM & L. TERENIUS. 1978.

Endorphins in human cerebrospinal fluid: Clinical correlations to some psychotic states. Acta Psychiatry Scand. **57:** 153–164.

77. LINDSTRÖM, L. H., R. EKMAN, H. WALLÉUS & E. WIDERLÖV. 1985. Delta sleep-inducing peptide in cerebrospinal fluid from schizophrenics, depressives and healthy volunteers. Prog. Neuropsychopharmacol. Biol. Psychiatry **9:** 83–90.

78. WIDERLÖV, E., L. H. LINDSTRÖM, G. BESEV, P. J. MANBERG, C. B. NEMEROFF, G. R. BREESE, J. S. KIZER & A. J. PRANGE, JR. 1982. Subnormal cerebrospinal fluid levels of neurotensin in a subgroup of schizophrenics: Normalization after neuroleptic treatment. Am. J. Psychiatry **139:** 1122–1126.

79. BISSETTE, G., E. WIDERLÖV, H. WALLÉUS, I. KARLSSON, K. EKLUND, A. FORSMAN & C. B. NEMEROFF. 1986. Alterations in cerebrospinal fluid concentrations of somatostatin-like immunoreactivity in neuropsychiatric disorders. Arch. Gen. Psychiatry **43:** 1148–1151.

80. FEIGHNER, J. P., E. ROBINS, S. B. GUZE, R. A. WOODRUFF, G. WINOKUR & R. MUNOZ. 1972. Diagnostic criteria for use in psychiatric research. Arch. Gen. Psychiatry **26:** 57–63.

# Dopamine Receptor Sensitivity Changes with Chronic Stimulants

TONG H. LEE, EVERETT H. ELLINWOOD, JR.,
AND J. KEN NISHITA

*Department of Psychiatry*
*Duke University Medical Center*
*Durham, North Carolina 27710*

## CHRONIC STIMULANT INTOXICATION SYNDROME: BEHAVIORALLY SIGNIFICANT MECHANISMS

In our early paradigms of the chronic stimulant intoxication syndrome, we considered a model consisting of at least two major stages.[1,2] The earlier stage was characterized by increasing suspiciousness and repetitive behavior in humans and constricted and intense stereotypy in animals. The later stage was characterized in humans by development of a psychotic–paranoid panic behavior or a hyperreactive, fearlike state with or without hallucinations and delusions. In animals this stage is marked by a tolerance to dopamine (DA), stereotyped behaviors, and a marked increase in bizarre behaviors (e.g., hyperreactivity to both real and nonexistent stimuli). We have attempted to distinguish the dosing regimens and underlying mechanisms that initiate the chronic-stimulant syndrome from those that maintain it.[3]

We now hypothesize that dosing chronicity is not the only factor contributing to the different initiating mechanisms involved with the two stages of the stimulant intoxication syndrome.[4] We have been interested in different dosing schedules as they relate to the residual sensitivity to stimulant-induced psychopathology and also how the altered state is implicated in the high rate of recidivism at certain stages of stimulant withdrawal. Within a week of amphetamine (AMPH) treatment the end-stage syndrome can be produced in laboratory animals, but these short-term paradigms have not produced the intense residual syndromes that evolve over a 2–3 month period, especially when moderate dosages are used for an extended priming period. The priming period could be clinically important, as it may function to establish the noncontingently reinforced behavior that gradually evolves into the chronic syndrome (including psychosis). However, we have seen a number of high-dose (continuous 1 gram or greater/day) AMPH users who maintained an escalated dose over a period of years but did not develop a chronic syndrome. This suggests that only the *lower dose priming* period may be an important factor in the development of the behavioral sensitization and/or conditioning that occurs so often in animal studies.[5] In contrast to the priming period, the continuous dosing schedule (which often follows the priming period in human abuse conditions) is associated with neurotoxic effects and the more bizarre behaviors and symptoms of the later stage of the chronic syndrome. One of the principal functions of our animal paradigms is to delineate the various mechanisms that are associated with the priming stage from those of the later stage of the chronic-stimulant process.

## STEREOTYPY AUGMENTATION STAGE:
## UNDERLYING MECHANISMS

Several mechanisms have been proposed to explain the augmentation of stereotypy by subsequent stimulant doses and/or by direct DA agonists such as apomorphine (APO).[6,7] The most parsimonious explanation of augmentation is postsynaptic alteration in the number or affinity of DA receptors. Unfortunately, the studies involving low-, moderate-, or high-dose chronic AMPH intoxication have not found consistent or sufficient receptor alterations to explain the behavioral data[8-11] This lack of evidence for postsynaptic receptor alteration, even following sensitization to APO doses sufficient to affect behavior, would argue for a downstream chronic change at the second messenger level or for a downstream interaction with outflow neurotransmitters (e.g., gamma-aminobutyric acid, acetylcholine, or serotonin). Presynaptic mechanisms have been demonstrated to affect behavior significantly following acute, moderately high doses of AMPH. [12,13] Antelman and Chiodo[14] reported a presynaptic subsensitivity following moderate doses of either intermittent or chronic AMPH intoxication. Most investigators have noted presynaptic DA subsensitivity on substantia nigra or ventral tegmental area (VTA) neuronal firing rates in only the early period following chronic stimulant dosing.[15,16] We have found that reserpine given concurrently with chronic AMPH does not block the ongoing AMPH response, but does block the development of AMPH-induced supersensitivity.[17] This finding is consistent with a presynaptic alteration.

There are reports demonstrating that animals become conditioned to the stimuli associated with the stimulant injection process when the doses are repeatedly administered.[5,18] Schiff[19] has demonstrated that the homovanillic acid response in the mesolimbic system also becomes conditioned to the injection process stimuli. Aversive stimuli that are paired with AMPH-induced stereotypy can totally block these AMPH-induced behaviors.[20] This AMPH-conditioned response appears to be partially a consequence of accidental conditioning specific to prepotent species-typical behaviors.[21,22] Devenport *et al.*[23] also have noted that lesions of the hippocampus facilitate the development of conditioned stereotypy. These data suggest that the augmentation process involves complex mechanisms that must be studied in intact animals rather than *in vitro*.

## MECHANISMS RELATED TO STEREOTYPY, TOLERANCE, AND
## EMERGENCE OF THE DYSKINETIC HYPERREACTIVE
## SYNDROME FOLLOWING SUSTAINED DOSING

Although long-term, high-dose stimulant dosing produces the most striking stereotypy tolerance/dyskinetic syndrome, paradigms using 1–2 weeks of sustained administration of high doses have provided equally important information on the nature of the mechanisms involved in the syndrome. Depletion of DA and its metabolites has repeatedly been observed.[24,27] A notable depletion of serotonin and tryptophan hydroxylase also has been reported, but this effect may be more specific for methylamphetamine than for dextroamphetamine.[28] Norepinephrine (NE) has been demonstrated to be depleted[24] and/or spared,[29,30] and extensive loss of DA reuptake sites also has been found.[31,32] None of the studies describing monoamine depletion in the striatum has established consistent findings for the nucleus accumbens, but any decrease in the mesoaccumbens is much less than that in the caudate.[33] These data suggest the possibility that on a functional basis there is a shift in the balance of activity from the nigrostriatal system to the mesolimbic system.

Steranka[34] demonstrated that amfonelic acid, a DA-reuptake blocker, can block the AMPH DA-depleting effects when given along with AMPH. This effect continued for as long as 8 hr after initiation of dosing. The effect of amfonelic acid suggests that a period of sustained AMPH is necessary, although it can be as short as one day. Another presynaptic mechanism operating at the level of the substantia nigra is the change from subsensitivity to supersensitivity of presynaptic somadendritic autoreceptors that govern the firing rate of the substantia nigra compacta (SNC) DA neurons. Seven days after withdrawal from chronic doses of AMPH, these SNC DA cells, but not VTA DA cells, are supersensitive to inhibition by very low doses of APO.[15,34]

## RECENT FINDINGS FROM OUR LABORATORY

We have recently completed a series of studies that systematically assessed somadendritic and terminal autoreceptors following chronic sustained administration of AMPH at 5 mg/day for seven days (15 mg/day using an Alzet minipump). We found that, other than moderate decreases in DA concentration, there was no indication of decreased DA transmission in the nigrostriatal or mesolimbic DA pathways under basal conditions. For example, there was no change in the level of impulse flow (i.e., number of impulses per minute) in the VTA or SNC cells either immediately after minipump removal or 7 days after. Furthermore, the DOPA/DA ratio, a general indicator of DA turnover rate, showed a time-dependent recovery increase over the 7 days following minipump removal.

Evidence of autoreceptor alterations were found when the system was perturbed with APO at low doses that activate presynaptic but not postsynaptic receptors. Immediately following minipump removal APO-induced inhibition of the terminal DA synthesis rate was decreased in both the striatum and olfactory tubercle. Decreased sensitivity of the somadendritic autoreceptor was also observed, as manifested in a shift to the right in the dose-response curve for APO inhibition in SNC firing rate. This decreased potency or subsensitivity of APO perturbation on all measures immediately following minipump removal was followed 7 days later by another set of changes. In the nigrostriatal system, impulse flow and terminal DA synthesis were supersensitive to inhibition by APO administration, yet no change in APO sensitivity was noted in terminal autoreceptors (as tested by L-DOPA accumulation with impulse flow blocked by gammabutyrolactone). More complex changes were observed in the olfactory tubercle at the 7-day withdrawal period; opposite changes in the potency of APO on DA synthesis were observed in the olfactory tubercle depending on whether or not impulse flow was blocked by gammabutyrolactone. Thus, in the olfactory tubercle subsensitivity was observed with gammabutyrolactone and supersensitivity without it (see FIG. 1). Furthermore, DA cells in the VTA also showed no significant overall change in sensitivity to inhibition of firing by APO. These results suggest that there are substantial sensitivity changes in the dynamic interrelationship of autoreceptors across the phases of AMPH withdrawal. This change over time in the balance of the DA system has important implications for clinical treatment, since the different withdrawal stages are sensitive to moderate pharmacological perturbations. Understanding the dynamic nature of these interrelationships may lead to an effective means of pharmacologically treating this withdrawal state and in preventing recidivism.

In summary, immediately postwithdrawal all indicators of autoreceptor activity appeared to be markedly subsensitive, while the system as a whole had returned to basal equilibrium showing little or no overall metabolic changes. The final effect of these changes may result from the balance of overall autoreceptor subsensitivity and

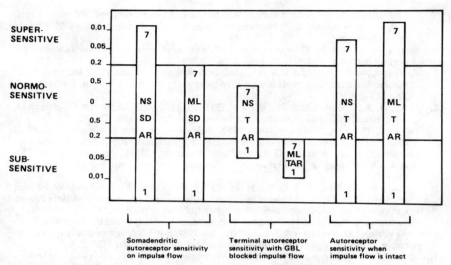

**FIGURE 1.** Schematic description of change in autoreceptor sensitivity from day-to-day post-AMPH withdrawal. NS = nigrostriatal; ML = mesolimbic; SD = somadendritic; T = terminal; AR = autoreceptor; 1 = Day; 7 = Day 7.

the decrease in the synthetic enzymes involved in DA synthesis. At 7 days postwithdrawal (a period frequently associated with increased agitation, irritability, and the emergence of "stimulant urges" in human stimulant abusers) the nigrostriatal system is noted to have supersensitivity of somadendritic autoreceptors and normosensitive terminal autoreceptors. At the same time, in the mesolimbic system the somadendritic autoreceptors are relatively normosensitive, yet the terminal autoreceptors remain subsensitive. An interesting item of conjecture is whether or not neurobiological manifestations occurring a week after withdrawal reflect the individual's sensitivity to conditioned drug cues that are possibly mediated by the mesolimbic-reinforcing system. The occurrence of subsensitivity of all autoreceptors in the immediate withdrawal phase deserves further exploration as one of the mechanisms involved with the period of "crash" hypersomnolence.

## REFERENCES

1.  ELLINWOOD, E. H., JR., A. SUDILOVSKY & L. NELSON. 1973. Evolving behavior in the clinical and experimental amphetamine psychosis. Am. J. Psychiatry **130:** 1088–1093.
2.  ELLINWOOD, E. H., JR. & A. SUDILOVSKY. 1973. Chronic amphetamine intoxication: Behavioral models of psychoses. *In* Psychopathology and Psychopharmacology. J. Cole *et al.*, Eds. Johns Hopkins Univ. Press. Baltimore, Md.
3.  ELLINWOOD, E. H., JR. & M. M. KILBEY. 1977. Chronic stimulant intoxication model of psychosis. *In* Animal Models in Psychiatry and Neurology. J. Hanin and E. Usdin, Eds. Pergamon Press. New York.
4.  DOUGHERTY, G. G., JR. & E. H. ELLINWOOD, JR. 1981. Amphetamine behavioral toxicity: Rotational behavior after chronic intrastriatal infusion. Biol. Psychiatry **16:** 479–488.
5.  POST, R. M. 1981. Central stimulants: Clinical and experimental evidence on tolerance and

sensitization. *In* Research Advances in Alcohol and Drug Problems, Vol. 6. Y. Israel, F. B. Glaser, H. Kalant, R. E. Popham, W. Schmidt, and R. G. Smart, Eds.: 1–65. Plenum Press. New York.

6. KILBEY, M. M. & E. H. ELLINWOOD, JR. 1977. Reverse tolerance to stimulant-induced abnormal behavior. Life Sci. **20:** 1063–1076.

7. KANENO S., A. WATANABE & R. TAKAHASHI. 1986. Alteration of striatal dopaminergic function implicated in methamphetamine-induced reverse tolerance in rat. Eur. J. Pharmacol. **123:** 287–294.

8. BURT, D. R., I. CREESE & S. H. SNYDER. 1977. Anti-schizophrenic drugs: Chronic treatment elevates dopamine receptor binding in brain. Science **196:** 326–328.

9. CONWAY, P. G. & N. J. URETSKY. 1982. Role of striatal dopaminergic receptors in amphetamine-induced behavioral facilitation. J. Pharmacol. Exp. Ther. **221:** 650–655.

10. NIELSEN, E. B., M. NIELSEN, G. ELLISON & C. BRAESTRUP. 1981. Decreased spiroperidol and LSD binding in rat brain after continuous amphetamine. Eur. J. Pharmacol. **66:** 149–154.

11. NIELSEN, E., M. NIELSEN & C. BRAESTRUP. 1983. Reduction of $^3$H-spiroperidol binding in rat striatum and frontal cortex by chronic amphetamine: Dose response, time course, and role of sustained dopamine release. Psychopharmacology **81:** 81–85.

12. HJORTH, S., A. CARLSSON, H. WILKSTROM, P. LINDBERG, D. SANCHEZ, U. HACKSELL, L. E. ARVIDSSON, U. SVENSSON & J. L. G. NILSSON. 1981. 3-PPP: A new centrally acting DA-receptor agonist with selectivity for autoreceptors. Life Sci. **28:** 1225–1238.

13. MUELLER, P. & P. SEEMAN. 1979. Presynaptic subsensitivity as a possible basis for sensitization by long-term dopamine mimetics. Eur. J. Pharmacol. **55:** 149–157.

14. ANTELMAN, S. M. & L. A. CHIODO. 1981. Dopamine autoreceptor subsensitivity: A mechanism common to the treatment of depression and the induction of amphetamine? Biol. Psychiatry **16:** 717–727.

15. ELLINWOOD, E. H., JR. & T. H. LEE. 1983. Effect of continuous systemic infusion of d-amphetamine on the sensitivity of nigral dopamine cells to apomorphine inhibition of firing rate. Brain Res. **273:** 379–383.

16. KAMATA, K. & G. V. REBEC. 1984. Long-term amphetamine treatment attenuates or reverses the depression of neuronal activity produced by dopamine agonists in the ventral tegmental area. Life Sci. **34:** 2419–2427.

17. DOUGHERTY, G. G. & E. H. ELLINWOOD, JR. 1984. The effect of reserpine on concurrent repeated administration of d-amphetamine. Psychopharmacology **82:** 327–329.

18. ELLINWOOD, E. H., JR. & M. M. KILBEY. 1980. Fundamental mechanisms underlying altered behavior following chronic administration of psychomotor stimulants. Biol. Psychiatry **15:** 749–757.

19. SCHIFF, S. R. 1982. Conditioned dopaminergic activity. Biol. Psychiatry **17:** 135–154.

20. BORBERG, S. 1974. Conditioning of amphetamine-induced behavior in the albino rat. Psychopharmacologia **34:** 191–198.

21. ELLINWOOD, E. H., JR. 1971. Accidental conditioning -lav 1 with chronic methamphetamine intoxication: Implications for theory of drug habituation. Psychopharmacologia **21:** 131–138.

22. ELLINWOOD, E. H., JR. & M. M. KILBEY. 1975. Amphetamine stereotypy: The influence of environmental factors and prepotent behavioral patterns on its topography and development. Biol. Psychiatry **10:** 3–16.

23. DEVENPORT, L. D., J. A. DEVENPORT & F. HOLLOWAY. 1981. Reward-induced stereotypy: Modulation by the hippocampus. Science **212:** 1288–1289.

24. SEIDEN, L. S., W. M. FISCHMAN & C. R. SCHUSTER. 1977. Changes in brain catecholamine induced by long-term methamphetamine administration in rhesus monkeys. *In* Cocaine and Other Stimulants. E. H. Ellinwood, Jr., and M. M. Kilbey, Eds. Plenum Press. New York.

25. GIBB, J. W. & M. E. MORGAN. 1978. Effects of methamphetamine on tyrosine hydroxylase activity in selected dopaminergic areas of the brain. Presented at the 11th Congress Collegium Internationale Neuropsychopharmacogicum. Vienna, Austria.

26. HOTCHKISS, A. J., M. E. MORGAN & J. W. GIBB. 1979. The long-term effects of multiple doses of methamphetamine on neostriatal tryptophan hydroxylase, tyrosine hydroxylase, choline acetyltransferase and glutamate decarboxylase activities. Life Sci. **25:** 1373–1378.

27. TRULSON, M. E. & B. L. JACOBS. 1979. Long-term amphetamine treatment decreases brain serotonin metabolism: Implication for theories of schizophrenia. Science **205**: 1295–1297.
28. HOTCHKISS, A. J. & J. W. GIBB. 1980. Long-term effects of multiple doses of methamphetamine on tryptophan hydroxylase and tyrosine hydroxylase activity in rat brain. J. Pharm. Exp. Ther. **214**: 257–262.
29. ELLISON, G., M. S. EISON, H. HUBERMAN & F. DANIEL. 1978. Long-term changes in dopaminergic innervation of caudate nucleus after continuous amphetamine administration. Science **201**: 276–278.
30. ELLISON, G., E. B. NIELSEN & M. LYON. 1981. Animal model of psychosis: Hallucinatory behaviors in monkeys during the late stage of continuous amphetamine intoxication. J. Psychiatr. Res. **16**: 13–22.
31. WAGNER, G. C., G. A. RICAURTE, L. S. SEIDEN, C. R. SCHUSTER, R. J. MILLER & H. WESTLEY. 1980. Long-lasting depletions of striatal dopamine and loss of dopamine uptake sites following repeated administration of methamphetamine. Brain Res. **181**: 151–160.
32. RICAURTE, G. A., C. R. SCHUSTER & L. S. SEIDEN. 1980. Long-term effects of repeated methylphenidate administration on dopamine and serotonin neurons in the rat brain: A regional study. Brain Res. **193**: 153–163.
33. LEE, T. H. & E. H. ELLINWOOD, JR. Sensitivity of terminal autoreceptors after a 7-day withdrawal. Submitted for publication.
34. STERANKA, L. R. 1982. Long-term decreases in striatal dopamine 3,4-dihydroxyphenylacetic acid and homovanillic acid after a single injection of amphetamine in iprindole-treated rats: Time-course and time-dependent interactions with amfonelic acid. Brain Res. **234**: 123–136.

# Mesocortical Dopaminergic Function and Human Cognition

DANIEL R. WEINBERGER,[a] KAREN FAITH BERMAN,[a]
AND THOMAS N. CHASE[b]

[a] *Clinical Brain Disorders Branch*
*Intramural Research Program*
*National Institute of Mental Health*
*William A. White Building*
*Saint Elizabeths Hospital*
*Washington, DC 20032*

[b] *Experimental Therapeutics Branch*
*National Institute of Neurological and*
*Communicative Disorders and Stroke*
*Bethesda, Maryland 20892*

## INTRODUCTION

The role of dopamine in human cortical function has been a subject of much speculation but surprisingly little research. There are a number of obvious difficulties in studying mesocortical dopaminergic activity in man. First and foremost, the system has not been accessible to direct, selective manipulation. As a result, most efforts to study it have resorted to one of three approaches: to measure metabolites of dopamine in the cortex at postmortem examination and to correlate the results with premortem clinical records,[1] to correlate peripheral measures [e.g., CSF homovanillic acid (HVA)] of dopamine metabolism during life with concurrent clinical ratings,[2] or to examine changes in cognitive function that follow treatment with dopamimetic agents.[3] While these approaches have yielded interesting data, they are indirect and may be prone to errors.

Another problem is that assumptions about mesocortical dopaminergic function that are based on experimentation in laboratory animals may not be applicable to humans. The dramatic development of the prefrontal cortex, in particular its dorsolateral aspect, is a hallmark of the human brain that makes comparisons to even the great apes limited.[4] The meaning of this evolutionary trend in terms of the importance of dopamine for cortical function is unknown. Mesocortical prefrontal dopaminergic projections, a principal component of the mesocortical dopamine system, could represent an important element in prefrontal evolution. On the other hand, mesocortical dopamine evolution might not have kept pace and may represent nothing more than a vestigial neurochemical system.

In this report, we describe our efforts to study human *prefrontal* dopaminergic function during life. Our research orientation derives from the work of Brozowski *et al.*[5] These investigators provided compelling data that dopaminergic activity in the prefrontal cortex of the rhesus monkey is involved in the expression of prefrontally mediated behavior, that is, cognition. They reported that chemical lesioning of the dorsolateral prefrontal cortex (DLPFC) (sulcus principalis) with 6-hydroxydopa-mine(6-OHDA) impaired behavior on delayed-response behavioral tasks that have become "acid tests" of DLPFC function in the monkey. In fact, their data suggest that dopamine depletion has almost as severe an impact on DLPFC function as does surgical ablation.

We have been pursuing the possibility of a human analogy of the experiment of Brozowski *et al.* There are several elements to this effort. First, we need to measure a behavior that can be considered a reflection of human DLPFC function. Then we need a technique for monitoring directly what is going on physiologically at the level of the DLPFC. Finally, we need a way of affecting dopaminergic activity. The behavior employed is the Wisconsin Card Sort Test; the technique for physiological monitoring is the Xenon inhalation regional cerebral blood flow (rCBF) method; and the means for bringing dopamine into the experiment is by studying patients with idiopathic Parkinson's disease. Patients with this illness have been found to have reductions in prefrontal dopaminergic metabolism of from 20% to 60% of normal.[1] In the discussion that follows each of these elements is described and an unexpected parallel is suggested between mesocortical dopaminergic function in Parkinson's disease and schizophrenia.

## A PREFRONTALLY MEDIATED BEHAVIOR: THE WISCONSIN CARD SORT TEST

Although it is an oversimplification to assume that any cognitive task involves only a finely demarcated cortical region, studies of patients with focal brain lesions suggest that performance on the Wisconsin Card Sort (WCS) is especially sensitive to the functional integrity of prefrontal cortex (PFC).[6] Moreover, even within the frontal lobe, poor performance on the WCS has localizing significance in that it correlates better with lesions of the dorsolateral PFC than with lesions in other prefrontal areas.[6] For these reasons, the WCS is widely regarded as the *sine qua non* of dorsolateral prefrontal cortical function in man. We have shown in a large sample of normal individuals that performance on the WCS is associated with an increase in cortical metabolism that is greatest in DLPFC.[7] The WCS is a relatively simple abstract reasoning, problem-solving test that involves achieving abstract sets, maintaining these sets, and then changing them depending on feedback that comes from the examiner. An automated version of the standard WCS was developed for our purposes. It is described in greater detail elsewhere.[7]

## AN *in Vivo* REGIONAL PHYSIOLOGICAL ASSAY: XENON rCBF

The method used for measuring prefrontal cortical activity during prefrontally mediated behavior is the noninvasive xenon inhalation regional cerebral blood flow (rCBF) technique developed by Obrist *et al.*[8] and modified by Deshmukh and Meyer.[9] The theoretical aspects and mathematics of this method have been described in detail.[8,9] Since, in the absence of a major disruption in cerebral autoregulation, blood flow to the cortex is determined primarily by neuronal metabolism, rCBF is an indirect but sensitive measure of cortical physiology.[10] Our rCBF system uses 32 extracranial radiation probes, monitoring 16 homologous regions for each hemisphere. To facilitate the administration of a cognitive task, subjects were studied while in a seated

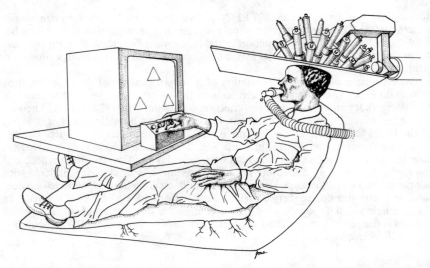

**FIGURE 1.** Drawing of subject undergoing a Xenon-133 inhalation rCBF procedure while taking an automated version of the test.

position. A schematic view of a subject undergoing an rCBF procedure while taking the WCS is shown in FIGURE 1.

In the studies to be described, each subject underwent three rCBF procedures. The first was during an eyes-closed resting state used primarily to acclimatize subjects to the testing environment and experience. The data for this condition will not be reported here. The second and third rCBF procedures were conducted during the performance of mental activation tasks that were presented in counterbalanced sequence to control for the possibility of an order effect. One task was the WCS. The other task was a simple automated number-matching (NM) procedure performed on the identical apparatus as in the WCS. The NM task served as an active baseline state against which rCBF during the WCS could be compared. In keeping with this latter purpose, the NM was conceived as an individualized control for aspects of the WCS rCBF experience other than DLPFC specific cognitive function, including eye scanning and visual stimulation and the emotional and psychological experience of taking a test during which rCBF is measured. In theory, these factors remained relatively constant from one task to another. We have previously found that by examining differences in rCBF between the NM and the WCS, those aspects of the WCS rCBF that are specific to the WCS, and probably to the DLPFC, may be better isolated.[7]

## PREFRONTAL rCBF AND COGNITIVE FUNCTION IN PARKINSON'S DISEASE

Although it has been reported that the concentration of dopamine metabolites is reduced in postmortem specimens of prefrontal cortex (as well as cingulate and temporal cortices) of patients with Parkinson's disease (PD),[1] the impact of this reduction on prefrontal function is unknown. However, the results of the experiment of

Brozowski et al.[5] suggest that reduced prefrontal cortical dopaminergic activity causes diminished prefrontal cognitive function, and many studies of cognitive function in Parkinson's disease have found that deficits in prefrontally linked problem-solving skills are common.[11,12] One of the tests that has often been cited as being difficult for PD patients is the Wisconsin Card Sort. This difficulty may be due to decreased dopamine afferentation of the prefrontal cortex, though other explanations have been proposed.[12]

We have studied prefrontal physiology and cognitive function simultaneously in a group of PD patients using the rCBF paradigm previously described. Ten patients (age range 54–76), most of whom had relatively mild disability [Hoehn and Yahr (reference 13) stages: I = 3 patients, II = 3 patients, III = 2 patients, IV = 1 patient] underwent the rCBF protocol. All patients were on standard doses of combination L-DOPA/carbidopa. Only two patients were considered on clinical examination to have evidence of cognitive impairment, and in both impairment was mild (cases with stages III and IV). Ten age- and sex-matched normal volunteer subjects served as controls.

Overall, mean brain metabolism was slightly lower ($.05 < p < .10$) in the patients, consistent with previous reports.[14,15] However, the pattern or distribution of rCBF did not differ significantly from the controls. The most interesting finding to emerge from this study is shown in FIGURE 2. The degree to which prefrontal activity increased during the WCS as compared with the NM baseline predicted fairly closely patients' performance on the WCS. This suggests that prefrontal physiological activity is a critical determinant of performance on this test in these patients. As is seen in FIGURE 2, a similar relationship between prefrontal physiology and cognitive function was not found in controls. In fact, we have never observed this relationship in normal control groups in any of our studies of prefrontal physiology during the WCS.

The finding that this relationship exists in PD patients, even in those who are not clinically demented, is not easily interpreted. In FIGURE 3, we hypothesize a sigmoidal relationship between prefrontal physiological activity and prefrontal cognitive function. Parkinson's disease patients are on the steep part of this curve where a small change in prefrontal physiology predicts a linearly related change in prefrontal cognitive function. In the controls, this tight coupling of physiology and function is not seen; perhaps because there is sufficient physiological redundancy. It is as if the controls are on the upper plateau section of the curve.

The possibility that dopaminergic activity is related to prefrontal function in these patients is suggested by several clinical correlations. The degree of DLPFC activation during the WCS over that during the NM task correlated with clinical ratings of those Parkinsonian symptoms most consistently linked to response to L-DOPA therapy, including overall disability score (Spearman rho = $-.80$, $p = .01$), stage of illness (rho = $-.86$, $p < .01$), rigidity (rho = $-.66$, $p = .05$), and bradykinesia (rho = $-.65$, $p < .06$), but not with tremor, illness duration, or age.

In summary, the same variable that correlated with prefrontally mediated cognition, that is, prefrontal physiological activation, correlated with clinical motor symptoms that are the result of diminished dopaminergic function. These results suggest that diminished dopaminergic function at the prefrontal cortical level could explain the loss of normal prefrontal physiological redundancy. Unfortunately, this is not the only possible interpretation of these data. In particular, it might be argued that altered prefrontal physiology is a secondary effect of diminished dopaminergic function in the striatum, especially in the caudate nucleus. Dopaminergic innervation of the striatum is reduced up to 90% in Parkinson's disease,[16] a much greater relative reduction than is found in the prefrontal cortex. Since a major projection of prefrontal cortex is to the caudate, loss of striatal dopaminergic function may have secondary repercussions for prefrontal behavior.

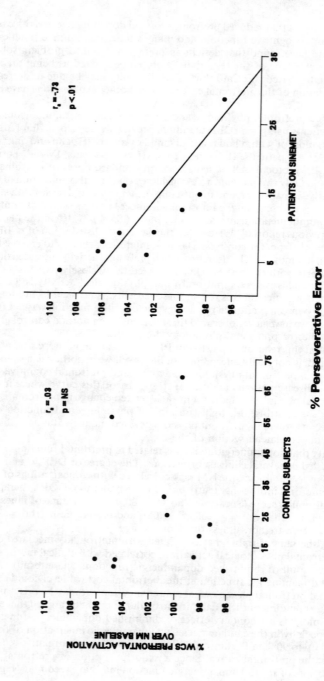

**FIGURE 2.** Relationship between prefrontal rCBF activation during the WCS and perseverative errors on the WCS in patients with Parkinson's disease and normal controls.

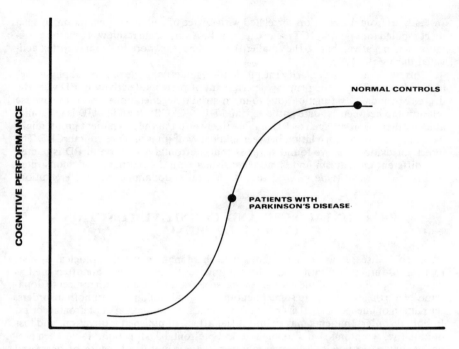

**FIGURE 3.** Hypothetical relationship between prefrontal physiological activation and prefrontal cognitive function.

We have been unable thus far to determine whether our findings in PD patients are the direct result of prefrontal dopaminergic deafferentation or are secondary to loss of nigro-striatal activity. However, data from a study of patients with Huntington's disease (HD) may shed some light on this question.

## PREFRONTAL rCBF AND COGNITIVE FUNCTION IN HUNTINGTON'S DISEASE

Recent studies have shown that in early Huntington's disease neuropathological changes are confined almost exclusively to the head of the caudate.[17] The fact that the cognitive deficits characteristically found in this illness are of the prefrontal type[18] suggests that caudate degeneration can have secondary (i.e., "upstream") effects on prefrontal function. Thus, based on the HD model, it might be predicted that if nigro-striatal degeneration is responsible for the prefrontal physiological–behavioral relationship seen in PD, then a similar relationship will be found in HD.

We studied 14 patients with mild to moderate HD with the same WCS rCBF protocol used to study PD.[19] The results were very different from those found in the PD patients. Prefrontal physiological activation did not correlate with performance on the WCS ($p > .6$). It also did not correlate with clinical ratings of disability ($p > .6$).

Instead, prefrontal activation correlated with degree of caudate degeneration, as seen on computed tomography (CT) scan (see FIG. 4). A surprising result was that the correlation was negative, that is, the smaller the caudate, the more prefrontal cortex activated during the WCS.

This observation may clarify the mechanism underlying the prefrontal physiological findings in PD. If the primary determinant of prefrontal activity in PD were the degree of caudate dysfunction (due to nigro-striatal degeneration), and if the inverse relationship between caudate pathology and DLPFC rCBF found in HD is generalizable to other disorders such as PD, a more likely result in the PD patient group might have been an inverse correlation between clinical symptoms and prefrontal rCBF. The direct correlation that we found suggests that prefrontal activation in PD is related to a different mechanism and is more consistent with the mechanism demonstrated by Brozowski *et al.* (*vide supra*),[5] that is, prefrontal dopaminergic deafferentation.

## PREFRONTAL rCBF AND COGNITIVE FUNCTION IN SCHIZOPHRENIA

Parkinson's disease has not been thought to share many neurophysiological or neurochemical similarities with schizophrenia. Indeed, these disorders are often cited as being on opposite ends of the neurochemical spectrum, especially with respect to dopamine. Nevertheless, there are some phenomenological similarities. In both disorders, the pattern of intellectual deficits most often implicates dysfunction of prefrontal cortex. In both disorders, patients may manifest flat affect, diminished motivation, and loss of initiative, symptoms that also might reflect prefrontal dysfunction.[4] It has been proposed that patients with PD may manifest these symptoms because of decreased

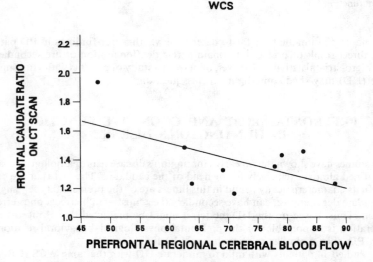

**FIGURE 4.** Relationship between prefrontal rCBF during the WCS and caudate atrophy on CT scan in patients with Huntington's disease ($r = .63, p < .05$). Lower frontal caudate ratio means *more* atrophy.

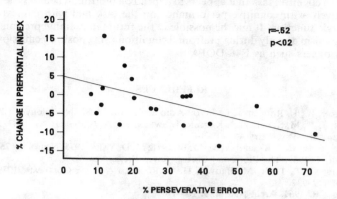

**FIGURE 5.** Relationship between relative prefrontal rCBF activation during WCS and perseverative errors on the WCS in patients with schizophrenia.

dopaminergic activity in the prefrontal cortex.[1] The possibility that the same mechanism may explain similar symptoms in schizophrenia is suggested by the results of rCBF studies in this disorder.

In a study of 20 medication-free patients with schizophrenia and 25 similarly aged normal control subjects,[7] the relationship between prefrontal rCBF during the WCS and performance on the WCS was similar to that previously described in the study of PD (see FIGURE 5), though the patients with schizophrenia did not manifest a normal rCBF pattern (they were hypometabolic prefrontally). In terms of the sigmoidal relationship proposed in FIGURE 3 (theoretically adjusted for age), this group might lie even lower on the linear segment than do the PD patients. We have examined the relationship between prefrontal cortical activation and prefrontal cortical cognitive function in a variety of neurological and psychiatric disorders. Only in PD and in schizophrenia have we found a direct relationship between physiology and cognitive function. If the pathophysiological mechanism for this relationship in PD is dopaminergic deafferentation, a similar mechanism may also explain the findings in schizophrenia.

In addition to the rCBF data, there is other circumstantial evidence suggesting that prefrontal dopaminergic activity may be reduced in schizophrenia. This includes reduced concentrations of dopamine metabolites in cerebrospinal fluid (see reference 20 for a discussion), improvement in so-called defect or negative symptoms after treatment with dopamimetic drugs, and reversal of reduced prefrontal rCBF following dopamimetic administration.[21] In fact, in a recent theoretical discussion about the pathogenesis of this disorder, it was proposed that reduced prefrontal dopaminergic activity is a critical element in the development of the illness.[20]

## SUMMARY

In summary, we have reviewed rCBF data in humans that suggest that mesoprefrontal dopaminergic activity is involved in human cognition. In patients with Parkinson's disease and possibly in patients with schizophrenia, prefrontal physiological activation during a cognitive task that appears to depend on prefrontal neural systems correlates positively with cognitive performance on the task and with clinical signs of dopaminergic function. It may be possible in the future to examine prefrontal dopamine metabolism directly during prefrontal cognition using positron emission tomography and tracers such as F-18 DOPA.

## REFERENCES

1. SCATTON, B., L. ROUQUIER, F. JAVOY-AGID & Y. AGID. 1982. Neurology 32: 1039–1040.
2. MANN, J. J., M. STANLEY, R. KAPLAN, J. SWEENEY & A. NEOPHYTIDES. 1983. J. Neurol. Neurosurg. Psychiatry 46: 905–910.
3. BOWEN, F. P., R. S. KAMIENNY, M. M. BURNS & M. D. YAHR. 1975. Neurology 25: 701–704.
4. FUSTER, J. 1980. The Prefrontal Cortex. Raven Press. New York.
5. BROZOWSKI, T. J., R. M. BROWN, H. E. ROSVOLD & P. S. GOLDMAN. 1979. Science 205: 929–932.
6. MILNER, B. 1963. Arch. Neurol. 9: 100–110.
7. WEINBERGER, D. R., K. F. BERMAN & R. F. ZEC. 1986. Arch Gen. Psychiatry 43: 114–124.
8. OBRIST, W. D., H. K. THOMPSON, H. S. WANG & W. E. WILKINSON. 1975. Stroke 6: 245–256.
9. DESHMUKH, V. D. & J. S. MEYER. 1978. Noninvasive Measurement of Cerebral Blood Flow. Prentice-Hall. Englewood Cliffs, N.J.
10. SKOLOFF, L. 1981. Fed. Proc., Fed. Am. Soc. Exp. Biol. 40: 2311–2316.
11. LEES, A. J. & E. SMITH. 1983. Brain 106: 257–270.
12. TAYLOR, A. E., A. SAINT-CYR & A. E. LANG. 1986. Brain 109: 845–883.
13. HOEHN, M. M. & M. D. YAHR. 1967. Neurology 17: 427–442.
14. BES, A., A. GUELL, N. FABRE, PH. DUPUE, G. VICTOR & G. GERAUD. 1983. J. Cereb. Blood Flow Metab. 3: 33–37.
15. WOLFSON, L. I., K. L. LEENDERS, L. L. BROWN & T. JONES. 1985. Neurology 35: 1399–1405.
16. HORNYKIEWICZ, O. 1982. Brain neurotransmitter changes in Parkinson's disease. In Movement Disorders. C. D. Marsden and S. Fahn, Eds.: 41–58. Butterworths. London.
17. VON SATTEL, J. P., R. H. MYERS, T. J. STEVENS, R. J. FERRANTE, E. D. BIRD & P. RICHARDSON, JR. 1985. J. Neuropath. Exp. Neurol. 44: 559–577.
18. JOSIASSEN, R. C., L. M. CURRY & E. L. MANCALL. 1983. Arch. Neurol. 40: 791–796.
19. WEINBERGER, D. R., K. F. BERMAN, M. IADAROLA, N. DRIESEN & R. F. ZEC. 1988. J. Neurol. Neurosurg. Psychiatry. 51: 94–104.
20. WEINBERGER, D. R. 1987. Arch. Gen. Psychiatry 44: 660–669.
21. GERAUD, G., M. C. ARNE-BES, A. GUELL & A. BES. 1987. J. Cereb. Blood Flow Metab. 7: 9–12.

# Plasma Homovanillic Acid as an Index of Central Dopaminergic Activity: Studies in Schizophrenic Patients

DAVID PICKAR, ALAN BREIER, AND JOHN KELSOE

*Section on Clinical Studies*
*Clinical Neuroscience Branch*
*National Institutes of Mental Health*
*Bethesda, Maryland 20892*

## INTRODUCTION

The dopamine hypothesis of schizophrenia, which proposes that enhanced CNS dopaminergic activity is causally related to schizophrenia, has been the most enduring etiologic hypothesis for this, the most severe of the mental illnesses. Even today, over a quarter of a century since the foundations of the hypothesis were first established, any new etiologic proposal must take into account the compelling evidence linking CNS dopamine function to the pathophysiology of schizophrenia. Advances in our understanding of CNS dopamine systems, however, have helped to refine the implications of initial observations and have altered our view of the mechanism of neuroleptic action. In this paper recent data using dopamine metabolite measurement strategies in schizophrenic patients are reviewed with emphasis on implications for neuroleptic mechanism of action. Specific relevance to mesocortical and mesolimbic dopamine system activities is discussed.

## NEUROLEPTICS AND CNS DOPAMINE SYSTEMS

The strongest evidence linking CNS dopamine systems to schizophrenia is the fact that all known antipsychotic drugs bind to non-adenyl cyclase dependent $D_2$ receptors and at least for a time reduce postsynaptic dopamine neurotransmission.[1] Further, the greater affinity for the receptor, the greater the "potency" of the drug.[2,3] Thus, chlorpromazine, whose effective antipsychotic dose range is approximately 400–1500 mg/day, has less affinity for $D_2$ receptors than does fluphenazine, whose typical antipsychotic doses are in the 15–40-mg/day range. These data, which link biochemical and clinical properties of neuroleptics drugs, provide the best support for the proposal that neuroleptic drugs produce antipsychotic effects by blockade of the postsynaptic receptor. The fact that the antipsychotic effects of neuroleptics develop over weeks or even months, whereas dopamine blockade and its clinical manifestation (e.g., extrapyramidal effects and increases in circulating levels of prolactin) occur within hours of drug administration, represents an important limitation to the receptor blockade model of neuroleptic drug action [3]

Over the past decade, preclinical studies have provided important new information impacting on our understanding of neuroleptic drug mechanisms and of the pathophysiology of schizophrenia. First, it is now known that the dopamine neurons that innervate the prefrontal cortex have electrophysiologic and pharmacologic properties that distinguish them from the subcortical nigro-striatal and mesolimbic dopamine systems.[5] As suggested by the studies of Pycock and co-workers,[6] in which lesion-diminished mesocortical dopamine neurons are associated with enhanced subcortical dopamine system activity, the mesocortical dopamine system likely modulates subcortical dopamine function. If the mesolimbic system mediates psychosis, as suggested by Stevens,[7] then mesocortical neurons may play a permissive role in its expression or even modify its clinical manifestations.

A second recent body of information regarding CNS dopamine systems that impacts on schizophrenia indicates electrophysiological[8,9] and biochemical[10] differences in dopamine neuronal response between short- and long-term neuroleptic administration. In nigro-striatal (Ag) and mesolimbic dopamine systems, neuroleptics first produce rapid increases in neuronal firing and in dopamine "turnover" (as reflected by the accumulation of dopamine metabolites); prolonged drug administration, however, is associated in these systems with markedly decreased patterns of neuronal firing and with reversal of initial increased turnover. It is thought that the reduction in electrical activity associated with prolonged neuroleptic administration is a result of "depolarization block."[8] Reversal of initial increases in dopamine turnover are thought to be the result of adaptive neuronal responses mediated through autoreceptor function.[11]

There are two particularly intriguing pharmacologic characteristics of mesocortical neurons: (1) in contrast to both nigro-striatal and mesolimbic systems, mesocortical neurons tend to show only a modest initial increase in activity in response to acute neuroleptic administration, and (2) neuroleptic-induced time-dependent changes are absent.[5] Although the underlying mechanism for these differences is unknown, it is thought that mesocortical neuronal lack of autoreceptors results in diminished adaptive response. In addition to these pharmacologic differences, mesocortical neurons are, among CNS dopamine systems, uniquely responsive to stress in animal models.[12,13]

## PLASMA HOMOVANILLIC ACID (HVA)
## AND NEUROLEPTIC RESPONSE

The measurement of dopamine metabolites in body fluids has been one of the most widely used strategies for studying underlying function of catecholamine systems in neuropsychiatric disorders. This approach is based on the understanding that metabolite production reflects neurotransmitter release and metabolism. We have measured plasma levels of the dopamine metabolite, homovanillic acid (HVA), in schizophrenic patients prior to and during controlled neuroleptic administration in order to study changes in dopaminergic system function that may accompany neuroleptic treatment.[14,15]

Under controlled double-blind conditions, fluphenazine administration (mean ± SEM mg/day: 30 ± 5) to young (mean ± SD years: 28 ± 2.8), chronically ill schizophrenic patients following and extended prior drug-free interval (mean ± SD drug-free days: 34 ± 6) produced time-dependent decreases in mean weekly levels (3 samples per week) of plasma HVA; as shown in FIGURE 1, significant decreases occurred after 3 weeks of continual fluphenazine administration.[15] A close association was seen between the course of change of nurses' ratings of psychosis and the fall in HVA when plasma HVA levels from all data points and corresponding ratings were compared (FIG. 2).[15] Consistent with these group data, individual patients showed good

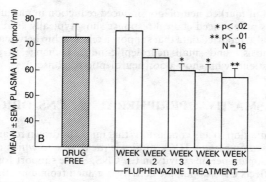

**FIGURE 1.** Neuroleptic-induced time-dependent decrease in mean weekly levels of plasma HVA in schizophrenic patients ($n = 16$).[15]

correlations between neuroleptic-induced reduction in plasma levels of HVA and neuroleptic-induced reduction in psychosis.[15] These data suggest that slow to develop reductions in presynaptic dopamine activity, as reflected by decrements in levels of plasma HVA, may more closely relate to the antipsychotic effects of neuroleptic drugs than does receptor blockade itself.

Our plasma HVA findings are compatible with those of the studies of Bowers *et al.*,[16] in which psychotic patients with more rapid antipsychotic response are found

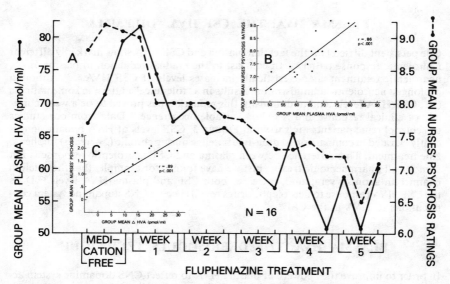

**FIGURE 2.** Levels of plasma HVA and corresponding nurses' psychosis ratings and their correlation during neuroleptic treatment ($n = 16$).[15]

to have a pattern of marked neuroleptic-induced reduction in plasma HVA, whereas patients with less pronounced clinical response show typically "flat" HVA response. Davis *et al.* have also reported data that support a relationship between levels of plasma HVA and psychosis[17] and small neuroleptic-induced change in plasma HVA in schizophrenic patients who show poor neuroleptic responses.[18]

## PLASMA HVA: PERIPHERAL vs. CNS ORIGINS

An important limitation to any conclusions that might be drawn regarding CNS dopamine activity based on plasma HVA studies is the degree to which circulating levels of HVA reflect dopaminergic activity in the CNS. Some support for the notion that plasma HVA reflects CNS dopamine activity is gained from animal studies in which pharmacologic probes that increase CNS dopamine turnover also increase plasma levels of HVA.[19,20] It has been estimated that between 40% and 60% of circulating levels of HVA are derived from brain in animal experiments;[21] similar values have been estimated to apply to humans.[22] The major nonbrain sources of levels of plasma HVA include the peripheral sympathetic nervous system, the adrenal medulla, and carotid body.[23] It is currently unproved that there are distinct dopaminergic neurons in the peripheral nervous system; peripherally derived dopamine metabolites are thus likely to be related to peripheral noradrenergic neuronal metabolic activity.[24]

Despite the fact that a significant portion of plasma HVA is peripherally derived, plasma HVA has proved a useful correlate of neuroleptic response and of psychotic symptoms. Moreover, the time-dependent nature of neuroleptic effects share similarity with some CNS dopamine systems. Nevertheless, important questions about the significance of the plasma HVA measure itself remain.

## PLASMA HVA: THE CSF HVA "DILEMMA"

One persistent difficulty is the fact that plasma and CSF HVA show markedly different neuroleptic response patterns. In contrast to the gradual reduction in plasma HVA, neuroleptic treatment characteristically increases levels of CSF HVA.[25,26] Although prolonged neuroleptic administration results in a "tolerance" pattern in some patients (i.e., CSF HVA levels tend to diminish), this reduction has proved to be a weak correlate of clinical response and is only a variable occurrence.[26] Data from our studies of schizophrenic patients are shown in FIGURE 3. CSF levels of HVA remain significantly elevated in comparison to drug-free baseline during chronic (>4 weeks) fluphenazine treatment. This difference between plasma and CSF neuroleptic response is not seen for all pharmacologic treatments; we have found, for example, that the calcium channel antagonist, verapamil, increases both CSF and plasma HVA levels.[27] Does the CSF HVA response to neuroleptic drugs reveal specific CNS dopamine system contributions to HVA in the CSF?

## PLASMA HVA: THE DEBRISOQUIN TECHNIQUE

In order to improve the "power" of plasma HVA to reflect CNS dopamine system activity, we and others[21,28] have administered the peripherally acting monoamine oxidase (MAO) inhibitor, debrisoquin. This strategy is based on the fact that HVA produc-

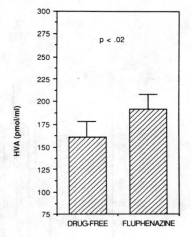

**FIGURE 3.** Neuroleptic-induced increase in CSF levels of HVA in schizophrenic patients (*n* = 20).

tion is dependent upon MAO activity; since debrisoquin does not enter the CNS,[29] it reduces only peripheral HVA production. The CNS "signal," therefore, is enhanced and the peripheral "signal" is reduced. FIGURE 4 shows CSF and plasma data from three schizophrenic patients in whom debrisoquin (40 mg/day) was administered when free from neuroleptic and through 4 weeks of neuroleptic treatment. Lumbar punctures were performed under three treatment conditions: neuroleptic-free prior to debrisoquin, neuroleptic-free during debrisoquin treatment, and during both fluphenazine and debrisoquin treatment. As seen in FIGURE 4, debrisoquin produced a substantial reduction in plasma levels of HVA without reducing CSF HVA, changes consistent with peripheral HVA reduction. Neuroleptic treatment was associated with a characteristic increase in CSF HVA; plasma levels of HVA showed the typical neuroleptic-induced decrease during neuroleptic treatment. Thus, even with enhancement of the CNS "signal," the fundamental difference between plasma and CSF response to neuroleptic treatment remains.

## CSF HVA: A REFLECTION OF MESOCORTICAL DOPAMINE ACTIVITY?

The traditional view that CSF HVA levels reflect nigro-striatal activity is based on the significant decrements in CSF HVA found in Parkinson's disease patients, the proximity of the striatum to cerebral ventricles, and the abundant amount of dopamine contained within striatal structures. Several lines of indirect evidence, however, suggest the possibility that mesocortical dopamine system activity may play a greater role in determining levels of CSF HVA than previously had been appreciated.

One of the principal differences between mesocortical and subcortical dopamine neurons is their inherent pattern of neuronal activity; basal firing rates are markedly high for mesocortical neurons.[5] Since the frontal cortex is of greater relative size in nonhuman and human primates in comparison to rodents, and since HVA itself is a reflection of neuronal activity, mesocortically derived HVA may under some conditions (e.g., when subcortical activity is relatively diminished) contribute significantly

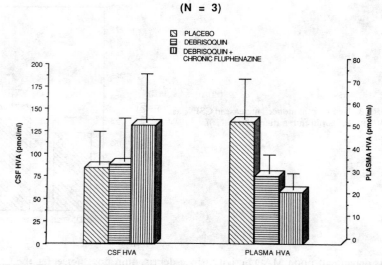

**FIGURE 4.** The effect of debrisoquin on neuroleptic-induced CSF and plasma HVA change in schizophrenic patients ($n = 3$).

to levels of HVA detected in CSF. Moreover, the lack of neuroleptic-induced time-dependent change in mesocortical neuronal function shares similarity with CSF HVA neuroleptic response patterns. Consistent with this notion are the reported associations between diminished levels of CSF HVA and evidence of cortical brain atrophy.[30-33] In particular, Doran et al.[34] have found that in schizophrenic patients lower levels of CSF HVA are associated with evidence of frontal cortical atrophy as seen by CT scan. Recent evidence from postmortem studies have also supported the hypothesis that CSF HVA reflects mesocortical activity. Elsworth et al.[35] have found in nonhuman primates that CSF HVA was significantly correlated with HVA in the dorsal prefrontal cortex but not with HVA in other cortical or subcortical regions. Similarly, Stanley et al.[36] have observed in human postmortem studies that CSF HVA is correlated with HVA in the frontal cortex.

Thus, data from preclinical, clinical, and postmortem studies provide some support for the hypothesis that CSF levels of HVA reflect mesocortical dopamine system activity. It should be appreciated, however, that the relative contributions of the different CNS dopamine systems to levels of CSF HVA, and for that matter to plasma HVA, may not be static. Illness, pharmacologic treatment, or other conditions (e.g., stress) may enhance or diminish one or the other system's contribution to levels of CSF HVA.

# SUMMARY

Despite the limitations of the dopamine hypothesis, compelling evidence remains that implicates dysfunction of CNS dopamine systems in the pathophysiology of schizophrenia. The longitudinal measurement of levels of plasma HVA has proved a useful tool in studying neuroleptic effects and has highlighted time-dependent effects as a potentially important facet of the mechanism of antipsychotic action of these drugs. Despite the good clinical correlates of plasma HVA levels, caution is needed in interpreting plasma levels of HVA with regard to CNS dopamine activity. The peripheral nervous system significantly contributes to levels of HVA that circulate in plasma. This issue is underscored by the fact that CSF HVA shows different neuroleptic response patterns than that seen in plasma. The administration of a peripherally acting MAO inhibitor to enhance the CNS "signal" in circulating levels of HVA does not resolve the "problem" of different CSF-plasma HVA neuroleptic response patterns. The possibility that mesocortical dopamine activity is reflected by CSF HVA is suggested by indirect evidence from clinical and preclinical studies. Future studies in which attempts are made at using both plasma and CSF HVA to enhance neurochemical and clinical correlates may help to advance our understanding of the contributions of specific CNS dopamine systems to schizophrenia.

## REFERENCES

1. CARLSSON, A. 1978. Am. J. Psychiatry **135:** 164–173.
2. CREESE, I., D. R. BURT & S. H. SNYDER. 1976. Science **192:** 481–483.
3. SEEMAN, P., T. LEE, M. CHAU-WONG & K. WONG. 1976. Nature **261:** 717–719.
4. PICKAR, D. 1986. Psychiatr. Clin. North Am. **9:** 35–48.
5. BANNON, M.J. & R. H. ROTH. 1983. Pharmacol. Rev. **35:** 53–68.
6. PYCOCK, C. J., R. W. KERWIN & C. J. CARTER. 1980. Nature **286:** 74–77.
7. STEVENS, J. R. 1973. Arch. Gen. Psychiatry **29:** 177–189.
8. BUNNEY, B. S. & A. A. GRACE. 1978. Life Sci. **23:** 1715–1728.
9. WHITE, J. F. & R. Y. WANG. 1983. Science **221:** 1054–1056.
10. ROTH, R. H. 1983. Neuroleptics: Functional chemistry. *In* Neuroleptics: Neurochemical, Behavioral and Clinical Perspectives. J. T. Coyle and S. J. Enna, Eds. Raven Press. New York.
11. ROTH, R. H. 1978. Commun. Psychopharmacol. **3:** 429–445.
12. THIERRY, A. M., J. P. TASSIN, G. BLANC & J. GLOWINSKI. 1976. Nature **263:** 242–244.
13. TAM, S.Y. & R. H. ROTH. 1985. Biochem. Pharmacol. **34:** 1595–1598.
14. PICKAR, D., R. LABARCA, M. LINNOILA, A. ROY, D. HOMMER, D. EVERETT & S. M. PAUL. 1984. Science **225:** 954–957.
15. PICKAR, D., R. LABARCA, A. R. DORAN, O. M. WOLKOWITZ, A. ROY, A. BREIER, M. LINNOILA & S. M. PAUL. 1986. Arch. Gen. Psychiatry **43:** 669–676.
16. BOWERS, M. B., M. SWIGAR, P. I. JATLOW & N. GOICOECHA. 1984. J. Clin. Psychiatry **6:** 248–251.
17. DAVIS, K. L., M. DAVIDSON, R. C. MOHS, K. S. KENDLER, V. M. DAVIS, C. A. JOHNS, Y. DENEGRIS & T. G. HORVATH. 1985. Science **227:** 1601–1602.
18. DAVIS, K. L. & M. DAVIDSON. 1987. Personal communication.
19. BACOPOULOS, N. G., S. E. HATTOX & R. H. ROTH. 1979. Eur. J. Pharmacol. **56:** 225–236.
20. KENDLER, K. S., G. R. HENINGER & R. H. ROTH. 1982. Life Sci. **30:** 2063–2069.
21. STERNBERG, D. E., G. R. HENINGER & R. H. ROTH. 1983. Life Sci. **32:** 2447–2452.
22. SWAN, A. C., *et al.* 1979. Life Sci. **27:** 1857–1862.
23. VAN LOON, G. R. 1983. Fed. Proc., Fed. Am. Soc. Exp. Biol. **42:** 3012–3018.
24. KOPIN, I. R. 1987. Personal communication.
25. SEDVALL, G., B. FYRO, H. NYBACK, F. H. WIESSEL & B. WODE-HELGODT. 1974. Psychiatry Res. **11:** 75–80.
26. BOWERS, M. B. & G. R. HENINGER. 1981. Psychiatry Res. **4:** 285–290.
27. PICKAR, D., O. M. WOLKOWITZ, A. R. DORAN, R. LABARCA, A. ROY, A. BREIER & P. K. NARANG. 1987. Arch. Gen. Psychiatry. **44:** 113–118.
28. DAVIDSON, M., A. B. GIORDANI, R. C. MOHS, T. B. HORVATH, B. M. DAVIS, P. POWCHIK & K. L. DAVIS. 1987. Arch. Gen. Psychiatry **44:** 189–190.
29. MEDINA, M. A., A. GIACHETTI & P. A. SHORE. 1969. Biochem. Pharmacol. **18:** 892–902.
30. NYBACK, H., F. A. WEIGEL, B. M. BERGGREN & T. HINDMARSH. 1982. Acta Psychiatry Scand. **65:** 403–414.

31. VAN KAMMEN, D. P., L. S. MANN, D. E. STERNBERG, M. SCHEININ, P. T. NINAN, S. R. MARDER, W. VAN KAMMEN, R. O. REIDER & M. LINNOILA. 1983. Science **220**: 974–977.
32. HOUSTON, J. P., J. W. MAAS, B. L. BOWDEN, S. A. CONTRERAS, K. L. MCINTYRE & M. A. A. JAVORS. 1986. Psychiatry Res. **19**: 207–214.
33. LASONCZY, M. F., S. I. SONG, R. C. MOHS, A. A. MATHE, M. DAVIDSON, B. M. DAVIS & K. L. DAVIS. 1986. Am. J. Psychiatry **143**: 1113–1118.
34. DORAN, A. R., J. BORONOW, D. R. WEINBERGER, O. M. WOLKOWITZ, A. BREIER & D. PICKAR. 1987. Neuropsychopharmacology **1**: 25–32.
35. ELSWORTH, J. D., D. J. LEAHY, R. H. ROTH & D. E. REDMOND. 1987. J. Neural Transm. **68**: 51–62.
36. STANLEY, M., L. TRASKMAN-BENDZ & K. DOROVINI-ZIS. 1985. Life Sci. **37**: 1279–1286.

# Interactions between Mesolimbic Dopamine Neurons, Cholecystokinin, and Neurotensin: Evidence Using *in Vivo* Voltammetry[a]

ANTHONY G. PHILLIPS,[b,c] CHARLES D. BLAHA,[c,d]
HANS C. FIBIGER,[d] AND ROSS F. LANE[d,e]

*Departments of Psychology,[c] Psychiatry[d]
and Chemistry[e]
University of British Columbia
Vancouver, B.C., Canada V6T 1Y7*

## INTRODUCTION

The study of peptidergic neurons has been an important facet of neuroscience for over thirty years. While neuropeptides may serve a host of specific physiological functions in the brain and body, their appearance in close proximity to and co-localization with classical transmitter substances, such as acetylcholine, norepinephrine, serotonin, or dopamine (DA), has directed attention toward possible functional interactions between these two classes of synaptic transmitters.[1] Of particular relevance to the present discussion is the evidence for modulatory actions of the octapeptide cholecystokinin (CCK8) and the tridecapeptide neurotensin (NT) on the electrophysiological, neurochemical, and behavioral correlates of the mesocorticolimbic DA systems.[2]

Immunocytochemical studies have identified moderately dense neuronal projections from the ventral mesencephalon to the periventricular region of the striatum and posteromedial nucleus accumbens, which contain both CCK8-like peptides and DA.[3] Detailed descriptions of the immunohistochemical distribution of NT have also confirmed the presence of this peptide in similar brain regions, including DA terminal areas in the nucleus accumbens, striatum, and central nucleus of the amygdala.[4,5] The loss of NT receptor binding after selective neurotoxic destruction of DA neurons in the ventral mesencephalon,[6] is consistent with the presence of NT receptors on DA perikarya in the ventral tegmental area (VTA) and substantia nigra.[6] As with CCK, NT and DA appear to be co-localized in neurons in the VTA.[7] Collectively, the immunohistochemical and receptor binding studies raise the possibility of modulation

[a] Initial studies on CCK–DA interactions were conducted at the Institute of Neuroscience, University of Oregon, Eugene, and were supported by U.S. Public Health Service Grants NS 13556 (R. F. L.) and MH 17148 (C. D. B.); all subsequent studies were conducted at the University of British Columbia, Vancouver, and were supported by a Medical Research Council Program Grant-23 (A. G. P. and H. C. F.).
[b] To whom correspondence should be addressed.

of DA release by these two neuropeptides. In this paper, evidence for such interactions is presented along with the results of recent *in vivo* electrochemical studies showing the inhibition of basal DA release in the nucleus accumbens by CCK8 and its enhancement by NT.

## ATTENUATION OF DOPAMINE RELEASE IN THE NUCLEUS ACCUMBENS BY PERIPHERAL OR CENTRAL ADMINISTRATION OF SULFATED CHOLECYSTOKININ OCTAPEPTIDE

Evidence from many sources suggests a functional interaction between CCK and mesencephalic DA neurons (for review, see references 2, 8). For example, recent electrophysiological studies have shown that the centrally active sulfated form of CCK octapeptide (CCK8-S), administered either intravenously (iv) or iontophoretically, may produce transient excitation followed by rapid (<1 min) long-term inactivation of neuronal firing in some DA/CCK cells.[9,10] These effects appear to be mediated by a direct action of CCK8-S on CCK receptors, since they can be blocked by pretreatment with the putative CCK receptor antagonist proglumide.[10,11] Additionally, measurements of local rates of glucose utilization, believed to reflect ongoing functional activity, are significantly decreased in both DA cell body and terminal regions of the rat brain following systemic injections of CCK8.[12] Neurochemical studies also point to a modulatory influence of CCK8-S on DA release; however, initial reports were contradictory. CCK8-S reportedly decreased[13] or had no effect[14] on basal efflux of [³H]DA from tissue slices of nucleus accumbens or striatum. Recent *in vivo* studies employing push–pull cannulation show that perfusion of CCK8-S directly into the nucleus accumbens enhanced the basal efflux of [³H]DA at low concentrations, but was ineffective at higher concentrations.[15] However, in contrast to these stimulatory effects of low concentrations of CCK8-S on the efflux of newly synthesized [³H]DA, local perfusion of CCK8-S attenuated the $K^+$-evoked release of endogenous DA in a concentration-dependent manner.[16]

Given the difficulties in the interpretation of data obtained from radio-labeled perfusion methodologies and *in vitro* techniques, we have examined the effects of systemic administration of CCK8-S on endogenous DA release in the nucleus accumbens using *in vivo* electrochemical techniques.[17-19] Experimental design and drug protocols are described in detail elsewhere.[20-23] Briefly, stearate-modified graphite paste working (recording) electrodes were implanted stereotaxically into the posteromedial nucleus accumbens of chloral hydrate anesthetized rats. As noted previously, this region of the nucleus accumbens appears to be innervated by neuronal processes containing high levels of both CCK and DA.[3] *In vivo* release of DA was monitored using repetitive chronoamperometry and linear sweep voltammetry with semidifferentiation.[18]

Intravenous administration of CCK8-S (0.5–8.0 µg/kg) produced a dose-related inhibition of DA release in the nucleus accumbens with an onset latency of 6–8 min independent of the dose injected.[20,21] TABLE 1 shows the time to reach maximum inhibition, total duration of action, and magnitudes of these effects. A representative example of a chronoamperometric recording showing the pronounced inhibitory effects of CCK8-S (4 µg/kg, iv) on baseline DA release levels in the nucleus accumbens is presented in FIGURE 1A. The specificity of action of CCK8-S was tested in the preceding paradigm by substituting CCK8-S with injections of relatively high doses (20 µg/kg) of the physiologically inactive nonsulfated form of the peptide (CCK8-US).[9,24] As shown in TABLE 1, in contrast to the marked inhibitory influence of CCK8-S, CCK8-US had

**TABLE 1.** Effects of Systemic Administration of Sulfated (S) and Unsulfated (US) Cholecystokinin Octapeptide on Dopamine Release in the Nucleus Accumbens

| Treatment | Dose (µg/kg) | Maximum Inhibition (%) | Time to Maximum Inhibition (min) | Total Duration of Action (min) |
|---|---|---|---|---|
| CCK8-S | 0.5 | 5 ± 4 | 15 | 30 |
| | 1 | 21 ± 3[a] | 20 | 60 |
| | 2 | 52 ± 6[a] | 35 | 120 |
| | 4 | 86 ± 5[a] | 40 | 160 |
| | 8 | 90 ± 5[a] | 40 | 220 |
| CCK8-US | 20 | No effect | — | — |
| PROG | 300 | No effect | — | — |
| PROG + CCK8-S | 300 4 | No effect | — | — |

NOTE: Values for maximum inhibition are presented as percentages of mean ± SEM decreases in DA release with respect to baseline ($n = 5$ per treatment).
[a] Significant difference from preinjection baseline values, $p < 0.001$. Note that proglumide (PROG) pretreatment blocks the effects of CCK8-S.

no effect on basal DA release. Furthermore, pretreatment with the putative CCK receptor antagonist proglumide (0.3 mg/kg, iv)[10,11] both blocked and reversed the inhibitory effects on DA release induced by a dose of 4 µg/kg of CCK8-S (TABLE 1; FIGURE 1B and 1C). Proglumide itself had no effect on DA release when administered alone. Collectively, these experiments with CCK8-US and proglumide provide strong support that specific CCK receptor sites[10,11,24] are involved in mediating the inhibitory action of CCK8-S on DA release in the nucleus accumbens.

A number of questions may be raised with respect to the direct effects of CCK8-S on central DA neurotransmission following systemic administration. First, there is considerable debate as to whether peripheral injections of small peptides can cross the blood–brain barrier (BBB) in sufficient quantity to exert physiological effects on the brain.[25,26] However, there have been a number of reports confirming that small peptides, including CCK-like peptides,[27] can indeed cross the BBB.[25,26,28] Second, despite the numerous behavioral and electrophysiological studies showing that peripherally administered CCK can alter central DA processes (for a review, see references 2, 8), the question remains as to whether these effects are produced via central as distinct from peripheral actions of the peptide, or by a combination of both. In this context, it is of interest to note that the effects of peripheral injections of CCK8-S on DA cell discharge remain unaltered after vagotomy, although these effects can be attenuated by lesions of the nucleus tractus solitarius (a site of vagal afferent input).[29]

In an attempt to resolve the issue of central versus peripheral actions of CCK8-S on DA release, we have employed central administration of the peptide via the lateral ventricle.[23] Intracerebroventricular (icv) administration of CCK8-S (1 to 100 ng) produced a dose-related *biphasic* excitatory-inhibitory effect on DA release in the nucleus accumbens. As shown in FIGURE 2, immediately following icv injections of CCK8-S (2.5 to 100 ng) chronoamperometric currents increased above preinjection baseline. The increases in the signals reached peak values within 7 min independent of the dose of CCK8-S employed. These peak increases were followed by a rapid decline to values below baseline. The threshold dose for these effects was 2.5 ng, although 1 ng produced a detectable effect on baseline measures. The inhibitory effects on DA release in the nucleus accumbens induced by CCK8-S (icv) at the doses of 10 to 100 ng, were

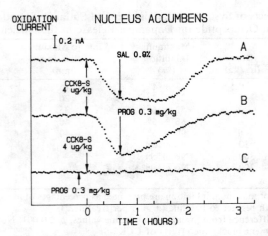

**FIGURE 1.** Time courses of the inhibitory effects of CCK8-S (4 µg/kg, iv) on DA release in the nucleus accumbens (**A**). Note that proglumide (PROG, 0.3 mg/kg, iv ) both reverses (**B**) and blocks (**C**) this inhibition by CCK8-S. Responses were obtained with chronoamperometry by applying a potential pulse for 1 sec from −0.10 V to +0.25 V vs. Ag/AgCl to the working electrode at 1 min intervals and measuring the oxidation current immediately before the end of each 1-sec pulse. For clarity, every second measurement taken is shown. Responses are representative from 4 animals per drug treatment. SAL: (0.9% saline, 0.4 ml/kg, iv).

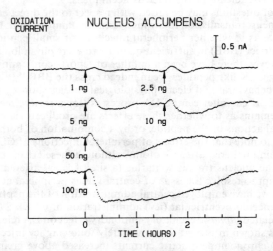

**FIGURE 2.** Time courses of the biphasic effects of various icv doses of CCK8-S on DA release in the nucleus accumbens. Chronoamperometry was performed here and in all subsequent experiments as described in the legend of FIGURE 1. All doses were injected over a 2-min period into the lateral ventricle, ipsilateral to the recording electrode in a 10-µl volume of 0.9% buffered saline, pH = 7.4. Responses are representative from 4 animals per drug treatment.

qualitatively similar to the effects observed following peripheral CCK8-S (2–8 µg/kg, iv) administration. Increasing the dose of CCK8-S lengthened the latencies to reach maximum levels of inhibition of DA release. In contrast to the effects of CCK8-S, injection of CCK8-US (100 ng, icv) produced no significant change in basal levels of DA release. In addition, peripheral administration of proglumide (0.3 mg/kg, iv), 10 min prior to CCK8-S, completely blocked the effects of CCK8-S at all icv doses tested while, again, having no effect on baseline DA release when administered alone.

Electrophysiological studies utilizing either iv or iontophoretic administration of CCK8-S have reported brief increases of discharge rates in identified mesencephalic DA neurons.[9,10,30] Given that the basal release of DA measured by the electrochemical methods employed here is an impulse-dependent process,[18] an initial phase of a CCK8-S-induced increase in DA release may be predicted. As previously shown, transient increases in DA release were observed following icv administration of low doses of CCK8-S (2.5–50 ng), but not with the iv (0.5–8 µg/kg) route of administration. Conceivably, high extracellular concentrations of CCK8-S produced by either route of administration may exert mainly inhibitory effects. Support for this suggestion comes from electrophysiological studies showing that high doses of CCK8-S (iv) completely abolish neuronal activity in some midbrain DA neurons without inducing a prior phase of excitation.[30] Alternatively, peripheral administration may preferentially activate inhibitory afferents to the VTA or nucleus accumbens.

## INTERACTIVE EFFECTS OF CHOLECYSTOKININ AND APOMORPHINE ON DOPAMINE NEUROTRANSMISSION

Focusing attention on the direct effects of CCK8-S on mesolimbic DA neurons permits the integration of the present neurochemical data with results of electrophysiological studies addressing the same questions. As mentioned previously, intravenous or iontophoretically applied CCK produce changes in some DA/CCK cells that rapidly lead to the cessation of spontaneous activity.[9,10,30] These electrophysiological data complement our results showing a predominant inhibition of spontaneous DA release in the nucleus accumbens after peripheral or central administration of CCK8-S. However, these results do not provide sufficient information as to the mechanism by which CCK8-S exerts its inhibitory effects on DA neurons. Low doses of the DA agonist apomorphine directly activate DA autoreceptors preferentially.[30,31] The consequences of such stimulation is hyperpolarization of the DA cell membrane potential leading to inhibition of spontaneous discharge[30,31] and concomitant decreases in basal DA release in DA nerve terminal regions[18,20,22] (FIG. 3C). Based on the results previously presented, CCK8-S could inhibit the release of DA by a mechanism similar to that of apomorphine and other direct-acting DA agonists. Contrary to this prediction, apomorphine (50 µg/kg, iv) administered during CCK8-S-induced (4 µg/kg, iv) inhibition of DA release, produced an immediate reversal of this inhibition. Baseline levels were reestablished within 15 to 20 min of treatment[20] (FIG. 3B). Administration of apomorphine (50 µg/kg, iv) alone caused a rapid decrease in the release of DA (FIG. 3C), in agreement with previous reports.[18,20,22]

In a further study, we examined whether peripheral injections of CCK8-S could similarly reverse the inhibitory influence of apomorphine on basal DA release in the nucleus accumbens.[22] As shown in FIGURE 3D, administration of CCK8-S (4 µg/kg, iv), near the time of maximum inhibition of DA release induced by apomorphine (50 µg/kg, iv) produced a temporary reversal of this inhibition by 46%. Also of interest

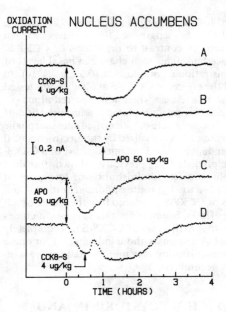

OXIDATION    NUCLEUS ACCUMBENS
CURRENT

**FIGURE 3.** Chronoamperometric recordings showing time courses of (**A**) the inhibitory effects of CCK8-S (4 µg/kg, iv) on DA release in the nucleus accumbens; (**B**) the reversal of this inhibition by apomorphine (APO, 50 µg/kg, iv); (**C**) the inhibitory effects of APO (50 µg/kg, iv) on DA release; and (**D**) the reversal of this inhibition by CCK8-S (4 µg/kg, iv). Note the second phase of inhibition induced by CCK8-S. Qualitatively similar responses were obtained with intravenous dose combinations of 25 µg/kg of APO and 1 µg/kg of CCK8-S.[22] Responses are representative from 4 to 5 animals per drug treatment.

was the observation that the reversal of apomorphine-induced inhibition of DA release by CCK8-S was followed by a second phase of attenuated DA release. This pattern of results is consistent with an initial CCK8-S-induced repolarization of DA cell membranes followed by a period of prolonged tonic depolarization (depolarization block) in DA neurons (see below).

Given the previous effects of apomorphine on the inhibitory influence of peripherally administered CCK8-S (see FIG. 3B), it was of considerable interest to examine the possible interactions between intravenous injections of apomorphine and centrally administered CCK8-S on DA release. As anticipated, apomorphine (50 µg/kg, iv) reversed the inhibitory effects on DA release in the nucleus accumbens produced by an icv injection of CCK8-S (100 ng). Baseline levels were reestablished within 15 to 20 min following the apomorphine challenge[23] (FIG. 4B). A similar pattern of results was observed with lower icv doses of CCK8-S (10 ng) and apomorphine (10 µg/kg, iv) (FIG. 5B). The reversal of the inhibitory effects of both peripheral and central administration of CCK8-S by intravenous injections of apomorphine lends support for the induction of depolarization block in these neurons by a similar mechanism(s).

The reversal of apomorphine-induced inhibition of DA release by CCK8-S is inconsistent with the suggestion that CCK and related peptides may potentiate the ability of apomorphine to inhibit DA neuronal activity by inducing DA autoreceptor supersensitivity,[32] as is the failure of sulpiride (a $D_2$ DA receptor antagonist) to block the inhibitory effects of CCK8-S on $K^+$-evoked release of DA in slices from the nucleus accumbens.[33] Recently, Crawley and colleagues[34] observed a facilitation of both DA-induced hyperlocomotion and apomorphine-induced stereotypy following CCK8-S administration into the nucleus accumbens. This potentiation of DA-mediated behaviors was attributed to an interaction between CCK and DA at postsynaptic receptors or presynaptic terminal sites in the nucleus accumbens. However, the neuronal mechanisms by which CCK potentiates the motor stimulant effects of DA agonists remain

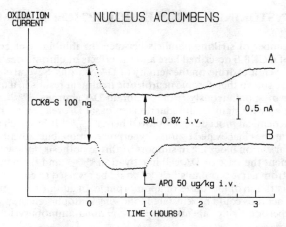

**FIGURE 4.** Time courses of **(A)** the inhibitory effects of CCK8-S (100 ng/10 µl, icv) on DA release in the nucleus accumbens and **(B)** reversal of this inhibition by apomorphine (APO, 50 µg/kg, iv). All icv injections of peptides were performed here and in subsequent experiments as described in the legend of FIGURE 2. Chronoamperometric records are representative from 4 animals per drug treatment. SAL: (0.9% saline, 0.4 ml/kg, iv).

to be determined. For example, CCK8-S facilitation of the postsynaptic action of DA has been called into question by recent electrophysiological studies. Iontophoretic application of CCK8-S and DA exerted independent and opposite effects on cell activity by depolarizing and hyperpolarizing the neuronal membranes of nucleus accumbens cells, respectively.[35] In addition, both compounds functionally antagonized each other in this brain region.

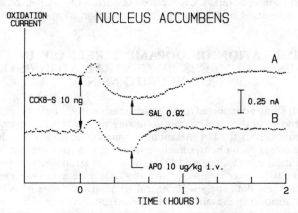

**FIGURE 5.** Time courses of **(A)** the biphasic excitatory-inhibitory effects of CCK8-S (10 ng/10 µl, icv) on DA release in the nucleus accumbens and **(B)** reversal of the inhibitory effects of CCK8-S by apomorphine (APO, 10 µg/kg, iv). Chronoamperometric records are representative from 4 animals per drug treatment. SAL: (0.9% saline, 0.4 ml/kg, iv).

## CHOLECYSTOKININ AND NEUROLEPTICS: A COMPARISON

There are a number of striking parallels between the inhibitory effects of acute administration of CCK8-S described here and the effects of chronic treatment with neuroleptic (antipsychotic) drugs on the activity of DA neurons. Several electrophysiological studies have shown that chronic neuroleptic treatment results in a marked decrease in the number of spontaneously firing midbrain DA neurons.[30,36-39] Such treatment also is associated with significant reductions in basal DA release, as measured by the *in vivo* electrochemical procedures employed here.[18,21,40,41] It has been postulated that these DA cells are not inactivated by tonic hyperpolarization, but rather by tonic depolarization (depolarization block).[36] In support of this hypothesis, following chronic neuroleptic treatment the state of DA cell inactivation [30,36-39] and the parallel reductions in DA release from nerve terminals[18,21,40,41] could be reversed to control levels by intravenous administration of low doses of apomorphine. In addition, normal spontaneous activity in DA neurons could be reinstated following iontophoretic application of other inhibitory hyperpolarizing agents, such as gamma-aminobutyric acid and DA itself.[30,36-39]

Although it is not possible to provide conclusive evidence of depolarization block in DA neurons using either extracellular electrophysiological or electrochemical techniques, recent intracellular recordings from identified midbrain DA cells demonstrated that after a chronic regimen of a neuroleptic the membrane potentials of inactivated DA neurons are significantly more depolarized than those in chronic vehicle-treated (control) rats. Under these conditions, apomorphine administration also has been shown to repolarize the cell membranes of these DA neurons and restore normal spontaneous activity.[30] Given these electrophysiological findings, the immediate reversal by apomorphine of the CCK8-S-induced decreases in DA release observed in our studies, and the comparable effects of apomorphine on the decreases in DA release seen in chronic neuroleptic-treated animals,[18,21,40,41] it may be conjectured that the inhibitory effects of CCK8-S can best be attributed to a condition resembling chronic neuroleptic-induced depolarization block. Strong support of this supposition comes from the fact that both intravenous and iontophoretic CCK-induced cessation of DA neuronal activity can be immediately reversed by intravenous administration of apomorphine.[9,10,30]

## STIMULATION OF DOPAMINE RELEASE IN THE NUCLEUS ACCUMBENS BY CENTRAL ADMINISTRATION OF NEUROTENSIN

Neurochemical studies conducted to date have consistently shown increases in DA synthesis and turnover in the rat forebrain following icv NT.[42,43] For example, increases in the concentrations of the DA metabolite homovanillic acid (HVA) have been observed in the nucleus accumbens, olfactory tubercle, and striatum. Additionally, central administration of NT increased DA synthesis in striatal tissue as evidenced by DOPA accumulation after treatment with the DOPA decarboxylase inhibitor NSD 1015. Together, these data suggested general stimulating effects of NT on both DA synthesis and turnover in mesolimbic and mesostriatal systems. However, there have been discrepancies between the implications of these neurochemical data and the results of psychopharmacological studies. Locomotor behavior elicited by systemic administration of DA agonists was attenuated by NT (icv), whereas DA agonist-induced stereotyped behavior was not.[44] Futhermore, injections of NT into the nucleus accumbens blocked locomotor behavior elicited by systemic amphetamine, while intrastriatal ad-

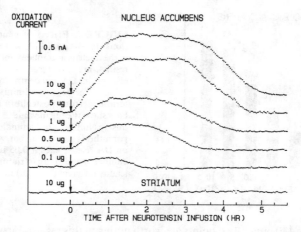

**FIGURE 6.** Chronoamperometric recordings depicting the time courses of the stimulatory effects of increasingly larger doses of neurotensin (NT, 0.1–10 μg/10 μl, icv) on DA release in the nucleus accumbens. Note the lack of effect in the striatum at a dose (10 μg) that produced a maximal effect in the nucleus accumbens. Administration of lower doses of NT also had no effect on basal DA release in the striatum. Data are representative from the number of animals per drug treatment shown in FIGURE 7.

ministration of NT failed to block amphetamine-induced stereotypy.[45] Therefore, these behavioral data suggested a selective action of NT on the mesolimbic DA system. Recently, we addressed the question of localized effects of icv NT on DA release in the rat forebrain *in vivo* and observed an enhancement in the nucleus accumbens but not the striatum over a dose range of 0.1–10 μg of NT.

*In vivo* electrochemical monitoring of extracellular DA concentrations in the posteromedial nucleus accumbens[17-19] revealed a dose-related increase in the release of DA immediately following icv administration of NT (FIG. 6). The threshold dose for this action of NT was 0.1 μg with a maximal effect observed at a dose of 10 μg (FIG. 7). Chronoamperometric measurements permitted precise temporal information on the onset latency, duration of peak effect, and total duration of action for each dose of NT tested. Onset latencies were uniformly observed to be 4–6-min postinjection across a dose range of 0.5 to 10 μg. Time to peak effect increased with progressively higher doses of NT (0.5–10 μg) and varied from 60 to 80 min. The duration of peak effects and total duration of action observed with the two highest doses of NT (5 and 10 μg) ranged from 1 to 1.5 and 4.5 to 5 hr, respectively (FIG. 6). In contrast, icv administration of NT had no effect on basal DA release in the anterodorsal striatum over the entire dose range tested, even with the dose of 10 μg, which increased DA release maximally in the nucleus accumbens (FIGS. 6 and 7).

The results of these *in vivo* electrochemical studies are in partial agreement with postmortem biochemical indices of DA activity in these dopaminergic terminal regions.[42,43] Previous studies report significant increases in the DA metabolite HVA in the nucleus accumbens following NT administration (30 μg/25 μl, icv), with peak changes occurring 60 min postinjection. In contrast to the present observations of a lack of an effect of NT on striatal DA release, significant elevations in HVA tissue concentrations have been observed in this structure with a duration of action persisting

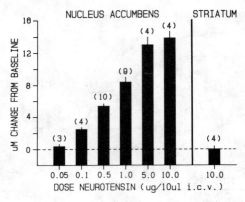

FIGURE 7. Effects of neurotensin injections (0.1–10 µg/10 µl, icv) on DA release in the nucleus accumbens and striatum. The results are expressed as the maximum change in DA concentration from basal values after peptide administration, as determined from postcalibration data. The bars show the mean value ± SEM for each dose. Number of animals is given in parenthesis above each bar. All dose effects on DA release except 0.05 µg (nucleus accumbens) and 10 µg (striatum) were significantly different ($p < 0.01$) from basal values.

for more than 120 min.[43] Two points are worth noting in this regard. First is the difference in the maximum dose of NT (10 µg vs. 30 µg, icv) employed. Conceivably, larger icv doses of NT (i.e., ⩾30 µg) than those employed currently may also yield detectable changes in DA release in the striatum. Second, biochemical analyses of NT in tissue samples microdissected from discrete forebrain DA regions, have shown important regional differences in the content of NT. For example, NT tissue concentrations in the nucleus accumbens have been reported to be four times greater than those found in the anterior striatum,[46] sites comparable to those employed in the present *in vivo* experiments. Of equal importance, the ratio for tissue concentrations of NT in the VTA versus substantia nigra is also approximately 4:1.[46] Such a disparity in regional NT tissue concentrations may well account for the greater sensitivity of mesolimbic DA neurons to the release promoting effects of NT.

## PHARMACOLOGICAL MODULATION OF NEUROTENSIN-INDUCED RELEASE OF DOPAMINE

Electrophysiological and psychopharmacological studies have provided evidence for a stimulatory influence of NT on DA neuronal activity[47] and DA mediated behaviors[48] when locally applied to DA cells in the ventral mesencephalon. Bilateral injections of NT into the VTA of the rat induced increases in locomotor activity.[48] This effect was attributed to increased release of DA in the nucleus accumbens produced by NT antagonism of DA autoreceptor inhibition in the VTA. A similar mechanism may account for the NT-induced release of DA in the nucleus accumbens we have observed. Previous studies have shown electrochemical baseline signals (both voltammetric and chronoamperometric) to be completely suppressed by administration of gamma-butyrolactone (GBL),[18] an agent known to block impulse flow in DA neurons. Studies of the effect of GBL on NT-induced changes in DA release in the nucleus accumbens confirm that these effects of NT are dependent on impulse activity. Administration of GBL (200 mg/kg, ip) produced an immediate reversal of the NT-induced (1 µg, icv) increases in DA release (FIG. 8B). Additionally, pretreatment with GBL (200 mg/kg, ip) 80 min prior to administration of NT (1 µg, icv), caused an inhibition of DA release and prevented the stimulatory effects of NT (FIG. 8C). A similar pattern of results was observed with presynaptic doses of apomorphine[48] (50 µg/kg, iv), known to hyperpolarize DA neurons.[30,31]

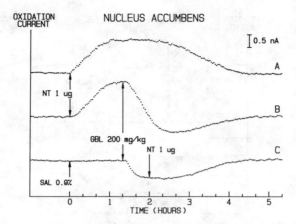

**FIGURE 8.** Chronoamperometric recordings showing (**A**) the stimulatory effects of neurotensin (NT, 1 μg/10 μl, icv) on DA release in the nucleus accumbens. Note that gamma-butyrolactone (GBL, 200 mg/kg, ip) both reverses (**B**) and blocks (**C**) this stimulatory effect of neurotensin. Responses are representative from 5 animals per drug treatment. SAL: (0.9% buffered saline icv).

These pharmacological data are consistent with the hypothesis that NT at low doses may enhance basal DA release by selectively increasing the activity of mesolimbic DA neurons. This action of NT, if confirmed, is opposite to its antagonism of DA neurotransmission at postsynaptic sites, as indicated by a variety of physiological and behavioral measures.[42] Although there are convincing arguments attributing these paradoxical effects of NT to a unitary mechanism that opposes the action of DA,[42] the question still remains as to whether either of these actions is physiologically relevant or merely pharmacological in nature.

The comparable pharmacology of NT and specific neuroleptic drugs is of considerable interest.[2,42] Both inhibit avoidance but not escape behavior, enhance the sedative effects of CNS depressants, and attenuate locomotor activity but not stereotypy elicited by indirect DA agonists. The last effect suggests a possible selective influence on the mesolimbic as distinct from the mesostriatal DA system. The present observations of a selective enhancement of DA release in the nucleus accumbens (at the doses tested), is a further endorsement of NT–mesolimbic DA interaction. There is evidence that atypical neuroleptic drugs (e.g., clozapine and thioridazine), largely devoid of extrapyramidal side effects, exert a selective influence on mesolimbic DA neurons, as measured electrophysiologically[37,39] or by *in vivo* electrochemistry.[18,41,50] Accordingly, as described in an accompanying paper in this volume,[49] we have compared NT and atypical neuroleptics using *in vivo* chronoamperometry at sites in the nucleus accumbens and striatum, alone, or under a variety of pharmacological conditions. The similarities between the data obtained with NT and clozapine were striking (see reference 49, fig. 1).

## ASYMMETRIC INTERACTIONS BETWEEN CHOLECYSTOKININ AND NEUROTENSIN

Our *in vivo* electrochemical data provide evidence that the neuropeptides CCK and NT exert opposing actions on DA release in the nucleus accumbens. These data and

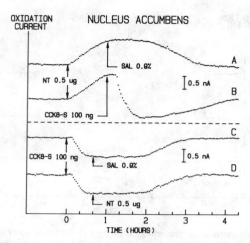

**FIGURE 9.** Chronoamperometric recordings showing (**A,B**) the reversal of the stimulatory effects of neurotensin (NT, 0.5 µg/10 µl, icv) on DA release in the nucleus accumbens by CCK8-S (100 ng/10 µl, icv). Note that neurotensin (0.5 µg/10 µl, icv) failed to reverse the inhibitory effects of CCK8-S (100 ng/10 µl, icv) on DA release in the nucleus accumbens (**C,D**). Responses are representative from 5 animals per drug treatment. SAL: (0.9% buffered saline icv).

the close proximity of these two peptides in the VTA and nucleus accumbens (Fallon *et al.*, this volume), raise the question as to whether each can functionally antagonize the action of the other on DA release. As may be seen in FIGURE 9, there is an intriguing asymmetry to their interaction. CCK8-S (100 ng, icv) antagonized the stimulatory effects of NT (0.5 µg, icv) on DA release (FIG. 9). This effect and the subsequent prolonged period of inhibited DA release are consistent with the putative ability of CCK to induce depolarization block in DA neurons.[20,22] In contrast, NT (0.5 µg, icv) could not reverse the inhibitory effects of CCK (100 ng, icv). This effect raises the possibility that NT depolarizes DA cell membranes, but not to the extent of inducing depolarization block.

## CONCLUSIONS

Interactions of CCK and NT with a population of DA neurons implicated in both the etiology and pharmacological treatment of schizophrenia has led to a number of hypotheses regarding the possible role of these neuropeptides as antipsychotic agents.[8,42,51] From our *in vivo* electrochemical studies, it is apparent that acute treatment with CCK8-S has a great deal in common with a chronic regimen of neuroleptics; in particular, the inhibition of DA release by an apparent mechanism of depolarization block. Given that chronic neuroleptic treatment is required for therapeutic efficacy, this similarity is a strong point in favor of CCK as a candidate antipsychotic compound.

As previously noted, there are also many compelling reasons for considering NT as an endogenous neuroleptic. To these we can now add its similarity to atypical neuroleptics in selectively stimulating the release of DA in the nucleus accumbens.[49] In view of previous comments regarding the prerequisite of chronic antipsychotic treatment regimens, it is perhaps premature to draw too close a comparison between the *acute* effects of NT and antipsychotic action of neuroleptics. An important task for future research will be to examine the effects of *chronic* NT treatment on the electrophysiology of DA neurons and *in vivo* release of DA in the mesocorticolimbic system. Prolonged excitation of DA neurons with chronic NT could possibly lead to the induction of a state of depolarization block, thus linking NT more closely to the antipsychotic action of neuroleptic drugs.

## ACKNOWLEDGMENT

The authors thank Valerie Chan for her skilled assistance in the preparation of this manuscript.

### REFERENCES

1. HOKFELT, T., O. JOHANSSON, A. LJUNGDAHL, J. M. LUNDBERG & M. SCHULTZBERG. 1980. Peptidergic neurons. Nature **284**: 515–521.
2. KALIVAS, P. W. 1985. Interactions between neuropeptides and dopamine neurons in the ventromedial mesencephalon. Neurosci. Biobehav. Rev. **9**: 573–587.
3. HOKFELT, T., L. SKIRBOLL, J. F. REHFELD, M. GOLDSTEIN, K. MARKEY & O. DANN. 1980. A subpopulation of mesencephalic dopamine neurons projecting to limbic areas contains a cholecystokinin-like peptide: Evidence from immunohistochemistry combined with retrograde tracing. Neuroscience **5**: 2093–2124.
4. UHL, G. R., J. P. BENNETT, JR. & S. H. SNYDER. 1979. Neurotensin-containing cell bodies, fibers and nerve terminals in the brainstem of the rat. Brain Res. **167**: 77–91.
5. JENNES, L., P. W. KALIVAS & W. E. STUMPF. 1982. Neurotensin: Topographical distribution in rat brain by immunohistochemistry. J. Comp. Neurol. **210**: 213–224.
6. PALACIOS, J. M. & M. J. KUHAR. 1981. Neurotensin receptors are located on dopamine-containing neurons in rat midbrain. Nature **294**: 587–589.
7. HOKFELT, T., B. J. EVERITT, E. THEODORSSON-NORHEIM & M. GOLDSTEIN. 1984. Occurrence of neurotensin-like immunoreactivity in subpopulations of hypothalamic, mesencephalic and medullary catecholamine neurons. J. Comp. Neurol. **222**: 543–559.
8. NAIR, N. P. V., S. LAL & D. M. BLOOM. 1986. Cholecystokinin and schizophrenia. *In* Psychiatric Disorders: Neurotransmitters and Neuropeptides, Vol. 65. J. M. Van Ree and S. Matthysse, Eds.: 237–258. Elsevier. New York.
9. SKIRBOLL, L. R., A. A. GRACE, D. W. HOMMER, J. REHFELD, M. GOLDSTEIN, T. HOKFELT & B. S. BUNNEY. 1981. Peptide-monoamine coexistence: Studies of the actions of cholecystokinin-like peptides on the electrical activity of midbrain dopamine neurons. Neuroscience **6**: 2111–2124.
10. BUNNEY, B. S., L. A. CHIODO & A. S. FREEMAN. 1985. Further studies on the specificity of proglumide as a selective cholecystokinin antagonist in the central nervous system. Ann. N.Y. Acad. Sci. **448**: 345–351.
11. CHIODO, L. A. & B. S. BUNNEY. 1983. Proglumide: Selective antagonism of excitatory effects of cholecystokinin in the central nervous system. Science **219**: 1449–1451.
12. LUCIGNANI, G., L. J. PORRINO & C. A. TAMMINGA. 1984. Effects of systemically administered cholecystokinin-octapeptide on local cerebral metabolism. Eur. J. Pharmacol. **101**: 147–151.
13. MARKSTEIN, R. & T. HOKFELT. 1984. Effects of cholecystokinin-octapeptide on dopamine release from slices of cat caudate nucleus. J. Neurosci. **4**: 570–575.
14. HAMILTON, M., M. J. SHEEHAN, J. DE BELLEROCHE & L. J. HERBERG. 1984. The cholecystokinin analogue, caerulein, does not modulate dopamine release or dopamine-induced locomotor activity in the nucleus accumbens. Neurosci. Lett. **44**: 77–82.
15. VOIGT, M. M., R. Y. WANG & T. C. WESTFALL. 1985. The effects of cholecystokinin on

      the *in vivo* release of newly synthesized [³H]dopamine from the nucleus accumbens of the rat. J. Neurosci. **5:** 2744–2749.

16. VOIGT, M. M. & R. Y. WANG. 1984. *In vivo* release of dopamine in the nucleus accumbens of the rat: Modulation by cholecystokinin. Brain Res. **296:** 189–193.

17. ADAMS, R. N. & C. A. MARSDEN. 1982. Electrochemical detection methods for monoamine measurements *in vitro* and *in vivo*. *In* Handbook of Psychopharmacology, Vol. 15. L. L. Iversen, S. D. Iversen, and S. H. Snyder, Eds.: 1–74. Plenum Press. New York.

18. LANE, R. F. & C. D. BLAHA. 1986. Electrochemistry *in vivo*: Application to CNS pharmacology. Ann. N.Y. Acad. Sci. **473:** 50–69.

19. BLAHA, C. D. & R. F. LANE. 1983. Chemically modified electrode for *in vivo* monitoring of brain catecholamines. Brain Res. Bull. **10:** 861–864.

20. LANE, R. F., C. D. BLAHA & A. G. PHILLIPS. 1986. *In vivo* electrochemical analysis of cholecystokinin-induced inhibition of dopamine release in the nucleus accumbens. Brain Res. **397:** 200–204.

21. LANE, R. F., C. D. BLAHA & A. G. PHILLIPS. 1987. Cholecystokinin-induced inhibition of dopamine neurotransmission: Comparison with chronic haloperidol treatment. Prog. Neuro-Psychopharmacol. Biol. Psychiatry **11:** 291–299.

22. BLAHA, C. D., A. G. PHILLIPS & R. F. LANE. 1987. Reversal by cholecystokinin of apomorphine-induced inhibition of dopamine release in the nucleus accumbens of the rat. Regulat. Peptides **17:** 301–310.

23. BLAHA, C. D., R. F. LANE & A. G. PHILLIPS. 1987. Application of *in vivo* electrochemistry to cholecystokinin-dopamine interactions in the ventral striatum. *In* The Basal Ganglia II: Structure and Function. M. Carpenter and A. Jayaraman, Eds.: 115–142. Plenum Press. New York.

24. WHITE, F. J. & R. Y. WANG. 1984. Interactions of cholecystokinin octapeptide and dopamine on nucleus accumbens neurons. Brain Res. **300:** 161–166.

25. KASTIN, A. J., J. E. ZADINA, W. A. BANKS & M. V. GRAF. 1984. Misleading concepts in the field of brain peptides. Peptides **5** (Suppl. 1): 249–253.

26. BANKS, W. A. & A. J. KASTIN. 1985. Permeability of the blood-brain barrier to neuropeptides: The case for penetration. Psychoneuroendocrinology **10:** 385–399.

27. STERN, J. J., C. A. CUDILLO & J. KRUPER. 1976. Ventromedial hypothalamus and short-term suppression of feeding by caerulein in male rats. J. Comp. Physiol. Psychol. **90:** 484–490.

28. KASTIN, A. J., C. NISSEN, A. V. SCHALLY & D. H. COY. 1979. Additional evidence that small amounts of a peptide can cross the blood-brain barrier. Pharmacol. Biochem. Behav. **11:** 717–719.

29. HOMMER, D. W., M. PALKOVITS, J. N. CRAWLEY, S. M. PAUL & L. R. SKIRBOLL. 1985. Cholecystokinin-induced excitation in the substantia nigra: Evidence for peripheral and central components. J. Neurosci. **5:** 1387–1392.

30. GRACE, A. A. & B. S. BUNNEY. 1986. Induction of depolarization block in midbrain dopamine neurons by repeated administration of haloperidol: Analysis using *in vivo* intracellular recording. J. Pharmacol. Exp. Ther. **238:** 1092–1100.

31. GRACE, A. A. & B. S. BUNNEY. 1985. Low doses of apomorphine elicit two opposing influences on dopamine cell electrophysiology. Brain Res. **333:** 285–289.

32. HOMMER, D. W. & L. R. SKIRBOLL. 1983. Cholecystokinin-like peptides potentiate apomorphine-induced inhibition of dopamine neurons. Eur. J. Pharmacol. **91:** 151–152.

33. VOIGT, M. M., R. Y. WANG & T. C. WESTFALL. 1986. Cholecystokinin octapeptides alter the release of endogenous dopamine from the rat nucleus accumbens *in vitro*. J. Pharmacol. Exp. Ther. **237:** 147–153.

34. CRAWLEY, J. N., J. A. STIVERS, L. K. BLUMSTEIN & S. M. PAUL. 1985. Cholecystokinin potentiates dopamine-mediated behaviors: Evidence for modulation specific to a site of co-existence. J. Neurosci. **5:** 1972–1983.

35. WANG, R. Y. & X.-T. HU. 1986. Does cholecystokinin potentiate dopamine action in the nucleus accumbens? Brain Res. **380:** 363–367.

36. BUNNEY, B. S. & A. A. GRACE. 1978. Acute and chronic haloperidol treatments: Comparison of effects of chronic administration on nigral dopaminergic activity. Life Sci. **23:** 1715–1728.

37.  CHIODO, L. A. & B. S. BUNNEY. 1983. Typical and atypical neuroleptics: Differential effects of chronic administration on the activity of A9 and A10 midbrain dopaminergic neurons. J. Neurosci. **8:** 1607–1619.
38.  WHITE, F. J. & R. Y. WANG. 1983. Comparison of the effects of chronic haloperidol treatment on A9 and A10 dopamine neurons in the rat. Life Sci. **32:** 983–993.
39.  WHITE, F. J. & R. Y. WANG. 1983. Differential effects of classical and atypical antipsychotic drugs on A9 and A10 dopamine neurons. Science **221:** 1054–1057.
40.  LANE, R. F. & C. D. BLAHA. 1987. Chronic haloperidol decreases dopamine release in striatum and nucleus accumbens *in vivo*: Depolarization block as a possible mechanism of action. Brain Res. Bull. **18:** 135–138.
41.  BLAHA, C. D. & R. F. LANE. 1987. Chronic treatment with classical and atypical antipsychotic drugs differentially decreases dopamine release in striatum and nucleus accumbens *in vivo*. Neurosci. Lett. **78:** 199–204.
42.  NEMEROFF, C. B. 1986. The interaction of neurotensin with dopaminergic pathways in the central nervous system: Basic neurobiology and implications for the pathogenesis and treatment of schizophrenia. Psychoneuroendocrinology **11:** 15–37.
43.  WIDERLOV, E., C. D. KILTS, R. B. MAILMAN, C. B. NEMEROFF, A. J. PRANGE, JR. & G. R. BREESE. 1982. Increases in dopamine metabolites in rat brain by neurotensin. J. Pharmacol. Exp. Ther. **222:** 1–6.
44.  JOLICOEUR, F. B., G. DE MICHELE & A. BARBEAU. 1983. Neurotensin affects hyperactivity but not sterotypy induced by pre- and post-synaptic dopaminergic stimulation. Neurosci. Biobehav. Rev. **7:** 385–390.
45.  ERVIN, G. N., L. S. BIRKEMO, C. B. NEMEROFF & A. J. PRANGE, JR. 1981. Neurotensin blocks certain amphetamine-induced behaviors. Nature **291:** 73–76.
46.  BISSETTE, G., C. RICHARDSON, J. S. KIZER & C. B. NEMEROFF. 1984. Ontogeny of brain neurotensin in the rat: A radioimmunoassay study. J. Neurochem. **43:** 283–287.
47.  ANDRADE, R. & G. K. AGHAJANIAN. 1981. Neurotensin selectively activates dopaminergic neurons in the substantia nigra. Soc. Neurosci. Abstr. **7:** 573.
48.  KALIVAS, P. W., S. K. BURGESS, C. B. NEMEROFF & A. J. PRANGE, JR. 1983. Behavioral and neurochemical effects of neurotensin microinjection into the ventral tegmental area. Neuroscience **8:** 496–505.
49.  BLAHA, C. D., A. G. PHILLIPS, H. C. FIBIGER & R. F. LANE. 1988. Effects of neurotensin on dopamine release in the nucleus accumbens: Comparisons with atypical antipsychotic drug action. This volume.
50.  LANE, R. F. & C. D. BLAHA. 1988. Effects of chronic neuroleptic administration on nigrostriatal and mesocorticolimbic dopamine release: Analysis using *in vivo* voltammetry. This volume.
51.  PHILLIPS, A. G., R. F. LANE & C. D. BLAHA. 1986. Inhibition of dopamine release by cholecystokinin: Relevance to schizophrenia. Trends Pharmacol. Sci. **7:** 126–129.

# Cholecystokinin, Dopamine, and Schizophrenia: Recent Progress and Current Problems[a]

REX Y. WANG

*Department of Psychiatry and Behavioral Science*
*State University of New York at Stony Brook*
*Stony Brook, New York 11794*

## INTRODUCTION

The presence of cholecystokinin (CCK), a gastrointestinal hormone,[1] has now been demonstrated in various areas of the central nervous system (CNS).[2-4] Studies utilizing biochemical methods have shown that the predominant form of CCK in the brain is the carboxy terminal octapeptide (CCK-8), and that CCK-8 exists mainly in the sulfated form (CCK-8S). Concentrations of CCK-8S are particularly high in the cerebral cortices and limbic structures, brain areas that have been associated with cognitive processes, emotion, and motivation. It is becoming apparent that CCK-8S may function as a neurotransmitter or neuromodulator in the CNS (for review, see Vanderhaeghen and Crawley[5]).

## COEXISTENCE OF CCK AND DA

In 1980, Hokfelt *et al.*[6] reported that CCK coexists with DA in a subset of mesencephalic dopamine (DA) neurons primarily in the ventral tegmental area (VTA or A10) and also in the medial and very lateral parts of the substantia-nigra pars compacta (SNC or A9) of rat and man, and that these CCK/DA neurons project primarily to the medial and caudal portions of the nucleus accumbens (N.Acc.) and olfactory tubercle. Since then, the discovery of the coexistence of CCK and DA has been confirmed by various investigators using both anatomical and biochemical techniques.[7-11] In addition, it has been shown that CCK might share the same storage sites as DA in some of the meso-N.Acc. terminals.[12,13] These findings are of particular interest in view of the suggested involvement of the A10 DA system in the pathophysiology of schizophrenia and the therapeutic action of antipsychotic drugs (APDs).[14-16]

According to the DA hypothesis of schizophrenia, a hyperactive DA system is responsible for at least some of the symptoms associated with this disease.[14-16] Recent studies have shown that atypical APDs such as clozapine and thioridazine, which have a lower

[a] This work was supported by U.S. Public Health Service Grants MH-41440, MH-41696, and MH-00378(RSDA).

potential for causing extrapyramidal side effects, preferentially act upon the A10 DA system, suggesting that the therapeutic actions of APDs may be related to the A10 mesolimbic regions rather than the A9 DA system. In addition, the sites of action of APDs are primarily on postsynaptic target neurons that receive DA projections, because lesions of these target neurons by ibotenic acid or kainic acid prevent the reduction of DA activity induced by chronic APD treatment.[17,18]

## INTERACTIONS BETWEEN CCK AND DA

To elucidate the functional role of CCK in the A10 DA system, we have been examining the interactions of CCK and DA in the rat N.Acc., a limbic structure that receives a topographically defined CCK/DA input from the VTA.

### Electrophysiological Studies

We have shown that application of CCK-8S by microiontophoresis (ionto-CCK-8S) markedly increases both the spontaneous and glutamate (GLUT) -induced firing rate of N.Acc. cells; in addition, ionto-CCK-8S activates a population of quiescent N.Acc. cells.[19-23] Interestingly, CCK-8S, but not GLUT (applied from the same micropipettes), preferentially activates cells in the medial N.Acc.[19-23] Similar to the GLUT, at high ejection current, CCK-8S often increases the firing rate of cells to the point of apparent depolarization inactivation (excessive depolarization such that the resting membrane potential is increased above the threshold and blocks the spike generating system).[19,20] Unsulfated CCK-8S (CCK-8US), which is biologically inactive in the peripheral system, appears to have little or no effect on N.Acc. cells when an equimolar concentration is applied.[19]

Intravenous or iontophoretic application of the putative CCK antagonist proglumide[24-26] prevents the activation produced by ionto-CCK, but not that produced by GLUT. In addition, scopolamine (iv) does not block the excitation induced by CCK-8S, suggesting that the blockade of CCK-8S by proglumide is not mediated indirectly via its reported antimuscarinic properties.[19] Proglumide also fails to change the excitatory effects of neurotensin upon DA cells in the midbrain, excitatory effects of substance P and inhibitory effects of Met-enkephalin on DA-sensitive prefrontal cortical neurons, or inhibitory effects of histamine in the sensorimotor cortex.[26] Combined, the results suggest that proglumide is a specific CCK antagonist in the CNS. However, it is clear that proglumide is by no means an ideal CCK antagonist, because it has been shown in some behavioral experiments that relatively high doses of proglumide are needed to block CCK-induced effects,[27-29] and that it does not bind to the recognition site of the CCK receptor.[30-32] Most recently, we have tested another CCK antagonist, lorglumide, an analog of proglumide, but with several orders of magnitude higher affinity to [125]I-CCK-8 binding sites than proglumide.[33] Lorglumide appears to be 10,000 times more potent than proglumide in blocking CCK-induced effects in the N.Acc. (FIG. 1). Moreover, the antagonizing effect of lorglumide is specific in that it fails to block the excitatory effect of GLUT and the inhibitory effects of substance P, somatostatin, neurotensin, and DA on N.Acc. cells.[34]

These results suggest that CCK is an extremely potent activator of neuronal activity, particularly in the dorsomedial N.Acc. This regional specificity of CCK-8S-induced excitation in the N.Acc. corresponds closely to previous findings indicating that the densities of CCK-like immunoreactivity[6] and autoradiographically visualized

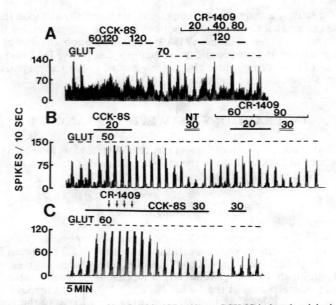

**FIGURE 1.** Antagonistic effects of lorglumide (CR1409) on CCK-8S-induced activity in the N.Acc. (**A**) Blockade of CCK-8S-induced excitation by iontophoretic application of lorglumide. Lorglumide had no effect on glutamate-induced activation. (**B**) Blockade of the facilitating action of CCK-8S on glutamate-induced activation by lorglumide. Neurotensin suppressed the glutamate-induced excitation. Lorglumide did not block neurotensin-induced suppression. (**C**) Blockade of CCK-8S-induced effect on glutamate activation by intravenous lorglumide (0.01, 0.02, 0.04, and 0.08 µg/kg at the times indicated by arrows). Lines and numbers above each cumulative-rate histogram represent the duration of iontophoretic current and the amount of current in nanoamperes. (Provided by X. T. Hu.)

CCK receptors[35,36] are considerably greater in the dorsomedial aspects of the N.Acc. Therefore, it seems likely that the excitatory effect of CCK-8S in the dorsomedial N.Acc. reflects endogenous physiological actions of this peptide. This possibility is further supported by the relative ineffectiveness of CCK-8US in activating N.Acc. cells and the fact that lorglumide potently blocks the excitatory effect of CCK-8S, but not that of GLUT. The latter two findings also suggest that the CCK receptors on N.Acc. cells resemble the so-called "pancreatic type."[34,37]

Ionto-DA markedly suppresses the spontaneous firing rate of N.Acc. neurons and the firing activity induced by either GLUT or CCK.[19,20] In addition, ionto-DA readily reverses the apparent depolarization inactivation produced by either CCK or GLUT, presumably by its hyperpolarizing actions.[19-23] When CCK-8S is ejected at lower currents onto the same cells, depolarization block fails to occur, and DA inhibits the CCK-8S-produced excitation (FIG. 2A). The effect of DA could be prevented or reversed by iontophoretic administration of the DA antagonist clozapine or haloperidol.[38,39] Therefore, the particular alteration in the activity of a given N.Acc. neuron during coadministration of CCK and DA depends upon the relative amounts of the two substances being administered. The results suggest that the response of a N.Acc. cell to DA and CCK is dependent upon the amount of DA and CCK being released from DA/CCK terminals.

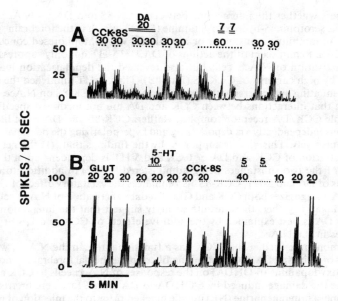

**FIGURE 2.** Comparison of the interactions of CCK-8S and dopamine (**A**) versus CCK-8S and serotonin (**B**) on N.Acc. cells. Low ejection currents of CCK-8S excited N.Acc. cells, whereas higher currents drove N.Acc. cells into depolarization block. Dopamine (**A**) and serotonin (**B**) inhibited the excitant effect of CCK-8S. They also reversed CCK-8S-induced depolarization block. (Provided by X. T. Hu.)

Our results represent the first direct electrophysiological evidence indicating a functional antagonism of CCK-8S and DA in the N.Acc., a limbic structure receiving dense topographic CCK/DA inputs from A10 CCK/DA neurons. Our findings are consistent with previous reports indicating that CCK-8S decreases DA release in the N.Acc.[40-43] and that CCK-8S exhibits the behavioral profile of APDs.[44-51] In contrast to these studies, however, Crawley *et al.*[52, 53] reported that CCK-8S, but not CCK-8US, injected directly into the N.Acc. enhanced DA-induced hyperlocomotion and apomorphine-induced stereotypy. Because this facilitation of DA receptor-mediated behavior by CCK-8S was not observed when CCK-8S was injected into the neostriatum, they suggested that the potentiation of DA by CCK-8S may be specific to the mesolimbic neurons where CCK-8S and DA coexist. This finding prompted us to reexamine the effects of CCK-8S and DA and their interactions on the physiological activities of N.Acc. neurons.

To determine whether CCK-8S would potentiate the inhibitory action of DA, CCK-8S was iontophoresed concurrently with DA on both spontaneously active and GLUT-activated N.Acc. neurons. The ejecting current of the CCK-8S barrel was adjusted so that CCK-8S, by itself, did not increase the cellular firing activity. Of the 19 N.Acc. neurons tested (14 spontaneously active and 5 GLUT-activated neurons), none showed any potentiation of DA-induced depressant effect by CCK.[20] In fact, in 15 cases (79%), CCK-8S reduced markedly the inhibitory effect of DA. These results are in agreement with our previous finding that CCK-8S functionally antagonizes DA-induced effects on N.Acc. cells.[19, 23] They fail to support the view that CCK-8S directly potentiates DA-induced action.

To assess whether the interactions between CCK-8S and DA on N.Acc. neurons are specific, serotonin [5-hydroxytryptamine (5-HT), which in the forebrain serves primarily as an inhibitory transmitter or modulator] was iontophoresed concomitantly with CCK-8S. Reminiscent of the actions of DA,[19,20] 5-HT not only suppressed CCK-induced activation of N.Acc. cells but also reversed the depolarization inactivation produced by high currents of CCK-8S (FIG. 2B). Thus, 5-HT mimicked the action of DA in attenuating and reversing the excitatory action of CCK-8S on N.Acc. neurons, indicating that interactions between CCK and DA are not mediated specifically via the possible CCK/DA receptor complex. Rather, CCK-8S and DA most likely exert their actions independently via depolarizing and hyperpolarizing the neuronal cell membrane, respectively. This view is supported by the findings that: (1) the net result of coadministration of CCK and DA or CCK and 5-HT is dependent upon the relative amounts of the two substances being administered,[19,20] (2) in addition to opposing the actions of DA and 5-HT, CCK-8S also enhances the excitatory effect of GLUT,[20,34] and (3) DA antagonizes both CCK and GLUT-induced activation of N.Acc. cells equally well.[19,20] Taken together, these results strongly suggest that the interaction between CCK and DA is best explained by the additive effects of CCK and DA at common target sites in the N.Acc.

To demonstrate further that CCK has a functional role in the N.Acc., we studied the effects of lesioning DA/CCK ascending fibers in the medial forebrain bundle (MFB) by 6-hydroxydopamine (6-OHDA) on the responses of N.Acc. cells to CCK and DA.[54] To confine the damage induced by 6-OHDA to DA fibers, rats were pretreated with desipramine, a norepinephrine (NE) uptake blocker, prior to the injection of 6-OHDA. Two other groups of rats were injected with either the vehicle or 5,7-dihydroxytryptamine (5,7-DHT, a relatively selective neurotoxin for serotoinergic systems) directly into the MFB and served as controls. Nomifensin (25 mg/kg, ip), a DA uptake blocker, was given 30 min prior to the injection of 5,7-DHT to prevent possible damage of DA systems from 5,7-DHT. The techniques of sucrose–potassium phosphate–glyoxylic acid histofluorescence,[55] and high-performance liquid chromatography-EC (HPLC-EC) were used for determining catecholamine histofluorescence and DA levels, respectively, in the N.Acc. to demonstrate the effectiveness of 6-OHDA in lesioning DA fibers.

In 6-OHDA rats, DA levels were reduced to 10% of controls, and there was a dramatic reduction of DA varicosities in the N.Acc.[54] In these rats, when compared to control rats, the dose-response curves for iontophoretically applied DA and CCK on N.Acc. neurons were shifted to the left; in contrast, the dose-response curves for 5-HT and GLUT were unchanged.[54] The sensitivity of N.Acc. cells to DA or CCK was unaffected in vehicle or 5,7-DHT pretreated rats (TABLE 1). Consistent with our results are the reports that lesions of DA cells increase the density of CCK binding sites in the N.Acc. of guinea pig[56] and enhance the behavioral responses of rats to CCK and DA agonists.[57] Thus, lesions of DA/CCK fibers by 6-OHDA are effective in inducing the development of denervation supersensitivity of N.Acc. cells to both CCK and DA. The results provide further evidence that CCK-8S coexists with DA; moreover, they indicate that CCK-8S has a functional role in the N.Acc.

## Effects of CCK on the Release of DA

By using knife cuts and kainic acid lesions, Hays et al.[58] demonstrated that approximately 25% of caudate CCK receptors lie on afferent axons and terminals, and that 75% of CCK receptors are located on neuronal cell bodies intrinsic to the caudate nucleus. Thus, it is possible that CCK, in addition to its action on N.Acc. cells, may modulate the release of DA via presynaptic receptors on CCK/DA terminals.

**TABLE 1.** Comparison of $ED_{80s}$ and $ID_{50s}$ of CCK-8S, DA, 5-HT, and GLUT on N.Acc. Neurons in 6-OHDA Pretreated and Various Control Rats

| Category of Rat | CCK-8S $ED_{80s}$ | DA $ID_{50s}$ | GLUT $ED_{80s}$ | 5-HT $ID_{50s}$ |
|---|---|---|---|---|
| Untreated | $29.2 \pm 4.9$ | $29.2 \pm 4.1$ | $25.7 \pm 2.3$ | $21.1 \pm 2.6$ |
| | ($n = 45$) | ($n = 34$) | ($n = 48$) | ($n = 9$) |
| Vehicle | $24.3 \pm 5.7$ | $24.3 \pm 5.7$ | $21.3 \pm 4.7$ | – |
| | ($n = 8$) | ($n = 7$) | ($n = 8$) | |
| 5,7-DHT | $27.7 \pm 3.6$ | $19.8 \pm 2.5$ | $26.7 \pm 3.4$ | $3.8 \pm 0.7^{a,b}$ |
| | ($n = 13$) | ($n = 21$) | ($n = 21$) | ($n = 12$) |
| 6-OHDA | $29.1 \pm 7.7$ | $24.9 \pm 7.3$ | $24.5 \pm 1.8$ | – |
| (Outside MFB) | ($n = 13$) | ($n = 10$) | ($n = 21$) | |
| 6-OHDA | $8.5 \pm 1.3^a$ | $8.9 \pm 0.2^a$ | $24.5 \pm 3.0$ | $25.0 \pm 6.3$ |
| (Inside MFB) | ($n = 40$) | ($n = 43$) | ($n = 41$) | ($n = 11$) |

NOTE: Values are given as the mean $\pm$ S.E.M. nanoamperes; $n$ represents the number of neurons.

$^a$ $p < 0.001$, compared to control groups (two-tailed $t$-test).
$^b$ $p < 0.01$, compred to 6-OHDA group (two-tailed $t$-test).

We have investigated the influence of CCK on the *in vivo* release of DA in the N.Acc. by using the technique of push–pull cannula local perfusion.[41,42] Continuous local perfusion for 4–5 hr at very slow rates caused a minimum of tissue damage. DA terminals within the perfused portion of the N.Acc. appeared to be functionally intact because: (1) ip injection of L-DOPA, the immediate precursor of DA, increased the release of endogenous DA, and (2) $^3$H-DA was continuously synthesized from locally administered $^3$H-tyrosine. This release was from a localized area only because no detectable DA was found in perfusates from an adjacent cortical area when 55-mM K$^+$ was applied. The K$^+$-induced release of DA was also found to be calcium-dependent, indicating that the process of release was physiological. In this system, CCK-8S, but not CCK-8US, attenuated the K$^+$-evoked release of DA in a dose-dependent fashion.[41,42]

In another study, we examined the action of CCK peptides on the basal and K$^+$-evoked release of $^3$H-DA, newly synthesized from $^3$H-tyrosine.[42] We chose to use newly synthesized $^3$H-DA as a marker of dopaminergic activity within the N.Acc. for two reasons: (1) the enhanced sensitivity afforded by radioisotopic techniques makes it possible to measure DA release under resting conditions, and (2) it appears that newly synthesized DA is preferentially released from nerve terminals.[59]

It appears that a large percentage of the $^3$H-DA released under resting conditions is dependent upon nerve impulse activity, since it was found that tetrodotoxin, absence of extracellular Ca$^{2+}$, and the inhibition of DA synthesis by alpha-methyl-$p$-tyrosine all decreased $^3$H-DA release by over 50%. In addition, the K$^+$-evoked release of $^3$H-DA was found to be almost completely dependent upon extracellular Ca$^{2+}$. These results indicate strongly that the release of $^3$H-DA is a physiological process.[42]

When CCK-8S was administered into the N.Acc., it was found to increase the basal levels of $^3$H-DA released at concentrations of $2 \times 10^{-8}$ and $2 \times 10^{-7}$ M. However, at $2 \times 10^{-6}$ M there was no longer an effect by this peptide. The CCK-8US was found to have no effect at a concentration that was maximally effective for the sulfated form (FIG. 3). In contrast to its effect on the basal release of $^3$H-DA, CCK-8S was found to attenuate the K$^+$-evoked release of $^3$H-DA from the N.Acc. in a concentration-dependent fashion from $2 \times 10^{-9}$ to $2 \times 10^{-6}$ M (FIG. 4). The CCK-8US had no effect on K$^+$-evoked release.[42]

To assess the possibility that the effect of CCK-8 on DA release is mediated by

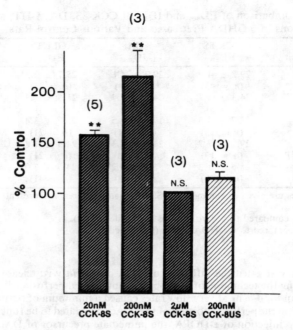

**FIGURE 3.** Effects of CCK-8 peptides on the basal release of newly synthesized $^3$H-DA. CCK-8 peptides were added to the superfusion buffer for 10 min at the indicated concentrations. At 20 nM, CCK-8S increased release to $155.8 \pm 5.8\%$ ($n = 5$) of control, whereas 200-nM CCK-8S increased release to $215.3 \pm 26\%$ ($n = 3$) of control. CCK-8S at 2 μM and CCK-8US at 200 nM had no effect on basal release. **Indicates values that are significantly different from that of control. $p < 0.01$ using a two-tailed Student's $t$-test. Numbers in parentheses are the number of animals tested. (From Voigt et al.[42] Reproduced by permission.)

long-loop feedback pathways, *in vitro* brain slice preparations were used. We observed that CCK-8S could enhance the resting release of DA from the posterior N.Acc.[43] This is very similar to what we have reported for CCK-8S action on the basal release of newly synthesized $^3$H-DA in the N.Acc. *in vivo*.[42] Since we removed the interconnections between the N.Acc. and other brain nuclei by performing this study *in vitro*, it would appear that this enhancing effect of CCK-8S on basal release of DA from the N.Acc. is the result of a direct action on presynaptic terminals or an indirect action mediated by local circuit neurons or axon collaterals of output neurons within the posterior N.Acc. In addition, as this effect was only observed in the posterior N.Acc. where most of the DA/CCK fibers terminate, it might be a phenomenon associated with CCK/DA coexistence. We also found that CCK-8S produced an attenuation of the K$^+$-evoked release of DA. Furthermore, proglumide, at a concentration of 500 μM, blocked the effect of CCK-8S on DA release.[43] The results are consistent with those from our push–pull cannula local perfusion study,[21] and they suggest that proglumide is much more effective in blocking the effect produced by CCK-8S on postsynaptic neurons than on presynaptic DA/CCK terminals. Is it possible that CCK receptors located on presynaptic DA terminals are different from those on postsynaptic neurons, as has been shown repeatedly for monoamines and perhaps also other transmitter

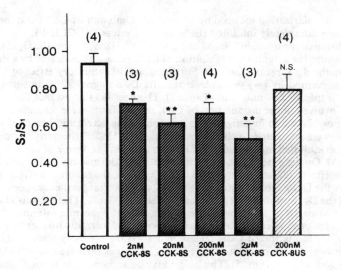

**FIGURE 4.** Effect of CCK-8 peptides on the $K^+$-evoked release of newly synthesized $^3H$-DA. CCK-8 peptides were added to the superfusion buffer during the $S_2$ period. Control value for $S_2/S_1$ was $0.93 \pm 0.06$. CCK-8S, when added to the buffer, attenuated release. $S_2/S_1$ values were: 2 nM, $0.71 \pm 0.03$; 20 nM, $0.61 \pm 0.05$; 200 nM, $0.66 \pm 0.06$; 2 µm, $0.52 \pm 0.08$. In contrast, CCK-8US had no significant effect on release ($0.78 \pm 0.09$). *, $p < 0.05$; **, $p < 0.02$ using a two-tailed Student's $t$-test. Numbers in parentheses are the number of animals tested. (From Voigt et al.[42] Reproduced by permission.)

systems? Different types of CCK receptors could explain the different potency of proglumide in our electrophysiological and release studies. In fact, there is evidence suggesting that at least two distinct CCK receptor subtypes exist in the brain.[32,37] Of course, more studies are needed to further characterize CCK receptor subtypes.

It has been postulated that CCK-8S may exert its effects by enhancing the ability of DA and DA agonists to inhibit DA transmission via DA autoreceptors,[60,61] which exhibit pharmacological characteristics of the DA $D_2$ receptor subtype.[62,63] This hypothesis was tested in one of our studies[43] and found not to be the case, since administration of the selective $D_2$ DA receptor antagonist sulpiride[64,65] did not block the inhibitory effect of CCK-8S on $K^+$-evoked DA release from slices of posterior N.Acc.[43] That DA autoreceptors are present in the posterior N.Acc. is suggested by the fact that sulpiride alone caused a marked enhancement of $K^+$-evoked DA release.[43]

## Effects of DA on the Release of CCK-LI

Since the great majority of CCK in the posterior medial N.Acc. coexists with DA, it is likely that DA might modulate the release of both DA and CCK via presynaptic autoreceptors localized on DA/CCK terminals. The effect of specific $D_2$ DA receptor agonists and antagonists on $K^+$-evoked release of CCK-like immunoreactivity (CCK-LI) was studied in tissue slices of the rat posterior N.Acc.[66] The results indicate that CCK-LI can be released from slices made from the posterior N.Acc. This release was evoked by depolarization induced by 55-mM $K^+$. Omission of $Ca^{2+}$ from the incubation medium completely inhibited the $K^+$-evoked release of CCK-LI.

Incubation of the tissue in 100 nM or 1 μM of LY 141865,[67] a specific $D_2$ DA receptor agonist, resulted in a significant inhibition of CCK release as indicated by a significant decrease in the $S_2/S_1$ ratio (TABLE 2). Furthermore, the inhibitory effect of LY 141865 could be prevented by (−)-sulpiride, a specific $D_2$ antagonist,[64,65] but not by SCH 23390,[68,69] a specific $D_1$ antagonist (TABLE 2). These results suggest that the $D_2$ receptor might be involved in the modulation of CCK release from nerve terminals present in the posterior N.Acc. To investigate this possibility, the active and inactive isomers of LY 141865 were presented to the tissue slices. LY 171555,[70] the active isomer of LY 141865, also inhibited the release of CCK, with the greatest degree of inhibition occurring at 1 nM. On the other hand, 1 nM of LY 181990,[70] the inactive isomer of LY 141865, had no significant effect on the release of CCK. Thus, the inhibitory effect on release of CCK by the $D_2$ agonist was stereospecific (TABLE 3). This further suggests that stimulation of the $D_2$ receptor might modulate the release of CCK. These results also showed LY 171555 to be 10 to 100 times more potent than the racemic mixture LY 141865. The reason for this increased potency is not known and warrants further investigation. Curiously, the inhibition of CCK release by LY 171555 was only present at the lower concentrations. As the concentration of LY 171555 was increased to 100 nM, the inhibitory effect was lost (FIG. 5). This effect may be an important homeostatic mechanism regulating the opposing effects of DA and CCK on N.Acc. neurons (see below).

## DA AND CCK INTERACTIONS: A MODEL

FIGURE 6 illustrates a working hypothesis for the dynamic interactions between DA and CCK at both pre- and postsynaptic levels in the N.Acc. It is clear that DA is the predominant transmitter of the DA/CCK neurons, since the amount of CCK released is only a very small fraction of the amount of DA (TABLE 4). However, CCK is an extremely potent activator in the N.Acc.; even a small amount of CCK at the synaptic cleft may disrupt normal DA function. To minimize the CCK interference, DA suppresses the release of CCK; and CCK itself enhances the basal release of DA, which

**TABLE 2.** Effects of $D_1$ or $D_2$ DA Receptor Antagonists on the Inhibition by 100 nM LY 141865 of $K^+$-Evoked Release of CCK-LI

| Treatment | n | $S_2/S_1$ | $B_2/B_1$ |
|---|---|---|---|
| Control | 11 | 0.77 ± 0.04[a] | 0.76 ± 0.10 |
| 100 nM LY 141865 | 10 | 0.41 ± 0.07 | 0.83 ± 0.12 |
| + 10 μM (−)-sulpiride | 9 | 0.75 ± 0.08[a] | 0.74 ± 0.10 |
| + 10 μM SCH 23390 | 11 | 0.47 ± 0.03 | 0.82 ± 0.16 |
| 10 μM (−)-sulpiride | 9 | 0.78 ± 0.10[a] | 0.80 ± 0.12 |
| 10 μM SCH 23390 | 6 | 0.79 ± 0.11[a] | 0.90 ± 0.07 |

NOTE: Results are expressed as the ratio of $S_2$ to $S_1$, which was consistent between experiments; the $S_1$ and $S_2$ values were determined by subtracting the previous basal release ($B_1$ and $B_2$) from the following $K^+$-evoked release. Values are given as the mean ± S.E.M.; $n$ represents the number of experiments.

[a] Significantly different from LY 141865, or LY 141865 plus SCH 23390 ($p < 0.05$, Duncan's multiple-range test).

**TABLE 3.** Stereospecificity of the Isomers of LY 141865 on Release of CCK-LI from the Posterior N.Acc.

| Treatment | $n$ | $S_2/S_1$ | $B_2/B_1$ |
|---|---|---|---|
| Control | 11 | $0.77 \pm 0.04$ | $0.76 \pm 0.10$ |
| 0.1 nM LY 171555 | 7 | $0.50 \pm 0.09^a$ | $0.73 \pm 0.12$ |
| 1 nM LY 171555 | 7 | $0.42 \pm 0.04^a$ | $0.74 \pm 0.10$ |
| 10 nM LY 171555 | 8 | $0.51 \pm 0.03^a$ | $0.79 \pm 0.16$ |
| 50 nM LY 171555 | 12 | $0.59 \pm 0.04^a$ | $0.74 \pm 0.11$ |
| 100 nM LY 171555 | 10 | $0.65 \pm 0.05$ | $0.93 \pm 0.14$ |
| 1 nM LY 181990 | 5 | $0.67 \pm 0.04^b$ | $0.68 \pm 0.11$ |

NOTE: LY 171555 is the active isomer and LY 18190 is the inactive isomer of LY 141865; $n$ represents the number of experiments.

[a] Significantly different from control ($p < 0.05$, Dunnett's $t$-test).
[b] Significantly different from 1 nM LY 171555 ($p < 0.01$, Student's $t$-test).

counteracts the excitatory action of CCK on N.Acc. cells. However, when DA neurons become hyperactive, and the synaptic cleft is flooded with DA (as mimicked by K⁺-evoked release), the inhibitory effect of DA on the release of CCK disappears. Due to disinhibition, more CCK-8S is released to counteract the hyperpolarizing action of DA on N.Acc. neurons. In addition, CCK no longer potentiates the release of DA. In fact, CCK, via either direct or indirect action, attenuates the evoked release of DA. This inhibition exhibits a more typical concentration-response curve, with greater inhibition of DA release occurring with increased CCK concentration. When the release of DA returns to normal, DA again inhibits the release of CCK. In essence, we hypothesize that CCK is an intrinsic and/or extrinsic mechanism (from those CCK cells not containing DA) that regulates DA activity. CCK is of particular importance in reducing DA hyperactivity when the DA autoregulatory mechanism may not be sufficient for attenuation of an overflow of DA. For example, it has been shown that stimulation causes the release of DA to increase 30- to 40-fold (TABLE 4), whereas the DA autoregulatory system reduces only about 50% of the DA activity.[63,71] Therefore, malfunctioning of such a dynamic interaction between DA and CCK might result in a DA dysregulation, which could be an important factor in the elaboration of schizophrenic symptoms.

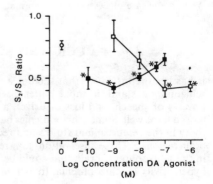

**FIGURE 5.** Effect of various concentrations of LY 141865 (□) and its active isomer LY 171555 (■) on the $S_2/S_1$ ratio of CCK-LI release from tissue slices of the posterior nucleus accumbens: * denotes that the $S_2/S_1$ ratio is significantly different from that of control (O). (From Martin *et al.*[66] Reproduced by permission.)

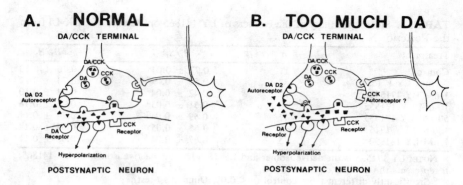

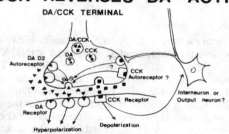

**FIGURE 6.** A model illustrating the dynamic interactions between DA and CCK at both pre- and postsynaptic levels in the N.Acc. (**A**) Under the normal condition, DA is the predominant transmitter because the amount of basal and K+-evoked release of CCK is only a very small fraction of that of DA. However, the very potent action of CCK may disrupt DA function. DA attenuates the release of CCK. On the other hand, CCK enhances the basal release of DA, which counteracts the excitatory action of CCK on the N.Acc. cells. (**B**) Whenever DA neurons become hyperactive or too much DA is released at the synaptic cleft, DA acts upon DA $D_2$ autoreceptors and attenuates its own release. In addition, DA no longer inhibits the release of CCK. (**C**) Due to disinhibition, more CCK is available at the synaptic cleft, causing a depolarization of the cell membrane of N.Acc. neurons and counteracting the hyperpolarizing effect produced by DA. In addition, CCK via either direct or indirect mechanisms, attenuates the evoked release of DA. When the release of DA is back to normal, DA again inhibits CCK release.

## CCK AND SCHIZOPHRENIA

It has been reported[72,73] that there is a reduction of CCK in the temporal cortex of schizophrenics and, in those patients with negative symptoms (affective flattening, poverty of speech, and loss of drive), a reduction of CCK in the hippocampus and amygdala as well. Some schizophrenics have a significant decrease in CCK immunoreactivity in the cerebrospinal fluid[74] and reduced numbers of CCK receptors in specific brain regions.[75] These observations may reflect a degeneration of CCK neuronal systems in the schizophrenic brain that could be functionally related to the hypothesis of DA hyperactivity in schizophrenia. In fact, in open clinical trials, both CCK and the chem-

**TABLE 4.** Comparison of Amounts of Dopamine and Cholecystokinin Released in Control Buffer vs. a High K$^+$ Buffer

|  | DA (pg/5 min) | CCK (pg/5 min) | DA/CCK |
|---|---|---|---|
| Basal release | 191 ± 13 | 11.4 ± 2.0 | 17 |
| 55 mM K$^+$ | 7534 ± 1233 | 38.9 ± 4.2 | 194 |

ically related decapeptide ceruletide were found to significantly modulate clinical symptoms of chronic schizophrenic patients who were resistant to neuroleptic treatment.[76-79]

In contrast to the results obtained from open clinical trials, more recent controlled clinical studies provide no evidence that systemic administration of CCK or caerulein modifies schizophrenic symptoms.[80-87] However, failure to observe a therapeutic effect for CCK-8S or caerulein could be due simply to insufficient amounts of these peptides passing the blood–brain barrier (BBB). Indeed, despite adequate caerulein drug levels in plasma, no definitive CNS effects of caerulein could be demonstrated;[87] neither EEG patterns of visual evoked potential nor plasma levels of prolactin or growth hormone were modified with caerulein. An elevation of prolactin level would be expected if sufficient amounts of CCK-8 or caerulein passed the BBB because in a previous study,[88] it was demonstrated that intraventricular, but not intravenous, administration of CCK-8 elevated plasma prolactin. Moreover, no $^{125}$I-CCK-8 was observed in the CSF following its intravenous injection.[89] Although it cannot be ruled out that a very small fraction of peripherally administered CCK-8 might cross the BBB,[90] the action of systemically injected CCK-8 appears to be mediated primarily by CCK receptors in the area postrema[37,91] and vagal afferents to the nucleus tractus solitarii.[92-95] Because peripherally circulating CCK is rapidly metabolized,[96,97] and it does not cross the BBB easily,[89,98] and because of the small number of schizophrenia patients in the clinical trials, the question of whether CCK-8 can reduce schizophrenic symptoms remains essentially untested at the present time. It should also be pointed out that none of the clinical trials to date have used an active placebo. As caerulein, CCK-8S, and CCK-33 all induce gastrointestinal symptoms, it is possible that such side effects may have "unblinded" the controlled investigations. To determine whether CCK has an antipsychotic action requires potent and selective CCK agonists that can readily cross the BBB. Alternatively, it might be fruitful to enhance the synthesis and release of CCK and to inhibit the degradation enzyme of CCK so that the amount of CCK at synaptic clefts will increase. In other words, it is desperately needed to understand the regulation of CCK biochemical metabolic machinery and pharmacology and physiology of CCK.

In an attempt to evaluate the role of CCK in potential DA activity,[52,53,60,61] Innis et al.[99] administered the putative CCK antagonist proglumide to schizophrenic patients in a double-blind placebo-controlled study. All patients were receiving concurrent neuroleptic medication, but were still significantly symptomatic. At doses of 1600 and 3200 mg/day, proglumide was without effect on the patients' psychosis ratings. In fact, the psychoses of two patients were deteriorated by proglumide. Because proglumide does not appear to have any antipsychotic properties, the results fail to support the view that CCK exerts its actions by potentiating DA activity. However, the selectivity and potency of proglumide as a CCK antagonist has been questioned.[27-32] In order to provide a definitive answer to the question whether CCK antagonists may block the possible DA-potentiating action of CCK and, therefore, may alleviate some schizophrenic symptoms, more potent and selective CCK antagonists should be tested.

## CCK AND ANTIPSYCHOTIC DRUGS

Following chronic treatment with the antipsychotic agent haloperidol, there was a significant increase in brain-specific $^{125}$I-labeled CCK binding sites.[56] Interestingly, in the guinea pig, the chronic haloperidol-induced increase of CCK binding was observed in the mesolimbic regions and frontal cortex, but not in the neostriatum.[56] Consistent with these findings is the report by Debonnel and de Montingny[100] showing that 3 to 5 weeks of haloperidol treatment induced a supersensitive response of N.Acc. neurons to CCK-8S; surprisingly, the response of N.Acc. cells to DA remained unchanged. By contrast, we have shown that N.Acc. neurons become supersensitive to both CCK-8S and DA following one-month treatment with either haloperidol or clozapine.[101] Taken together, the results from these studies suggest that CCK may have an important role in the therapeutic action of APDs. Support for this view comes from a recent study[102] showing that iv injection of proglumide but not naloxone reversed the depolarization block of DA activity produced by chronic haloperidol treatment. We have demonstrated that lorglumide administered iv or injected directly into the medial N.Acc. reverses chronic haloperidol-induced depolarization inactivation of midbrain DA cells.[103] Lorglumide injected into other brain regions, such as the neostriatum and lateral part of N.Acc., was without effect. These results suggest that CCK receptors in the medial N.Acc. form an important link for maintaining chronic haloperidol-induced effect on DA cells and that CCK is involved in the therapeutic action of APDs.

## CONCLUSIONS

Since the discovery of the coexistence of DA and CCK in the subpopulation of mesencephalic DA neurons, research into the interaction between DA and CCK has been flourishing. The results so far indicate that CCK and DA interact intimately at both pre- and postsynaptic levels in the N.Acc. Our results indicate that CCK functionally antagonizes DA.

In order to clarify further the role of CCK and DA as coexisting neurotransmitters or neuromodulators and the role of CCK in the central nervous system in general, it is necessary to have specific and potent CCK antagonists. Most recently, a new generation of CCK receptor antagonists, including lorglumide, L-364,718, and CCK analogues, which have degrees of selectivity for different CCK receptor subtypes, has been developed.[104] Studies are on-going in various laboratories to identify and characterize subclasses of CCK receptors. With the availability of specific CCK antagonists, it can be expected that the research into the pharmacological and physiological actions of CCK will be greatly advanced. Moreover, it is warranted to examine further the potential therapeutic utility of CCK agonists and antagonists in the management of psychiatric disorders.

## ACKNOWLEDGMENTS

Special thanks to Jane Blanchard and Judith Shivak for preparation of this manuscript.

## REFERENCES

1. Ivy, A. C. & E. Oldberg. 1928. A hormone mechanism for gall-bladder contraction and evacuation. Am. J. Physiol. **86:** 599–613.

2. BEINFELD, M. C., D. K. MEYER, R. L. ESKAY, R. T. JENSEN & M. J. BROWNSTEIN. 1981. The distribution of cholecystokinin immunoreactivity in the central nervous system of the rat as determined by radiommunoassay. Brain Res. **212:** 51-57.

3. INNIS, R. B. & S. H. SNYDER. 1980. Distinct cholecystokinin receptors in brain and pancreas. Proc. Natl. Acad. Sci. U.S.A. **77:** 6917-6921.

4. VANDERHAEGHEN, J. J., J. C. SIGNEAU & W. GEPT. 1975. New peptide in the vertebrate CNS reacting with gastrin antibodies. Nature **257:** 604-605.

5. VANDERHAEGHEN, J. J. & J. N. CRAWLEY, Eds. 1985. Neuronal Cholecystokinin. Ann. N.Y. Acad. Sci. **448**.

6. HOKFELT, T., L. SKIRBOLL, J. F. REHFELD, M. GOLDSTEIN, K. MARKEY & O. DANN. 1980. A subpopulation of mesencephalic dopamine neurons projecting to limbic areas contains a cholecystokinin-like peptide: Evidence from immunohistochemistry combined with retrograde tracing. Neurosci. **5:** 2093-2124.

7. FALLON, J. H, R. HICKS & S. E. LOUGHLIN. 1983. The origin of cholecystokinin terminals in the basal forebrain of the rat: Evidence from immunofluorescence and retrograde tracing. Neurosci. Lett. **37:** 29-35.

8. GILLES, C., F. LOTSTRA & J. J. VANDERHAEGHEN. 1983. CCK nerve terminals in the rat striatal and limbic areas originate partly in the brain stem and partly in telencephalic structures. Life Sci. **32:** 1683-1690.

9. MARLEY, P. D., P. C. EMSON & J. F. REHFELD. 1982. Effect of 6-hydroxydopamine lesions of the medial forebrain bundle on the distribution of cholecystokinin in rat forebrain. Brain Res. **252:** 382-385.

10. STUDLER, J. M., H. SIMON, F. CESSELIN, J. C. LEGRAND, J. GLOWINSKI & J. P. TASSIN. 1981. Biochemical investigation on the localization of the cholecystokinin octapeptide in dopaminergic neurons originating from the ventral tegmental area of the rat. Neuropeptides **2:** 131-139.

11. ZABORSZKY, L., G. F. ALHEID, M. C. BEINFELD, L. E. EIDEN, L. HEIMER & M. PALKOVITS. 1985. Cholecystokinin innervation of the ventral striatum: A morphological and radioimmunological study. Neuroscience **14:** 427-453.

12. LOOPUIJT, L. D. & D. VAN DER KOOY. 1985. Simultaneous ultrastructural localization of cholecystokinin- and tyrosine hydroxylase-like immunoreactivity in nerve fibers of the rat nucleus accumbens. Neurosci. Lett. **56:** 329-334.

13. STUDLER, J. M., M. REIBAUD, G. TRAMU, G. BLANC, J. GLOWINSKI & J. P. TASSIN. 1984. Pharmacological study on the mixed CCK/DA meso-nucleus accumbens pathway: Evidence for the existence of storage sites containing the two transmitters. Brain Res. **298:** 91-97.

14. STEVENS, J. R. 1973. An anatomy of schizophrenia? Arch. Gen. Psychiat. **29:** 177-189.

15. WHITE, F. J. & R. Y. WANG. 1983. Differential effects of classical and atypical antipsychotic drugs on A9 and A10 dopamine neurons. Science **221:** 1054-1057.

16. CHIODO, L. A. & B. S. BUNNEY. 1983. Typical and atypical neuroleptics: Differential effects of chronic administration of the activity of A9 and A10 midbrain dopaminergic neurons. J. Neurosci. **3:** 1607-1619.

17. BUNNEY, B.S. & A. A. GRACE. 1978. Acute and chronic haloperidol treatment: Comparison of effects on nigral dopaminergic cell activity. Life Sci. **23:** 1715-1728.

18. WHITE, F. J. & R. Y. WANG. 1983. Comparison of the effects of chronic haloperidol treatment on A9 and A10 dopamine neurons in the rat. Life Sci. **32:** 983-993.

19. WHITE, F. J. & R. Y. WANG. 1984. Interactions of cholecystokinin octapeptide and dopamine on nucleus accumbens neurons. Brain Res. **300:** 161-166.

20. WANG, R. Y. & X.-T. HU. 1986. Does cholecystokinin potentiate dopamine action in the nucleus accumbens? Brain Res. **380:** 363-367.

21. WANG, R. Y., F. J. WHITE & M. M. VOIGT. 1984. Cholecystokinin, dopamine and schizophrenia. Trends in Pharmacol. Sci. **5:** 436-438.

22. WANG, R. Y. & F. J. WHITE. 1985. Electrophysiological effects of cholecystokinin on central dopaminergic systems. *In* Endocoids. H. Lal, F. LaBella, and J. Lane, Eds. 95-103. Alan Liss. New York.

23. WANG, R. Y., F. J. WHITE & M. M. VOIGT. 1985. Interactions of CCK and dopamine in the nucleus accumbens. Ann. N.Y. Acad. Sci. **448:** 352-360.

24. CHIODO, L. A. & B. S. BUNNEY. 1983. Proglumide: Selective antagonism of excitatory effects of cholecystokinin in central nervous system. Science 219: 1449–1451.
25. HAHNE, W. F., R. T. JENSEN, G.F. LEMP & J. D. GARDNER. 1981. Proglumide and benzotript: Members of a different class of cholecystokinin receptor antagonists. Proc. Natl. Acad. Sci. U.S.A. 78: 6304–6308.
26. BUNNEY, B. S., L. A. CHIODO & A. S. FREEMAN. 1985. Further studies on the specificity of proglumide as a selective cholecystokinin antagonist in the central nervous system. Ann. N.Y. Acad. Sci. 448: 345–351.
27. COLLINS, S., D. WALKER, P. FORSYTH & L. BELBECK. 1983. The effects of proglumide on cholecystokinin-, bombesin-, and glucagon-induced satiety in the rat. Life Sci. 32: 2223–2229.
28. CRAWLEY, J. N., J. A. STIVERS, D. W. HOMMER, L. R. SKIRBOLL & S. M. PAUL. 1986. Antagonists of central and peripheral behavioral actions of cholecystokinin octapeptide. J. Pharmacol. Exp. Ther. 236: 320–330.
29. HSIAO, S., G. KATSUURA & S. ITOH. 1984. Cholecystokinin tetrapeptide, proglumide and open-field behavior in rats. Life Sci. 34: 2165–2168.
30. GAUDREAU, P., R. QUIRION, S. ST.-PIERRE & C. B. PERT. 1983. Characterization and visualization of cholecystokinin receptors in rat brain using ³H-pentagastrin. Peptides 4: 755–762.
31. LIN, C. W. & T. MILLER. 1985. Characterization of cholecystokinin receptor sites in guinea-pig cortical membranes using ¹²⁵I-bolton hunter-cholecystokinin octapeptide. J. Pharmacol. Exp. Ther. 232: 775–780.
32. WENNOGLE, L. P., D. J. STELL & B. PETRACK. 1985. Characterization of central cholecystokinin receptors using a radioiodinated octapeptide probe. Life Sci. 36: 1485–1492.
33. MAKOVEC, F., R. CHISTE, M. RANI, M. A. PACINI, I. SETRIKAR & L. A. ROVATI. 1985. New glutaramic acid derivatives with potent competitive and specific cholecystokinin-antagonistic activity. Arzneim. Forsch. 35: 1048–1051.
34. WANG, R. Y., R. J. KASSER & X. T. HU. 1988. Cholecystokinin receptor subtypes in the rat nucleus accumbens. In Cholecystokinin Antagonists. R. Y. Wang and R. Schoenfeld, Eds. Alan Liss. New York. In press.
35. VAN DIJK, A., J. G. RICHARDS, A. TRZECIAK, D. GRILLESSEN & H. MOHLER. 1984. Cholecystokinin receptors: Biochemical demonstration and autoradiographical localization in rat brain and pancreas using [³H]cholecystokinin 8 as radioligand. J. Neurosci. 4: 1021–1033.
36. ZARBIN, M. A., R. B. INNIS, J. K. WAMSLEY, S. H. SNYDER & M. J. KUHAR. 1983. Autoradiographic localization of cholecystokinin receptors in rodent brain. J. Neurosci. 5: 877–906.
37. MORAN, T. H., P. H. ROBINSON, M. S. GOLDRICH & P. R. McHUGH. 1986. Two brain cholecystokinin receptors: Implications for behavioral actions. Brain Res. 362: 175–179.
38. HAND, T. H., X.-T. HU & R. Y. WANG. 1987. Differential effects of typical and atypical antipsychotic drugs on the activity of dopamine neurons and their postsynaptic target cells. In Neurophysiology of Dopaminergic Systems: Current Status and Clinical Perspectives. L. A. Chiodo and A. S. Freeman, Eds. Lake Shore. Detroit, Mich.
39. HU, X.-T. & R. Y. WANG. 1986. Differential effects of haloperidol and clozapine in the rat neostriatum and nucleus accumbens: Microiontophoretic studies. Neurosci. Abstr. 12: 1389.
40. FUXE, K., K. ANDERSSON, V. LOCATELLI, L. F. AGNATI, T. HOKFELT, L. SKIRBOLL & V. MUTT. 1980. Cholecystokinin peptides produce marked reduction of dopamine turnover in discrete areas in the rat brain following intraventricular injection. Eur. J. Pharmacol. 67: 329–331.
41. VOIGT, M. M. & R. Y. WANG. 1984. In vivo release of dopamine in the nucleus accumbens of the rat: Modulation by cholecystokinin. Brain Res. 296: 189–193.
42. VOIGT, M. M., R. Y. WANG & T. C. WESTFALL. 1985. The effects of cholecystokinin on in vivo release of dopamine from the nucleus accumbens of the rat. J. Neurosci. 5: 2744–2749.
43. VOIGT, M. M., R. Y. WANG & T. C. WESTFALL. 1986. Cholecystokinin-octapeptides alter

the release of endogenous dopamine from rat nucleus accumbens *in vitro*. J. Pharmacol. Exp. Ther. **237:** 147–153.

44. COHEN, S. L., M. KNIGHT, C. A. TAMMINGA & T. N. CHASE. 1982. Cholecystokinin effects on conditioned avoidance behavior, stereotypy and catalepsy. Eur. J. Pharmacol. **83:** 213–222.

45. KELLY, P. H., P. W. SEVIOUR & S. D. IVERSEN. 1975. Amphetamine and apomorphine responses in the rat following 6-OHDA lesions of the nucleus accumbens septi and corpus striatum. Brain Res. **94:** 507–522.

46. SCHNEIDER, L. H., J. E. ALPERT & D. S. IVERSEN. 1983. CCK-8 modulation of mesolimbic doapmine: Antagonism of amphetamine-stimulated behaviors. Peptides **4:** 749–753.

47. VACCARINO, F. J. & G. F. KOOB. 1984. Microinjections of nanogram amounts of sulfated cholecystokinin octapeptide into the rat nucleus accumbens attenuates brain stimulation reward. Neurosci. Lett. **52:** 61–66.

48. VAN REE, J. M., O. GAFFORI & D. DE WIED. 1983. In rats the behavioral profile of CCK-8-related peptides resembles that of antipsychotic agents. Eur. J. Pharmacol. **93:** 65–78.

49. ZETLER, G. 1981. Central effects of ceruletide analogues. Peptides, Suppl. 2, **2:** 65–99.

50. ZETLER, G. 1983. Neuroleptic-like effects of ceruletide and cholecystokinin octapeptide: Interactions with apomorphine, methylphenidate and picrotoxin. Eur. J. Pharmacol. **94:** 261–270.

51. ZETLER, G. 1985. Antistereotypic effects of cholecystokinin octapeptide (CCK-8), ceruletide and related peptides on apomorphine-induced gnawing in sensitized mice. Neuropharmacology **24:** 251–259.

52. CRAWLEY, J. N., D.W. HOMMER & L. R. SKIRBOLL. 1984. Behavioral and neurophysiological evidence for a facilatory interaction between coexisting transmitters: Cholecystokinin and dopamine. Neurochem. Int. **6:** 755–760.

53. CRAWLEY, J. N., J. A. STIVERS, L. K. BLUMSTEIN & S. M. PAUL. 1985. Cholecystokinin potentiates dopamine-mediated behaviors: Evidence for modulation specific to a site of co-existence. J. Neurosci. **5:** 1972–1983.

54. HU, X.-T. & R. Y. WANG. 1985. Denervation supersensitivity to cholecystokinin and dopamine in the rat nucleus accumbens: Microiontophorectic studies. Neurosci. Abstr. **11:** 743.

55. DE LA TORRE, J. C. 1980. Standardization of the sucrose-potassium phosphate-glyoxylic acid histofluorescence method for tissue monoamines. Neurosci. Lett. **17:** 339–340.

56. CHANG, R. S. L., V. J. LOTTI, G. E. MARTIN & T. B. CHEN. 1983. Increase in brain [125]I-cholecystokinin (CCK) receptor binding following chronic haloperidol treatment, intracisternal 6-hydroxydopamine or ventral tegmental lesions. Life Sci. **32:** 871–878.

57. HSIAO, S., G. KATSUURA & S. ITOH. 1985. Altered responding to cholecystokinin and dopaminergic agonist following 6-hydroxydopamine treatment in rats. Behav. Neurosci. **99:** 853–860.

58. HAYS, S. E., D. K. MEYER & S. M. PAUL. 1981. Localization of cholecystokinin receptors on neuronal elements in rat caudate nucleus. Brain Res. **219:** 208–213.

59. BESSON J. J., A. CHERAMY, P. FELTZ & J. GLOWINSKI. 1969. Release of newly-synthesized dopamine from dopamine-containing terminals in the striatum of the rat. Proc. Natl. Acad. Sci. U.S.A. **62:** 741–748.

60. HOMMER, D. W. & L. R. SKIRBOLL. 1983. Cholecystokinin-like peptides potentiate apomorphine-induced inhibition of dopamine neurons. Eur. J. Pharmcol. **91:** 151–152.

61. HOMMER, D. W., G. STONER, J. N. CRAWLEY, S. M. PAUL & L. R. SKIRBOLL. 1986. Cholecystokinin-dopamine coexistence: Electrophysiological actions corresponding to cholecystokinin receptor subtype. J. Neurosci. **6:** 3039–3043.

62. LEHMANN, J., M. BRILEY & S. Z. LANGER. 1983. Characterization of dopamine autoreceptor and ³H-spiperone binding sites with classical and novel dopamine receptor agonists. Eur. J. Pharmacol. **88:** 11–26.

63. WHITE, F. J. & R. Y. WANG. 1984. Pharmacological characterization of dopamine autoreceptors in the rat ventral tegmental area: Microiontophoretic studies. J. Pharmacol. Exp. Ther. **231:** 275–280.

64. GARAU, L., S. GOVONI, E. STEFANINI, M. TRABUSCHI & P. F. SPANO. 1978. Dopamine receptors: Pharmacological and anatomical evidence indicates two distinct dopamine receptor populations are present in rat striatum. Life Sci. **23:** 1745–1753.

65. JENNER, P. & C. D. MARSDEN. 1983. Substituted benzamide drugs as selective neuroleptic agents. Neuropharmacology. **20:** 1285–1293.
66. MARTIN, J. R., M. C. BEINFELD & R. Y. WANG. 1986. Modulation of cholecystokinin release from posterior nucleus accumbens by D-2 dopamine receptor. Brain Res. **397:** 253–258.
67. TSURUTA, K., E. A. FREY, C. W. GREWE, T. E. COTE, R. L. ESKAY & J. W. KEBABIAN. 1981. Evidence that LY-141865 specifically stimulates the D-2 dopamine receptor. Nature **292:** 463–465.
68. HYTELL, J. 1983. SCH23390 — The first selective dopamine D-1 antagonist. Eur. J. Pharmacol. **91:** 153–154.
69. IORIO, L. C., A. BARNETT, F. H. LEITZ, V. P. HOUSER & C. A. KORDUBA. 1983. SCH23390, a potential benzazepine antipsychotic with unique interactions on dopamine systems. J. Pharmacol. Exp. Ther. **226:** 462–468.
70. WONG, D. T., F. P. BYMASTER, L. R. REID, R. W. FULLER, K. W. PERRY & E. C. KORN-FELD. 1983. Effect of a stereospecific D2-dopamine agonist on acetylcholine concentration in corpus striatum of rat brain. J. Neural Transm. **58:** 55–67.
71. ZETTERSTROM, T. & U. UNGERSTEDT. 1984. Effects of apomorphine on the *in vivo* release of dopamine and its metabolite, studied by brain dialysis. Eur. J. Pharmacol. **97:** 29–36.
72. FERRIER, I. N., G. W. ROBERTS, T. J. CROW, E. C. JOHNSTONE, D. G. C. OWENS, Y. C. LEE, D. O'SHAUGHNESSY, T. E. ADRIAN, J. M. POLASK & S. R. BLOOM. 1983. Reduced cholecystokinin-like and somatostatin-like immunoreactivity in limbic lobe is associated with negative symptoms in schizophrenia. Life Sci. **33:** 475–482.
73. ROBERTS, G., I. N. FERRIER, Y. LEE, T. J. CROW, E. C. JOHNSTONE, D. B. C. OWENS, A. J. BACARASE-HAMILTON, G. MCGREGOR, D. O'SHAUGHNESSEY, J. M. POKAK & S. R. BLOOM. 1983. The limbic lobe and schizophrenia. Brain. Res. **288:** 199–211.
74. VERBANCK, P. M. P., F. LOTSTRA, C. GILLES, P. LINKOWSKI, J. MENDLEWICZ & J. J. VANDERHAEGHEN. 1984. Reduced cholecystokinin immunoreactivity in the cerebrospinal fluid of patients with psychiatric disorders. Life Sci. **34:** 64–72.
75. FARMERY, S. M., F. OWEN, M. POULTER & T. J. CROW. 1985. Reduced high affinity cholecystokinin binding in hippocampus and frontal cortex of schizophrenic patients. Life Sci. **36:** 473–477.
76. MOROJI, T., N. WATANABE, N. AOKI & S. ITOH. 1982. Antipsychotic effects of caerulein, a decapeptide chemically related to cholecystokinin octapeptide, on schizophrenia. Int. Pharmacopsychiatry **17:** 255–273.
77. NAIR, N. P. V., D. M. BLOOM & J. N. NESTOROS. 1982. Cholecystokinin appears to have antipsychotic properties. Prog. Neuro-Psychopharmacol. Biol. Psychiatry **6:** 509–512.
78. BLOOM, D. M., N. P. V. NAIR & G. SCHWARTZ. 1983. CCK-8 in the treatment of chronic schizophrenia. Psychopharmacol. Bull. **19:** 361–363.
79. VAN REE, J. M., W. M. A. VERHOEVEN, G. J. GRONWER & D. DE WIED. 1984. Ceruletide resembles antipsychotics in rats and schizophrenic patients. Neuropsychobiology **12:** 4–8.
80. ALBUS, M., M. ACKENHEIL, U. MUNCH & D. NABER. 1984. Ceruletide: A new drug for the treatment of schizophrenic patients? Arch. Gen. Psychiatry **41:** 528.
81. HOMMER, D. W., D. PIKAR, A. ROY, P. NINAN, J. BORONOW & S. M. PAUL. 1984. The effects of ceruletide in schizophrenia. Arch. Gen. Psychiatry **41:** 617–619.
82. ITOH, H., Y. SHIMAZONO, Y. KAWAKITA, Y. KUDO, Y. SATOH & R. TAKAHASHI. 1986. Clinical evaluation of ceruletide in schizophrenia: A multiinstitutional cooperative double-blind controlled study. Psychopharmacol. Bull. **22:** 123–128.
83. LOTSTRA, F., P. VERBANCK, J. MENDLEWICZ & J. J. VANDERHAEGHEN. 1984. No evidence of antipsychotic effect of caerulein in schizophrenic patients free of neuroleptics: A double-blind cross-over study. Biol. Psychiatry **19:** 877–882.
84. MATTES, J. A., W. HOM, J. M. ROCHFORD & M. ORLOSKY. 1985. Ceruletide for schizophrenia: A double-blind study. Biol. Psychiatry **20:** 533–538.
85. MATTES, J. A., W. HOM & J. M. ROCHFORD. 1985. A high dose double-blind study of ceruletide in the treatment of schizophrenia. Am. J. Psychiatry **142:** 1482–1484.
86. PESELOW, E., B. ANGRIST, A. SUDILOVSKY, J. CORWIN, J. SIEKIERSKI, F. TRENT & J. ROTROSEN. 1987. Double blind controlled trials of cholecystokinin octapeptide in neuroleptic-refractory schizophrenia. Psychopharmacology **91:** 80–84.

87. TAMMINGA, C. A., R. L. LITTMAN & L. D. ALPHS. 1986. Cholecystokinin: A neuropeptide in the treatment of schizophrenia. Psychopharmacol. Bull. **22:** 129–132.
88. TANIMOTO, K., C. A. TAMMINGA, M. KNIGHT & T. N. CHASE. 1985. Intraventricular cholecystokinin octapeptide elevates plasma prolactin. Neurosci. Abstr. **11:** 1298.
89. PASSARO, E., JR., H. DEBAS, W. OLDENDORF & T. YAMADA. 1982. Rapid appearance of intraventricularly administered neuropeptides in the peripheral circulation. Brain Res. **241:** 338–340.
90. HOMMER, D. W., M. PALKOVITS, J. N. CRAWLEY, S. M. PAUL & L. R. SKIRBOLL. 1985. Cholecystokinin-induced excitation in the substantia nigra: Evidence for peripheral and central components. J. Neurosci. **5:** 1387–1392.
91. NEWTON, B. W. & B. E. MALEY. 1985. Cholecystokinin-octapeptide-like immunoreactivity in the area postrema of the rat and cat. Reg. Peptides **13:** 31–40.
92. ANIKA, S. M., T. R. HOUPT & K. A. HOUPT. 1977. Satiety elicited by cholecystokinin in intact and vagotomized rats. Physiol. Behav. **19:** 761–766.
93. CRAWLEY, J. N. & J. S. SCHWABER. 1984. Abolition of the behavioral effects of cholecystokinin following bilateral radiofrequency lesions of the parvocellular subdivision of the nucleus tractus solitarius. Brain Res. **295:** 289–299.
94. CRAWLEY, J. N., J. Z. KISS & E. MEZEY. 1984. Bilateral midbrain transections block the behavioral effects of cholecystokinin on feeding and exploration in rats. Brain Res. **322:** 316–321.
95. SMITH, G. P., C. JEROME, B. J. CUSHIN, R. ETERNO & K. J. SIMANSKY. 1981. Abdominal vagotomy blocks the satiety effect of cholecystokinin in the rat. Science **213:** 1036–1037.
96. KOULISCHER, D., L. MORODER & M. DESCHODT-LANCKMAN. 1982. Degradation of cholecystokinin octapeptide, related fragments and analogs by human and rat plasma in vitro. Reg. Peptides **4:** 127–139.
97. DESCHODT-LANCKMANN, M., D. B. NGOC, M. NOYER & J. CHRISTOPHE. 1981. Degradation of cholecystokinin-like peptides by a crude rat membrane synaptosomal fraction; a study by high pressure liquid chromatography. Reg. Peptides **2:** 15–30.
98. STEEL, D. J., P. L. WOOD & B. PETRACK. 1986. Evidence for a direct central action of cholecystokinin in regulation of cerebellar function. Neurosci. Abstr. **12:** 153.
99. INNIS, R. B., B. S. BUNNEY, D. S. CHARNEY, L. H. PRICE, W. M. GLAZER, D. E. STERNBERG, A. L. RUBIN & G. R. HENINGER. 1986. Does the cholecystokinin antagonist proglumide possess antipsychotic activity? Psychiatr. Res. **18:** 1–8.
100. DEBONNEL, G. & C. DE MONTIGNY. 1986. Long-term haloperidol treatment induces a supersensitivity to cholecystokinin but not to dopamine in the rat nucleus accumbens. Neurosci. Abstr. **12:** 1319.
101. HU, X.-T. & R. Y. WANG. 1987. Supersensitivity to dopamine and cholecystokinin of nucleus accumbens cells following chronic treatment with haloperidol or clozapine. Neurosci. Abstr. **13:** 915.
102. CHIODO, L. A. & B. S. BUNNEY. 1987. Population response of midbrain dopaminergic neurons to neuroleptics: Further studies on time course and nondopaminergic neuronal influences. J. Neurosci. **7:** 629–633.
103. JIANG, L. H., R. J. KASSER & R. Y. WANG. 1988. Cholecystokinin antagonist lorglumide reverses chronic haloperidol induced effects on dopamine neurons. Submitted for publication in Brain Res.
104. WANG, R. Y. & R. SCHOENFELD, Eds. 1988. Cholecystokinin Antagonists. Alan Liss. New York. In press.

# Modulation of Mesolimbic Dopaminergic Behaviors by Cholecystokinin

JACQUELINE N. CRAWLEY

*Unit on Behavioral Neuropharmacology*
*Clinical Neuroscience Branch*
*National Institute of Mental Health*
*Bethesda, Maryland 20892*

## INTRODUCTION

Since the discovery of neuropeptides that appear to act as neurotransmitters in the mammalian central nervous system,[31,62] several neuropeptides have been proposed as modulators of dopaminergic function in the mesolimbic pathway. Substance P, cholecystokinin (CCK), enkephalin, and dynorphin have been identified in the ventral tegmental area,[18] with receptors for these and other peptides also present in the ventral tegmental area.[50] Of these, Hökfelt and co-workers discovered that a large population of ventral tegmental neurons appear to contain both cholecystokinin and dopamine,[32,34] that a smaller population of neurons appear to contain both neurotensin and dopamine,[29] and that a smaller population of neurons appears to contain cholecystokinin, neurotensin, and dopamine (Fallon, this volume). The finding that cholecystokinin octapeptide sulfate (CCK-8S) coexists with dopamine (DA) in the mesolimbic pathway aroused great interest in the possibility that a peptide such as CCK could be involved in the etiology of schizophrenia, and that novel antipsychotic treatments could be developed based on CCK-related compounds. Neuroscientists, biological psychiatrists, and pharmaceutical companies initiated studies on the possible interactions between CCK and DA, using a variety of available techniques. The results to date remain somewhat contradictory, often controversial, but continually provocative. This paper attempts to integrate the current findings into a more cohesive interpretation of mechanisms of CCK–DA interactions.

The coexistence of CCK and DA in the mammalian mesolimbic pathway has been confirmed by several independent laboratories.[17,32,47,65] Immunocytochemical studies of adjacent sections show that in the caudal region of the ventral tegmental area of the rat, as much as 80–90% of the dopamine-containing neurons also contain CCK-like immunoreactivity, with an average of 40% of all ventral tegmental neurons that contain DA also containing CCK.[30] Immunofluorescence double labeling combined with retrograde tracing, lesions of the mesolimbic pathway with 6-hydroxydopamine,[32,47,65] and depletion of the mesolimbic neurons with reserpine or α-methyl-paratyrosine,[64] have confirmed a parallel decrease of tyrosine hydroxylase immunoreactivity and CCK-like immunoreactivity in ventral tegmental neurons and in the terminal field of the medial posterior nucleus accumbens. In the rat, CCK appears to coexist with DA in the ventral tegmental area (A10) and in the medial portion of the substantia nigra pars compacta (A9), but few neurons in the lateral portion of the substantia nigra and none in the substantia nigra pars reticulata region contained CCK.[33] Local microinjection of colchicine into the substantia nigra–ventral tegmental area produced a distribution of CCK–DA coexistence in the lateral substantia nigra and caudate nucleus, as well as in the ventral tegmental neurons and in the medial posterior nucleus accumbens, suggesting that low levels of CCK may also be present in dopamine-containing neurons of the nigrostriatal pathway of the rat.[60] In the cat, CCK appears to coexist with DA to a lesser extent in the medial ventral tegmental area, but to a considerable extent in portions of the substantia nigra pars compacta and pars lateralis, suggesting a considerable population of CCK–DA neurons in the nigrostriatal pathway, as compared to the mesolimbic pathway, in this species.[33] In the monkey and in the mouse, CCK appears to coexist with DA only in the ventral tegmental area.[30] In the guinea pig, no coexistence of CCK and DA was detected.[30]

Indirect evidence on vesicular localization of CCK, using reserpine depletion, suggests that CCK is stored in two types of presynaptic vesicles, mixed CCK–DA vesicles, and vesicles containing only CCK.[64]

CCK appears to modulate the release of DA, as measured by both *in vitro* tissue slice preparations and *in vivo* push–pull and voltammetry studies. In 1980, Fuxe and co-workers[22] reported that intraventricular administration of 1-nmol CCK-7 or of CCK-8 reduced the turnover of DA in the caudate nucleus and in the anterior nucleus accumbens of the rat. These are the regions in which CCK is present, but not coexisting within the same neuron, as DA. No effects of 1-nmol CCK on DA turnover were seen in the posterior nucleus accumbens of the olfactory tubercle, where CCK–DA coexistence is reported. In another study using slices from rat brain, 0.1- and 1.0-μM CCK-8S enhanced the resting release of DA from the posterior nucleus accumbens without affecting DA release from the anterior nucleus accumbens, while 1-nm CCK inhibited potassium-stimulated DA release from both regions of the nucleus accumbens.[72] In slices from cat caudate nucleus, where CCK and DA were reported to coexist, sulfated but not unsulfated CCK octapeptide inhibited electrically stimulated release of DA in concentrations of CCK as low as 10 fmol.[46] These effects of CCK on DA turnover were not replicated *in vivo* by Widerlov and co-workers,[75] who found no effect of 10 μg CCK-8S administered intraventricularly on DA metabolites in the nucleus accumbens, olfactory tubercle, or striatum of the rat. Hamilton and co-workers[26] also reported no effect of caerulein administered *in vivo* at concentrations of 1 nmol to 100 μmol on DA release from slices from the nucleus accumbens. These contradictory data on the effects of CCK on DA release may relate to (1) choice of tissue, that is, anatomical regions containing terminals where CCK and DA coexist versus regions where they do not coexist, and (2) method of release, that is, the level of neuronal activation attained by the various methods of stimulation, may determine which pools of DA are affected by CCK. The most recent studies on release, using *in vivo* voltammetry, suggest that doses of 2.5–100 ng CCK, administered intraventricularly, initially stimulate DA release, then produce a prolonged inhibition of DA release, in the posterior nucleus accumbens[43] (Phillips, this volume).

Corollary studies on the effects of DA on CCK release, by Meyer and co-workers,[5,49] reported that dopamine $D_2$ receptor agonists enhanced the release of CCK induced by veratridine or potassium from the caudate–putamen of the rat, while $D_1$ receptor agonists inhibited CCK release.[48]

Chronic infusion with the dopamine receptor antagonist, haloperidol, was found to increase concentrations of CCK in both the striatum and the nucleus accumbens–olfactory tubercle region.[20] However, others have been unable to replicate these effects of chronic neuroleptic treatment on concentrations of CCK.[23,25]

Interactions between CCK and DA at the level of receptors supports a modulatory role for CCK that is dependent on concentration of CCK and anatomical site. Striatal $D_2$ receptors were found to show a decrease in $B_{max}$ and an increase in $K_d$,[21] while olfactory tubercle $D_2$ receptors increased in $B_{max}$, following treatment of homogenates with 1-μM CCK-8S.[53] Conversely, CCK-8S, infused into the lateral ventricle of the rat, 2 ng/hr, for 24 hr to 14 days, increased the $B_{max}$ of $D_2$ receptors in both the nucleus accumbens and the striatum.[15] Chronic infusion of haloperidol significantly increased [125]I-CCK-33 binding in nucleus accumbens, olfactory tubercle, and frontal cortex, but not in striatum, in both guinea pig and mice,[2] and increased the ability of caerulein to stimulate $^3$H-spiperone binding.[70] Increased CCK binding was also found in the nucleus accumbens, olfactory tubercle, and cortex, following unilateral ventral tegmental lesions or intracisternal 6-hydroxydopamine lesions.[2] Taken together, these early studies suggest that, in the regions of CCK–DA coexistence, loss of DA could increase the number of CCK binding sites, while increased CCK input could increase DA antagonist binding.

The second messenger for CCK receptors in the brain remains unknown, although the effector system for peripheral CCK is known to be the phosphatidyl inositol hydrolysis cascade.[14] Therefore, studies of CCK–DA interactions at the level of effector systems are limited to investigations of CCK modulating DA-linked adenylate cyclase. Studler and co-workers [63] reported that CCK (0.3–1 μM) potentiated DA-stimulated adenylate cyclase in the posterior part of the nucleus accumbens, where CCK and DA coexist, while CCK (0.3–1 μM) inhibited DA-stimulated adenylate cyclase in the anterior part of the nucleus accumbens, where CCK and DA do not exist, in the rat. This functional study emphasizes the importance of comparing CCK–DA interactions in anatomical sites of coexistence, versus in sites where CCK and DA are found in separate neurons.

Neurophysiological studies of extracellular single-unit neuronal activity in the ventral tegmental area and in the substantia-nigra pars compacta of the rat have reported an increase in firing rate and bursting activity when CCK was administered, intravenously at doses of 1–16 μg/kg, while CCK was without effect in the zona reticulata, where CCK immunoreactivity is not seen[19,61] (Bunney, this volume). Microiontophoresis of 10 μg/ml CCK at 20 or 40 nA current also increased the firing rate and bursting activity of the same neurons.[61] In some cells, the higher doses of CCK produced depolarization inactivation, which could be reversed with apomorphine.[19,61] CCK was similarly found to excite neurons in the nucleus accumbens in the rat[74] and rabbit.[11] However, when CCK was coadministered in combination with DA, or with DA agonists such as apomorphine, CCK potentiated the inhibitory actions of DA in the ventral tegmentum and medial substantia nigra pars compacta region.[19,35,36] CCK also potentiated DA inhibition, in the caudal portion of the nucleus accumbens, of an evoked response from the hippocampal fimbria of the rabbit.[11] However, microiontophoresis of CCK into the nucleus accumbens of the rat was reported to block DA-inhibition of firing in the nucleus of the rat.[74] Studies in the nucleus accumbens have not been undertaken by other laboratories to date. This may be due to the fact that dopamine-sensitive neurons of the nucleus accumbens are not spontaneously firing, but must be activated by an excitatory agent such as glutamate. Pharmacological activation of postsynaptic neurons may confound interpretation of CCK–DA interactions, similar to the conflicting interpretations of the CCK–DA release studies in resting versus stimulated tissue slices.

## BEHAVIORAL STUDIES

Behavioral researchers were in an ideal position to study the functional significance of the CCK–DA coexistence in the mesolimbic pathway for two reasons: (1) established behavioral paradigms had identified hyperlocomotion elicited by dopamine and its agonists in the mesolimbic pathway, and had identified stereotyped sniffing and grooming elicited by dopamine and its agonists in the nigrostriatal pathway in the rat; and (2) the anatomy of the CCK–DA coexistence showed specificity to the mesolimbic pathway in the rat, such that the nigrostriatal pathway could serve as a parallel control for CCK–DA interactions that were not a function of coexistence.

In the first studies, doses of CCK in the microgram range were injected centrally in conjunction with peripheral administration of amphetamine or apomorphine. Schneider and co-workers[59] found that 1.25-μg CCK-8S significantly reduced rearing behavior stimulated by amphetamine, when CCK was microinjected into the ventral tegmental area or into the nucleus accumbens. CCK had no significant effect on amphetamine-induced hyperlocomotion at this dose, and unsulfated CCK-8 had no effect on any behavioral action of amphetamine at the 1.25-μg dose. Weiss and co-workers[73] and Van Ree and co-workers[69] subsequently confirmed the ability of lower doses of CCK (20 ng), microinjected into the nucleus accumbens, to block amphetamine-induced hyperlocomotion.

Widerlov and co-workers[75] investigated the effects of CCK-8S on spontaneous loco-motion and rearing, and on amphetamine-induced hyperlocomotion and apomorphine-induced stereotypies. Doses of 5-μg or 25-μg CCK intraventricularly had no effect on spontaneous locomotion or rearing, or on amphetamine-induced locomotion or apomorphine-induced rearing. Administration of CCK into the ventral tegmental area reduced rearing and locomotion at a dose of 10.2 μg, but had no effect at doses of 0.34 μg and 3.4 μg. No change in locomotion or rearing was noted for CCK adminis-tration into the nucleus accumbens at doses of 3.4–10 μg.

Hamilton and co-workers[25] reported that a dose of 1 μg of the CCK analog, caerulein, had no effect on spontaneous locomotion or on DA-induced hyperlocomotion, when microinjected alone or in combination with DA into the nucleus accumbens.

Ellinwood and co-workers[16] reported that the CCK analog, caerulein, potentiated apomorphine-induced behavior at a dose of 0.3 μg intraventricularly, while inhibiting apomorphine-induced behaviors at a dose of 0.8 μg intraventricularly.

Van Ree and co-workers[69] investigated the behavioral effects of CCK-8S, CCK-8US, and caerulein on several paradigms over a range of low doses. Microinjection into the nucleus accumbens of 1–10-ng CCK or its analogs increased spontaneous sniffing and potentiated apomorphine-induced sniffing. Doses of 1-pg–10-ng CCK, microinjected into the nucleus accumbens, were found to block apomorphine-induced hypomotility. This was the only study that reported significant effects of CCK and its analog administered alone, and the only study that found significant effects of un-sulfated CCK, in the mesolimbic pathway. The time course studied in the spontaneous and apomorphine-induced locomotion and stereotypy experiments was 25–45 minutes. CCK-8S was found to block amphetamine-induced hyperlocomotion at doses of 1 ng and 10 ng into the nucleus accumbens. As in other studies, in the caudate nucleus, CCK-8S, CCK-8US, or caeruletide at a dose of 10 ng, had no effect alone or in combi-nation with apomorphine or amphetamine on locomotion or stereotypy. In tests of one-trial passive avoidance responses, a standard test for neuroleptic drug activity, high doses of all three analogs, 3 μg and 10 μg administered subcutaneously, significantly facilitated retention. Unilateral microinjection of 0.3 pg of all three analogs into the nucleus accumbens significantly attenuated passive avoidance responding, interpretable as an antipsychotic action. The time course studied in the spontaneous and apomor-phine-induced locomotion and stereotypy experiments was 25–45 minutes after pep-tide injection. Lane and co-workers[43] (Phillips, this volume) reported that over this time period, release of DA from the posterior nucleus accumbens is inhibited by CCK.

Our laboratory initiated a comprehensive analysis of the behavioral effects of

CCK–DA interactions, based on the results of the studies previously reported. Our understanding of the literature of 1982–1984 was that microgram doses of CCK had no effect alone on spontaneous locomotion or stereotypies, but could block some components of apomorphine or amphetamine-induced stereotypies or locomotion, when microinjected into either the nucleus accumbens or ventral tegmental area. CCK appeared to have no action alone or in conjunction with these dopaminergic agents when administered into the caudate nucleus. Lower doses of CCK appeared to inhibit apomorphine-induced hypomotility and amphetamine-induced hypermotility, and to inhibit passive avoidance behaviors, when microinjected into the nucleus accumbens, 25–45 minutes before testing. The important issues to be clarified appeared to be:

(1) Dose of CCK: linear or biphasic dose-response curve.
(2) Location of microinjection (posterior nucleus accumbens, anterior nucleus accumbens, caudate nucleus, ventral tegmentum): are interactions specific to sites of coexistence.
(3) Time course after injection: correlation with half-life of CCK *in vivo*.
(4) Effects of CCK on spontaneous behaviors alone versus in conjunction with dopaminergic agonists.
(5) Activity of unsulfated CCK, CCK analogs, CCK antagonists: which CCK receptor subtype.

To address these issues, CCK-8S, or CCK-8US, was microinjected into the medial posterior nucleus accumbens, into the anterior nucleus accumbens, into the caudate nucleus, or into the ventral tegmentum immediately before testing, alone or in combination with DA, or in combination with systemically administered apomorphine or amphetamine, over a dose range from 20 pg to 4 μg.

CCK administered alone was found to have no effect on locomotion or stereotypy.[7] At doses from 20 pg to 2 μg, CCK had no effect on ambulation or stereotyped sniffing when microinjected bilaterally into the medial–posterior nucleus accumbens or into the caudate nucleus. When given in combination with dopaminergic agonists, CCK significantly potentiated stereotyped sniffing induced by apomorphine (0.2 mg/kg, sc 15 min before CCK microinjection), and hyperlocomotion induced by DA (20 μg, simultaneous injected with CCK into the medial–posterior nucleus accumbens), at doses of CCK from 20 pg to 200 ng (20 fmol–200 pmol).[7,8] The dose-response curve was biphasic, with doses below 20 pg and above 400 ng having no significant effect on apomorphine-induced stereotyped sniffing, or on DA-induced hyperlocomotion.

To further test the biphasic nature of the dose-response curve by which CCK potentiated DA-induced hyperlocomotion, especially in light of the earlier work done in the microgram range of CCK, we recently tested 4-μg CCK, microinjected alone or in combination with DA 20 μg, bilaterally into the medial–posterior nucleus accumbens. Using the standard microinjection volume of 0.2 μl per injection site, 4-μg CCK was at the upper limit of its solubility, and therefore the maximum dose tested. FIGURE 1 illustrates this more complete dose-response curve for CCK on DA-induced hyperlocomotion. The high doses of 2-μg and 4-μg CCK had no effect on DA-induced hyperlocomotion. This data point supports our original finding of a dose-response curve in which low and high doses were without effect, while doses in the range of picogram to nanogram CCK potentiated DA-induced hyperlocomotion. This lack of effect of high range of CCK doses is consistent with previous reports, such as Widerlov *et al.*,[75] in which only high doses of CCK were tested, and no behavioral interaction between CCK and DA-ergic agents were reported. It is possible that microgram quantities of CCK are causing some percentage of neurons to go into depolarization block,[19,61,74]

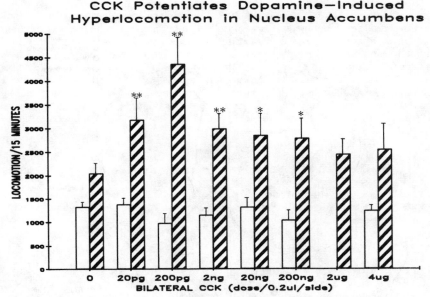

**FIGURE 1.** Saline, dopamine, cholecystokinin octapeptide sulfate (CCK-8S), or dopamine + cholecystokinin, was bilaterally microinjected in a volume of 0.2 μl over a period of 1 min into the medial posterior nucleus accumbens of the rat, stereotaxic coordinates 1.2 mm anterior to bregma, 1.2 mm bilateral to the midline, and 5.7 mm ventral to the surface of the skull. Immediately after microinjection, rats were placed in a Digiscan photocell activity monitor for 15 min. Ambulatory locomotion scores revealed a significant potentiation of dopamine-induced hyperlocomotion by CCK 20 pg–200 ng, while no effect of CCK administered alone on locomotion was observed at any dose. Data are presented as mean + standard error of the mean. $N = 5 - 8$ for each dose of each treatment. *White bars* represent treatments of saline + increasing doses of CCK. *Striped bars* represent dopamine (10 μg) + increasing doses of CCK. *The two bars on the left* are treatment groups of saline (*white*) and dopamine (*striped*), without CCK, representing the standard increase in locomotion observed with this dose of dopamine. ANOVA for CCK alone: $F_{(5,25)} = 1.41$, not significant. ANOVA for dopamine + CCK: $F_{(6,48)} = 4.46$, $p < 0.01$; Newman–Keuls test for significance of individual means, * $p < 0.05$ for dopamine + CCK 20 ng, dopamine + CCK 200 ng, as compared to dopamine + saline, ** $p < 0.01$ for dopamine + CCK 20 pg, dopamine + CCK 200 pg, dopamine + CCK 2 ng, as compared to dopamine + saline.[7] A biphasic dose-response curve was obtained, with CCK doses of 2 μg and 4 μg showing no effect on dopamine-induced hyperlocomotion.

cancelling out some percentage of neurons that are responding to DA and potentiated by the applied CCK.

Location of the CCK microinjection site was found to be critical to the functional interaction of CCK with DA. In the caudate nucleus, CCK had no effect alone and no effect in combination with apomorphine on stereotyped sniffing.[7] However, CCK potentiated apomorphine-induced stereotypy when CCK was microinjected into the nucleus accumbens.[7] In addition, CCK microinjected into the nucleus accumbens, but not into the caudate nucleus, shifted the dose-response curve for apomorphine-induced stereotypy to the left.[8] The ability of CCK to potentiate APO-induced stereotypy in

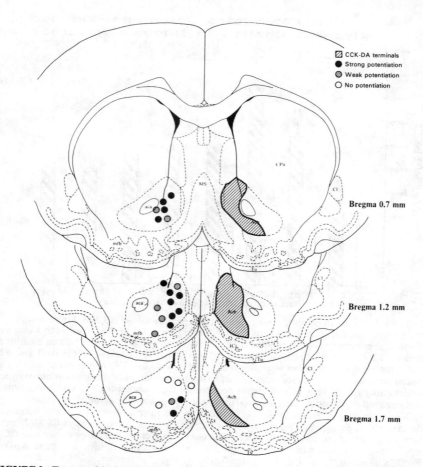

**FIGURE 2.** Topographical analysis of nucleus accumbens sites at which cholecystokinin (CCK) potentiates dopamine-induced hyperlocomotion in the rat. Rats cannulated bilaterally at seven sites within the nucleus accumbens (1 mm rostral, 1 mm caudal, 1 mm lateral, 1 mm medial, 1 mm ventral, and 1 mm dorsal, to the site described in the legend to FIG. 1), were administered saline, dopamine (20 µg), or dopamine (20 µg + CCK 1 ng), and tested for locomotor activity, as previously described. No significant differences were seen between locomotor scores for saline treatment (780 + 202) or for dopamine treatment (1565 + 356) among the seven sites. The *shaded areas* on the right represent the anatomical region within the nucleus accumbens in which CCK and dopamine are co-localized in terminals from ventral tegmental neurons.[32,34] The *filled black circles* on the left represent microinjection sites at which CCK elicited strong potentiation of DA-induced hyperlocomotion (ambulatory locomotion scores >2200). *Hatched circles* represent microinjected sites at which CCK elicited weak potentiation of DA-induced hyperlocomotion (ambulatory locomotion scores between 1500 and 2200). *Open circles* represent sites at which CCK elicited no potentiation of DA-induced hyperlocomotion (ambulatory scores < 1500). Significant reductions in CCK-potentiation of DA-induced hyperlocomotion were found at sites 1 mm rostral, 1 mm lateral, and 1 mm medial to the standard medial posterior nucleus accumbens site.[9]

the nucleus accumbens may be due to the postulated feedback pathway from the nigro-striatal to the mesolimbic pathway.[6]

Immunocytochemical studies previously cited found that CCK coexists with DA in the medial–posterior nucleus accumbens, but not in the anterior nucleus accumbens or caudate nucleus. We therefore tested the hypothesis that the modulatory role of CCK on DA-mediated behaviors is limited to regions in which CCK and DA coexist, by microinjecting CCK into either the medial–posterior nucleus accumbens or into sites surrounding this region. FIGURE 2 reflects the significant correlation obtained between anatomical sites within the nucleus accumbens where CCK and DA coexist and the anatomical sites where CCK potentiated DA-induced hyperlocomotion.[9]

Since the neurophysiological studies had shown that CCK potentiates DA-inhibition of neuronal firing in the ventral tegmental cell bodies, and since Widerlov and co-workers[75] had reported that microgram doses of CCK inhibited rearing and locomotion, we recently tested the interaction of CCK and DA on locomotor behavior when microinjected into the ventral tegmental area. At stereotaxic coordinates of AP 6.3-mm posterior to bregma, bilaterally 0.5 mm from the midline, and 7.9 mm from the surface of the skull, 10-μg DA was found to significantly inhibit locomotion, as compared to saline controls, as previously reported.[56] As shown in FIGURE 3, CCK potentiated the hypolocomotion induced by DA at the ventral tegmental area site. Doses of CCK tested to date include 1 ng, 10 ng, and 100 ng, with a more complete dose-response curve in progress. These doses had no effect on locomotion when administered alone into the ventral tegmental area. The ability of CCK to potentiate the inhibitory actions of DA in the ventral tegmental area is consistent with the neurophysiological findings, and consistent with the hypothesis that CCK interacts with DA in a facilitatory manner.

Application of analogs and antagonists of CCK-8S provided a useful approach to investigate the receptor mechanisms through which CCK might potentiate DA-induced hyperlocomotion. We found that unsulfated CCK-8, microinjected into the medial posterior nucleus accumbens, had no effect on apomorphine-induced stereotypy or on DA-induced hyperlocomotion, at doses equivalent to or 1000 times greater than the doses of CCK-8S that were active in our paradigms.[8–10] These findings are consistent with all previous reports showing behavioral inactivity of CCK-8US, except that of Van Ree and co-workers[69] previously discussed above. CCK-4, which shows opposite effects of CCK-8US on some paradigms,[38] also had no effect on DA-induced hyperlocomotion when microinjected into the nucleus accumbens.[10] Neither CCK-8US nor CCK-4 blocked the actions of CCK-8S, suggesting that these two analogs do not act as antagonists of CCK-8S in the present paradigms. Receptor binding studies have shown that binding affinities for $^{125}$I-CCK-33, $^{125}$I-CCK-8, $^{3}$H-CCK-8, $^{3}$H-CCK-5, and $^{3}$H-CCK-4, are all within a tenfold range.[24,27,40,42,57,58,68] This behavioral finding of specificity for CCK-8S therefore suggests that the site through which CCK potentiates dopamine-induced hyperlocomotion is not the high-affinity central-type receptor. In addition, antagonists of CCK, which are potent at the peripheral CCK receptor but relatively inactive at the central, high-affinity CCK receptor, for example, proglumide and benzotript, effectively blocked the actions of CCK-8S on potentiating DA-induced hyperlocomotion when the antagonists were administered systemically (FIG. 4), as well as into the nucleus accumbens.[10] These antagonist studies lend further support to the notion that the behavioral actions of CCK on potentiating DA in the nucleus accumbens are not mediated by the high-affinity central-type CCK receptor. A peripheral-type CCK receptor has been described in circumventricular brain regions, including the posterior hypothalamic nucleus, interpeduncular nucleus, area postrema, and nucleus tractus solitarius.[51] The pharmacology of this receptor type appears to match the phar-

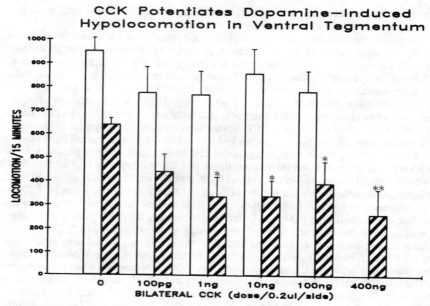

**FIGURE 3.** Rats were administered saline, dopamine (10 µg), doses of CCK, or dopamine (10 µg) + doses of CCK, into the ventral tegmental area, at stereotaxic coordinates 6.3 mm posterior to bregma, 0.5 mm bilateral to the midline, and 7.9 mm from the surface of the skull, and immediately tested for ambulatory locomotion as described in the legend to FIGURE 1. Data are presented as mean + standard error of the mean. $N = 6 - 8$ for each dose of each treatment. *White bars* represented treatments of CCK administered alone, showing no significant effect on locomotion as compared to saline treated vehicle controls, ANOVA F (4,15) = 0.16, not significant. *Striped bars* represent CCK administered in combination with dopamine, showing a significant potentiation by CCK of the locomotor inhibition induced by dopamine, ANOVA F (6,49) = 14.82, $p \ll 0.01$, Newman–Keuls * $p < 0.05$ for DA + CCK 1 ng, DA + CCK 10 ng, DA + CCK 100 ng, as compared to DA: ** $p < 0.01$ for DA + CCK 400 ng, as compared to DA.

macology of our behavioral effects of CCK. However, Moran and co-workers[51] did not detect measurable levels of their "peripheral-type" CCK receptor in the nucleus accumbens.

Since the doses of CCK reported by Schneider and co-workers,[59] Van Ree and co-workers,[69] and Weiss and co-workers[73] produced a decrease in amphetamine-induced hyperlocomotion when CCK was microinjected into the nucleus accumbens, we recently replicated the paradigms of these investigators to determine the actions of CCK on amphetamine-induced hyperlocomotion. As seen in FIGURE 5, our data are consistent with the previous findings that CCK inhibits amphetamine-induced hyperlocomotion. In thinking about the difference between DA-induced hyperlocomotion and amphetamine-induced hyperlocomotion, one might ascribe the differences in CCK actions to the different sites of action of DA and amphetamine. Amphetamine acts primarily by causing release of DA from presynaptic terminals.[41] Several peptides have been shown to affect release of DA.[3] Release studies previously cited suggest that low concentrations of CCK inhibit release of DA from presynaptic terminals. CCK may therefore be acting to pharmacologically antagonize the ability of amphetamine to

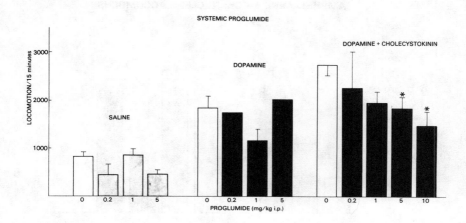

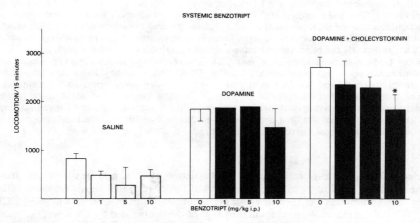

**FIGURE 4.** Systemic administration of the CCK receptor antagonists, proglumide and benzotript, blocked the ability of CCK to potentiate dopamine-induced hyperlocomotion, but had no effect alone on baseline locomotion or dopamine-induced hyperlocomotion. Antagonists or saline were administered intraperitoneally, 5 min before microinjection of saline, dopamine (20 µg), or dopamine (20 µg) + CCK (1 ng) into the medial posterior nucleus accumbens, immediately before testing for locomotor activity, as described in the legend to FIGURE 1. Proglumide significantly attenuated the CCK potentiation of DA-induced hyperlocomotion at doses of 5 mg/kg and 10 mg/kg (*$p < 0.05$, as compared to saline ip + DA + CCK intraaccumbens, by t-test analysis). Benzotript significantly attenuated the CCK potentiation of DA-induced hyperlocomotion at a dose of 10 mg/kg, ip (* $p < 0.05$, as compared to saline ip + DA + CCK intraaccumbens). At these doses, proglumide and benzotript had no significant effects on DA-induced hyperlocomotion, suggesting that endogenous CCK does not play a significant role in the increase in locomotion induced by DA applied exogenously into the nucleus accumbens.

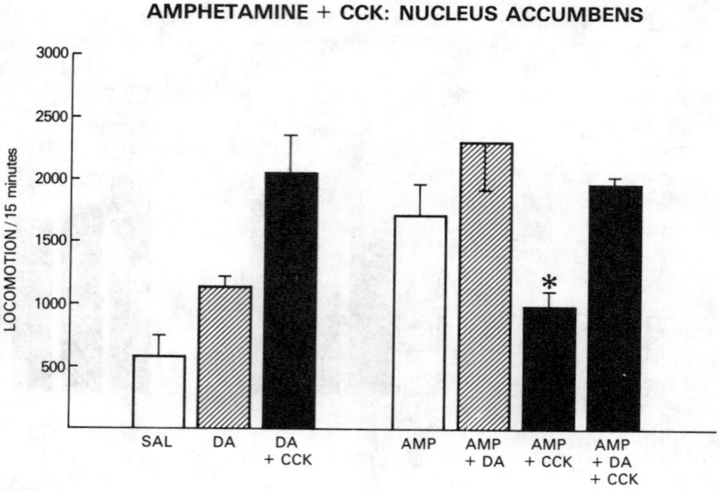

AMPHETAMINE + CCK: NUCLEUS ACCUMBENS

**FIGURE 5.** Amphetamine sulfate, 5 µg, or saline was microinjected alone or in combination with dopamine (20 µg), CCK (2 ng), or dopamine (20 µg) + CCK (2 ng), into the medial–posterior nucleus accumbens, immediately before testing for locomotor activity, as described in the legend to FIGURE 1. *The three bars on the left* illustrate the previously observed dopamine-induced hyperlocomotion and the CCK potentiation of dopamine-induced hyperlocomotion. Amphetamine microinjected into the nucleus accumbens induced hyperlocomotion, as previously described.[56] CCK significantly inhibited amphetamine-induced hyperlocomotion (* $p < 0.05$, $t = 2.23$, $df = 10$). Combining dopamine (20 µg) with CCK (1 ng) and amphetamine (5 µg) produced locomotor scores equivalent to dopamine (20 µg) + CCK (1 ng + saline). These data support the findings cited in the text that CCK inhibits the release of endogenous dopamine. Since amphetamine induces release of endogenous dopamine, CCK may oppose the releasing action of amphetamine on the presynaptic dopamine terminal in the nucleus accumbens. Exogenously applied DA + CCK may act on a postsynaptic receptor to override the effects of amphetamine + CCK on the presynaptic release mechanism.

release DA from presynaptic terminals. This action of CCK may be dissociable from the ability of CCK to potentiate the effects of DA at its postsynaptic receptor in the nucleus accumbens. As seen in FIGURE 5, administration of amphetamine + CCK + DA yielded locomotion scores in the range of those obtained for CCK + DA. These data suggest that the action of CCK in potentiating DA at a postsynaptic site can override the action of CCK on blocking DA release by amphetamine at a presynaptic site.

The studies previously described appear to reconcile several controversies in the literature on CCK–DA interactions on rodent behavior. CCK appears to potentiate DA-mediated behaviors, while having no actions alone, in the picogram to nanogram range. Potentiation is seen within 15 min after peptide microinjection, while inhibition is seen at later time points, consistent with *in vivo* release studies[43] (Phillips, this volume). Microgram doses that may have interesting pharmacological actions, but are less likely to be as physiologically relevant, appear to have no effect on postsynaptic DA-mediated behaviors in the mesolimbic pathway, perhaps due to the summation of neuronal activity in which some DA-inhibited neurons are potentiated by CCK, while some enter depolarization inactivation at high doses of CCK. Facilitatory actions of CCK appear to be restricted to the posterior medial region of the nucleus accumbens, where CCK and DA coexist in terminals derived primarily from the ventral tegmental area and medial substantia-nigra in the rat. In addition, as described in the preceding paragraph and shown in FIGURE 5, the actions of amphetamine may differ from the actions of microinjected DA, such that CCK could antagonize the ability of amphetamine to release presynaptic DA while potentiating the ability of DA to inhibit postsynaptic neurons. The actions of low doses of apomorphine, which induce hypolocomotion, are also thought to be presynaptic. Therefore, the reported finding that CCK blocks apomorphine-induced hypolocomotion while potentiating apomorphine-induced stereotypy[69] may also relate to the pre- versus postsynaptic site of action of the dopaminergic agent.

In addition to effects of CCK on mesolimbic DA-mediated motor behaviors, interesting studies on the role of CCK in mesolimbic brain stimulation and self-administration of drugs into the mesolimbic pathway have recently been reported. Hoebel and Ausili[28] reported that 400 ng/µl CCK was self-administered into the nucleus accumbens in a manner similar to self-administration of amphetamine, and blocked by dopamine receptor antagonists. This study supports a facilitatory role for CCK on DA receptors in the nucleus accumbens. De Witte and co-workers[13] reported that 150 pmol, approximately 150 ng, of CCK microinjected into the medial–posterior nucleus accumbens potentiated intracranial self-stimulation when the electrodes were implanted into the posterolateral area of the hypothalamus. Vaccarino and Koob[67] reported that nanogram doses of CCK microinjected into the nucleus accumbens antagonized intracranial self-stimulation when the electrodes were implanted in the ventral tegmentum. This controversy may relate to site of CCK microinjection. Vaccarino and Koob[67] administered CCK into the dorsal and anterior nucleus accumbens (3.2 mm anterior to bregma), while De Witte and co-workers[13] administered CCK into the ventral–posterior nucleus accumbens (1.2 mm anterior to bregma). The posterior nucleus accumbens site (1.2 mm anterior to bregma) was the area in which CCK potentiated DA-induced hyperlocomotion in the studies previously described (FIG. 2). The opposite behavioral effects of CCK in the anterior versus the posterior nucleus accumbens may relate to recent biochemical studies of CCK on DA-stimulated adenylate cyclase in the nucleus accumbens. As previously described, Studler and co-workers[63] found that CCK potentiated DA-stimulated adenylate cyclase in the posterior portion of the nucleus accumbens, but CCK inhibited DA-stimulated adenylate cyclase in the anterior nucleus accumbens. This finding may explain the variability in behavioral effects of CCK previously described, that is, the ability of CCK to inhibit intracranial self-stimulation in the anterior nucleus accumbens, but to potentiate intracranial self-stimulation in the posterior nucleus accumbens.[13,67]

The facilitatory action of CCK on DA-mediated behaviors is a function in search of a receptor. Our current thinking is that CCK potentiates DA-induced hyperlocomotion in the posterior nucleus accumbens via a receptor site that is linked to the DA receptor, such that the peptide can increase the functional response to DA transmission. Considering the distribution of terminals within the nucleus accumbens that contain both CCK and DA, it appears that the potentiating effects of CCK on DA function are restricted to the postsynaptic sites receiving the terminals of this coexistence.

## CLINICAL TRIALS

The discovery of CCK in DA pathways that have been implicated in the pathophysiology of schizophrenia raised the idea that CCK, its analogs, or its antagonists might be developed as antipsychotic drugs. Verbanck and co-workers[71] reported reduced CCK immunoreactivity in the cerebrospinal fluid of untreated schizophrenics, suggesting that a loss of CCK in the brain was a part of the psychopathology of the disease. The first pilot clinical trials of CCK were conducted in 1982. Moroji and co-workers[52] administered ceruletide, 0.3 μg/kg or 0.6 μg/kg, intramuscularly, in a single injection, to schizophrenic patients receiving various neuroleptic drugs. Of the 20 patients, 16 showed reductions in auditory hallucinations and improvement in negative mood state, with improvements persisting for three weeks after injection. Nair and co-workers[54] similarly found therapeutic efficacy of CCK in neuroleptic-resistent schizophrenic patients. However, subsequent studies using placebo-controlled, double-blind crossover protocols, have failed to replicate the antipsychotic activity of CCK.[1,37,45,66] Contrary to uncontrolled studies, therefore, CCK and caerulein, administered intramuscularly in well-controlled experimental designs, failed to produce significant antipsychotic effects.

These clinical studies are difficult to interpret in terms of the potential for CCK to act as an antipsychotic, because of the problems inherent in using a peptide as a drug. First, CCK does not cross the blood–brain barrier in measurable quantities.[55] Second, CCK is quickly degraded by metabolic enzymes *in vivo*.[12,44] Third, the high dose of CCK that might be necessary to circumvent these limitations when the peptide is given intramuscularly, will cause gastric distress due to the effects of CCK on its gut receptors. This problem could conceivably be circumvented by administering low doses of a peripheral CCK receptor antagonist in combination with a centrally selective CCK agonist. For these reasons, both the positive results of the pilot studies, and the negative results of the controlled studies, cannot be used as conclusive evidence for or against the efficacy of CCK-related drugs as antipsychotics.

The basic research just described could predict that either CCK analogs or antagonists could act as antipsychotics. High doses of CCK, which may not be physiologically relevant, can induce depolarization inactivation of DA neurons, inhibit DA release, and block DA-mediated behaviors. These data lend support to the development of nonpeptide analogs of CCK that cross the blood–brain barrier, are not rapidly degraded, and act at the high-affinity central CCK binding site. On the other hand, CCK enhanced the release of DA in some studies, increased DA-stimulated adenylate cyclase in the posterior nucleus accumbens, and low doses of CCK potentiated DA-mediated behaviors in the posterior nucleus accumbens. These data lend support to the development of nonpeptide antagonists of CCK that cross the blood–brain barrier, are not rapidly degraded, and act on an as yet unidentified CCK binding site that potentiates DA-stimulation of adenylate cyclase in the posterior nucleus accumbens.

CCK antagonists that are relatively selective, but not potent, for peripheral effects of CCK, have been shown to block the ability of CCK to potentiate DA-induced hyperlocomotion in the nucleus accumbens,[10] and to antagonize the excitatory effects of CCK in the ventral tegmental–substantia-nigra area.[4] One clinical trial of a CCK antagonist has been performed to date. Innis and co-workers[39] administered proglumide in doses of 1600 mg/day or 3200 mg/kg to four schizophrenic patients being treated with either haloperidol or chlorpromazine, for an average of 26 days. Double-blind, placebo-controlled psychiatric nurses' ratings found no significant effects of proglumide on the patients' psychosis ratings. However, this study employed a small number of patients (4) and a drug that is noted for its peripheral rather than its central CCK receptor selectivity. Several more potent CCK antagonists are currently under development, some of which may be selective for the central rather than the peripheral CCK receptor. Both CCK agonists and antagonists need to be tested alone and in combination with standard DA receptor antagonists. While controlled clinical trials are extremely difficult in schizophrenic patients, the basic research findings make a strong case for testing centrally selective CCK-related drugs for antipsychotic activity. The hope of researchers in this field is that peptides such as CCK, which act primarily as modulators of DA function, and act primarily in the mesolimbic rather than the nigrostriatal pathway, will be efficacious either alone or in combination with reduced doses of DA receptor antagonists, as therapeutic antipsychotics at low risk for the development of tardive dyskinesias.

## REFERENCES

1.  ALBUS, M., K. VON GELLHORN, U. MUNCH, D. NABER & M. ACKENHEIL. 1986. A double-blind study with ceruletide in chronic schizophrenic patients: Biochemical and clinical results. Psychiatry Res. **19**: 1–7.

2.  CHANG, R. S. L., V. J. LOTTI, G. E. MARTIN & T. B. CHEN. 1983. Increase in brain $^{125}$I-cholecystokinin (CCK) receptor binding following chronic haloperidol treatment, intracisternal 6-hydroxydopamine or ventral tegmental lesions. Life Sci. **32**: 871–878.

3.  CHESSELET, M. F. 1984. Presynaptic regulation of neurotransmitter release in the brain: Facts and hypothesis. Neuroscience **12**: 347–375.

4.  CHIODO, L. A. & B. S. BUNNEY. 1982. Proglumide: Selective antagonism of excitatory effects of cholecystokinin in central nervous system. Science **219**: 1449–1451.

5.  CONZELMANN, V., A. HOLLAND & D. K. MEYER. 1984. Effects of selective dopamine D-receptor agonists on the release of cholecystokinin-like immunoreactivity from rat neostriatum. Eur. J. Pharmacol. **101**: 119–125.

6.  COSTALL, B. R., J. NAYLOR, J. G. CANNON & T. LEE. 1977. Differentiation of the dopamine mechanisms mediating stereotyped behavior and hyperactivity in the nucleus accumbens and caudate-putamen. J. Pharm. Pharmacol. **29**: 337–342.

7.  CRAWLEY, J. N., J. A. STIVERS, L. K. BLUMSTEIN & S. M. PAUL. 1985. Cholecystokinin potentiates dopamine-mediated behaviors: Evidence for modulation specific to a site of coexistence. J. Neurosci. **5**: 1972–1983.

8.  CRAWLEY, J. N., D. W. HOMMER & L. R. SKIRBOLL. 1984. Behavioral and neurophysiological evidence for a facilatory interaction between co-existing transmitters: Cholecystokinin and dopamine. Neurochem. Int. **6**: 755–760.

9.  CRAWLEY, J. N., D. W. HOMMER & L. R. SKIRBOLL. 1985. Topographical analysis of nucleus accumbens sites at which cholecystokinin potentiates dopamine-induced hyperlocomotion. Brain Res. **355**: 337–341.

10. CRAWLEY, J. N., J. A. STIVERS, D. W. HOMMER, L. R. SKIRBOLL & S. M. PAUL. 1986. Antagonists of central and peripheral behavioral actions of cholecystokinin octapeptide. J. Pharmacol. Exp. Ther. **236**: 320–330.

11. DEFRANCE, J. F., R. W. SIKES & R. B. CHRONISTER. 1984. Effects of CCK-8 in the nucleus accumbens. Peptides **5**: 1–6.

12. DESCHODT-LANCKMAN, M., N. D. BVI, M. NOYER & J. CHRISTOPHE. 1981. Degradation of cholecystokinin-like peptides by a crude rat brain synaptosomal fraction: A study by high pressure liquid chromatography. Regul. Peptides **2**: 15–30.

13. DE WITTE, P., C. HEIBREDER, B. ROQUES & J. J. VANDERHAEGHEN. 1987. Opposite effects of cholecystokinin octapeptide (CCK-8) and tetrapeptide (CCK-4) after injection into the caudal part of the nucleus accumbens or into its rostral part and the cerebral ventricles. Neurochem. Int. **10**: 473–479.

14. DOWNES, C. P. 1982. Receptor-stimulated inositol phospholipid metabolism in the central nervous system. Cell Cal. **3**: 413–428.

15. DUMBRILLE-ROSS, A. & P. SEEMAN. 1984. Dopamine receptor elevation by cholecystokinin. Peptides **5**: 1207–1212.

16. ELLINWOOD, E. H., K. ROCKWELL & N. WAGONER. 1983. Apomorphine behavioral effect is facilitated by dibutyryl/cAMP and inhibited by caerulein. Psychopharmacol. Bull. **19**: 352–354.

17. FALLON, J. H., R. HICKS & S. E. LOUGHLIN. 1983. The origin of cholecystokinin terminals in the basal forebrain of the rat: Evidence from immunofluorescence and retrograde tracing. Neurosci. Lett. **37**: 29–35.

18. FALLON, J. H. & S. E. LOUGHLIN. 1985. Substantia nigra. *In* The Rat Nervous System, Chap. 9, Vol. 1, Forebrain and Midbrain. G. Paxinos, Ed. Academic Press. New York.

19. FREEMAN, A. S. & B. S. BUNNEY. 1987. Activity of A9 and A10 dopaminergic neurons in unrestrained rats: Further characterization and effects of apomorphine and cholecystokinin. Brain Res. **405:** 46–55.

20. FREY, P. 1986. Cholecystokinin octapeptide levels in rat brain are changed after chronic neuroleptic treatment. Eur. J. Pharmacol. **95:** 87–92.

21. FUXE, K., L. F. AGNATI, F. BENEFENATI, M. CIMMINO, S. ALGERI, T. HOKFELT & V. MUTT. 1981. Modulation by cholecystokinins of 3H-spiroperidol binding in rat striatum: Evidence for increased affinity and reduction in number of binding sites. Acta Physiol. Scand. **113:** 567–569.

22. FUXE, K., K. ANDERSSON, V. LOCATELLI, L. F. AGNATI, T. HOKFELT, L. SKIRBOLL & V. MUTT. 1980. Cholecystokinin peptides produce reduction of dopamine turnover in discrete areas in the rat brain following intraventricular injection. Eur. J. Pharmacol. **67:** 329–331.

23. GAUDREAU, P., J. N. CRAWLEY & R. QUIRION. 1986. Effects of chronic haloperidol treatment on brain cholecystokinin receptors in rat. Abstract 230.12, Society for Neuroscience.

24. GAUDREAU, P., R. QUIRION, S. ST-PIERRE & C. B. PERT. 1983. Tritium-sensitive film autoradiography of [³H]cholecystokinin-5/pentagastrin receptors in rat brain. Eur. J. Pharmacol. **87:** 173–174.

25. GYSLING, K. & M. C. BEINFELD. 1984. Failure of chronic haloperidol treatment to alter levels of cholecystokinin in the rat brain striatum and olfactory tubercle-nucleus accumbens area. Neuropeptides **4:** 421–423.

26. HAMILTON, M., M. J. SHEEHAN, J. DEBELLEROCHE & L. G. HERBERG. 1984. The cholecystokinin analogue, caerulein, does not modulate dopamine release or dopamine-induced locomotor activity in the nucleus accumbens of rat. Neurosci. Lett. **44:** 77–82.

27. HAYS, S. E., M. C. BEINFELD, R. T. JENSEN, F. K. GOODWIN & S. M. PAUL. 1980. Demonstration of a putative receptor site for cholecystokinin in rat brain. Neuropeptides **1:** 53–62.

28. HOEBEL, B. G. & E. AUSILI. 1984. Cholecystokinin self-injection in the nucleus accumbens and block with proglumide. Abstract 203.7, Society for Neuroscience.

29. HÖKFELT, T., B. J. EVERITT, E. THEODORSSON-NORHEIM & M. GOLDSTEIN. 1984. Occurrence of neurotensinlike immunoreactivity in subpopulations of hypothalamic, mesencephalic and medullary catecholamine neurons. J. Comp. Neurol. **222:** 543–559.

30. HÖKFELT, T., V. R. HOLETS, W. STAINES, B. MEISTER, T. MELANDER, M. SCHALLING, M. SCHULTZBERG, J. FREEDMAN, H. BJORKLUND, L. OLSON, B. LINDH, L. G. ELFVIN, J. M. LUNDBERG, J. A. LINDGREN, B. SAMUELSSON, B. PERNOW, L. TERENIUS, C. POST, B. EVERITT & M. GOLDSTEIN. 1986. Coexistence of neuronal messengers — An overview. *In* Progress in Brain Research, Chap. 4, Vol. 68. T. Hökfelt, K. Fuxe, and B. Pernow, Eds. Amer. Elsevier. New York.

31. HÖKFELT, T., O. JOHANSSON & M. GOLDSTEIN. 1984. Chemical anatomy of the brain. Science **225:** 1326–1334.

32. HÖKFELT, T., J. F. REHFELD, L. SKIRBOLL, B. IVEMARK, M. GOLDSTEIN & K. MARKEY. 1980. Evidence for coexistence of dopamine and CCK in mesolimbic neurons. Nature **285:** 476–478.

33. HÖKFELT, T., L. SKIRBOLL, B. J. EVERITT, B. MEISTER, M. BROWNSTEIN, T. JACOBS, A. FADEN, S. KUGA, M. GOLDSTEIN, R. MARKSTEIN, G. DOCKRAY & J. REHFELD. 1985. Distribution of cholecystokinin-like immunoreactivity in the nervous system with special reference to coexistence with classical neurotransmitters and other neuropeptides. *In* Neuronal Cholecystokinin. J. J. Vanderhaeghen and J. N. Crawley, Eds. Ann. N.Y. Acad. Sci. **448:** 255–274.

34. HÖKFELT, T., L. SKIRBOLL, J. F. REHFELD, M. GOLDSTEIN, K. MARKEY & O. DANN. 1980. A subpopulation of mesencephalic dopamine neurons projecting to limbic areas contains a cholecystokinin-like peptide: Evidence from immunohistochemistry combined with retrograde tracing. Neuroscience **5:** 2093–2124.

35. HOMMER, D. W. & L. R. SKIRBOLL. 1983. Cholecystokinin-like peptides potentiate apomorphine-induced inhibition of dopamine neurons. Eur. J. Pharmacol. **91:** 151–152.

36. HOMMER, D. W., M. PALKOVITS, J. N. CRAWLEY & S. M. PAUL. 1985. Cholecystokinin-

induced excitation in the substantia nigra: Evidence for peripheral and central components. J. Neurosci. **5:** 1387–1392.

37. HOMMER, D. W., D. PICKAR, A. ROY, P. NINAN, J. BORONOW & S. M. PAUL. 1984. The effects of ceruletide in schizophrenia. Arch. Gen. Psychiatry **41:** 617–619.

38. HSIAO, S., G. KATSUURA & S. ITOH. 1984. Cholecystokinin tetrapeptides, proglumide and open-field behavior in rats. Life Sci. **34:** 2165–2168.

39. INNIS, R. B., B. S. BUNNEY, D. S. CHARNEY, L. H. PRICE, W. M. GLAZER, D. E. STERBERG, A. L. RUBIN & G. R. HENINGER. 1986. Does the cholecystokinin antagonist proglumide possess antipsychotic activity? Psychiatry Res. **18:** 1–7.

40. INNIS, R. B. & S. H. SNYDER. 1980. Cholecystokinin receptor binding in brain and pancreas: Regulation of pancreatic binding by cyclic and acyclic guanine nucleotides. Eur. J. Pharmacol. **65:** 123–124.

41. IVERSEN, S. D. & L. L. IVERSEN. 1981. Behavioral Pharmacology. Oxford Univ. Press. London/New York.

42. KNIGHT, M., C. A. TAMMINGA, L. STEARDO, M. E. BECK, P. BARONE & T. N. CHASE. 1984. Cholecystokinin-octapeptide fragments: Binding in brain cholecystokinin receptors. Eur. J. Pharmacol. **105:** 49–55.

43. LANE, R. F., C. D. BLAHA & A. G. PHILLIPS. 1986. In vivo electrochemical analysis of cholecystokinin-induced inhibition of dopamine release in the nucleus accumbens. Brain Res. **397:** 200–204.

44. LONOVICS, J., F. HAJNAL, P. MARA, I. SZABO & V. VARRO. 1979. Investigation of cholecystokinin octapeptide splitting enzyme in the dog kidney. Acta Hepato-Gastroenterol. **26:** 222–226.

45. LOTSTRA, F., P. VERBANCK, J. MENDLEWICZ & J. J. VANDERHAEGHEN. 1984. No evidence of antipsychotic effect of caerulein in schizophrenic patients free of neuroleptics: A double-blind cross-over study. Biol. Psychiatry **19:** 877–882.

46. MARKSTEIN, R. & T. HÖKFELT. 1984. Effect of cholecystokinin-octapeptide on dopamine release from slices of cat caudate nucleus. J. Neurosci. **4:** 570–575.

47. MARLEY, P. D., P. C. EMSON & J. F. REHFELD. 1982. Effect of 6-hydroxydopamine lesions of the medial forebrain bundle on the distribution of cholecystokinin in rat forebrain. Brain Res. **252:** 382–385.

48. MEYER, D. K., A. HOLLAND & U. CONZELMANN. 1984. Dopamine D-1 receptor stimulation reduced neostriatal cholecystokinin release. Eur. J. Pharmacol. **104:** 387–388.

49. MEYER, D. K. & J. KRAUSS. 1983. Dopamine modulates cholecystokinin release in neostriatum. Nature **301:** 338–340.

50. MOODY, T. W., Ed. 1986. Neural and Endocrine Peptides and Receptors. Plenum. New York.

51. MORAN, T. H., P. H. ROBINSON, M. S. GOLDRICH & P. R. McHUGH. 1986. Two brain cholecystokinin receptors: Implications for behavioral actions. Brain Res. **362:** 175–179.

52. MORAJI, T., N. WATANABE, N. AOKI & S. ITOH. 1982. Antipsychotic effects of ceruletide (caerulein) on chronic schizophrenia. Arch. Gen. Psychiatry **39:** 485–486.

53. MURPHY, R. B. & D. I. SCHUSTER. 1982. Modulation of 3H-dopamine binding by cholecystokinin octapeptide (CCK-8). Peptides **3:** 539–543.

54. NAIR, N. P. V., D. M. BLOOM, J. N. NESTOROS & G. SCHWARTZ. 1983. Therapeutic efficacy of cholecystokinin in neuroleptic-resistant schizophrenic subjects. Psychopharmacol. Bull. **19:** 134–136.

55. PASSARO, E., H. DEBAS, W. OLDENDORF & T. YAMADA. 1982. Rapid appearance of intraventricularly administered neuropeptides in the peripheral circulation. Brain Res. **241:** 335–340.

56. PIJNENBURG, A. J. J., W. M. M. HONIG, J. A. M. VAN DER HEYDEN & J. M. VAN ROSSUM. 1976. Effects of chemical stimulation of the mesolimbic dopamine system upon locomotor activity. Eur. J. Pharmacol. **35:** 45–58.

57. PRAISSMAN, M., P. A. MARTINEZ, C. F. SALADINO, J. M. BERKOWITZ, A. W. STEGGLES & J. A. FINKELSTEIN. 1983. Characterization of cholecystokinin binding sites in rat cerebral cortex using a 125-I-CCK-8 probe resistant to degradation. J. Neurochem. **40:** 1406–1413.

58. SAITO, A., I. D. GOLDFINE & J. A. WILLIAMS. 1981. Characterization of receptors for cholecystokinin and related peptides in mouse cerebral cortex. J. Neurochem. **37:** 483–490.

59. SCHNEIDER, L. H., J. E. ALPERT & S. D. IVERSEN. 1983. CCK-8 modulation of mesolimbic dopamine: Antagonism of amphetamine-stimulated behaviors. Peptides **4:** 749–753.

60. SEROOGY, K. B., K. DANGARAN, S. LIM & J. H. FALLON. 1985. Innervation of forebrain structures by ventral mesencephalic neurons containing both cholecystokinin- and tyrosine hydroxylase-like immunoreactivities: A fluorescent triple-labeling study. Abstract 47.8, Society for Neuroscience.

61. SKIRBOLL, L. R., A. A. GRACE, D. W. HOMMER, J. REHFELD, M. GOLDSTEIN, T. HÖKFELT & B. S. BUNNEY. 1981. Peptide-monoamine coexistence: Studies of the actions of cholecystokinin-like peptide on the electrical activity of midbrain dopamine neurons. Neuroscience 6: 2111–2124.

62. SNYDER, S. H. 1980. Brain peptides as neurotransmitters. Science 209: 976–983.

63. STUDLER, J. M., M. REIBAUD, D. HERVE, G. BLANC, J. GLOWINSKI & J. P. TASSIN. 1986. Opposite effects of sulfated cholecystokinin on DA-sensitive adenylate cyclase in two areas of the rat nucleus accumbens. Eur. J. Pharmacol. 126: 125–128.

64. STUDLER, J. M., M. REIBAUD, G. TRAMU, G. BLANC, J. GLOWINSKI & J. P. TASSIN. 1984. Pharmacological study on the mixed CCK-8-DA meso-nucleus accumbens pathway: Evidence for the existence of storage sites containing the two transmitters. Brain Res. 298: 91–97.

65. STUDLER, J. M., H. SIMON, F. CESSELIN, J. C. LEGRAND, J. GLOWINSKI & J. P. TASSIN. 1981. Biochemical investigation on the localization of the cholecystokinin octapeptide in dopaminergic neurons orginating from the ventral tegmental area of the rat. Neuropeptides 2: 131–139.

66. TAMMINGA, C. A., R. L. LITTMAN & L. D. ALPHS. 1986. Cholecystokinin: A neuropeptide in the treatment of schizophrenia. Psychopharmacol. Bull. 22: 129–132.

67. VACCARINO, F. J. & G. F. KOOB. 1984. Microinjections of nanogram amounts of sulfated cholecystokinin octapeptide into the rat nucleus accumbens attenuates brain stimulation reward. Neurosci. Lett. 52: 61–66.

68. VAN DIJK, A., J. G. RICHARDS, A. TRZECIAK, D. GILLESSEN & H. MOHLER. 1984. Cholecystokinin receptors: Biochemical demonstration and autoradiographical localization in rat brain and pancreas using [³H] cholecystokinin-8 as radioligand. J. Neurosci. 4: 1021–1033.

69. VAN REE, J. M., O. GAFFORI & D. DeWEID. 1983. In rats, the behavioral profile of CCK-8 related peptides resembles that of antipsychotic agents. Eur. J. Pharmacol. 93: 63–78.

70. VASAR, E., M. MAIMETS, A. NURK & L. ALLIKMETS. 1984. Caerulein stimulates [³H]-spiperone binding in vivo after long-term haloperidol administration. Psychopharmacol. Bull. 20: 4: 691–692.

71. VERBANCK, P. M. P., F. LOTSTRA, C. GILLES, P. LINKOWSKI, J. MENDLEWICZ & J. J. VANDERHAEGHEN. 1984. Reduced cholecystokinin immunoreactivity in the cerebrospinal fluid of patients with psychiatric disorders. Life Sci. 34: 67–72.

72. VOIGHT, M., R. Y. WANG & T. C. WESTFALL. 1986. Cholecystokinin octapeptides alter the release of endogenous dopamine from the rat nucleus accumbens in vitro. J. Pharmacol. Exp. Ther. 237: 147–153.

73. WEISS, F., J. C. HORVITZ, J. G. MANN & A. ETTENBERG. 1986. Intra-accumbens injections of CCK block the hyperlocomotion and potentiate the stereotypy produced by amphetamine. Abstract 400.10, Society of Neuroscience.

74. WHITE, F. J. & R. Y. WANG. 1984. Interactions of cholecystokinin octapeptide and dopamine on nucleus accumbens neurons. Brain Res. 300: 161–166.

75. WIDERLOV, E., P. W. KALIVAS, M. H. LEWIS, A. J. PRANGE & G. R. BREESE. 1983. Influence of cholecystokinin on central monoaminergic pathways. Regul. Peptides 6: 99–109.

# Neurotensin and the Mesocorticolimbic Dopamine System[a]

GARTH BISSETTE[b] AND CHARLES B. NEMEROFF[b,c,d]

*Departments of Psychiatry[b] and Pharmacology[c] and the*
*Center for Aging and Human Development[d]*
*Duke University Medical Center*
*Durham, North Carolina 27710*

Considerable evidence supports the view that neurotensin (NT), a neuropeptide neurotransmitter, is intimately involved in the regulation of the mesocorticolimbic dopamine system. In the 15 years that have elapsed since the initial isolation,[1] sequencing,[2] and characterization[3] of NT from bovine hypothalamus by Carraway and Leeman, remarkable progress has been achieved in our understanding of the physiological actions of this neuropeptide. This work was first summarized in the proceedings of a New York Academy of Sciences symposium on neurotensin held in 1981. By this time, the major criteria for the neurotransmitter status of NT were firmly established. Neurotensin is unevenly distributed within the central nervous system and is also found in high concentration in the ileum and pancreas in all mammalian species examined. Neurotensin is released from neurons by depolarizing stimuli in a calcium-dependent manner, is preferentially localized within the synaptosomal fraction after density gradient centrifugation, is degraded by specific brain peptidases, and acts upon specific high-affinity receptors. In addition, electrophysiological studies indicate that iontophoretically applied NT alters the firing rate of neurons in several CNS locations. Within the brains of rats[4-12] and humans,[13-15] NT is found in high concentration in regions known to contain dopamine (DA) cell bodies and terminals, including the substantia nigra, ventral tegmental area (VTA), caudate nucleus, nucleus accumbens, and olfactory tubercles. Recently, a putative NT pathway with cell bodies in the VTA and terminals in the nucleus accumbens has been described in the rat using NT immunohistochemistry coupled with retrograde tracers.[16] Neurons in the ventral tegmental area (A10) containing tyrosine hydroxylase, the rate-limiting enzyme for catecholamine synthesis and shown to be present in dopamine neurons, have also been found to contain NT by immunohistochemistry;[16,17] this is also true in the substantia nigra (A9) and retrorubral area (A8).[17] Within the VTA, almost all the cells staining for NT were also shown to contain tyrosine hydroxylase. In contradiction to these findings, several lines of evidence indicate that at best only a small minority of dopamine-containing neurons also contain NT. The use of 6-hydroxydopamine (6-OHDA) (with desmethylimipramine to protect noradrenergic neurons) is a standard laboratory technique to produce specific lesions of brain dopamine systems. Successful depletion of 95 to 99% of brain dopamine from such regions as the VTA–substantia nigra, the caudate nucleus, nucleus accumbens, olfactory tubercles, and frontal cortex does not significantly reduce NT concentrations of these regions[18] (FIG. 1). Goedert *et al.*[19] have also failed to observe any reduction in immunoreactive NT concentrations after 6-OHDA lesions. In

[a] This work was supported by a grant from the Schizophrenia Research Foundation of the Scottish Rite and the National Institute of Mental Health MH-39415.

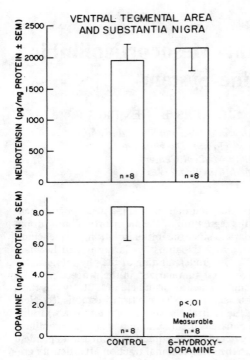

**FIGURE 1.** Intracisternal 6-hydroxydopamine destroys dopamine but not neurotensin in rat ventral tegmentum and substantia nigra. Adult male Sprague-Dawley rats (280–300 g) were pretreated with desmethylimipramine (30 mg/kg, ip) one hour before intracisternal injection of 6-hydroxydopamine (200 μg in 0.05% ascorbic acid) under ether anesthesia. This treatment was repeated one week later. Controls received desmethylimipramine and ascorbic acid vehicle. Rats were allowed to recover 6 weeks before decapitation, brain removal, and dissection. Neurotensin was measured by radioimmunoassay and dopamine was measured by high-pressure liquid chromatography with electrochemical detection.

patients with idiopathic Parkinson's disease, associated with a greater than 70% depletion of striatal dopamine, there are no significant alterations in NT concentration in such DA terminal and cell body regions as the frontal cortex, nucleus accumbens, striatum, VTA, or substantia nigra[20] (FIG. 2). Thus, either the neurons that contain NT and dopamine are resistant to both 6-OHDA and the pathologic changes due to Parkinson's disease or their contribution to the total population of dopamine neurons is quite small. However, our laboratory has recently examined NT concentrations in mice treated with another dopamine neurotoxin, MPTP. Significant depletions of NT were observed in several dopamine terminal areas (see abstract by Levant *et al.* in this volume).

It has been clearly demonstrated with autoradiographic methods that dopamine perikarya also contain NT receptors.[19,21,22] These VTA and nigral NT receptors have been shown to be decreased in Parkinson's disease.[23] Moreover, 6-OHDA lesions of the VTA have been shown to produce decreases in the number of NT receptors in the VTA, substantia nigra, and striatum.[24]

Activation of NT receptors on midbrain dopamine neurons stimulates their electrical activity.[25] Intraventricular injection of NT increases DA turnover, as measured by increased concentrations of homovanillic acid (HVA) and dihydroxyphenylacetic acid (DOPAC) in the nucleus accumbens, striatum, and olfactory tubercles.[26–30] Direct bilateral application of NT into the VTA increases DA turnover in mesolimbic projection terminals (nucleus accumbens and olfactory tubercles) as well in the VTA projection to the diagonal band.[31]

Behaviors mediated by the A10 mesolimbic dopamine projections of the VTA in-

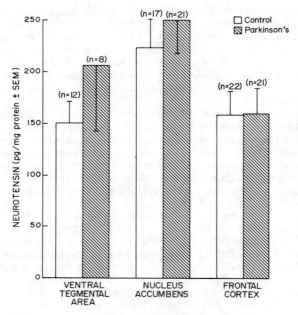

**FIGURE 2.** Neurotensin concentrations in mesolimbicocortical brain regions from Parkinson's disease patients and controls. Brain tissue dissected from patients dying with Parkinson's disease (greater than 70% depletion of caudate dopamine) or age- and sex-matched non-Parkinson's controls were received frozen and were extracted and radioimmunoassayed for neurotensin. See Bissette *et al*.[20] for details.

clude locomotion and rearing while nigro-striatal projections of the A9 dopamine cell bodies mediate grooming and stereotypical behavior. These concepts were elegantly elucidated by Creese and Iversen[32] using the behavioral response to *d*-amphetamine in the rat. Ventricular infusion of NT has been shown to decrease both locomotor activity in mice[33] and open field exploratory behavior in rats.[34,35] Injection of NT directly into the nucleus accumbens decreases spontaneous locomotor activity[36] and produces a dose-dependent antagonism of DA-induced locomotion and rearing.[37] However, when injected directly into the VTA, NT increases locomotion, rearing, and sniffing,[38] which is associated with increased DA turnover in the nucleus accumbens.[31] This effect on DA turnover is sensitized by daily VTA application of NT.[39] Moreover, the increase in locomotion seen after NT injection into the VTA is blocked by concomitant NT infusion into the nucleus accumbens.[40] Thus ventricular application of NT has the same effect of decreasing locomotion as does direct infusion of NT into the mesolimbic dopamine terminal region of the nucleus accumbens, while injection of NT into the cell body region (VTA) of this dopamine projection effectively activates this system, resulting in increased turnover and increased locomotion. The behavioral effects of indirect DA agonists on mesolimbic terminal regions can be blocked by NT administration. Intracerebral NT blocks locomotion induced by methylphenidate, amphetamine, and cocaine,[41] but not the locomotion induced by scopolamine or caffeine.[42] Similar to haloperidol, NT administered into the nucleus accumbens blocks the locomotion and rearing produced by relatively low doses of *d*-amphetamine, while NT injected into the caudate nucleus is, unlike haloperidol, unable to block the stereotypic behavior seen after a larger dose of $d$-amphetamine.[43] Thus NT applied to the ventricles or the nucleus accumbens seems to block the behavioral effects of mesolimbic dopamine circuit activation, but NT does not alter behavior mediated by the nigrostriatal dopamine projections when applied to the caudate nucleus.

There are many other similarities between NT and antipsychotic drugs in terms of the pharmacological and neurochemical effects, as well as some decided differences. Several current reviews are available.[44-47]

Both centrally administered NT and systemically administered antipsychotic drugs increase DA turnover in the nucleus accumbens, olfactory tubercles, and striatum. In addition, both the peptide and neuroleptics induce hypothermia, potentiate ethanol, and barbiturate sedation, produce catalepsy and muscle relaxation, decrease locomotor activity, and inhibit avoidance but not escape behavior during a conditioned active avoidance response. Unlike neuroleptics, NT does not displace agonists or antagonists from the DA receptor, and does not block stereotypic behavior induced by $d$-amphetamine.

Govani et al.[48] were the first to demonstrate significantly increased concentrations of NT in the nucleus accumbens and striatum of rats treated for three weeks with a variety of clinically effective antipsychotic compounds. Clinically ineffective phenothiazines were not able to alter NT concentrations after chronic administration. Kilts et al.[49] have extended these findings using a micropunch dissection and have surveyed 38 brain regions for alterations in NT concentration after chronic treatment with haloperidol or clozapine. Both neuroleptics significantly increased NT concentrations in the nucleus accumbens and decreased NT concentrations in the anterior cingulate and medial prefrontal cortices as well as in the bed nucleus of the stria terminalis when compared to controls. Haloperidol increased NT concentrations in the caudate nucleus and putamen, while clozapine, which is purported to be without extrapyramidal effects,[50] did not. Recently, we have treated rats chronically with (+) or (−) butaclamol and then measured NT concentrations in rat brain regions.[51] The isomers of butaclamol both exhibit equal actions at acetylcholine, histamine, and noradrenergic receptors, but only (−) butaclamol displaces dopamine from $D_2$ receptors and possesses clinical antipsychotic potency. Chronic treatment of rats with (+) butaclamol or haloperidol (1 mg/kg) produced increased NT concentrations in the nucleus accumbens, striatum, and olfactory tubercles, when compared to rats treated with (−) butaclamol or vehicle (TABLE 1). Thus, the ability of antipsychotic drugs to increase NT concentrations in the nucleus accumbens may predict clinical efficacy, while the increase in the caudate nucleus may predict extrapyramidal side-effect liability.

**TABLE 1.** Effects of Chronic Treatment with (+)Butaclamol and (−)Butaclamol on Neurotensin Concentrations in the Anterior Caudate Nucleus and the Nucleus Accumbens

| Treatment[a] | Neurotensin Concentration (pg/mg protein)[b] | |
| --- | --- | --- |
| | Anterior Caudate | Nucleus Accumbens |
| Vehicle | 90.8 ± 15 | 209 ± 16 |
| (+)Butaclamol (1 mg/kg) | 137.1 ± 13[c] | 340 ± 22[c] |
| (−)Butaclamol (1 mg/kg) | 101.5 ± 12 | 207 ± 33 |

[a] Vehicle, (+)butaclamol, or (−)butaclamol were administered daily for 14 days.

[b] Values represent the $X \pm$ SEM.

[c] Significantly different ($p < 0.05$) than vehicle-treated controls using ANOVA and Newman–Keuls test.

The many similarities in the actions of NT and neuroleptic drugs raised the question of potential involvement of NT in schizophrenia. Schizophrenia is currently believed to involve hyperactivity of the mesocorticolimbic dopamine pathway.[52] The extent of neuropeptide involvement in this disease is described in detail in a chapter by Bissette *et al.*[53] Widerlov *et al.*[54] reported reduced CSF concentration of NT in a subgroup of drug-free schizophrenic patients when compared to normal controls. In a second study of drug-free patients, we again observed significantly reduced CSF NT levels in the schizophrenic group, but not in depressed patients or anorexic/bulemics,[55] lending some specificity to the finding of decreased NT in the CSF of schizophrenics. Increased concentrations of immunoreactive NT were measured in the frontal cortex (Brodmann's area[10]) in schizophrenics compared to controls; no changes were observed in the nucleus accumbens or other cortical areas (Brodmann's area 12 and 28).[56] Substantia nigra from both neuroleptic-treated rats and schizophrenic patients have been found to exhibit increased numbers of NT receptors.[57] It is not known whether the increase in NT receptor number in schizophrenic patients is due to neuroleptic drug treatment or to the disease itself, as no tissues are available from drug-free schizophrenics. Obviously, clinical trials of NT in the treatment of schizophrenia would appear to be warranted. However, because NT cannot cross the blood–brain barrier, such trials either await analogs that can cross, or novel CNS delivery strategies.

Neurotensin has many actions that are only now beginning to be fully appreciated. The possible uses of this endogenous compound in the treatment of schizophrenia hold great promise. The intimate involvement of this peptide in the regulation of the mesocorticolimbic dopamine system is now apparent and further research will undoubtedly add to the burgeoning data base.

## REFERENCES

1. CARRAWAY, R. & S. E. LEEMAN. 1977. Regional and subcellular distribution of brain neurotensin. Life Sci. **19:** 1827–1832.
2. CARRAWAY, R. & S. E. LEEMAN. 1975. The amino acid sequence of a hypothalamic peptide, neurotensin. J. Biol. Chem. **250:** 1907–1911.
3. CARRAWAY, R. & S. E. LEEMAN. 1976. Characterization of radioimmunoassayable neurotensin in the rat: Its differential distribution in the central nervous system, small intestine, and stomach. J. Biol Chem. **251:** 7045–7052.
4. UHL, G. R. & S. H. SNYDER. 1977. Regional and subcellular distribution of brain neurotensin. Life Sci. **19:** 1827–1832.
5. KOBAYASHI, R. M., M. R. BROWN & W. VALE. 1977. Regional distribution of neurotensin and somatostatin in rat brain. Brain Res. **126:** 584–588.
6. KAHN, D., G. M. ABRAMS, E. A. ZIMMERMAN, R. CARRAWAY & S. E. LEEMAN. 1980. Neurotensin neurons in the rat hypothalamus: An immunocytochemical study. Endocrinology **107:** 47–54.
7. JENNES, L., W. E. STUMPF & P. W. KALIVAS. 1982. Neurotensin: Topographical distribution in rat brain by immunohistochemistry. J. Comp. Neurol. **210:** 211–224.
8. ROBERTS, G. W., P. L. WOODHAUS, J. M. POLAK & T. J. CROW. 1982. Distribution of neuropeptides in the limbic system of the rat: The amygdala complex. Neuroscience **7:** 99–131.
9. EMSON, P. C., M. GOEDERT, P. HORSFIELD, F. RIOUX & S. PIERRE. 1982. The regional distribution and chromatographic characterization of neurotensin-like immunoreactivity in the rat central nervous system. J. Neurochem. **28:** 992–999.
10. GOEDERT, M., P. W. MANTYH, S. P. HUNT & P. C. EMSON. 1983. Mosaic distribution of neurotensin-like immunoreactivity in the cat striatum. Brain Res. **274:** 176–179.
11. REINECKE, M., R. E. CARRAWAY, S. FALKEMER, G. E. FEURLEY & W. G. FORSSMAN. 1980.

Occurrence of neurotensin-immunoreactive cells in the digestive tract of lower vertebrates and deuterostomian invertebrates. Cell Tissue Res. **212:** 173–183.

12. ANDERSON, C. M., G. BISSETTE, C. B. NEMEROFF & C. D. KILTS. 1984. Microtopographic distribution of neurotensin and catecholamine concentrations at the level of individual rat brain nuclei. Soc. Neurosci. Abstr. **10:** 437.

13. COOPER, P. E., M. H. FERNSTROM, O. P. RORSTAD, S. E. LEEMAN & J. B. MARTIN. 1981. The regional distribution of somatostatin, substance P and neurotensin in human brain. Brain Res. **218:** 218–232.

14. MANBERG, P. J., W. W. YOUNGBLOOD, C. B. NEMEROFF, M. ROSSOR, L. L. IVERSEN, A. J. PRANGE, JR. & J. S. KIZER. 1982. Regional distribution of neurotensin in the human brain. J. Neurochem. **38:** 1777–1780.

15. GHATEI, M. A., S. R. BLOOM, H. LANGEVIN, G. P. MCGREGOR, Y. C. LEE, T. W. ADRIAN, D. J. O'SHAUGHNESSY, M. A. BLANK & L. O. UTTENTHAL. 1984. Regional distribution of bombesin and seven other regulatory peptides in the human brain. Brain Res. **293:** 101–109.

16. KALIVAS, P. W. & J. S. MILLER. 1984. Neurotensin neurons in the ventral tegmental area project to the medial nucleus accumbens. Brain Res. **300:** 157–160.

17. HOKFELT, T., B. J. EVERITT, E. THEODORSSON-NORHEIM & M. GOLDSTEIN. 1984. Occurrence of neurotensin-like immunoreactivity in subpopulations of hypothalamic, mesencephalic, and medullary catecholamine neurons. J. Comp. Neurol. **222:** 543–559.

18. BISSETTE, G., J. JENNES, A. J. PRANGE, JR., G. R. BREESE & C. B. NEMEROFF. 1983. Neurotensin and dopamine are not co-localized in rat brain. Soc. Neurosci. Abstr. **9:** 290.

19. GOEDERT, M., K. PITTAWAY & P. C. EMSON. 1984. Neurotensin receptors in the rat striatum: Lesion studies. Brain Res. **299:** 164–168.

20. BISSETTE, G., C. B. NEMEROFF, M. W. DECKER, J. S. KIZER, Y. AGID & F. JAVOY-AGID. 1985. Alterations in regional brain concentrations of neurotensin and bombesin in Parkinson's disease. Ann. Neurol. **17:** 324–329.

21. PALACIOS, J. M. & M. J. KUHAR. 1981. Neurotensin receptors are located on dopamine-containing neurons in rat midbrain. Nature **294:** 587–589.

22. QUIRION, R., P. GAUDREAU, S. ST. PIERRE, F. RIOUX & C. PERT. 1982. Autoradiographic distribution of [³H]neurotensin receptors in rat brain. Peptides **3:** 757–763.

23. UHL, G. R., P. J. WHITEHOUSE, K. L. PRICE, W. W. TOURTELOTTE & M. J. KUHAR. 1984. Parkinson's disease: Depletion of substantia nigra neurotensin receptors. Brain Res. **299:** 164–168.

24. HERVE, D., J. P. TASSIN, J. M. STUDLER, C. DANA, P. KITABGI, J. P. VINCENT, J. GLOWINOSKI & W. ROSTENE. 1986. Dopaminergic control of $^{125}$I-labeled neurotensin binding site density in corticolimbic structures of the rat brain. Proc. Natl. Acad. Sci. U.S.A. **83:** 6203–6207.

25. ANDRADE, R. & G. K. AGHAJANIAN. 1981. Neurotensin selectively activates dopamine neurons in the substantia nigra. Soc. Neurosci. Abstr. **7:** 573.

26. GARCIA-SEVILLA, J. A., T. MAGNUSSON, A. CARLSON, J. LEBAN & K. FOLKERS. 1978. Neurotensin and its amide analogue [Gln⁴]-neurotensin: Effects on brain monoamine turnover. Naunyn-Schmiedeberg's Arch. Pharmacol. **305:** 213–218.

27. RECHES, A., R. E. BURKE, D. JIANG, H. R. WAGNER & S. HAHN. 1982. The effect of neurotensin on dopaminergic neurons in rat brain. Ann. N.Y. Acad. Sci. **400:** 420–421.

28. RECHES, A., R. E. BURKE, D. H. JIANG, H. R. WAGNER & S. HAHN. 1983. Neurotensin interactions with dopaminergic neurons in rat brain. Peptides **4:** 43–48.

29. WIDERLOV, E., C. D. KILTS, R. B. MAILMAN, C. B. NEMEROFF, T. J. MCCOWN, A. J. PRANGE, JR. & G. R. BREESE. 1982. Increase in dopamine metabolites in rat brain by neurotensin. J. Pharmacol. Exp. Ther. **222:** 1–6.

30. NEMEROFF, C. B., D. LUTTINGER, D. E. HERNANDEZ, R. B. MAILMAN, G. A. MASON, S. K. DAVIS, E. WIDERLOV, G. D. FRYE, C. D. KILTS, K. BEAUMONT, G. R. BREESE & A. J. PRANGE, JR. 1983. Interactions of neurotensin with brain dopamine systems: Biochemical and behavioral studies. J. Pharmacol. Exp. Ther. **225:** 337–345.

31. KALIVAS, P. W., L. JENNES & J. S. MILLER. 1985. A catecholaminergic projection from the ventral tegmental area to the diagonal band of Broca: Modulation by neurotensin. Brain Res. **326:** 229–238.

32. CREESE, I. & S. D. IVERSEN. 1975. The pharmacological and anatomical substrates of the amphetamine response in the rat. Brain Res. **83:** 419–436.

33. MEISENBURG, G. & W. H. SIMMONS. 1985. Motor hyperactivity induced by neurotensin and related peptides in mice. Pharm. Biochem. Behav. **22:** 189–193.
34. RINKEL, G. J. E., E. C. HOEKE & J. B. VAN WIMERSMA-GREIDANAUS. 1983. Elective tolerance to behavioral effects of neurotensin. Pharmacol. Behav. **31:** 467–470.
35. ELLIOT, P. J., J. CHAN, Y. M. PARKER & C. B. NEMEROFF. 1986. Behavioral effects of neurotensin in the open field: Structure-activity studies. Brain Res. **381:** 259–265.
36. GRIFFITHS, E. C., P. SLATER & V. A. D. WEBSTER. 1981. Behavioral interaction between neurotensin and thyrotropin releasing hormone in rat central nervous system. J. Physiol. **320:** 90.
37. KALIVAS, P. W., C. B. NEMEROFF & A. J. PRANGE, JR. 1984. Neurotensin microinjection into the nucleus accumbens antagonizes dopamine-induced increase in locomotion and rearing. Neuroscience **11:** 919–930.
38. KALIVAS, P. W., C. B. NEMEROFF & A. J. PRANGE, JR. 1981. Increase in spontaneous motor activity following infusion of neurotensin into the ventral tegmental area. Brain Res. **229:** 525–529.
39. KALIVAS, P. W. & S. TAYLOR. 1985. Behavioral and neurochemical effect of daily injections with neurotensin into the ventral tegmental area. Brain Res. **358:** 70–76.
40. ELLIOT, P. E. & C. B. NEMEROFF. 1986. Repeated neurotensin administration in the ventral tegmental area: Effects on baseline and d-amphetamine-induced locomotor activity. Neurosci. Lett. **68:** 239–244.
41. KALIVAS, P. W., C. B. NEMEROFF & A. J. PRANGE, JR. 1982. Neuroanatomical site specific modulation of spontaneous motor activity by neurotensin. Eur. J. Pharmacol. **78:** 471–474.
42. SKOOG, K. M., S. T. CAIN & C. B. NEMEROFF. 1986. Centrally administered neurotensin suppresses locomotor hyperactivity induced by d-amphetamine but not by scopolamine or caffeine. Neuropharmacology **25:** 777–782.
43. ERVIN, G. N., L. S. BIRKEMO, C. B. NEMEROFF & A. J. PRANGE, JR. 1981. Neurotensin blocks certain amphetamine behaviors. Nature **291:** 73–76.
44. NEMEROFF, C. B. 1980. Neurotensin: Perchance an endogenous neuroleptic? Biol. Psychiatry **15:** 283–302.
45. NEMEROFF, C. B. 1986. The interaction of neurotensin with dopaminergic pathways in the central nervous system: Basic neurobiology and implications for the treatment of schizophrenia. Psychoneuroendocrinology **11:** 15–37.
46. NEMEROFF, C. B. & S. T. CAIN. 1985. Neurotensin-dopamine interactions in the central nervous stem. Trends Pharmacol. Sci. **6:** 201–205.
47. NEMEROFF, C. B., A. J. PRANGE, JR., D. LUTTINGER, D. E. HERNANDEZ, R. A. KING & S. K. BURGESS. 1981. Similarities and differences in the effects of centrally administered neurotensin and neuroleptics. Psycopharmacol. Bull. **17:** 145–147.
48. GOVANI, S., J. S. HONG, H.-Y. T. YANG & E. COSTA. 1980. Increase of neurotensin content elicited by neurolepics in nucleus accumbens. J. Pharmacol. Exp. Ther. **215:** 413–417.
49. KILTS, C. D., C. ANDERSON, G. BISSETTE, T. ELY & C. B. NEMEROFF. 1988. Differential effects of antipsychotic drugs on the neurotensin content of discrete rat brain nuclei. Biochem. Pharmacol. **37:** 1547–1554.
50. RUPNIAK, N. M. J., S. MANN, M. D. HALL, P. JENNER & C. D. MARSDEN. 1984. Comparison of the effects on striatal DA receptor function of chronic administration of haloperidol, clozapine or sulpiride to rats for up to 12 months. In Catecholamines: Neuropharmacology and CNS-Theoretical Aspects. E. Usdin, S. Carlsson, A. Dahlstrom, and J. Engels, Eds. Alan Liss. New York.
51. BISSETTE, G., W. T. DAUER, C. D. KILTS, L. O'CONNOR & C. B. NEMEROFF. 1986. Effect of d-amphetamine and dopamine receptor antagonists on neurotensin concentrations in microdissected rat brain regions. Soc. Neurosci. Abstr. **12:** 33.
52. SNYDER, S. H. 1982. Schizophrenia. Lancet. **ii:** 970–974.
53. BISSETTE, G., C. B. NEMEROFF & A. V. P. MACKAY. 1986. Neuropeptides in schizophrenia. Prog. Brain Res. **66:** 161–174.
54. WIDERLOV, E., L. H. LINDSTROM, G. BESEV, P. J. MANBERG, C. B. NEMEROFF, G. R. BREESE, J. S. KIZER & A. J. PRANGE, JR. 1982. Subnormal CSF levels of neurotensin in a subgroup of schizophrenic patients: Normalization after neuroleptic treatment. Am. J. Psychiatry **139:** 1122–1126.
55. MANBERG, P. J., C. B. NEMEROFF, G. BISSETTE, A. J. PRANGE, JR. & R. H. GERNER. 1983.

Cerebrospinal fluid levels of neurotensin-like immunoreactivity in normal controls and in patients with affective disorder, anorexia nervosa and premenstrual syndrome. Soc. Neurosci. Abstr. **9:** 1054.

56.  NEMEROFF, C. B., W. YOUNGBLOOD, P. J. MANBERG, A. J. PRANGE, JR. & J. S. KIZER. 1983. Regional brain concentrations of neuropeptides in Huntington's chorea and schizophrenia. Science **221:** 972–975.

57.  UHL, G. R. & M. J. KUHAR. 1984. Chronic neuroleptic treatment enhances neurotensin receptor binding in human and rat substantia nigra. Nature **309:** 350–352.

# Enkephalin Modulation of A10 Dopamine Neurons: A Role in Dopamine Sensitization[a]

PETER W. KALIVAS,[b] PATRICIA DUFFY,
ROGER DILTS, AND RAYMOND ABHOLD

*Department of Veterinary and Comparative
Anatomy, Pharmacology, and Physiology
College of Veterinary Medicine
Washington State University
Pullman, Washington 99164–6520*

## INTRODUCTION

Many lines of evidence support the possibility that the opioid pentapeptides Met- and Leu-enkephalin have a neurotransmitterlike function in the mammalian central nervous system.[1] A neurotransmitter role for enkephalin in modulating the mesocorticolimbic dopamine (DA) system at the level of the dopaminergic perikarya in the A10 region is indicated by many anatomical studies. A moderate density of enkephalinergic fibers and a few perikarya are present in the A10 DA region.[2,3] The A10 also contains a moderate and low density of mu and delta opioid receptors, respectively.[4,5] On the basis of these anatomical studies, a number of behavioral, neurochemical, and electrophysiological studies have been initiated to study a potential enkephalin–DA interaction in this brain region. Microinjection of enkephalin analogues into the A10 region of rats produces an increase in spontaneous motor activity that is antagonized by pretreatment with DA receptor antagonists.[6-8] Furthermore, the increased motor activity following intra-A10 injection with enkephalin analogues is associated with increased DA metabolism in the nucleus accumbens (a major mesolimbic DA terminal field).[8] Finally, iontophresis of opioids was found to facilitate the spontaneous activity of DA neurons, but was inhibitory on spontaneously active non-DA neurons.[9] Because only the inhibitory action was naloxone reversible and peripherally administered morphine excited DA neurons in a naloxone-reversible manner, it has been proposed that the electrophysiological activation of DA neurons is mediated indirectly through disinhibition.[9,10]

In this article we describe our recent anatomical, behavioral, and neurochemical work that further characterizes the interaction between enkephalin and the mesocorticolimbic DA system. In addition, it has recently been shown that daily administration of opioids into the A10 region produces a progressive increase in the motor stimulant effect of subsequent acute intra-A10 injection of opioids.[11-13] We have recently characterized some neurochemical components of this behavioral sensitization to opioids

[a] This work was supported in part by National Institutes of Health Grants MH-40817 and DA-03906 and in part by a grant from the Scottish Rite Schizophrenia Foundation.
[b] To whom correspondence should be sent.

that indicate it may be mediated by alterations in mesocorticolimbic DA function. These data, as well as data demonstrating a role for endogenous enkephalin in the capacity of stress to augment the behavioral effects of opioids is discussed.

## ANATOMY

Johnson *et al.* provided the first study focusing on the proximity of enkephalin terminals to the A10 DA neurons.[2] It has been more recently shown that a few enkephalinergic perikarya are also found in the A10 region.[3,14] In an effort to determine the origin of the enkephalinergic fibers in the A10, we have retrogradely labeled neurons by injecting horseradish peroxidase into the A10 region, and double-labeling cells for enkephalin immunoreactivity using methods modified from Bowker *et al.*[15,16] It was found that enkephalinergic neurons having ascending projections into the A10 region were located in the dorsal raphe, dorsal tegmental nucleus, parabrachial nuclei, and the pedunculopontine region, including the cuniform nucleus. This later projection from the pedunculopontine region is of special interest, since it provides a closure of the established mesolimbic output pathway that goes from the nucleus accumbens to the ventral pallidum to the pedunculopontine region.[17,18] Thus, this enkephalinergic projection is a substrate whereby the activity of A10 DA neurons projecting to the nucleus accumbens can be modulated depending upon the output through the pedunculopontine region.

Both mu and delta opioid receptors are located in the A10 region.[4,5] To determine if the mu receptors are located on DA perikarya in the A10 region, unilateral injection of 6-hydroxydopamine to lesion DA perikarya or quinolinic acid to lesion all intrinsic neurons was made into the A10, and mu-receptor density measured using light microscopic receptor autoradiography. The details of this study are described elsewhere in this volume.[5] Using $^{125}$I-DAGO [Tyr-D-Ala-Gly-N-MePhe-Gly(ol)] as the mu opioid receptor ligand, it was found that 6-hydroxydopamine lesions that markedly decreased $^{125}$I-Tyr$_3$-neurotensin binding did not alter DAGO binding. However, the quinolinic acid lesions produced a 50–70% depletion of DAGO receptors, in addition to decreasing neurotensin binding. These data demonstrate that the mu opioid receptors are not located on the DA perikarya, but are to a great extent present on non-dopaminergic perikarya in the A10 region. These data are consistent with the electrophysiological data previously described, indicating that activation of the A10 DA neurons by opioids is produced via disinhibition.[9,10] One possibility is that the mu opioid receptors are located on GABAergic neurons within the A10 that provide a tonic inhibitory influence on the A10 DA neurons.

## BEHAVIORAL AND NEUROCHEMICAL EFFECTS OF ENKEPHALIN IN THE A10

Many laboratories have demonstrated that acute microinjection of enkephalin analogues into the A10 region produces an increase in spontaneous motor activity, and that this effect is blocked by intraaccumbens or peripheral administration of DA receptor antagonists.[6-8] FIGURE 1b demonstrates the motor stimulant effect produced by injection of the mu-receptor agonist, DAGO, into the A10 region. FIGURE 1b also shows that an equimolar dose of the delta receptor agonist, DPEN ([D-Pen$^{2,5}$]-enkephalin), was ineffective. Using a complete dose-response analysis we have demonstrated that the mu-receptor agonist is approximately 1000-fold more potent than the delta agonist,

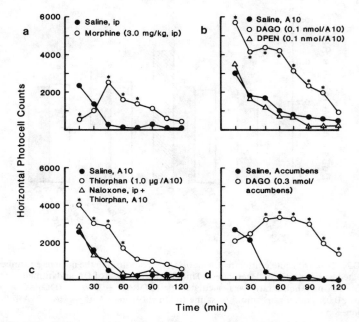

**FIGURE 1.** Effect of acute opioid treatment on horizontal motor activity in the rat. All rats were adapted to the photocell apparatus for 60 min prior to injection with opioid. * $p < 0.05$, comparing saline to opioid treatment using a one-way analysis of variance (ANOVA) followed by a Newman–Keuls test.

and that this potency difference does not involve differences in the rate of elimination of the microinjected enkephalin analogue from the A10 region.[19] Furthermore, the motor stimulant effect of DAGO was blocked by pretreatment with the selective mu-1 receptor antagonist, naloxonazine,[20] arguing that the mu-1 isoreceptor is mediating a major portion of the activation of A10 DA neurons previously demonstrated with mixed mu and delta opioid agonists.[19] This conclusion is supported by the fact that DAGO was more potent than DPEN at increasing DA metabolism in the nucleus accumbens after injection into the A10 region (FIG. 2). This neurochemical effect of DAGO was also attenuated by pretreatment with naloxonazine.[19]

FIGURE 1c shows that a motor stimulant effect can be produced by inhibition of enkephalin metabolism in the A10 region. Thiorphan is a dipeptidyl carboxypeptidase inhibitor that has been shown to enhance the recovery of enkephalins released from depolarized brain slices and to produce naloxone-reversible antinociception and other opioidlike behavioral effects when given centrally.[21] As described in a recent study in our laboratory, the motor stimulant effect produced by intra-A10 injection of thiorphan was blocked by pretreatment with naloxone or the DA receptor antagonist, haloperidol.[22] These data argue that enhancement of endogenous enkephalin neurotransmission in the A10 region by inhibiting enkephalin metabolism can activate the mesocorticolimbic DA system. This conclusion is supported by the neurochemical data in FIGURE 2 showing that thiorphan increases DA metabolism in the nucleus accumbens. This effect of thiorphan was also blocked by pretreatment with naloxone.[22]

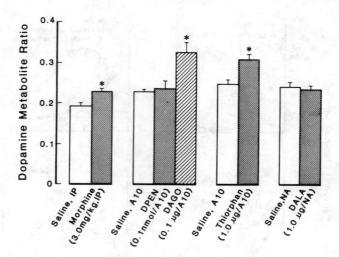

**FIGURE 2.** Effect of acute opioid treatment on DA metabolism in the nucleus accumbens. Rats were injected with the opioid, decapitated 30 min later, and levels of DA and its metabolites measured. The DA metabolite ratio was calculated as: (DOPAC + HVA) / (DOPAC + HVA + DA). * $p < 0.05$, comparing opioid to saline treatment using a one-way ANOVA followed by a Newman–Keuls test.

FIGURE 1d shows that enkephalin analogue injection into the nucleus accumbens also produces a motor stimulant effect. However, it has been shown that this action is not blocked by pretreatment with DA receptor antagonists into the nucleus accumbens,[8,23] arguing that the behavioral hyperactivity is not mediated by augmenting the release of DA from terminals in the accumbens. This is supported by the data in FIGURE 2 demonstrating that intraaccumbens injection of enkephalin analogue does not alter DA metabolism in the nucleus accumbens.[8] FIGURE 1a demonstrates that peripheral administration of morphine also elicits a motor stimulant response.[24,25] It is interesting that the time course of the behavioral response to peripheral morphine resembles that of intraaccumbens, and not intra-A10 injection of enkephalin. The possibility that the behavioral stimulant effect of peripheral morphine results more from an action in the nucleus accumbens than in the A10 region was demonstrated by Amalric and Koob,[26] who found that intraaccumbens injection of opioid antagonist more potently blocked the motor stimulant effect of peripheral heroin administration than did intra-A10 injection of antagonist.

## SENSITIZATION TO DAILY ENKEPHALIN INJECTION INTO THE A10

Joyce and Iversen[11] first observed that daily injection of morphine into the A10 region resulted in a progressive enhancement in the motor stimulant effect of acute intra-A10 morphine. This effect has since been replicated with both morphine and enkephalin analogues.[12,13] FIGURE 3b shows that daily DAGO injection into the A10 region produces a sensitization of the motor stimulant effect. This effect persists for at least two weeks,

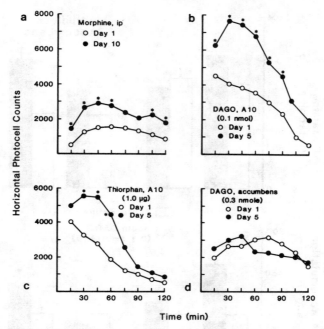

**FIGURE 3.** Effect of daily opioid treatment on horizontal motor activity. The data obtained on the first and last day of opioid treatment are compared. In general, on all intervening days the daily opioid injection was made in the home cage. Rats were adapted to the photocell apparatus for 60 min prior to injection with opioid. * $p < 0.05$, comparing the first day of opioid treatment to the last day, using a repeated measures ANOVA followed by a Newman–Keuls test.

and is blocked by pretreatment with naloxone.[13] FIGURE 3c shows that behavioral sensitization can also be produced by daily injection of thiorphan into the A10 region.[22] FIGURE 3 also shows that daily peripheral administration of morphine, but not daily injection of DAGO into the nucleus accumbens produces behavioral sensitization. Likewise, intraaccumbens injection of morphine did not produce behavioral sensitization.[27] Thus, unlike the acute behavioral stimulant effect of peripheral morphine that appears to be mediated predominately in the nucleus accumbens,[26] behavioral sensitization to daily morphine injections may be mediated by an action in the A10 region. This conclusion is supported by the fact that daily intra-A10, but not daily intraaccumbens, pretreatment with naltrexone methobromide abolished the development of behavioral sensitization following daily peripheral morphine injection.[25]

The possibility that behavioral sensitization to intra-A10 injection of DAGO is mediated by an alteration in DA neurotransmission in the mesocorticolimbic DA system is supported by the fact that rats pretreated with daily injections of DAGO demonstrate a greater increase in DA metabolism and DOPA accumulation in the nucleus accumbens in response to an acute challenge with DAGO than did rats pretreated with daily saline (FIG. 4). In contrast, the effect of acute DAGO on DA metabolism and DOPA accumulation in the A10 region was absent in rats pretreated daily with DAGO. These data argue that the behavioral sensitization to intra-A10 administration of DAGO is mediated by an increase in DA neurotransmission in the nucleus accumbens. Fur-

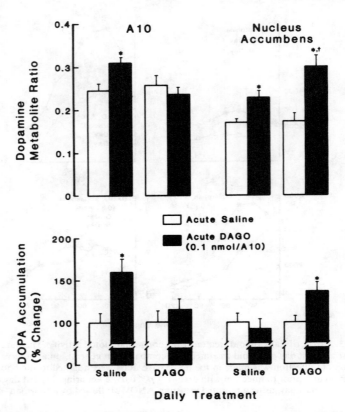

**FIGURE 4.** Effect of daily DAGO treatment on the capacity of acute DAGO injection to alter DA metabolism or dopa accumulation. Rats were pretreated with 5 daily injections of DAGO (0.1 nmole/A10) or saline, and injected acutely with saline or DAGO 2 weeks later. The DA metabolite ratio was calculated as described in the legend for FIGURE 2. For DOPA accumulation, rats were pretreated with NSD-1015 (100 mg/kg, ip), given DAGO or saline 5 min later, and decapitated 25 min afterwards. DOPA was measured using HPLC-EC. * $p < 0.05$, comparing the effect of acute DAGO with acute saline, using a one-way ANOVA followed by a Newman–Keuls test. + $p < 0.05$, comparing saline and DAGO daily treatments within the same acute treatment group.

thermore, this increase in dopaminergic activity in the accumbens may result from a decrease in DA neurotransmission in the A10 region that would produce less stimulation of somatodendritic autoreceptors, and thereby diminish the negative regulation normally occurring during stimulation of the A10 DA neurons by injection of DAGO. A similar neurochemical profile was observed in rats sensitized to peripheral morphine administration.[25] The effect of peripheral morphine on DOPA accumulation in the nucleus accumbens was significantly augmented in rats pretreated daily with morphine, and the stimulation of DA metabolism and DOPA accumulation in the A10 by acute morphine injection was significantly blunted in rats pretreated daily with morphine (FIG. 5).

A final series of experiments employing *in vitro* release of endogenous DA from

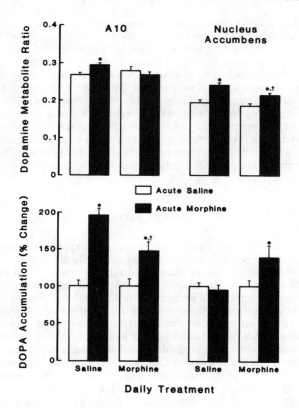

**FIGURE 5.** Effect of daily morphine treatment on the capacity of acute morphine injection to alter DA metabolism or DOPA accumulation. See FIGURE 4 legend for further details.

tissue slices of the A10 and A9 regions and the nucleus accumbens supports the possibility that behavioral sensitization to daily peripheral and intra-A10 administration of opioids is mediated by a decrease in DA neurotransmission in the DA perikarya. These findings are discussed in detail elsewhere in this volume.[28] Rats were pretreated with daily injection of enkephalin analogue into the A10 region or morphine, ip, and it was found that tissue slices containing the DA perikarya released less DA in response to potassium-induced depolarization. In contrast, no consistent effect was observed in the DA terminal fields examined on potassium-induced release of DA. These data argue that a decrease in the release of somatodendritic DA in opioid-sensitized rats may be the primary alteration mediating the increase in DA release in the terminal fields.

## ROLE OF ENKEPHALIN IN THE A10 IN CROSS-SENSITIZATION WITH STRESS

We have recently demonstrated that daily exposure to mild footshock stress (i.e., producing no vocalization or behavioral indications of pain) enhances the motor stimulant effect of enkephalin analogue injection into the A10 region.[29] Conversely, daily intra-A10 injection of enkephalin analogue into the A10 region significantly potentiated the capacity of acute footshock to elevate DA metabolism in the nucleus accumbens and septum, but not in the prefrontal cortex. More recently we investigated the possibility that this cross-sensitization between intra-A10 injection of enkephalin analogue and footshock stress in mediated by the release of endogenous enkephalin into the A10 region.[30] Supporting this possibility, it was shown that daily pretreatment with naltrexone methobromide into the A10 region prior to exposure to daily footshock prevented the augmentation of the motor stimulant effect of intra-A10 injection of enkephalin analogue. Furthermore, it was observed that footshock produced a time-dependent decrease in the level of immunoreactive Met-enkephalin in the medial A10 region, which may be indicative of a footshock-induced increase in release and metabolism of Met-enkephalin.[30]

## CONCLUSIONS

The data previously outlined argue strongly that enkephalin is a physiological neuromodulator of the mesocorticolimbic DA system at the level of the DA perikarya in the A10 region. Not only is the anatomical substrate present that could support such a role for enkephalin, but inhibition of enkephalin metabolism in the A10 increases DA neurotransmission. Furthermore, mild footshock releases enkephalin in the A10 region that increases DA neurotransmission. The mu opioid receptor appears to be mediating the activation of the DA neurons, and the studies employing 6-hydroxydopamine lesions and quinolinic acid lesions of the A10 coupled with light microscopic receptor autoradiography demonstrate that the mu opioid receptors are not located directly on the DA neurons, but are found on non-DA neurons intrinsic to the A10 region.[5] These anatomical data are consistent with the electrophysiological evidence arguing that opioid activation of the A10 DA neurons is mediated indirectly via disinhibition.[9,10] Based upon these data we propose the model in FIGURE 6 as a

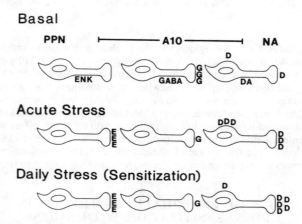

**FIGURE 6.** Model of how acute and chronic stress-induced release of enkephalin into the A10 DA region alters dopaminergic neurotransmission in the nucleus accumbens. D = dopamine; E = enkephalin; G = GABA; PPN = pedunculopontine nucleus; NA = nucleus accumbens.

mechanism by which enkephalin activates the A10 DA neurons, and by which behavioral sensitization to enkephalin is produced. It is proposed that enkephalin acts via inhibiting a gamma-aminobutyric acid (GABA) interneuron located in the A10, thereby releasing the DA neuron from tonic GABAergic inhibition. Under resting conditions the enkephalin release is minimal or absent, allowing maximal tonic GABAergic inhibition. However, during acute stress enkephalin is released that inhbits GABA release, and thereby increases DA neurotransmission. The increase in somatodendritic DA release stimulates autoreceptors moderating the excitatory effect of disinhibition on neuronal activity and the resulting release of DA in the nucleus accumbens. However, in rats sensitized by daily stress or opioid administration the disinhibition of the DA perikarya by stress-induced release of enkephalin does not result in as marked an increase in somatodendritic DA release. This would produce less stimulation of somatodendritic autoreceptors, leading to an increase in neuronal firing frequency and enhanced DA release in the terminal fields. While this model remains unproved, it is consistent with the data presented in this article, and provides a framework in which to formulate and test hypotheses regarding the modulatory role of enkephalin on mesocorticolimbic DA neurotransmission, and the role enkephalin has in producing alterations in DA neurotransmission that may underlie behavioral sensitization to opioids and stress.

## REFERENCES

1.  MILLER, R. J. 1983. The enkephalins. *In* Handbook of Psychopharmacology, Vol. 18. L. L. Iversen, S. D. Iversen, and S. H. Snyder, Eds.: 107–208.
2.  JOHNSON, R. P., M. SAR & W. E. STUMPF. 1980. A topographic locoalization of enkephalin on the dopamine neurons of the rat substantia nigra and ventral tegmental area demonstrated by combined histofluorescence-immunocytochemistry. Brain Res. **194:** 566–571.
3.  KHACHATURIAN, H., M. E. LEWIS & S. J. WATSON. 1983. Enkephalin systems in diencephalon and brainstem of the rat. J. Comp. Neurol. **220:** 310–320.
4.  MOSKOWITZ, A. S. & R. R. GOODMAN. 1984. Light microscopic autoradiographic localization of opioid binding sites in the mouse central nervous system. J. Neurosci. **4:** 1331–1342.
5.  DILTS, R. P. & P. W. KALIVAS. 1988. Localization of mu opioid and neurotensin receptors within the A10 region of the rat. This volume.
6.  KELLEY, A. E., L. STINUS & S. D. IVERSEN. 1980. Interactions between D-Ala-Met-enkephalin, A10 dopaminergic neurones, and spontaneous behavior in the rat. Behav. Brain Res. **1:** 3–24.
7.  BROEKKAMP, C. L. E., A. G. PHILLIPS & A. T. COOLS. 1979. Stimulant effects of enkephalin injection into the dopaminergic A10 area. Nature **278:** 560–562.
8.  KALIVAS, P. W., E. WIDERLOV, D. STANLEY, G. BREESE & A. J. PRANGE, JR. 1983. Enkephalin action on the mesolimbic system: A dopamine-dependent and a dopamine-independent increase in locomotor activity. J. Pharmacol. Exp. Ther. **227:** 229–237.
9.  GYSLING, K. & R.Y. WANG. 1983. Morphine-induced activation of A10 dopamine neurons in rat brain. Brain Res. **277:** 119–127.
10. HOMMER, D. W. & A. PERT. 1983. The action of opiates in the rat substantia nigra: An electrohysiological analysis. Peptides **4:** 603–608.
11. JOYCE, E. M. & S. D. IVERSEN. 1979. The effect of morphine applied locally to mesencephalic dopamine cell bodies on spontaneous motor activity in the rat. Neurosci. Lett. **14:** 207–212.
12. VEZINA, P. & J. STEWART. 1984. Conditioning and place-specific sensitization increases activity induced by morphine in the VTA. Pharmacol. Biochem. Behav. **20:** 925–934.
13. KALIVAS, P. W., S. TAYLOR & J. S. MILLER. Sensitization to repeated enkephalin administration into the ventral tegmental area of the rat. I. Behavioral characterization. J. Pharmacol. Exp. Ther. **235:** 537–543.
14. KALIVAS, P. W. 1985. Interactions between neuropeptides and dopamine neurons in the ventromedial mesencephalon. Neurosci. Biobehav. Rev. **9:** 573–587.
15. BOWKER, R. M., H. W. M. STEINBUSCH & J. D. COULTER. 1981. Serotonergic and pep-

tidergic projections to the spinal cord demonstrated by a combined retrograde HRP histochemical and immunocytochemical staining method. Brain Res. **211:** 412–417.

16.  KALIVAS, P. W. & J. S. MILLER. 1984. A neurotensin pathway from the ventral tegmental area to the medial nucleus accumbens. Brain Res. **300:** 157–160.

17.  MOGENSON, G. J., D. L. JONES & C. Y. YIM. 1980. From motivation to action: Functional interface between the limbic system and the motor system. Prog. Neurobiol. **14:** 69–97.

18.  GARCIA-RILL, E. 1986. The basal ganglia and locomotor region. Brain Res. Rev. **11:** 47–63.

19.  LATIMER, L. G., P. DUFFY & P. W. KALIVAS. 1987. Mu opioid receptor involvement in enkephalin activation of dopamine neurons in the ventral tegmental area. J. Pharmacol. Exp. Ther. **241:** 328–337.

20.  PASTERNAK, G. W. 1986. Multiple mu opiate receptors: Biochemical and pharmacological evidence for multiplicity. Biochem. Pharmacol. **35:** 361–364.

21.  SCHWARTZ, J.-C., J. COSTENTIN & J.-M. LECONTE. 1985. Pharmacology of enkephalin inhibitors. Trends Pharmacol. Sci. **6:** 472–476.

22.  KALIVAS, P. W. & R. RICHARDSON-CARLSON. 1986. Endogenous enkephalin modulation of dopamine neurons in ventral tegmental area. Am. J. Physiol. **251:** R243–R249.

23.  PERT, A. & C. SIVIT. 1977. Neuroanatomical focus for morphine and enkephalin-induced hypermotility. Nature **265:** 645–647.

24.  BABBINI, M. & W. M. DAVIS. 1972. Time-dose relationships for locomotor activity effects of morphine after acute or repeated treatment. Br. J. Pharmacol. **46:** 213–224.

25.  KALIVAS, P. W. & P. DUFFY. 1987. Sensitization to repeated morphine injection in the rat: Possible involvement of A10 dopamine neurons. J. Pharmacol. Exp. Ther. **241:** 204–212.

26.  AMALRIC, M. & G. F. KOOB. 1985. Low doses of methylnaloxonium in the nucleus accumbens antagonize hyperactivity induced by heroin in the rat. Pharmacol. Biochem. Behav. **23:**411–415.

27.  VEZINA, P., P. W. KALIVAS & J. STEWART. 1987. Sensitization occurs to the locomotor effects of morphine and the specific mu opioid receptor agonist, DAGO, administered repeatedly to the ventral tegmental area but not to the nucleus accumbens. Brain Res. In press.

28.  DUFFY, P. & P. W. KALIVAS. 1988. Inhibition of endogenous dopamine release from the ventromedial mesencephalon after daily cocaine or morphine. This issue.

29.  KALIVAS, P. W., R. RICHARDSON-CARLSON & G. VAN ORDEN. 1986. Cross-sensitization between footshock stress and enkephalin-induced motor activity. Biol. Psychiatry **21:** 939–950.

30.  KALIVAS, P. W. & R. ABHOLD. 1987. Enkephalin release into the ventral tegmental area in response to stress: Modulation of mesocortical dopamine. Brain Res. **414:** 339–348.

# Behavioral Evidence for Differential Neuropeptide Modulation of the Mesolimbic Dopamine System

ANN E. KELLEY[a] AND MARTINE CADOR[b]

[a]Department of Psychology
Harvard University
Cambridge, Massachusetts 02138

[b]Psychobiologie des Comportements Adaptatifs
INSERM U. 259
Université de Bordeaux
33077 Bordeaux, France

## INTRODUCTION

The mesolimbic dopamine (DA-A10) system, which originates in the ventral tegmental area (VTA) and projects to limbic forebrain regions, plays a integral role in mediating several important aspects of behavior. The DA-A10 neurons have been shown to be involved in such diverse functions as facilitation of motor output, reinforcement, sensory, and attentional processes. Parallel anatomical studies have revealed multiple networks of neuropeptide-containing nerve fibers and terminals in the vicinity of these DA cell bodies and terminals. As expected from what is known about the behavioral functions of the DA-A10 system, peptidergic manipulation of these neurons has marked effects on behavior. For example, several neuropeptides when injected into the VTA produce a general behavioral activation. However, given the multiplicity of functions ascribed to the DA neurons and the striking diversity of peptidergic innervation associated with them, it would seem likely that their differential peptidergic modulation may constitute the substrate of different behavioral processes. The main objective of our experiments has been to evaluate this hypothesis and to attempt to dissociate locomotor effects of VTA-peptide stimulation from effects on other aspects of behavior.

## MESOLIMBIC DOPAMINE AND BEHAVIOR

In order to provide a theoretical framework for investigation of such behavioral processes, it is worthwhile to briefly review some of the major concepts that have emerged from experimental investigation of the mesolimbic DA system. Perhaps the most accepted and well-documented finding is that dopamine depletion in the nucleus accumbens and surrounding ventromedial striatum blocks the locomotor response to amphetamine.[1,2] This finding led to the hypothesis that increased DA release in the accumbens region was responsible for the motor activational properties of psychostimulants. A logical extension of this hypothesis was that mesolimbic dopamine was necessary for the normal motor expression of heightened arousal states.[3] Rats with specific 6-hydroxydopamine (6-OHDA) lesions of the DA-A10 neurons are found to be less active in situations associated with a high level of arousal, such as a novel environment, in the absence of any major motor deficit.[4] The construct of "motivational arousal" arose to account for a number of behavioral findings. Certain ethologically significant behaviors, such as hoarding and displacement (adjunctive) behaviors, which occur during a state of enhanced motivation, are specifically dependent on DA release in the accumbens region.[5,6]

Mesolimbic dopamine is linked to another motivational construct, reinforcement, through research on psychostimulant drugs. An impressive array of data provides support for the notion that the rewarding or hedonic properties of amphetamine, cocaine, and possibly opiate drugs are mediated through increased activity of DA-A10 neurons.[7,8] Thus one could summarize these emergent concepts by saying that activation of DA-A10 neurons, particularly those projecting to the nucleus accumbens, is associated with an appetitive motivational state characterized behaviorally by increased output of approach responses, and subjectively by positive affect. It is of interest to note that many years ago Hebb[9] and Bindra[10] developed theories that linked arousal and positive affect. It is an appealing notion that the mesolimbic dopamine system may constitute the brain substrate for this linkage.

## NEUROPEPTIDES AND MODULATION OF VTA DOPAMINE NEURONS

One way of approaching the study of the behavioral functions of this system is to investigate the substances that might regulate its activity. Mapping studies have demonstrated networks of peptide-containing nerve terminals in the VTA, site of the DA-A10 cell bodies. The anatomical proximity, as well as several lines of evidence summarized below, provide support for a functional interaction between neurons containing certain peptides and those containing dopamine. The best characterized peptides in this regard are the tachykinins, Met-enkephalin, and neurotensin (NT), which are also the peptides that we have studied closely. However, it should be noted that the VTA contains other neuropeptides that warrant further study, such as somatostatin, calcitonin-gene related peptide, dynorphin, and cholecystokinin.[11,12]

### Tachykinins

Immunohistochemical mapping has revealed that substance P (SP) and the related tachykinin neurokinin- (substance K) (NKA) are localized in the VTA, and their common precursor and close codistribution indicates that they are both probably synthesized within the same neurons.[13,14] Autoradiographic binding studies indicate that binding sites for SP are relatively sparse in the VTA and substantia nigra, whereas binding sites for NKA are in greater density.[13,15]

Electrophysiological results with studies of the tachykinins in the dopaminergic regions are somewhat discrepant. Originally Davies and Dray[16] showed that substantia nigra neurons were excited by SP applied microinotophoretically, although DA neurons were not strictly identified in this study. Pinnock and colleagues showed that SP and SP N-terminal fragments excited neurons in the zona reticulata, but had only weak effects in compacta (most probably dopaminergic) cells.[17] Aghajanian and colleagues have also found negative effects of SP in the substantia nigra, but in contrast, NKA was found to strongly depolarize dopaminergic cells in the substantia nigra.[18]

Neurochemical approaches have suggested evidence for a tachykinin–DA interaction in the midbrain. Earlier experiments in the cat demonstrated that intranigral infusions of SP caused increased DA release in the ipsilateral striatum.[19] SP injected into VTA increases dopamine metabolism (indicated by the DOPAC/DA ratio) in the nucleus accumbens, but this effect is variable and a much greater and more consistent effect is observed in the frontal cortex.[20,21] In contrast to SP, NKA injected into VTA does not affect DA metabolism in the frontal cortex, but does alter the nucleus accumbens DA metabolism.[14] Such findings suggest that SP and NKA may be interacting selectively with different subpopulations of DA neurons.

## Neurotensin

Neurotensinlike immunoreactivity is found in high amounts surrounding the DA neurons of the substantia nigra and VTA.[22] Indeed, the distributions of both NT-like immunoreactivity and NT receptor binding in these regions strikingly resemble the distribution of the midbrain DA neurons. For neurotensin, evidence for a functional interaction with DA is more convincing than for the tachykinins. It appears that a large majority of NT receptors are *localized* on DA neurons in both the nigra and the VTA.[23,24] Quirion and colleagues showed that a selective unilateral 6-OHDA lesion of DA neurons resulted in the complete disappearance of NT-receptor binding on the lesioned side.[24] In Parkinsonian brains, NT receptors are also reduced in the substantia nigra.[25,26]

The suggested interaction between NT and DA is of an excitatory nature. Andrade and Aghajanian[27] first showed that NT selectively depolarized DA neurons of the substantia nigra, and Pinnock replicated these findings.[28] Little is known about effects of NT applied iontophoretically to VTA neurons.

Neurochemical analysis has revealed that NT injected into VTA elicits a marked augmentation of DA turnover in the nucleus accumbens, but not in the striatum.[29] On the other hand, Napier and colleagues found that DA metabolism in the striatum is augmented after NT injections into the substantia nigra.[30]

## Opioids

The VTA contains a moderate density of Met-enkephalinlike immunoreactivity that appears to overlap with the distribution of DA neurons.[31,32] Recently it was demonstrated that dynorphin-B-like immunoreactivity is present in considerable amounts in the VTA.[12] Autoradiographically labeled opiate binding sites are also present, and are primarily the μ and δ type,[33] although the presence of dynorphin suggests that the k receptor may also be of physiological relevance in the dopaminergic regions. Evidence for localization on DA neurons is not as clear as for NT receptors. In one report, 6-OHDA lesion of the nigro-striatal pathway decreased opiate receptor binding by only 20%.[34] Electrophysiological analysis provides consistent findings, although it is still not clear whether opiates act directly on DA neurons or through an interneuron. Morphine, the prototypical μ agonist, excites dopaminergic neurons whether administered systemically or directly iontophoresed.[35,36] Most investigators have found the excitatory effect to be naloxone reversible. Since opiates have inhibitory neuronal effects in nearly all systems studied, it has generally been hypothesized that the excitatory effects on DA cells are indirectly mediated. A recent experiment showed that morphine and a k receptor agonist had opposite effects on the firing rate of dopamine cells in the nigra.[37] The k agonist inhibited DA cells, suggesting that naturally occurring dynorphin may act quite differently from enkephalin in this region. In another study, dynorphin inhibited zona reticulata cells but had no effect on compacta cells.[38] Little is known about the electrophysiological effects of enkephalinlike compounds in the VTA; however, as discussed below, enkephalin and morphine have very similar effects behaviorally when administered in this area.

There is support from neurochemical findings for opioid peptides facilitating DA activity. When injected into VTA, D-ala-Met-enkephalinamide (D-ALA), a long-lasting synthetic analog of Met-enkephalin, produces marked increases in dopamine metabolites in the nucleus accumbens.[39]

### Behavioral Effects of VTA Injection of Neuropeptides

The preceding account would suggest that all three classes of peptides interact in a facilitory fashion with mesolimbic DA neurons, although the precise circuitry and involvement of other neurotransmitters has yet to be elucidated. Considering the hypothesized role of the DA-A10 neurons in spontaneous motor activity, it would be expected that application of these peptides into the VTA would enhance locomotor activity. Indeed, analysis of locomotor activity has been the technique of choice in studies of the mesolimbic DA system, because this variable is very sensitive to drug or neurotransmitter manipulations of this system. Systemic administration of amphetamine or direct injection of this drug into the nucleus accumbens produces marked increases in locomotion and rearing, behaviors indicative of heightened behavioral arousal. It is therefore of interest to examine the behavioral profile of peptide-induced activation of the DA-A10 system.

When injected into the VTA, tachykinins, neurotensin, and opioids all produce dose-related, DA-dependent increases in spontaneous motor activity. SP infused into the VTA results in increased activity that is blocked by either a 6-OHDA lesion of the nucleus accumbens or by neuroleptic blockade of the accumbens.[40–43] The behavioral effect of NT infusion into VTA is also enhanced locomotor activity, which is dependent on the functioning of mesolimbic DA neurons.[29,44] Further, morphine injected into VTA was found to result in enhanced activity,[45] and after this original finding it was soon after reported that enkephalin, enkephalin analogs, and endorphins produced similar effects.[46,47] All the opiate-induced behavioral effects were found to be naloxone-reversible and blocked by DA lesion or DA pharmacological blockade.

Thus at first glance it would appear that all three classes of peptides produce the same behavioral consequences, and may act in a similar manner physiologically. However, the main thesis of this paper is that in fact these three different substances are acting very differently in their interactions with dopaminergic neurons. This hypothesis has emerged from a series of studies in which we conducted a detailed behavioral investigation of neuropeptide effects in the VTA. These studies were done in collaboration with Drs. L. Stinus and M. Le Moal at the University of Bordeaux. We have employed several behavioral paradigms that are designed to measure behavioral processes other than general motor activity, and find increasing evidence for differential interaction of these peptides with DA.

Before considering the two behavioral paradigms that reveal the greatest differences, fixed-interval operant responding and feeding behavior, it is worthwhile to observe the comparisons made in TABLE 1. Here the profiles of locomotion, open field behavior, and exploratory behavior after VTA infusion of peptides are provided. The

**TABLE 1.** Summary of Behavioral Profiles Elicited by Different Neuropeptides Injected into VTA

| Peptide | Locomotor Activity | Behavioral Profiles Open-Field Profile | Investigatory Behavior |
|---|---|---|---|
| Tachykinins (SP, NKA) | ↑ | ↑ Square crossings<br>↑ Rearing<br>↑ Center activity | ↑ Hole-poke responses<br>↓ Duration of responses (motor acceleration) |
| Neurotensin | ↑ | Slightly ↑ square crossings, but ↑ rearing primary effect | ↑ Hole pokes (small effect).<br>No effect on duration |
| Opioids (Met-enkephalin, dynorphin) | ↑ | ↑ Square crossings<br>↑ Rearing | ↑ Hole pokes<br>↓ Duration of responses |
| Amphetamine (for comparison) | ↑ | ↑ Square crossings<br>↑ Rearing<br>↑ Center activity | ↑ Hole pokes<br>↓ Duration of responses |

NOTE: Behavioral effects of systemic amphetamine are provided for comparison.

first suggestion of differential behavioral effects resulted from the latter two categories of behavior. An open field analysis enables qualitative assessment of motor activity. Unlike automatic recording of general motor activity, one can make observations about specific categories or patterns of behavior. TABLE 1 shows that the patterns of activity after VTA injections of tachykinins, neurotensin, opioids, and systemic amphetamine was found to be quite similar, characterized by increases in square crossings and rearing, and increased activities in the center of the open field. NT had a somewhat more pronounced effect on rearing than on square crossing. Exploratory behavior was measured in a circular apparatus equipped with holes around the wall, and hole investigation was automatically recorded. It can be noted that SP, D-ALA, and amphetamine all potently *increased* the frequency of hole-poke responses, but *decreased* the average duration of responses.[69,70,72] In other words, there is a marked acceleration in the production of investigatory responses. NT infused into VTA induces a small increase in hole investigation and does not affect average duration.[68] This was the first indication that the topography of behavioral responses differed somewhat among the various peptides.

## NEUROPEPTIDES AND OPERANT BEHAVIOR

The use of operant techniques provides a different approach to the analysis of behavioral effect of peptides. The strength of operant techniques lies in the opportunity for the experiment to control the output of behavior and to quantitatively assess many aspects of this behavior. We undertook a study in which the effects of VTA infusion of SP, NKA, NT, and D-ALA on operant responding for food reward were investigated.[48] In an operant chamber, rats were trained on a fixed-interval 40-sec schedule of reinforcement. A fixed-interval (FI) schedule was chosen, since a considerable amount is known about how dopaminergic drugs, such as amphetamine and neuroleptics, affect fixed-interval performance.

### Method

A brief summary of the method used is provided here; for further experimental details the reader is referred to our original study.[48] Hungry rats were trained to stable baseline performance under an FI 40-sec schedule. In this schedule, the first lever-press after each 40-sec interval is rewarded. In this procedure rats quickly learn the temporal discrimination, and their baseline performance shows the typical FI "scallop": low rates early in the interval, and progressively higher rates later in the interval. The responding is very stable over days, as is the "quarter-life." The quarter-life is a quantitative index of the temporal pattern of responding (for further description see the note to TABLE 2). When performance had stabilized, different groups of rats were administered differing doses of either SP, NKA, NT or D-ALA, and the effect on the pattern of responding was measured. In addition to analyzing raw data with analysis of variance, we conducted rate-dependency analyses in which the drug effect is measured in terms of its effect on the baseline rate of responding.[49]

### Results and Discussion

The effect of SP and NKA are shown in FIGURES 1 and 2. Responding across the interval is shown on the left side of the graph (the intervals are divided into ten 4-sec

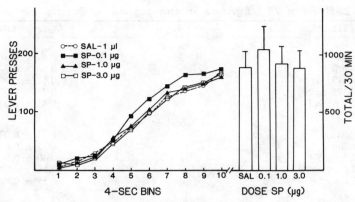

**FIGURE 1.** Effect of substance P injected into VTA on fixed-interval responding. *Left*: Data points represent means across all intervals for each bin. *Right*: Total number of responses for test session (mean + S.E.M.). (From Kelley *et al.*[48] Reproduced by permission.)

time-bins), and total responding for the whole session, irrespective of time-bin, is shown on the right side. None of the doses of SP had any measurable effects on operant responding. Although NKA did not affect total responding, there were several significant dose × time-bin interactions. The lowest dose of NKA had the tendency to increase rates of responding throughout the second half of the interval. The middle dose increased rates around the middle of the interval, but had the tendency to decrease rates toward the end. The highest dose did not differ significantly from saline control, although its profile resembled that of the middle dose of NKA. Neither the effects

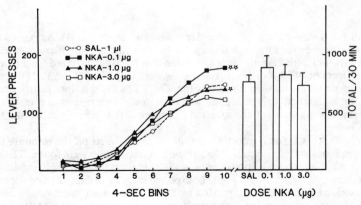

**FIGURE 2.** Effect of neurokinin-α injected into VTA on fixed-interval responding. *Left*: Data points represent means across all intervals for each bin. *Right*: Total number of responses for test session (mean + S.E.M.). ★ $p < 0.05$, ★ $p < 0.01$ (dose × bin interaction with respect to saline). (From Kelley *et al.*[48] Reproduced by permission.)

**TABLE 2.** Effect of VTA Injection of Neuropeptides on Quarter-Life

| Treatment | Quarter-Life[a] |
|---|---|
| *Neurotensin* | |
| Control | 0.64 ± 0.08 |
| saline | 0.62 ± 0.07 |
| 0.0175 µg NT | 0.62 ± 0.07 |
| 0.175 µg NT | 0.72 ± 0.05 |
| 0.5 µg NT | 0.63 ± 0.07 |
| *Substance P* | |
| Control | 0.62 ± 0.03 |
| saline | 0.59 ± 0.04 |
| 0.1 µg SP | 0.60 ± 0.03 |
| 1.0 µg SP | 0.58 ± 0.03 |
| 3.0 µg SP | 0.58 ± 0.02 |
| *Neurokinin-α* | |
| Control | 0.62 ± 0.01 |
| saline | 0.64 ± 0.02 |
| 0.1 µg NKA | 0.66 ± 0.02 |
| 1.0 µg NKA | 0.60 ± 0.01 |
| 3.0 µg NKA | 0.58 ± 0.05 |
| *D-ALA-Met-enkephalin* | |
| Control | 0.69 ± 0.02 |
| saline | 0.68 ± 0.03 |
| 0.01 µg D-ALA | 0.65 ± 0.02 |
| 0.1 µg D-ALA | 0.61 ± 0.02[b] |
| 1.0 µg D-ALA | 0.54 ± 0.02[b] |

[a] The index of quarter-life is a measure of the temporal pattern of responding. It is the proportion of the interval during which the first one-quarter of the total number of responses in that interval is made. If responding is constant throughout the interval, the quarter-life equals one-fourth of the interval, that is, 0.25. If responding is accelerated throughout the interval, the quarter-life is considerably higher. Values represent mean ± S.E.M.
[b] $p < 0.01$.

of SP nor NKA were significantly rate-dependent (see reference 48). As expected from lack of significance for rate-dependency, the quarter-life measure was not affected by either tachykinin, although the data suggested that NKA tends to reduce it (TABLE 2).

The effects of NT on operant responding were very clear (FIG. 3). NT produced a dose-dependent decrease in operant responding. The highest dose nearly abolished responding altogether. This reduction was monotonic with regard to rate, that is, all rates of responding were equally affected (for more detail, see reference 48). Quarter-life was not affected.

Finally, D-ALA infused into VTA produced clear effects on the response profile, as shown in FIGURE 4. Significant dose × time-bin interactions were found. The middle dose of D-ALA-enhanced response rates, and the highest dose strongly enhanced low rates but decreased high rates. As would be expected from these data, the rate-dependency analysis yielded significant effects, that is, D-ALA increased low baseline rates and had no effect on or decreased high rates (see FIG. 5). Quarter-life was markedly affected by D-ALA (see TABLE 2). D-ALA produced a dose-dependent decrement in this index, indicating that D-ALA-treated animals distributed their responses more evenly throughout the interval.

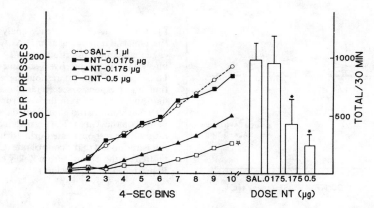

**FIGURE 3.** Effect of neurotensin injected into VTA on fixed-interval responding. *Left*: Data points represent means across all intervals for each bin. *Right*: Total number of responses for test session (mean + S.E.M.). ★ $p < 0.05$, * $p < 0.05$, dose × bin interaction with respect to saline. (From Kelley *et al.*[48] Reproduced by permission.)

The data from these experiments provided the first evidence that the behavioral response to VTA injection of several peptides that are putative neuromodulators in that region can be differentiated. The results with D-ALA are perhaps most easily interpreted. The profile of fixed-interval performance after opioid peptide stimulation of VTA is strikingly similar to that produced by systemic administration of *d*-amphetamine. The rate-dependent effects of amphetamine are well documented in several species,[49] and quarter-life is decreased.[48,50] One study showed that the rate-dependent ef-

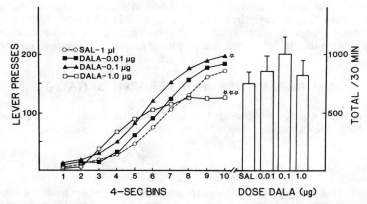

**FIGURE 4.** Effect of D-ALA-Met-enkephalinamide injected into VTA on fixed-interval responding. *Left*: Data points represent means across all intervals for each bin. *Right*: Total number of responses for test session (mean + S.E.M.). ★ $p < 0.05$, ★ ★ ★ $p < 0.001$, dose × bin interaction with respect to saline. (From Kelley *et al.*[48] Reproduced by permission.)

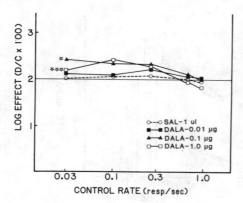

**FIGURE 5.** Rate-dependency analysis of fixed-interval responding after D-ALA-Met-enkephalinamide injection into VTA. The interval is divided into five 8-sec time-bins. Local control rates of responding across time-bins (responses/sec averaged over the half-hour session) were derived from two different control (no injection) days and plotted on the X-axis. The logarithm of the ratio of the response rate during drug administration (D) to the control rate (C) was plotted on the Y-axis. (From Kelley et al.[48] Reproduced by permission.)

fects of amphetamine are dependent on DA release in the nucleus accumbens.[51] Thus, although we have not shown directly that the effects of D-ALA on operant behavior are dependent on dopamine, the simplest explanation for the effects is that D-ALA produces a similar state to that of amphetamine (most likely low to moderate doses of amphetamine).

The effects of the tachykinins were unlike those induced by D-ALA in that there were no rate-dependent effects nor changes in quarter-life. SP, in doses that induce locomotor activation, does not affect the pattern of responding. However, the result with NKA deserves further investigation, since this peptide appears to alter the shape of the response curve in a manner that in some ways is similar to D-ALA.

Neurotensin produced quite unexpected effects. Paradoxically, the profile of fixed-interval performance after VTA infusion of this peptide resembles that of neuroleptics.[52] Neuroleptics induce a monotonic decrease in the rate of responding. It is unlikely that the reduction in responding was due to "overactivation" or stereotypy, since even a rather low dose reduced responding, and upon observation there was no indication of stereotyped behaviors. Casual observation indicated that neurotensin-treated animals were not active in these conditions, but were engaged in a bizarre, prostrate posture interspersed with bursts of movement. Thus at the same doses that induce locomotor activity in other testing conditions, neurotensin reduces operant responding for food.

## NEUROPEPTIDES AND FEEDING BEHAVIOR

A second set of experiments provided support for differential effects of peptides injected into VTA on feeding, which had not been previously studied.

### Method

Details of the methology employed are provided in our recent study.[54] In these experiments, the effects of VTA injection of several doses of either SP, NT, or D-ALA were assessed on a number of feeding parameters. During a 30-min test in the home cage, the latency to eat, total food intake, food spillage, number of eating bouts, and duration of eating were measured by direct observation, with the aid of a computer-

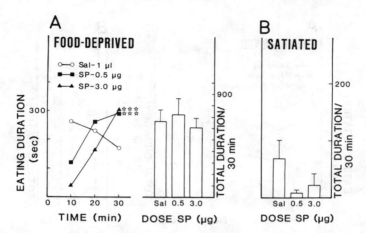

**FIGURE 6.** Effect of substance P injection into VTA on feeding behavior in both food-deprived (**A**) and satiated (**B**) conditions. For the food-deprived condition, both the time course and the totals over the session are shown. ★ ★ ★ $p < 0.001$, dose × time interaction with respect to saline. (From Cador *et al.*[54] Reproduced by permission.)

controlled event recorder. Similar measures were taken for drinking. Feeding was measured in both satiated and food-deprived (18-hr) conditions.

## Results and Discussion

The results from these tests can be observed in FIGURES 6–8. SP infused into the VTA had no overall effect on feeding during the total 30-min test for either condition, but did produce significant dose × time interactions for the food-deprived condition. FIGURE 6A shows that SP-treated rats show less feeding in the beginning of the session, and more feeding in the end when compared with saline-injected rats. As can be expected from this finding, the latency to eat was dose-dependently increased by SP (see TABLE 3). There was no effect of SP in the satiated condition (FIG. 6B).

NT infused into VTA had a potent inhibitory effect on feeding (FIG. 7). It can be observed that in satiated rats, NT produced a dose-dependent reduction in feeding duration. TABLE 3 indicates that NT significantly increased the latency to feed and reduced gram intake of food. Several rats that received the higher dose of NT did not eat throughout the session, although they had been food deprived for 18 hours. Drinking also tended to be inhibited by NT; the higher dose significantly reduced number of drinking bouts and total duration of drinking.[54] [It should be noted, however, that in water-deprived rats, NT did not reduce water intake in a similar test (unpublished findings).] NT had no effect on feeding behavior in satiated rats, as would be expected by the very low baseline of feeding in these rats.

In contrast to NT, D-ALA infused into VTA produced an enhancement of feeding in both satiated and food-deprived animals. FIGURE 8 shows the effect of D-ALA on duration of feeding over the 30 min in both conditions. TABLE 4A shows that in the satiated condition, the latency to feed was reduced by D-ALA in a dose-dependent manner. Food intake in grams was increased, although not significantly. The number

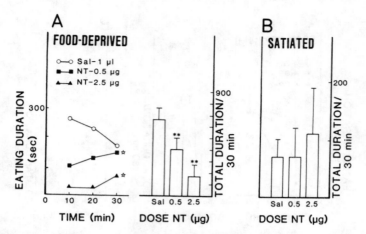

**FIGURE 7.** Effect of neurotensin injection into VTA on feeding behavior in both food-deprived (**A**) and satiated (**B**) conditions. For the food-deprived condition, both the time course and the totals over the session are shown. ★ ★ ★ $p < 0.001$, dose × time interaction with respect to saline. (From Cador *et al.*[54] Reproduced by permission.)

of eating bouts was increased by D-ALA. In food-deprived animals (TABLE 4B), gram intake was significantly increased by both doses of D-ALA.

These findings indicate that microinjections of different peptides that occur endogenously in the VTA have differential effects on feeding behavior. The increased latency to feed and the temporal effect for duration of feeding induced by SP is most

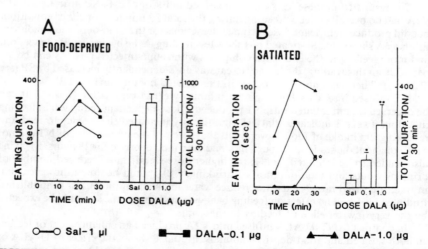

**FIGURE 8.** Effect of D-ALA-Met-enkephalin injection into VTA on feeding behavior in both food-deprived (**A**) and satiated (**B**) conditions. The time course and the totals over the session are shown. * $p < 0.05$, ** $p < 0.01$, ★ $p < 0.05$, dose × time interaction with respect to saline. (From Cador *et al.*[54] Reproduced by permission.)

**TABLE 3.** Effect of Neuropeptides Injected into VTA on Feeding Behavior in Food-Deprived (18-hr) Rats

| Treatment | Latency to Eat (sec) | Food Intake (g) | Number of Eating Bouts |
|---|---|---|---|
| Sal (6) −1 μl | 67 ± 35 | 3.6 ± 0.7 | 19.1 ± 3.0 |
| SP (7) −0.5 μg | 118 ± 18 | 3.8 ± 0.6 | 18.0 ± 6.8 |
| SP (7) −3.0 μg | 578 ± 218[a] | 2.8 ± 0.3 | 14.4 ± 5.5 |
| NT (6) −0.5 μg | 616 ± 256[a] | 1.9 ± 0.6[b] | 12.9 ± 3.7 |
| NT (6) −2.5 μg | 1153 ± 325[a] | 1.3 ± 0.7[b] | 9.9 ± 4.7 |

NOTE: Values in parentheses indicate number of rats in each group. Data represent mean ± S.E.M.
[a] $p < 0.01$.
[b] $p < 0.05$.

simply explained by a behavioral competition between the feeding response and the strong motor activation induced by SP. Indeed, as expected, SP-treated rats were observed to be very active in the first part of the session. Most other aspects of food intake, such as total intake and number of bouts, were not significantly changed. To our knowledge, SP has not been found to be implicated in any aspects of feeding behavior.

NT inhibited food intake and duration of eating. We hypothesized that a behavioral competition hypothesis could not account for this effect, as the NT-treated rats, paradoxically, were very often observed to be still (in an odd posture similar to that observed in the operant experiments). It is possibly that NT inhibits feeding as part of a satiety system, as NT injections into the hypothalamus also potently inhibit feeding.[55]

**TABLE 4A.** Effect of D-ALA-[Met]enkephalin Injection into Ventral Tegmental Area on Ingestive Behaviors in Satiated Rats

| Treatment | Latency to Eat | Food Intake | Number of Eating Bouts |
|---|---|---|---|
| Sal (7)       −1 μl | 1734 ± 43 | 0.10 ± 0.06 | 1.14 ± 0.73 |
| D-ALA (9) −0.1 μg | 1086 ± 190[a] | 0.49 ± 0.17 | 3.33 ± 0.91 |
| D-ALA (14)−1.0 μg | 799 ± 162[b] | 0.62 ± 0.23 | 10.93 ± 2.44[b] |

NOTE: Newman–Keuls test. Numbers in parentheses indicate number of animals in each group. Data represent mean ± S.E.M.
[a] $p < 0.05$.
[b] $p < 0.01$.

**TABLE 4B.** Effect of D-ALA-[Met]enkephalin Injection into the Ventral Tegmental Area on Ingestive Behaviors in Food-Deprived Rats

| Treatment | Latency to Eat | Food Intake | Number of Eating Bouts |
|---|---|---|---|
| Sal (7)       −1 μl | 93 ± 22 | 2.04 ± 0.52 | 23.1 ± 4.5 |
| D-ALA (9) −0.1 μg | 148 ± 101 | 4.0 ± 0.42[a] | 25.2 ± 5.3 |
| D-ALA (14)−1.0 μg | 112 ± 29 | 3.99 ± 0.48[a] | 24.8 ± 2.8 |

NOTE: Newman–Keuls test.
[a] $p < 0.05$.

However, more experiments are needed in order to clarify possible mechanisms involved in this effect.

In contrast to both SP and NT, opioid peptide stimulation of VTA facilitated feeding. This effect is in agreement with recent findings that showed that both morphine, enkephalin analogs, and dynorphin injected into VTA enhance feeding.[56] In our experiments, the rats were observed to be very activated. However, in contrast to SP, D-ALA-induced activation was not incompatible with feeding. In the satiated rats the activity was focused on the food pellets; often the animals were observed to rear up with food pellets in the mouth. There are several interpretations for these findings. It may be that opiate receptor stimulation of the VTA elicits feeding in a specific manner, as a large number of reports implicate endogenous opiate mechanisms in feeding and satiety.[53] On the other hand, D-ALA-treated rats may feed because of nonspecific motivational effects, in a manner similar to that induced by electrical hypothalamic stimulation.[59] This may explain the behavior of satiated rats; however, the increase in feeding in food-deprived rats, which is remarkable considering the already elevated baseline of feeding, suggests that regulatory mechanisms may also be involved.

## GENERAL DISCUSSION

The results provide the first evidence that the behavioral effects injections of tachykinins, neurotensin, and opioids, at doses that have a stimulatory effect on locomotor behavior, can be differentiated. As outlined in the introduction, all three of these classes of neuropeptides are found in nerve terminals in the VTA, and previous work has convincingly shown that they produce increased locomotor stimulation and stimulate dopamine metabolism in DA terminal areas. Therefore from previous work it might be assumed that all these substances are acting on DA neurons in a similar fashion; however, the present study suggests this is not the case. Although we have not shown directly in the present experiments that that dopamine is involved in the effects, it is important to discuss the putative role of DA-A10 neurons, since there is evidence from other experiments that DA is critically involved.

The response to D-ALA is perhaps the most clearly interpreted. All the available data from our laboratory and others suggest that opioid stimulation of the VTA induces an appetitive motivational state via activation of DA-A10 neurons, most likely those projecting to nucleus accumbens. Further, this state is very similar to the behavioral state induced by low doses of amphetamine, or direct application of amphetamine into the nucleus accumbens. Enkephalin injections into the VTA are highly reinforcing, both in the place-conditioning test and the self-administration paradigm.[57,58] Enkephalin stimulation of VTA facilitates approach responses, such as locomotion, rearing, and hole investigation, and the profiles of exploratory behavior after VTA injection of DALA or systemic amphetamine are remarkably similar.[70,72]

In the context of motivation theory, Bindra developed a model that attempted to explain the interaction of arousal, environment stimuli, and certain types of behavior.[10] Bindra proposed that a wide variety of "incentive" stimuli could elicit responses in a nonspecific manner. Bindra cited experiments in which incentive stimuli such as food-associated cues or novelty could affect the general activity or exploratory tendencies of the animal. Bindra proposed a hypothetical neural substrate for such an "energizing" function:

> This state of enhanced neural activity in parts of the appetitive motivation system may be described as a positive incentive motivational state; it may be thought of as a state

that promotes a variety of appetitive, environmentally-oriented approach response tendencies. (p. 13)

It is proposed that the mesolimbic DA neurons projecting to accumbens are a critical part of this system, and that opioid-peptide-containing nerve terminals within the VTA are an additional link in the system. The origin of the Met-enkephalin within VTA is unknown, but it is interesting to speculate that the lateral hypothalamus, which is known to project to VTA, may send enkephalinergic projections to VTA. Stimulation of the lateral hypothalamus produces nonspecific approach responses (including feeding),[59,60] and is potently rewarding, and these effects are mediated through mesolimbic dopamine activation.[61,62] In summary, activation of this putative motivational system, whether at the level of the lateral hypothalamus, VTA opiate receptors, or nucleus accumbens, enhances motor responses associated with a positive affective state.

Evaluation of the neurotensin-induced behavioral state is more problematic. This does not appear to be a classic "amphetaminelike" state, and stands in marked contrast to D-ALA-induced effects. Indeed, on the basis of the operant and feeding studies, the behavioral effects resemble those of antidopaminergic drugs (neuroleptics). There is little evidence that NT induces an "appetitive" motivational state, although NT stimulation of the VTA has been reported to be reinforcing in the place-conditioning and self-administration paradigms.[63,64] Our group found no evidence for VTA injections of NT in doses ranging from 0.01 to 2.5 µg to be reinforcing in the place-conditioning test (unpublished findings). These paradoxical effects must be clarified with further behavioral experiments. In terms of neurochemical mechanisms, there is no question that NT interacts with midbrain dopamine systems, but the nature of that interaction is far from clear. It has been suggested that NT may induce increased synthesis and accumulation of DA in nerve terminals, but may actually decrease impulse flow and DA release.[65] In support of this hypothesis, unilateral injection of NT into the substantia nigra induced a marked increase in striatal dopamine metabolism on the same side, but did not induce any rotation.[30] However, if amphetamine was given in conjunction with nigral NT injections, or even 20 hours after the nigral injection, contralateral turning was observed. NT may have long-term, multiphasic effects on DA cell activity.

Substance P and neurokinin-α elicit similar locomotor and open-field profiles, but there is evidence that although these two substances may be co-localized, they may be selectively released and may interact with different subpopulations of DA-A10 neurons. SP is found to act more potently on DA neurons projecting to the prefrontal cortex,[14,71] and footshock stress depletes SP levels but not NKA levels in VTA.[66] When injected into VTA, NKA affects DA metabolism in nucleus accumbens but leaves the frontal cortex metabolism unchanged.[14] NKA is more potent than SP in inducing locomotor activity.[13,67] Thus, the behavioral profile of NKA may be more closely aligned with that elicited by D-ALA, a suggestion supported by the results with operant behavior.

A summary of these speculations is provided in FIGURE 9. Two hypothetical models are provided that could explain the differential behavioral effects, and that offer speculation concerning the physiological roles of the endogenous peptide systems in the VTA. Model 1 suggests that different peptides in this region interact selectively with different DA-A10 subpopulations. As previously suggested, for example, SP, when released, may activate cortical DA neurons, while NKA would bind to receptors on neurons projecting to accumbens. Alternatively, different neuropeptides could activate different subpopulations of DA neurons projecting to the same region. Model 2 suggests that all these peptides may influence the same subset of DA-A10 neurons, but that differential postsynaptic effects account for the behavioral differentiation.

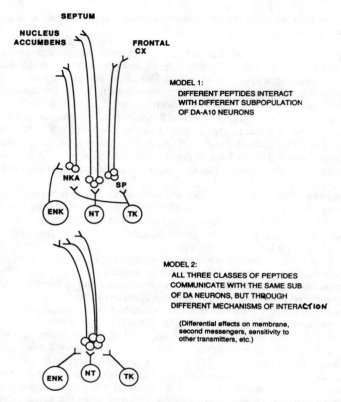

**FIGURE 9.** Two hypothetical models that may explain the differential behavioral effects of different neuropeptides infused into the region of the DA-A10 cell bodies. See text for discussion.

Given the wide range of unconventional neuronal effects that peptides have (such as altering the postsynaptic response to other neurotransmitters), there are many possibilities for variation in the interaction between peptide-containing nerve terminals and DA cell bodies, such as interaction with different second messenger systems or varying short- and long-term effects. Information gained from further investigation of both the behavioral state and neuronal changes induced by these peptides may elucidate the relative contributions of these models in explaining the differential behavioral effects described here.

## REFERENCES

1.  KELLY, P. H., P. SEVIOUR & S. D. IVERSEN. 1976. Amphetamine and apomorphine responses in the rat following 6-OHDA lesions of the nucleus accumbens septi and corpus striatum. Brain Res. **94:** 507–522.
2.  KOOB, G. F., L. STINUS & M. LE MOAL. 1981. Hyperactivity and hypoactivity produced by lesions to the mesolimbic dopamine system. Behav. Brain. Res. **3:** 341–359.

3. ROBBINS, T. W. & B. J. EVERITT. 1982. Functional studies of the central catecholamines. Int. Rev. Neurobiol. **23:** 303–365.
4. KELLEY, A. E., M. CADOR & L. STINUS. 1987. Exploration and its measurement: A psychopharmacological perspective. *In* Neuromethods: Psychopharmacology, Vol. 13. A. A. Boulton, G. B. Baker, and A. J. Greenshaw, Eds. Humana Press. Clifton, N. J. In press.
5. ROBBINS, T. W. & G. F. KOOB. 1980. Selective disruptions of displacement behavior by lesions of the mesolimbic dopamine system. Nature **285:** 409–412.
6. KELLEY, A. E. & L. STINUS. 1985. Disappearance of hoarding behavior after 6-hydroxydopamine lesions of the mesolimbic dopamine neurons and its reinstatement with L-dopa. Behav. Neurosci. **99:** 531–545.
7. STEWART, J., H. DE WIT & R. EIKELBOOM. 1984. Role of unconditioned and conditioned drug effects in the self-administration of opiates and stimulants. Psychol. Rev. **91:** 251–268.
8. BOZARTH, M. A. 1986. Neural basis of psychomotor stimlulant and opiate reward: Evidence suggesting the involvement of a common dopaminergic system. Behav. Brain Res. **22:** 107–116.
9. HEBB, D. O. 1955. Drives and the CNS (Conceptual Nervous System). Psych. Rev. **62:** 243–254.
10. BINDRA, D. 1968. Neuropsychological interpretation of the effects of drive and incentive-motivation on general activity and instrumental behavior. Psychol. Rev. **75:** 1–22.
11. DEUTCH, A. Y. & R. H. ROTH. 1987. Calcitonin gene-related peptide in the ventral tegmental area: Selective modulation of prefrontal cortical dopamine metabolism. Neurosci. Lett. **74:** 169–174.
12. FALLON, J. H. & F. M. LESLIE. 1986. Distribution of dynorphin and enkephlin peptides in the rat brain. J. Comp. Neurol. **249:** 293–336.
13. KALIVAS, P. W., A. DEUTCH, J. E. MAGGIO, P. MANTYH & R. H. ROTH. 1985. Substance P and substance K in the ventral tegmental area. Neurosci. Lett. **57:** 241–246.
14. DEUTCH, A. Y., J. E. MAGGIO, M. BANNON, P. W. KALIVAS, S. Y. TAM, M. GOLDSTEIN & R. H. ROTH. 1985. Substance K and substance P differentially modulate mesolimbic and mesocortical systems Peptides **6:** 113–122.
15. MANTYH, P. W., J. E. MAGGIO & S. P. HUNT. 1984. The autoradiographic distribution of kassinin and substance K binding sites is different from the distribution of substance P binding sites in rat brain. Eur. J. Pharmacol. **102:** 361–364.
16. DAVIES, J. & A. DRAY. 1976. Substance P in the substantia nigra. Brain Res. **107:** 623–627.
17. PINNOCK, R. D., G. N. WOODRUFF & M. J. TURNBULL. 1983. Actions of substance P, MIF, TRH and related peptides in the substantia nigra, caudate nucleus and nucleus accumbens. Neuropharmacology **22:** 687–696.
18. INNIS, R. B., R. ANDRADE & G. K. AGHAJANIAN. 1985. Substance K excites dopaminergic and non-dopaminergic neurons in rat substantia nigra. Brain Res. **335:** 381–383.
19. CHERAMY, A., A. NIEOULLON, R. MICHELOT & J. GLOWINSKI. 1977. Effects of intranigral application of dopamine and substance P on the in vivo release of newly synthesized $^3$H-dopamine in the ipsilateral caudate nucleus of the cat. Neurosci. Lett. **4:** 105–109.
20. KALIVAS, P. W. 1985. Interactions between neuropeptides and dopamine neuron in the ventromedial mesencephalon. Neurosci. Biobehav. Rev. **9:** 573–587.
21. IVERSEN L. L., P. J. ELLIOTT, M. J. BANNON, J. E. ALPERT & S. D. IVERSEN. 1983. Interaction of substance P with dopaminergic neurones in brain. *In* Substance P: Proceedings of the International Symposium. P. Skrabanek and D. Powell, Eds.: 43–44. Boole Press, Dublin.
22. UHL, G. R., M. J. KUHAR & S. H. SNYDER. 1977. Neurotensin: Immunohistochemical localization in rat central nervous system. Proc. Natl. Acad. Sci. U.S.A. **74:** 4059–4063.
23. PALACIOS, J. M. & M. KUHAR. 1981. Neurotensin receptors are located on dopamine containing neurones in rat midbrain. Nature **294:** 587–589.
24. QUIRION, R., C. C. CHIVCEH, H. D. EVERIST & A. PERT. 1985. Comparative localization of neurotensin receptors on nigrostriatal and mesolimbic dopaminergic terminals. Brain Res. **327:** 385–389.
25. UHL, G. R., P. J. WHITEHOUSE, D. L. PRICE, W. W. TOURTELOTTE & M. J. KUHAR. 1984. Parkinson's disease: Depletion of substantia nigra neurotensin receptors. Brain Res. **308:** 186–190.
26. AGID Y., M. RUBERG, B. DUBOIS, F. JAVOY-AGID. 1984. Biochemical Substrates of Mental

Disease. *In* Advances in Neurology, Vol. 40. R. G. Hassler and J. F. Christ. Raven. New York.

27. ANDRADE, R. & G. K. AGHAJANIAN. 1981. Neurotensin selectively activates dopaminergic neurons of the substantia nigra. Soc. Neurosci. Abstr. **7:** 573.

28. PINNOCK, R. D. 1985. Neurotensin depolarizes substantia nigra dopamine neurones. Brain Res. **338:** 151–154.

29. KALIVAS, P. W., P. W. BURGESS, C. B. NEMEROFF & A. J. PRANGE, JR. 1983. Behavioral and neurochemical effects of neurotensin microinjection into the ventral tegmental area. Neuroscience **8:** 225–238.

30. NAPIER, T. C., D. A. GAY, K. L. HULEBAK & G. R. BREESE. 1985. Behavioral and biochemical assessment of time-related changes in globus pallidus and striatal dopamine induced by intranigrally administered neurotensin. Peptides **6:** 1057–1068.

31. UHL, G. R., R. R. GOODMAN, M. J. KUHAR, S. R. CHILDERS & S. H. SNYDER. 1979. Immunohistochemical mapping of enkephalin-containing cell bodies fibers and nerve terminals in the brain stem of the rat. Brain Res. **166:** 75–94.

32. JOHNSON, R. P., M. SAR & W. E. STUMPF. 1980. A topographic localization of enkephalin on the dopamine neurons of the rat substantia nigra and ventral tegmental area demonstrated by combined histofluorescence-immunohistochemistry. Brain Res. **194:** 556–571.

33. MOSKOWITZ, A. S. & R. R. GOODMAN. 1984. Light microscope autoradiographic localization of μ and δ opioid binding sites in the mouse central nervous system. J. Neurosci. **4:** 1331–1342.

34. LLORENS-CORTES, C., H. POLLARD & J. C. SCHWARTZ. 1979. Localization of opiate receptors in substantia nigra: Evidence by lesion studies. Neurosci. Lett. **12:** 321–326.

35. GYSLING, K. & R. U. WANG. 1983. Morphine-induced activation of A10 dopamine neurons in the rat. Brain Res. **277:** 119–127.

36. MATTHEWS, R. T. & D. C. GERMAN. 1984. Electrophysiological evidence for excitation of rat ventral tegmental area dopamine neurons by morphine. Neuroscience **11:** 617–625.

37. WALKER J. M., L. A. THOMPSON, J. FRASCELLA & M. W. FRIEDERICH. 1987. Opposite effects of μ and k opiates on the firing rate of dopamine cells in the substantia nigra of the rat. Eur. J. Pharmacol. **134:** 53–59.

38. LAVIN, A. & M. GARCIA-MUNOZ. 1985. Electrophysiological changes in substantia nigra after dynorphin administration. Brain Res. **369:** 298–302.

39. KALIVAS, P. W., E. WIDELOV, D. STANLEY, G. BREESE & A. J. PRANGE, JR. 1983. Enkephalin action on the mesolimbic system: A dopamine dependent and a dopamine independent increase in locomotor activity. J. Pharm. Exp. Ther. **227:** 229–237.

40. STINUS, L., A. E. KELLEY & S. D. IVERSEN. 1978. Increased spontaneous activity following substance P infusion into A10 dopaminergic area. Nature **276:** 616–618.

41. KELLEY, A. E., L. STINUS & S. D. IVERSEN. 1979. Behavioural activation induced in the rat by substance P infusion into the ventral tegmental area: Implication of dopaminergic A10 neurones. Neurosci. Lett. **11:** 335–339.

42. EISON, A. S., J. E. ALPERT, M. J. BANNON & S. D. IVERSEN. 1986. Selective activation of mesolimbic and mesocortical dopamine metabolism in rat brain by infusion of a stable substance P analogue into the ventral tegmental area. Brain Res. **363:** 145–147.

43. ELLIOTT, P. J. & S. D. IVERSEN. 1986. Behavioral effects of tachykinins and related peptides. Brain Res. **381:** 68–76.

44. ELLIOTT, P. J. & C. B. NEMEROFF. 1986. Repeated neurotensin administration in the ventral tegmental area: Effects on baseline and d-amphetamine induced locomotor activity. Neurosci. Lett. **68:** 239–244.

45. JOYCE, E. & S. D. IVERSEN. 1979. The effect of morphine applied locally to mesenscephalic dopamine cell bodies on spontaneous motor activity in the rat. Neurosci. Lett. **14:** 207–212.

46. KELLEY, A. E., L. STINUS & S.D. IVERSEN. 1980. Interactions between D-ala-Met-enkephalin, A10 dopaminergic neurones and spontaneous behavior in the rat. Behav. Brain Res. **1:** 3–24.

47. BROEKKAMP, C. L. E., A. G. PHILLIPS & A. T. COOLS. 1979. Stimulant effects of enkephalin injection into the dopaminergic A10 area. Nature (London) **278:** 560–562.

48. KELLEY, A. E., M. CADOR, L. STINUS & M. LE MOAL. 1987. Neurotensin, substance P, neurokinin-α and enkephalin: Injection into ventral tegmental area in the rat produces differential effects on operant responding. Psychopharmacology. In press.

49. DEWS, P. B. & G. R. WENGER. 1977. Rate-dependency of the behavioral effects of amphetamine. *In* Advances in Behavioral Pharmacology, Vol. 1. T. Thompson and P. B. Dews, Eds.: 167–227. Academic Press, New York.
50. BYRD, L. D. 1973. Effects of d-amphetamine on schedule-controlled key pressing and drinking in the chimpanzee. J. Pharmacol. Exp. Ther. **185:** 633–641.
51. ROBBINS, T. W., D. C. S. ROBERTS & G. F. KOOB. 1983. Effects of d-amphetamine and apomorphine upon operant behavior and schedule-induced licking in rats with 6-hydroxydopamine-induced lesions of the nucleus accumbens. J. Pharmacol. Exp. Ther. **224:** 662–673.
52. WAGNER, G. C., D. B. MASTERS & A. TOMIE. 1984. Effects of phencyclidine, haloperidol, and naloxone on fixed-interval performance in rats. Psychopharmacology **84:** 32–38.
53. MORLEY, J. E., B. A. GOSNELL & A. S. LEVINE. 1984. The role of peptides in feeding. Trends Pharmacol. Sci. **10:** 468–471.
54. CADOR, M., A. E. KELLEY, M. LE MOAL & L. STINUS. 1986. Ventral tegmental area infusion of substance P, neurotensin and enkephalin: Differential effects on feeding behavior. Neuroscience **18:** 659–669.
55. STANLEY, B. G., B. G. HOEBEL & S. F. LEIBOWITZ. 1983. Neurotensin: Effects of hypothalamic and intravenous injections on eating and drinking in rats. Peptides **4:** 493–500.
56. JENCK, F., A. GRATTON & R. A. WISE. 1986. Opposite effects of ventral tegmental and periaqueductal gray morphine injections on lateral hypothalamic stimulation-induced feeding. Brain Res. **399:** 24–32.
57. PHILLIPS, A. G., F. G. LEPIANE & H. C. FIBIGER. 1983. Dopaminergic mediation of reward produced by direct injection of enkephalin into the ventral tegmental area. Life Sci. **33:** 2505–2511.
58. BOZARTH, M. A. & R. A. WISE. 1980. Intracranial self-administration of morphine into the ventral tegmental area. Life Sci. **28:** 551–555.
59. VALENSTEIN, E. S. 1969. Behavior elicited by hypothalamic stimulation: A prepotency hypothesis. Brain Behav. Evol. **2:** 295–316.
60. STELLAR, J. R., F. H. BROOKS & L. E. MILLS. 1979. Approach and withdrawal analysis of the effects of hypothalamic stimulation and lesions in rats. J. Comp. Physiol. Psych. **93:** 446–466.
61. STELLAR, J. R., A. E. KELLEY & D. CORBETT. 1983. Effects of peripheral and central dopamine blockade on lateral hypothalamic self-stimulation: Evidence for both reward and motor deficits. Pharmacol. Biochem. Behav. **18:** 433–442.
62. MOGENSON, G. J. 1982. Studies of the nucleus accumbens and its mesolimbic dopaminergic afferents in relation to ingestive behaviors and reward. *In* Neural Basis of Feeding and Reward. B. G. Hoebel and D. Novin, Eds.: 275–287. Haer Institute, Brunswick, Me.
63. GLIMCHER, P. W., A. A. GIOVINO & B. G. HOEBEL. 1987. Neurotensin self-injection in the ventral tegmental area. Brain Res. **403:** 147–150.
64. GLIMCHER, P. W., R. MARGOLIN & G. C. HOEBEL. 1984. Neurotensin: A new "reward" peptide. Brain Res. **291:** 119–124.
65. EVERIST, H. D., C. C. CHIEUH & A. PERT. Effects of neurotensin on dopaminergic activity following intranigral or intrastriatal injections. 1983. Soc. Neurosci. Abstr. **9:** 716.
66. BANNON, M. J. 1986. Mild footshock stress dissociates substance P from substance K and dynorphin from Met- and Leu-enkephalin. Brain Res. **381:** 393–396.
67. TAKANO, Y., Y. TAKEDA, K. YAMADA & H. KAMIYA. 1986. Substance K, a novel tachykinin injected bilaterally into the ventral tegmental area of rats increases behavioral response. Life Sci. **37:** 2507–2514.
68. CADOR, M., A. E. KELLEY, M. LE MOAL & L. STINUS. 1985. Behavioral analysis of the effect of neurotensin injected into the ventral mesencephalon on investigatory and spontaneous motor behaviour in the rat. Psychopharmacology **85:** 187–196.
69. KELLEY, A. E., M. CADOR & L. STINUS. 1985. Behavioural analysis of the effect of substance P injected into the ventral mesencephalon on investigatory and spontaneous motor behavior in the rat. Psychopharmacology **85:** 37–46.
70. KELLEY, A. E., M. WINNOCK & L. STINUS. 1986. Amphetamine, apomorphine, and investigatory behavior in the rat: Analysis of the structure and pattern of responses. Psychopharmacology **86:** 66–74.

71. IVERSEN, S. D. 1982. Behavioural effects of substance P through dopaminergic pathways in the brain. *In* Substance P in the Nervous System. Ciba Foundation Symposium 91.: 307–318. Pitman, London.
72. CADOR, M., A. E. KELLEY, M. LE MOAL & L. STINUS. 1987. Behavioral analysis of the effect of d-ala-Met-enkephalin injected into the ventral mesencephalon on investigatory and spontaneous motor behavior in the rat. Brain Res. Submitted for publication.

# Neuroleptic Binding to Human Brain Receptors: Relation to Clinical Effects[a]

ELLIOTT RICHELSON

*Departments of Psychiatry and Pharmacology*
*Mayo Clinic and Foundation*
*Rochester, Minnesota 55905*

## INTRODUCTION

Results from both biochemical and neurophysiological research on neuroleptics have led to a better understanding of how these drugs cause many of their adverse effects and possibly their therapeutic effects. From these studies it is known that neuroleptics have many actions at many different sites in the nervous system. In fact, chlorpromazine, the principal neuroleptic, was found to have such a large number of actions by researchers at Rhone-Poulenc in France that it received the trade name "Largactyl."

## NEUROLEPTICS AND NEUROTRANSMITTER RECEPTORS

Receptors are the cellular recognition sites for neurotransmitters, hormones, and many drugs. They are generally membrane-bound proteins on the outside surface of the cell and have the remarkable property of being able to recognize specific molecular structures. During neurotransmission there is a release of the chemical neurotransmitter from the nerve ending. The neurotransmitter then diffuses across the synapse to stimulate the receptor. Recognition (binding) of an activator (agonist) of a receptor leads to a complex biological response within the cell as a result of the coupling of the agonist–receptor complex to an effector (for example, an ion channel). All known neurotransmitters are receptor agonists. Neuroleptics are antagonists of several different neurotransmitter receptors. An antagonist is a compound that binds to a receptor but does not activate it, thereby preventing the neurotransmitter from stimulating its receptor.

How tightly a neurotransmitter or antagonist binds to a receptor is measured in terms of affinity, and the affinity of a neuroleptic for a particular receptor may be predictive of the likelihood that the drug will cause certain adverse effects in patients. Drug-receptor affinities commonly are determined by radioligand binding techniques[1] that usually make use of a radioactively labeled drug (the radioligand) to measure directly the binding of a compound to a receptor site. Biological responses resulting from receptor stimulation [for example, the formation of cyclic adenosine monophosphate (AMP)] can also be utilized to determine affinities of drugs.

[a] This work was supported in part by the Mayo Foundation and in part by U.S. Public Health Service Grant MH27692.

The affinity is a constant for a given drug and receptor, and for many receptors it appears to be a constant regardless of the species or the tissue from which the receptors are derived. By obtaining the affinities for a series of drugs, one can rank them according to their potency of blockade at a particular receptor site. In addition, by comparing the affinities for a single drug at several different receptors, one can determine at which receptor the drug is most potent.

Most radioligand binding studies have used receptors from animal tissue. To be certain that the data are applicable to humans, in recent years, we have used normal human brain tissue obtained at autopsy as the source of receptors for our radioligand binding assays. Here, we present our results for a series of neuroleptics at the following receptors of human brain: dopamine $D_2$, muscarinic acetylcholine, histamine $H_1$, $\alpha_1$- and $\alpha_2$-adrenergic, and serotonin $S_1$ and $S_2$.

## INTERACTIONS WITH THE DOPAMINE $D_2$ RECEPTOR

For many years it has been considered that catecholamines are involved in the etiology of schizophrenia and that neuroleptics cause many of their effects — both therapeutic and adverse — by antagonizing dopamine receptors. Thus, attention has been focused on these receptors and the first biochemical model was the dopamine-stimulated adenylate cyclase system.[2] In homogenates of brain from areas rich in dopamine (for example, the caudate nucleus), dopamine at low concentrations stimulates the synthesis of cyclic AMP. Thus, the effector for this dopamine receptor (called "$D_1$" because it was the first to be discovered) is adenylate cyclase that, when activated, causes the synthesis of cyclic AMP from adenosine triphosphate (ATP). Cyclic AMP is called a "second messenger," the first being the neurotransmitter, and brings about a biological change within the cell.

This effect of dopamine at the $D_1$ receptor is competitively antagonized by low concentrations of antipsychotic drugs, and there is a reasonable agreement between the potency of a neuroleptic as an inhibitor of dopamine-sensitive adenylate cyclase and the potency as an antipsychotic agent.[2]

However, there is one major discrepancy that relates to the potency of haloperidol and structurally related compounds. These drugs are clinically many times more potent than chlorpromazine but less potent than chlorpromazine is in this in vitro system. Thus, this model for the dopamine receptor was not predictive of the clinical potency of all neuroleptics, and researchers therefore searched for other models.

With a radioactively labeled neuroleptic as a radioligand, another dopamine receptor ($D_2$) was identified by direct binding assays. Correlations between the average daily clinical dose for controlling schizophrenia and neuroleptic affinities for $D_2$ receptors of calf,[3] rat,[4] and human[5] caudate nucleus are excellent. Caudate nucleus, rather than limbic tissue, has been used in most studies because it is a much richer source of $D_2$ receptors, making experimentation easier. However, neuroleptic affinities in the caudate are similar if not identical to their respective affinities in limbic structures.[5] Thus, these data (TABLE 1) strongly suggest that neuroleptics cause their therapeutic effects by antagonizing the dopamine $D_2$ receptor and that this assay can be used to screen for new neuroleptics that antagonize the dopamine receptor. It should be noted, however, that because of the side effects resulting from dopamine receptor blockade, neuroleptics without this property are needed.

These binding data showing that all neuroleptics antagonize the $D_2$ receptor are the basis for an assay to measure neuroleptics in blood.[6] This radioreceptor assay is similar to a radioimmunoassay, except that instead of using an antibody to recognize

**TABLE 1.** Affinities[a] of Some Antipsychotics for Several Neurotransmitter Receptors of the Human Brain[5,7]

| Compound | Dopamine $D_2$ | Histamine $H_1$ | Adrenergic $\alpha_1$ | $\alpha_2$ | Muscarinic | Serotonin $S_1$ | $S_2$ |
|---|---|---|---|---|---|---|---|
| **Antipsychotics** | | | | | | | |
| d-Butaclamol[b] | 116 | 0.26 | 1.8 | 0.32 | 0.0083 | 0.13 | 250 |
| Chlorpromazine | 5.3 | 11 | 38 | 0.13 | 1.4 | 0.031 | 71 |
| Clozapine[b] | 0.56 | 36 | 11 | 0.62 | 8.3 | 0.056 | 63 |
| Fluphenazine | 125 | 4.8 | 11 | 0.064 | 0.053 | 0.0025 | 0.53 |
| Haloperidol | 25 | 0.053 | 16 | 0.026 | 0.0042 | 0.036 | 2.8 |
| Loxapine | 1.4 | 20 | 3.6 | 0.042 | 0.22 | 0.034 | 59 |
| Mesoridazine | 5.3 | 55 | 50 | 0.062 | 1.4 | 0.20 | 21 |
| Molindone | 0.83 | 0.00081 | 0.040 | 0.16 | 0.00026 | 0.083 | 0.020 |
| Perphenazine | 71 | 12 | 10 | 0.20 | 0.067 | 0.028 | 18 |
| Prochlorperazine | 14 | 5.3 | 4.2 | 0.059 | 0.18 | 0.017 | 6.7 |
| Promazine | 0.62 | 50 | 17 | 0.11 | 0.67 | 0.0083 | 6.3 |
| Spiperone[b] | 625 | 0.21 | 83 | 0.15 | 0.037 | 0.31 | 260 |
| Thioridazine | 3.8 | 6.2 | 20 | 0.12 | 5.6 | 0.29 | 4.5 |
| cis-Thiothixene | 222 | 17 | 9.1 | 0.50 | 0.034 | 0.071 | 0.77 |
| Trifluoperazine | 38 | 1.6 | 4.2 | 0.038 | 0.15 | 0.0043 | 7.1 |
| **Reference Compounds** | | | | | | | |
| Diphenhydramine | | 7.1 | | | | | |
| Phentolamine | | | 6.7 | 2.3 | | | |
| Atropine | | | | | 42 | | |
| Methysergide | | | | | | | 15 |

[a] $10^{-7} \times 1/K_d$, in which $K_d$ is the equilibrium dissociation constant in molarity. A larger number indicates greater affinity and, hence, greater blockade of a given receptor.
[b] Not available for clinical use in the United States.

the radioactive tracer and the drug (antigen), it uses dopamine receptors. Like a radioimmunoassay, this radioreceptor assay is very sensitive, but unlike a radioimmunoassay, it is not at all specific. That is, the radioreceptor assay for neuroleptics detects dopamine receptor binding activity in a sample, but alone cannot identify the compound(s) causing the activity. However, this lack of specificity has the advantage of measuring not only the parent compound but also active metabolites, since these metabolites would also antagonize the $D_2$ receptor. It is possible, however, that a metabolite could be formed that blocks the dopamine receptor but because of its structure, would not penetrate into the brain. This situation would cause problems in relating blood levels of neuroleptic binding activity to clinical response or to toxic effects.

In TABLE 1 are listed the data from our laboratory[5,7] on the affinities of neuroleptics for the dopamine $D_2$ receptor of the human brain, along with data for several other putative neurotransmitter receptors (histamine $H_1$, $\alpha_1$- and $\alpha_2$-adrenergic, muscarinic, serotonin $S_1$ and $S_2$ receptors) as determined in radioligand binding assays with normal tissue obtained at autopsy. Compounds are listed alphabetically.

At the dopamine $D_2$ receptor, the most potent compound is the butyrophenone spiperone, which is not currently available in this country for clinical use. This drug is more than 1000-fold more potent than the weakest compound, clozapine, which is also not available for use in the United States. The rank order of neuroleptics is predictive of the likelihood that these compounds will cause certain endocrinological and extrapyramidal side effects as is discussed in more detail below. For example, thiothixene will more likely cause a Parkinsonian-like picture than will promazine. As discussed below, intrinsic antimuscarinic activity of the drug also plays a part in the incidence of extrapyramidal side effects of neuroleptics.

Elevated serum levels of prolactin that result from neuroleptic blockade of the dopamine receptors in the pituitary[8] can subsequently cause galactorrhea, menstrual changes,[9] and sexual dysfunction.[10] For a time there was some concern that these elevated levels of prolactin would also cause breast cancer in patients on chronic neuroleptic treatment.[11] This hypothesis led to the consideration by the Food and Drug Administration (FDA) that neuroleptics should not be prescribed. Fortunately, the evidence does not support this hypothesis.[12]

The extrapyramidal side effects of neuroleptics can be divided into those of early onset (acute dyskinesia, akathisia, and Parkinsonism) and those of late onset (tardive dyskinesia and, rarely, the rabbit syndrome). The early onset problems occur within the first 10 weeks of therapy and are always reversible. The only relatively common late onset extrapyramidal side effect is tardive dyskinesia, which is by definition caused by neuroleptics and is not always reversible. Tardive dyskinesia is characterized by abnormal involuntary, persistent movements of the tongue, lips, facial, and sometimes trunk muscles. The rabbit syndrome, a rare extrapyramidal side effect occurring late, although clinically similar to tardive dyskinesia, is distinguished from this disorder by its responsiveness to treatment with antimuscarinic agents. Again, the available clinical data seem to suggest that neuroleptics with low affinity for the dopamine $D_2$ receptor will have low propensity to cause these extrapyramidal problems.

In addition to the dopamine $D_2$ receptor, many other biogenic amine receptors in human brain can be identified by radioligand binding techniques. Neuroleptics interact in a significant way with histamine $H_1$, $\alpha$-adrenergic, muscarinic, and serotoninergic receptors.

## INTERACTIONS WITH HISTAMINE RECEPTORS

Neuroleptics also antagonize receptors for histamine, which has many different effects on various cell types and very likely serves as a neurotransmitter. This biogenic amine causes its effects by activation of two different receptors ($H_1$ and $H_2$), which are distinguished by their differential sensitivities to agonists and antagonists. Classically, the histamine $H_1$ receptor mediates anaphylactic and allergic reactions, and the histamine $H_2$ receptor mediates stimulation of gastric acid secretion. In brain, histamine receptors are thought to be involved with a number of functions including arousal ($H_1$) and the regulation of appetite ($H_1$).[13]

Currently, only the histamine $H_1$ receptor can be identified with certainty by radioligand binding techniques, and [3H]doxepin, a tricyclic antidepressant with very high affinity for the histamine $H_1$ receptor,[14] is an excellent ligand for this purpose. Neuroleptics competitively antagonize the histamine $H_1$ receptor of human brain and many are potent at doing so. In fact, half of the drugs that we studied are more potent than the classic histamine $H_1$ antagonist diphenhydramine (TABLE 1). Mesoridazine is the most potent drug at these receptors and molindone is essentially devoid of activity. Contrary to earlier data, neuroleptics are weak antagonists of the histamine $H_2$ receptor (data not shown).[15]

The antihistaminic ($H_1$) property of these drugs likely relates to their ability to cause sedation and drowsiness. Because sedation is the most common side effect of histamine $H_1$ antagonists, they are used clinically as sedative-hypnotics. In addition, neuroleptics with high affinity for the histamine $H_1$ receptor will potentiate the actions of central depressant drugs that also cause sedation and drowsiness (in most cases by other mechanisms). Histamine may also be involved with blood pressure regulation, and therefore this antihistaminic property of neuroleptics may relate to their hypotensive effects.

In addition, histamine $H_1$-receptor blockade by neuroleptics and other compounds may play a role in the appetite-stimulating effects of these drugs. A switch to a drug that is less potent as an antihistamine (TABLE 1) may alleviate this problem. In fact, use of molindone, which is a very weak antihistamine (TABLE 1), results in significant weight loss in severely ill hospitalized schizophrenics who had been treated with other neuroleptics.[16]

## INTERACTIONS WITH α-ADRENERGIC RECEPTORS

There are also two subclassifications of α-adrenergic receptors — $\alpha_1$ and $\alpha_2$ — and neuroleptics competitively antagonize each (TABLE 1). These receptors are located both in the central and in the peripheral nervous systems and may play important roles in the regulation of blood pressure. Prazosin hydrochloride (Minipress), an antihypertensive drug, is a potent antagonist of the $\alpha_1$ receptor; and clonidine hydrochloride (Catapres), also an antihypertensive agent, stimulates the $\alpha_2$ receptor.

Neuroleptics are much more potent at blocking $\alpha_1$- than $\alpha_2$-adrenoceptors (TABLE 1). Most are more potent at blocking the $\alpha_1$-adrenoceptor than the nonselective α-antagonist phentolamine (TABLE 1), which is more potent than any neuroleptic at the $\alpha_2$-adrenoceptor. Thus, all neuroleptics except molindone in clinical practice will likely cause significant blockade at the $\alpha_1$-adrenoceptor. This may cause postural hypotension, dizziness, and a reflex form of tachycardia (TABLE 2). If tolerance to these effects does not occur, then the patient should be given a trial with a drug with lower affinity at the $\alpha_1$-adrenoceptor (TABLE 1).

At the $\alpha_2$-adrenoceptor of the human brain, clozapine is the most potent and haloperidol is the least potent of the neuroleptics as antagonists of this receptor (TABLE 1). In general, these drugs are relatively and absolutely weak at these receptors, so that their effects on the $\alpha_2$-adrenoceptor in clinical practice should be minimal except perhaps for a few drugs such as clozapine and cis-thiothixene. Although a side effect associated with blockade of the $\alpha_2$-adrenoceptor is unknown, this property may reduce the effectiveness of those antihypertensive agents that are thought to work by ultimately stimulating the $\alpha_2$-adrenoceptor (clonidine, guanabenz, and methyldopa).

## INTERACTIONS WITH THE MUSCARINIC ACETYLCHOLINE RECEPTOR

The vast majority of acetylcholine receptors are muscarinic in the brain, where they are thought to be involved with memory and motor functions among other things.[17] Furthermore, there exist at least two different subtypes of the muscarinic receptor,[18] called $M_1$ and $M_2$, which have different regional distributions within the human brain.[19] In the periphery, some important functions of this receptor are the control of gastrointestinal motility and micturition. Neuroleptics competitively antagonize the muscarinic receptor in the human brain[5,19] with no apparent selectivity for the different subtypes of this receptor. Potency of these drugs based upon their affinities (TABLE 1) shows that clozapine is the most potent and molindone the least potent at blocking

**TABLE 2.** Side Effects and Drug–Drug Interactions of Neuroleptics Due to Receptor Blockade

| Receptor | Possible Clinical Consequences |
|---|---|
| Dopamine $D_2$ receptor | • Extrapyramidal movement disorders (dystonia, Parkinsonism, akathisia, tardive dyskinesia, rabbit syndrome)<br>• Endocrine changes (prolactin elevation causing galactorrhea, gynecomastia, menstrual changes, sexual dysfunction) |
| Histamine $H_1$ receptor | • Potentiation of central depressant drugs<br>• Sedation drowsiness<br>• Weight gain<br>• Hypotension |
| Muscarinic receptor | • Blurred vision<br>• Dry mouth<br>• Sinus tachycardia<br>• Constipation<br>• Urinary retention<br>• Memory dysfunction |
| $\alpha_1$-Adrenergic receptor | • Potentiation of the antihypertensive effect of prazosin (Minipress)<br>• Postural hypotension, dizziness<br>• Reflex tachycardia |
| $\alpha_2$-Adrenergic receptor | • Blockade of the antihypertensive effects of clonidine (Catapres), guanabenz (Wytensin), and $\alpha$-methyldopa (Aldomet) |
| Serotonin $S_2$ receptors | • Ejaculatory disturbances<br>• Hypotension<br>• Prevention of migraine headaches |

the muscarinic receptor. For the phenothiazines the potency of blockade of the muscarinic receptor correlates with the type of side chain as follows: piperidine > aliphatic >> piperazine.

Although no antipsychotic drug is more potent than the classic antimuscarinic drug atropine at blocking the muscarinic receptor, clinically significant muscarinic receptor blockade will occur in patients given the drugs that have the highest affinity for this receptor (TABLE 1) due to the high doses and, therefore, high receptor levels achieved in clinical practice. Atropine is used at 1 mg or less, reflecting its high affinity for the muscarinic receptor, whereas a drug like thioridazine is used at 50 or more times that amount. In terms of receptor pharmacology, a drug with a relatively low affinity for a receptor can achieve the same degree of receptor blockade as a drug of relatively high affinity, but in order to do so the lower affinity drug needs to be present at a higher concentration at the receptor site.

The antimuscarinic property of these drugs may result in several different types of side effects (TABLE 2). For example, it may cause memory dysfunction (possibly a result of blocking $M_1$ receptors[20]) or urinary retention. Again, low affinity for the muscarinic receptor (TABLE 1) suggests a low propensity to cause antimuscarinic side effects. Thus, by choosing a drug low on the list (TABLE 1), these side effects should be minimized.

As mentioned previously, this property may also have a salutary effect on reducing the incidence of extrapyramidal side effects of neuroleptics.[21,22] Thus, drugs with potent antimuscarinic effects (e.g., clozapine and thioridazine) are less likely to cause these problems.

## INTERACTIONS WITH SEROTONIN $S_1$ AND $S_2$ RECEPTORS

Serotonin receptors exist in at least two subtypes labeled $S_1$ and $S_2$. Neuroleptics competitively antagonize each, with their most potent interactions at the $S_2$ receptor (TABLE 1).[7] The clinical relevance[23] of antagonism of serotonin receptors is uncertain in part because of our lack of knowledge of what functions these receptors have in humans. Ketanserin, a potent serotonin $S_2$ receptor antagonist, is used clinically outside the United States to treat hypertension. Then, perhaps the blood pressure lowering effects of some neuroleptics may be mediated by this property. In addition, serotonin appears to be involved in contraction of vascular smooth muscle and this action may be involved in the pathophysiology of vascular headaches that are treated by such drugs as methysergide.[24] Some neuroleptics may therefore be useful in the treatment of migraine. However, because of the serious extrapyramidal side effect of tardive dyskinesia, these drugs should be used with extreme caution in nonpsychotic patients.

## SUMMARY

TABLE 2 summarizes the potential clinical consequences of neurotransmitter receptor blockade by neuroleptics. These pharmacological effects of neuroleptics at receptors in brain and elsewhere in the body are likely responsible for therapeutic and certain adverse effects as well as some drug–drug interactions. Data presented here should allow the physician a rational basis for selecting neuroleptics to minimize these unwanted effects in patients.

## REFERENCES

1. RICHELSON, E. 1984. Studying neurotransmitter receptors: Binding and biological assay. *In* Neuroreceptors in Health and Disease, Vol. 10. J. Marwaha and W. J. Anderson, Eds.: 4–19. Karger. Basel.
2. KEBABIAN, J. W., G. L. PETZOLD & P. GREENGARD. 1972. Dopamine sensitive adenylate cyclase in caudate nucleus of rat brain, and its similarity to the "dopamine receptor." Proc. Natl. Acad. Sci. U.S.A. **69:** 2145–2149.
3. SEEMAN, P., T. LEE, M. CHAU-WONG & K. WONG. 1976. Antipsychotic drug doses and neuroleptic/dopamine receptors. Nature. **261:** 717–719.
4. CREESE, A., D. R. BURT & S. H. SNYDER. 1976. Dopamine receptor binding predicts clinical and pharmacological potencies of antischizophrenic drugs. Science. **192:** 481–483.
5. RICHELSON, E. & A. NELSON. 1984. Antagonism by neuroleptics of neurotransmitter receptors of normal human brain in vitro. Eur. J. Pharmacol. **103:** 197–204.
6. CREESE, I. & S. H. SNYDER. 1977. A simple and sensitive radioreceptor assay for antischizophrenic drugs in blood. Nature. **270:** 180–182.
7. WANDER, T. J., A. NELSON, H. OKAZAKI & E. RICHELSON. 1987. Antagonism by neuroleptics of serotonin 5-HT$_{1a}$ and 5-HT$_2$ receptors of normal human brain in vitro. Eur. J. Pharmacol. **143:** 279–282.
8. SACHAR, E. J. 1978. Neuroendocrine responses to psychotropic drugs. *In* Psychopharmacology: A Generation of Progress. M. A. Lipton, A. DiMascio, and K. F. Killam, Eds.: 499–507. Raven Press. New York.

9. CAUFRIEZ, A. 1985. Menstrual disorders associated with hyperprolactinemia. Hormone Res. **22:** 209–214.
10. BUVAT, J., A. LEMAIRE, M. BUVAT-HERBAUT, J. C. FOURLINNIE, A. RACADOT & P. FOSSATI. 1985. Hyperprolactinemia and sexual function in men. Hormone Res. **22:** 196–203.
11. SCHYVE, P. M., F. SMITHLINE & H. Y. MELTZER. 1978. Neuroleptic-induced prolactin level elevation and breast cancer. Arch. Gen. Psychiatry. **35:** 1291–1301.
12. GOODE, D. J., W. T. CORBETT, H. M. SCHEY, S. H. SUH, B. WOODIE *et al.* 1981. Breast cancer in hospitalized psychiatric patients. Am. J. Psychiatry. **138:** 804–806.
13. TAYLOR, J. E. & E. RICHELSON. 1981. Histamine receptors in neural tissue. *In* Neurotransmitter Receptors, Part 2, Series B, Vol. 10. H. I. Yamamura & S. Enna, Eds.: 71–100. Chapman & Hall. London.
14. KANBA, S. & E. RICHELSON. 1984. Histamine $H_1$ receptors in human brain labeled with [3H]doxepin. Brain Res. **304:** 1–7.
15. KANBA, S. & E. RICHELSON. 1983. Antidepressants are weak competitive antagonists of histamine $H_2$ receptors in dissociated tissue from the guinea pig hippocampus. Eur. J. Pharmacol. **94:** 313–318.
16. GARDOS, G. & J. O. COLE. 1977. Weight reduction in schizophrenics by molindone. Am. J. Psychiatry **134:** 302–304.
17. MCKINNEY, M. & E. RICHELSON. 1984. The coupling of the neuronal muscarinic receptor to responses. Ann. Rev. Pharmacol. Toxicol. **24:** 121–146.
18. BIRDSALL, N. J. M. & E. C. HULME. 1983. Muscarinic receptor subclasses. Trends Pharmacol. Sci. **4:** 459–463.
19. LIN, S. C., K. OLSON, H. OKAZAKI & E. RICHELSON. 1986. Studies on muscarinic binding sites in human brain identified with [³H]pirenzepine. J. Neurochem. **46:** 274–290.
20. CAULFIELD, M. P., G. A. HIGGINS & D. W. STRAUGHAN. 1983. Central administration of the muscarinic receptor subtype-selective antagonist pirenzepine selectively impairs passive avoidance learning in the mouse. J. Pharm. Pharmacol. **35:** 131–132.
21. MILLER, R. J. & C. R. HILEY. 1974. Anti-muscarinic properties of neuroleptics and drug-induced Parkinsonism. Nature. **248:** 596–597.
22. SNYDER, S., D. GREENBERG & H. I. YAMAMURA. 1974. Antischizophrenic drugs and brain cholinergic receptors—Affinity for muscarinic sites predicts extrapyramidal effects. Arch. Gen. Psychiatry **31:** 58–61.
23. PEROUTKA, S. J. & S. H. SNYDER. 1980. Relationship of neuroleptic drug effects at brain dopamine, serotonin, α-adrenergic, and histamine receptors to clinical potency. Am. J. Psychiatry **137:** 1518–1522.
24. PEROUTKA, S. J. 1984. Vascular serotonin receptors. Biochem. Pharmacol. **33:** 2349–2353.

# Dopamine Neuronal Tracts in Schizophrenia: Their Pharmacology and *in Vivo* Glucose Metabolism

CAROL A. TAMMINGA,[a] G. HOWARD BURROWS,[b]
THOMAS N. CHASE,[b] LARRY D. ALPHS,[a] AND
GUNVANT K. THAKER[a]

[a]*Maryland Psychiatric Research Center*
*Department of Psychiatry*
*University of Maryland*
*Baltimore, Maryland 21228*

[b]*Experimental Therapeutics Branch*
*National Institute of Neurological and Communicative Disorders*
*and Stroke*
*Baltimore, Maryland 20892*

## INTRODUCTION

Much is already known and many new observations have been reported in this journal, about distinguishing biologic characteristics of mesencephalic dopamine (DA) -containing neuronal tracts in the mammalian brain. It is now clear that the major dopaminergic pathways have distinct modulatory transmitters, different cotransmitters, separate autoregulatory and activation mechanisms, and unique functional roles. These biologic differences have prompted the speculation that the systems can be selectively modulated pharmacologically in humans for different therapeutic indications. This strategy would seem to mimic nature's own differential activation of specific DA systems for distinct behavioral functions, for example, mesocortical dopaminergic activation in response to footshock stress.[1]

Nevertheless, the successful application of these preclinical observations to the development of improved pharmacotherapies for dopamine-related illnesses requires a more complete understanding of the physiology of these tracts in man. It is necessary to know the major functions (or sets of functions) subserved by each of the DA-mediated pathways in humans. It would also be desirable to know whether biologic changes in any of the dopaminergic tracts accompany the illness itself or whether the pharmacologic effect exerted through the tract is nonspecific. Then, as a corollary, the disease characteristics or the therapeutic actions, if any, subserved by the distinct dopaminergic pathways might become clear.

The answer to each of these questions has direct relevance to schizophrenia, a mental disorder characterized by cognitive and affective distortions, and loss of reality orientation. The illness may be etiologically and/or pathophysiologically heterogeneous.[2]

The single most widely replicated and generally accepted biologic observation about schizophrenia is the therapeutic response of its psychotic symptoms to antidopaminergic treatments.[3] Thus has derived the tight association between schizophrenia and DA pharmacology over the years. Although DA antagonists improve schizophrenic symptoms, there is little to support the hypothesis that dopamine-mediated transmission is abnormal in the illness: plasma and CSF measures of DA and its metabolites show no consistent alterations;[4] plasma levels of DA-regulated hormones like prolactin remain normal;[5,6] postmortem analysis of DA, its metabolites, and related enzyme systems are elevated in certain brain areas, but purportedly only in response to chronic neuroleptic drug treatment.[7-9] The lack of a consistent picture of DA system dysfunction in schizophrenia suggests that antidopaminergic treatments may be nonspecific in their attenuation of psychosis. But, recent *in vivo* receptor studies could indicate primary DA receptor changes in schizophrenia,[10] again suggesting DA system dysfunction in the illness. Whether pathophysiologically involved or only therapeutically relevant in the illness, the "localization" of the antidopaminergic action that mediates psychosis improvement may be important to the understanding of the illness.

## DOPAMINE-RELATED PHARMACOLOGY OF SCHIZOPHRENIA: WHERE ARE NEUROLEPTICS ANTIPSYCHOTIC?

Psychotic symptoms improve with neuroleptic drugs, an effect thought to be mediated by blockade of DA receptors.[11] Symptomatic improvement begins soon after initiation of drug treatment and gradually progresses to full or maximal benefit over 2–8 weeks. Other drugs that modify DA-mediated transmission, including DA synthesis inhibitors,[12] DA storage depletors,[13] and DA autoreceptor agonists,[14] also improve psychosis. Among the unknown response characteristics in this process is the actual brain area where DA receptor blockade exerts its antipsychotic effect. It has often been assumed that this must involve mesolimbic and/or mesocortical areas because of the primary cognitive functions of the limbic and frontal cortex contrasted with the suspected motor functions associated with the striatum. But what is already known about striatal modulation of cortical function[15,16] would encourage a full examination of the options.

Chronic administration of neuroleptic drugs induces changes in the number and affinity of DA receptors in the striatum of experimental animals.[17] This has also been confirmed in the human brain.[9] In rat striatum, traditional neuroleptic drugs (e.g., haloperidol) increase $D_2$ but not $D_1$ receptors, whereas atypical neuroleptics (e.g., clozapine) modify $D_1$ but not $D_2$ receptors.[18] However, essentially no alterations occur in DA-receptor number or affinity in the limbic areas of the rat brain with chronic neuroleptic exposure.[19] Thus, since no clear clinical evidence supports the existence of a late-onset supersensitivity phenomenon in psychotic symptoms, this would suggest that localization of neuroleptic-induced psychosis improvement may occur in limbic areas of the brain, outside the striatal terminal fields. In contrast, since there are late-developing motor symptoms associated with chronic neuroleptic treatment, these are likely mediated by the striatal DA receptor changes.

Dopamine autoreceptors appear to be present on only nigrostriatal and selected mesolimbic DA-containing neurons.[1] These receptors can be stimulated to diminish DA synthesis and/or release by low doses of apomorphine or by selective DA autoreceptor agonists.[20,21] Since this action reduces dopamine-mediated transmission, it would be predicted to produce an antipsychotic action. And, indeed, low doses of apomorphine do have antipsychotic actions,[22] as do other autoreceptor agonists like N-propylnorapomorphine (TABLE 1). Thus, it is tempting to suggest that DA terminal

**TABLE 1.** *N*-propylnorapomorphine Effect in Schizophrenia: Neuroleptic Nonresponders *vs.* Neuroleptic Responders

| | 0 mg | 5 mg | 10 mg | 15 mg | 20 mg | 30 mg | 40 mg |
|---|---|---|---|---|---|---|---|
| Neuroleptic responder[a] | −0.4[b](2.6) | −2.6(1.5) | −0.6(6.3) | −6.7(3.8) | −5.3(5.2) | −0.4(1.1) | −5.3(3.1) |
| Neuroleptic nonresponder | −2.9(.4) | +1.9(6.8) | +3.8(10) | −1.4(3.7) | +5(9.6) | −0.75(1.1) | +3.8(3.9) |

[a] A neuroleptic responder was defined as a schizophrenic having greater than a 50% symptom response to haloperidol with optimal dose treatment delivered over at least 4 weeks.

[b] Change from that day's baseline in Brief Psychiatric Rating Scale (BPRS) rating at 2 hours and 4 hours after NPA administration. Mean (SD).

areas, innervated by autoreceptor-regulated neurons, are involved in mediating the antipsychotic effects of functional DA antagonists.

An examination of the action of drugs that selectively modify different DA tracts provides another approach to the localization of DA-containing brain areas related to psychosis. Cholecystokinin octapeptide (CCK-8) is a neurally active peptide colocalized with DA in some but not all of its neuronal tracts. Those DA neurons that contain CCK-8 project in the rat to the dorsomedial striatum, nucleus accumbens, and sparsely to the frontal cortex.[23] Thus, either a direct action of CCK-8 on psychotic symptoms or a modification of a neuroleptic effect would implicate these areas in psychosis. CCK-8 has been studied in schizophrenia[24,25] and in Parkinson's disease[26] without consistent evidence of clinical efficacy. Despite demonstrable CCK-8 blood levels in a group of schizophrenic patients, no alteration in blindly rated psychosis scores was found by these investigators in the patients compared with placebo response (TABLE 2). The interpretation of these data is complicated by the question of CNS penetrability. In the experimental monkey, intravenous injection of [³H]CCK-8 did not result in the presence of any of the [³H]CCK-8 in the ventricular fluid of that chronically cannulated animal at times up to 30 min after iv injection (M. Knight and C. Tamminga, unpublished data). Also, there are no measureable CNS changes with systemic CCK-8 administration in humans, including motor alterations, vital sign change, and change in evoked potential response.[25] Thus, it is probable that CCK-8 fails to enter the brain in concentrations sufficient to modify DA-mediated transmission, hence leaving the initial question of its action in psychosis unanswered. A pharmacologic probe, effective in modifying cholecystokinin function upon systemic administration, is needed to explore this question effectively.

In summary, autoreceptor agonists, which are antipsychotic in schizophrenia, appear to act only in nigro-striatal and mesolimbic DA tracts. DA receptor supersensitivity, while present in the striatal terminal areas, cannot be demonstrated in the limbic regions, consistent with the lack of tardive symptoms in cognitive and affective (contrasted with motor) functions. Unfortunately, a relatively selective mesolimbic DA system cotransmitter CCK-8 has failed to be a useful probe as yet because of its lack of CNS penetrability. Thus, these circumstantial data would focus attention on the mesolimbic DA system as the tract mediating the neuroleptic-induced antipsychotic action.

## IMAGING OF DA TERMINAL AREAS IN SCHIZOPHRENIA

Using the ${}^{11}$C-$N$-methylspiperone (${}^{11}$C-NMSP) tracer with PET, DA receptors in the human striatum appear to be increased in number.[10] Although, results derived from

**TABLE 2.** Cholecystokinin-8 Analogue (Caerulein) Effect[b] in Schizophrenia

| Placebo | | | Caerulein | | |
|---|---|---|---|---|---|
| Hour | Total | Psychosis | Hour | Total | Psychosis |
| 0[a] | 54(14) | 9.5(6) | 0 | 53(17) | 9.5(6) |
| 4 | 50(13) | 8.3(5) | 4 | 55(18) | 9.7(5) |
| 24 | 53(13) | 10.3(7) | 24 | 53(16) | 9.0(6) |

[a] Hours after receiving 0.3 µg/kg caerulein; $n = 5$.

[b] Mean BPRS score (mean, SD), calculated as total score (Total) and as psychosis subscale score (Psychosis), at baseline and two different time points after caerulein administration (4 hr and 24 hr).

the use of a different tracer has produced conflicting findings,[27] this is a particularly provocative finding, because the results were present in not only previously treated schizophrenic patients but also in neuroleptic-naive schizophrenics. Unfortunately, an examination of DA receptor characteristics in other brain areas remains difficult and complex because of the lack of DA receptor specificity of the probe, [11]C-NMSP. But this information is clearly relevant to understand the implications of DA receptor alterations to schizophrenic symptoms.

The [18]FDG tracer technique, with PET, can provide information about glucose metabolism in schizophrenia in all DA terminal areas. The metabolic rate of glucose in a given brain area is generally taken to represent the integrated neuronal activity of the terminals in that region.[28] Thus, without expecting information pertinent to a specific transmitter, the local neuronal activity in the distinct DA terminal areas can be studied as an integral of glucose utilization in that particular brain area.

We have recently studied eleven right-handed patients with schizophrenia (age, sex) in comparison with eleven normal controls (age, sex). All study subjects were free from any medication for at least four weeks and had active psychotic symptoms. PET scans were conducted under resting conditions in a quiet, dimly lit room, with the subjects' ears plugged and eyes patched.[29] All subjects were unmedicated and kept fasting during the preceding 5–6 hours. [18]F-deoxyglucose (FDG; 5 mCI) was administered as an intravenous bolus. Serial, "arterialized" venous blood samples were obtained from the opposite arm for the determination of plasma FDG and glucose levels as a function of time. Scanning (NINCDS NeuroPET; resolution approximately 6 mm, full width at half maximum) began 30 min after isotope injection. Images were reconstructed and local metabolic rates for glucose calculated as previously described.[30] The entire brain was imaged by means of 7–42 horizontal sections parallel to the canthomeatal plane. Four sections at levels 32, 64, 83, 92 mm inferior to the cerebral vertex[31] were selected for detailed analysis. Glucose utilization in cortical brain areas, presumably containing DA terminal areas and subcortical nuclei with prominent DA projections was calculated using a Vax Image Analyzing System by an investigator blind to the identity of the PET image. PET slices were matched to the atlas plane by distance from the top of the brain and by the distribution of the PET-defined structures; areas selected for analysis were identified in the atlas and the corresponding area located on the corresponding PET slice. The Image Analyzing System was based on LISPIX, a processing system composed of a FORTRAN library of pixel-level operations driven by LISP.[32]

There were no differences in absolute glucose utilization in any of the areas evaluated between the left and and the right sides of the brain in schizophrenic patients or normal controls. In the frontal and temporal cortex, no differences in glucose consumption were apparent between schizophrenic and normal subjects (TABLE 3). Neither were there any changes in these areas in the relative metabolic rate (brain area/cerebellum). However, in some areas of brain, which were all located in the limbic system, CNS glucose utilization appeared diminished. In the hippocampus, a 27% decrease in metabolism occurred ($p < 0.001$); in the anterior cingulate cortex the decrease was 26% ($p < 0.008$); and in the amygdala area, the reduction was 18% ($p < 0.05$). Moreover, the relative glucose utilization values (brain area/cerebellum) in these particular areas were all significantly reduced in schizophrenic patients as well.

## CONCLUSIONS

The pharmacologic and imaging data, while providing some evidence to maintain a broad interest in the different DA terminal areas as they may be related to schizophrenia,

**TABLE 3.** Glucose Utilization in DA Tracts in Human Brain: Schizophrenic vs. Normal

| Area | Schizophrenic (μmoles/100 gm/min) ($n = 11$) | Normal (μmoles/100 gm/min) ($n = 11$) | |
|---|---|---|---|
| Frontal Cortex | | | |
| Superior | 9.7 ± 2.0 | 11.2 ± 2.8 | NS |
| Middle | 10.5 ± 2.1 | 12.8 ± 3.8 | NS |
| Inferior | 10.9 ± 2.7 | 11.2 ± 2.6 | NS |
| Temporal Cortex | | | |
| Superior | 9.5 ± 2.2 | 10.3 ± 2.1 | NS |
| Middle | 9.1 ± 2.3 | 9.5 ± 2.5 | NS |
| Inferior | 7.3 ± 2.3 | 7.8 ± 1.6 | NS |
| Anterior cingulate cortex | 9.6 ± 1.9 | 12.9 ± 3.2 | 0.008 |
| Hippocampal cortex | 6.9 ± 1.6 | 9.5 ± 1.7 | 0.001 |
| Amygdala area | 5.9 ± 1.1 | 7.2 ± 1.4 | 0.05 |
| Caudate | 10.2 ± 2.3 | 11.9 ± 3.6 | NS |
| Globus pallidus | 10.3 ± 2.6 | 12.5 ± 4.2 | NS |
| Brain stem (SN level) | 7.7 ± 1.3 | 8.7 ± 1.6 | NS |

Mean ± SD, left side.

do suggest some increased focus on limbic structures and their afferent DA pathways in the pathophysiology of the disease. This would lead to consideration of the mesolimbic pathways as being pivotal in the mediation of psychosis and/or the antipsychotic effect of neuroleptic drugs. This emphasis on the limbic system is suggested both by the pharmacologic data and by the glucose metabolism results reported in this study. Lack of autoreceptors on mesocortical DA neurons would tend to discourage interest in this track as functionally relevant in schizophrenia. And, lack of "tardive" manifestation of psychosis would tend to argue against the nigrostriatal system in this capacity. While these pieces of evidence are quite circumstantial, they are consistent with our own *in vivo* clinical findings that suggest a metabolic abnormality in schizophrenia in the limbic area of the brain; here the reduction in metabolism occurs in the hippocampus in the anterior cingulate cortex, and the amygdala. These *in vivo* metabolic findings in the limbic system of schizophrenics are consistent with published morphometric findings in postmortem samples from hippocampus and anterior cingulate[33,34] and with postmortem volume measurements in schizophrenic brains.[35] Finally, a dysfunction of neuronal groups in these regions is consistent with the complex behavioral symptoms in the illness.

## REFERENCES

1. BANNON, M. J., M. E. WOLF & R. H. ROTH. 1983. Pharmacology of dopamine neurons innervating the prefrontal, cingulate and piriform cortices. Eur. J. Pharmacol. **91:** 119–125.
2. CARPENTER, W. T., D. W. HEINRICHS & A. M. I. WAGMAN. Deficit and non-deficit forms of schizophrenia. Submitted for publication in Am. J. Psychiatry.
3. TAMMINGA, C. A. & J. GERLACH. 1987. New neuroleptics and experimental antipsychotics in schizophrenia. *In* Psychopharmacology: The Third Generation of Progress. H. Y. Meltzer, Ed.: 1129–1140. Raven Press. New York.
4. BOWERS, M. B., JR. 1974. Central dopamine turnover in schizophrenic syndromes. Arch. Gen. Psychiatry **31:** 50–54.
5. GUREN, P. H., E. J. SACHAR, G. LANGER, N. ALTMAN, M. LEIFER, A. FRANTZ & F. S.

HALPERN. 1978. Prolactin responses to neuroleptics in normal and schizophrenic subjects. Arch. Gen. Psychiatry **35:** 108-116.

6. TAMMINGA, C. A., R. C. SMITH, G. PANDEY, L. A. FROHMAN & J. M. DAVIS. 1977. A neuroendocrine study of supersensitivity in tardive dyskinesia. Arch. Gen. Psychiatry **34:** 1199-1203.

7. BIRD, E. D., E. G. S. SPOKES & L. L. IVERSEN. 1979. Increased dopamine concentration in limbic areas of brain from patients dying with schizophrenia. Brain **102:** 347-360.

8. CROW, T. J., H. F. BAKER, A. J. CROSS, M. H. JOSEPH, R. LOFTHOUSE, A. LONGDEN, F. OWEN, G. J. RILEY, V. GLOVER & W. S. KILLPACK. 1979. Monoamine mechanisms in chronic schizophrenia: Postmortem neurochemical findings. Br. J. Psychiatry **134:** 249-256.

9. MACKAY, A. V. P., L. L. IVERSEN, M. ROSSER, E. SPOKES, E. BIRD, A. ARREGUI, I. CREESE & S. H. SNYDER. 1982. Increased brain dopamine and dopamine receptors in schizophrenia. Arch. Gen. Psychiatry **39:** 991-997.

10. WONG, D. F., H. N. WAGNER, L. E. TUNE, R. F., DANNALS, G. D. PEARLSON, J. M. LINKS, C. A. TAMMINGA, E. P. BROUSSOLLE, H. T. RAVERT, A. A. WILSON, J. K. THOMAS TOUNG, J. MALAT, J. A. WILLIAMS, L. A. O'TUAMA, S. H. SNYDER, M. J. KUHAR & A. GJEDDE. 1986. Positron emission tomography reveals elevated D2 dopamine receptors in drug-naive schizophrenics. Science **234:** 1558-1563.

11. CARLSSON, A. & M. LINDQVIST. 1969. Central and peripheral monoaminergic membrane-pump blockade by some addictive analgesics and antihistamines. J. Pharm. Pharmacol. **21:** 460-464.

12. WALINDER, J., A. SKOTT, A. CARLSSON & B. E. ROOS. 1976. Potentiation by metyrosine of thioridazine effects in chronic schizophrenics. A Long-term trial using double-blind crossover technique. Arch. Gen. Psychiatry **33:** 501-505.

13. GILMAN, A. G., L. S. GOODMAN & A. GILMAN, EDS. 1980. Goodman and Gilman's The Pharmacological Basis of Therapeutics, 6th ed. p. 392. Macmillan. New York.

14. TAMMINGA, C. A., M. D. GOTTS, G. K. THAKER, L. D. ALPHS & N. L. FOSTER. 1986. Dopamine agonist treatment of schizophrenia with N-propylnorapomorphine. Arch. Gen. Psychiatry **43:** 398-402.

15. CARLSSON, A. 1987. The role of dopamine in normal and abnormal behavior. Presented at the International Congress for Schizophrenia Research, Clearwater, Fla.

16. KORNHUBER, J. & M. E. KORNHUBER. 1986. Presynaptic dopaminergic modulation of cortical input to the striatum. Life Sci. **39:** 669-674.

17. CLOW, A., A. THEODOROU, P. JENNER & C. D. MARSDEN. 1980. Cerebral dopamine function in rats following withdrawal from one year of continuous neuroleptic administration. Eur. J. Pharmacol. **63:** 145-157.

18. RUPNIAK, N. M. J., M. D. HALL, S. MANN, S. FLEMINGER, G. KILPATRICK, P. JENNER & C. D. MARSDEN. 1985a. Chronic treatment with clozapine, unlike haloperidol, does not induce changes in striatal D-2 receptor function in the rat. Biochem. Pharmacol. **34:** 2755-2763.

19. RUPNIAK, N. M. J., M. D. HALL, E. KELLY, S. FLEMINGER, G. KILPATRICK, P. JENNER & C. D. MARSDEN. 1985b. Mesolimbic dopamine function is not altered during continuous chronic treatment of rats with typical or atypical neuroleptic drug. J. Neural Transm. **62:** 249-266.

20. KEHR, W., A. CARLSSON, M. LINDQVIST, T. MAGNUSSON & C. ATACK. 1972. J. Pharm. Pharmacol. **24:** 744-747.

21. CARLSSON, A. 1976. Some aspects of dopamine in the basal ganglia. *In* The Basal Ganglia, M. D. Yahr, Ed.: 181-190. Raven Press. New York.

22. TAMMINGA, C. A., M. H. SCHAFFER, R. C. SMITH & J. M. DAVIS. 1978. Schizophrenic symptoms improve with apomorphine. Science **200:** 567-568.

23. HOKFELT, T., L. REHFELD, B. SKIRBOLL, M. IVEMARK, M. GOLDSTEIN & K. MARKEY. 1980. Evidence for coexistence of dopamine and CCK in mesolimbic neurones. Nature **285:** 476-478.

24. MOROJI, N., N. WATANABE, N. AOKI & S. ITOH. 1982. Antipsychotic effects of caerulein in chronic schizophrenia. Arch. Gen. Psychiatry **39:** 485.

25. TAMMINGA, C. A., R. L. LITTMAN, L. D. ALPHS, T. N. CHASE, G. K. THAKER & A. M.

WAGMAN. 1986. Neuronal cholecystokinin and schizophrenia: Pathogenic and therapeutic studies. Psychopharmacology **88:** 387–391.

26.  CHASE, T. N., P. BARONE, G. BRUNO, S. L. COHEN, J. JUNCOS, M. KNIGHT, S. RUGGERI, L. STEARDO & C. A. TAMMINGA. 1985. Cholecystokinin-mediated synaptic function and the treatment of neuropsychiatric disease. *In* Neuronal Cholecystokinin, J. J. Vanderhagen and J. W. Crawley, Eds.: 553–561. Ann. N.Y. Acad. Sci.

27.  FARDE, L., F. A. WIESEL, H. HALL, C. HOLLDIN, S. STONE-ELANDER & G. SEDVALL. 1987. No $D_2$ receptor increase in PET study of schizophrenia. Arch. Gen. Psychiatry. **44:** 671.

28.  SOKOLOFF, L., M. REIVICH, C. KENNEDY, M. H. DES ROSIERS, C. S. PATLAK, K. D. PETTIGREW, O. SAKURADA & M. SHINOHARA. 1977. The [14C] deoxyglucose method for the measurement of local cerebral glucose utilization: Theory, procedure, and normal values in the conscious and anesthetized albino rat. J. Neurochem. **28:** 897–916.

29.  FOSTER, N. L., T. N. CHASE, L. MANSI, R. BROOKS, P. FEDIO, N. J. PATRONAS & G. DICHIRO. 1984. Cortical abnormalities in Alzheimer's disease. Ann. Neurol. **16:** 649–654.

30.  DICHIRO, G., R. A. BROOK, N. J. PATRONAS, D. BAIRAMIAN, P. L. KORNBLITH, B. H. SMITH, L. MANSI & J. BARKER. 1984. Issues in the *in vivo* measurement of glucose metabolism of human central nervous system tumors. Ann. Neurol. **15:** 138–146.

31.  AQUILONIUS, S. M. & S. A. ECKERNAS. 1980. A Colour Atlas of the Human Brain Adapted to Computed Tomography. Raven Press. New York.

32.  KIRSCH, R. A. 1971. Computer determination of the constituent structure of biological images. Comput. Biomed. Res. **4:** 315–328.

33.  BOGERTS, B., E. MEERTZ & R. SCHONFELDT-BAUSCH. 1985. Basal ganglia and limbic system pathology in schizophrenia: A morphometric study. Arch. Gen. Psychiatry. **42:** 784–791.

34.  BENES, F. M. & E. D. BIRD. 1987. An analysis of the arrangement of neurons in the cingulate cortex of schizophrenic patients. Arch. Gen. Psychiatry. **44:** 608–616.

35.  BROWN, R., N. COLTER, J. A. A. CORSELLIS, T. J. CROW, C. D. FIRTH, J. JAGOE, E. C. JOHNSTONE & L. MARSH. 1986. Postmortem evidence of structure brain changes in schizophrenia. Arch. Gen. Psychiatry. **43:** 36–42.

# MPTP Effects on Dopamine Neurons

IRWIN J. KOPIN

*National Institute of Neurological and Communicative Disorders
and Stroke
National Institutes of Health
Bethesda, Maryland 20892*

## INTRODUCTION

The demonstration that there are marked differences in the concentrations of dopamine in different brain areas (see review by Carlsson[1]) provided the basis for considering dopamine to be a neurotransmitter, as well as a precursor for norepinephrine and epinephrine. With the development of fluorescent histochemistry for identifying catecholamine-containing structures, immunohistochemical methods for localizing catecholamine biosynthetic enzymes, and various retrograde and anterograde tracing techniques, it has become possible to identify dopamine-containing neurons and trace their projections throughout the central nervous system (see text by Cooper *et al.*[2]). Such anatomical studies have defined brain dopaminergic pathways, while complementary physiological, biochemical, and pharmacological studies have demonstrated functional differences among the dopaminergic pathways.

Neurotoxins that selectively destroy catecholamine-containing neurons have provided useful tools for evaluating the roles attributed to these neurons. Recently, it was discovered that 1-methyl-4-phenyl-1,2,3,6-tetrahydropyridine (MPTP) causes destruction of selected dopaminergic neurons. Although MPTP was commercially available and used in industry as a chemical intermediate, its toxic properties were not appreciated until it was recognized that MPTP was responsible for the rapid development of a severe Parkinsonism syndrome after its self-administration by drug abusers.[3,4] The compound was a contaminant of an illicitly produced analogue of meperidine, 1-methy-4-phenyl-4-propionoxypiperidine (MPPP) formed as the result of dehydration (instead of proprionylation) of the precursor of this compound (FIG. 1). Systemic administration to primates [5-7] of MPTP is followed almost immediately by acute transient symptoms that have little relationship to the chronic Parkinsonian syndrome that develops subsequently, over the course of 7–14 days. These observations elicited wide interest in MPTP-toxicity as a means for producing an animal model of Parkinson's disease[5-7] and as a clue to mechanisms that might be involved in the pathogenesis of the spontaneously occurring movement disorder. Behavioral and biochemical effects, as well as the disposition and metabolism, of MPTP have been examined in a wide variety of species, *in vivo* and *in vitro*. It is the purpose of this review to summarize briefly current knowledge about MPTP toxicity and to describe the impact this discovery has had on the directions of research on brain dopaminergic systems.

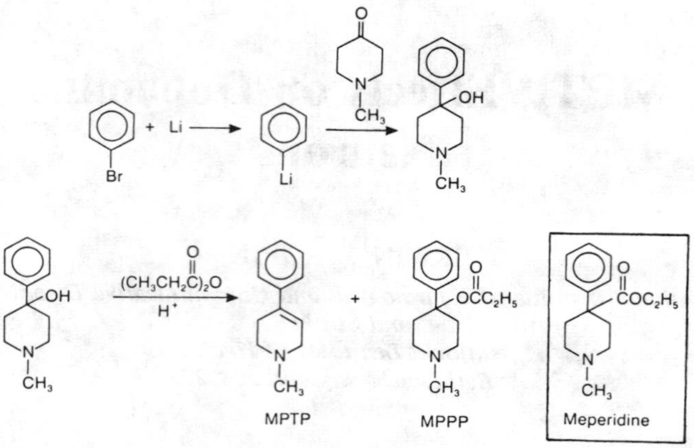

**FIGURE 1.** Formation of 1-methyl-4-phenyl-1,2,3,6-tetrahydropyridine (MPTP) as a side reaction product of the illicit synthesis used to produce the Meperidine analogue 1-methyl-4-phenyl-4-propionoxypyridine (MPPP). The structure of meperidine is shown in the rectangle.

## Acute Behavioral and Biochemical Effects of MPTP

In almost all species in which the effects of MPTP have been examined, the drug produces acute transient behavioral changes. The effects were first observed in rats soon after MPTP was first encountered.[3] Within seconds after intravenous administration of 10–20 mg/kg MPTP, there appear patterns of behavior reminiscent of the "serotonin-syndrome" characterized by hunched posture, splayed hind limbs, erect (Straub) tail, profuse salivation, piloerection, proptosis, and retropulsion with clonic movements of the forelegs.[8,9] This syndrome can be prevented or reversed by administration of a serotonin antagonist, methysergide; marked hyperactivity replaces the "serotonin syndrome." In guinea pigs, a similar syndrome is produced after subcutaneous administration of MPTP, but head jerks are more prominent and the effects last for 4 to 6 hours. In these species MPTP may have some slight effects on motor activity beyond the first day, but they generally show little if any signs of motor impairment. Large repeated doses of MPTP (up to 50 mg/kg) have been used in mice to produce partial destruction of brain dopaminergic neurones; these doses produce transient immobility but no striking differences in motor behavior after recovery from the initial effects. In monkeys, the acute effects of doses (0.2–0.6 mg/kg) of MPTP that have chronic toxic effects are initially relatively mild, but higher doses required in some primate species cause acute tremors, postural changes (including erect tail), and rotary eye movement.

Humans who have taken MPTP report a burning sensation at the injection site, a metallic or medicinal taste, blurred or dimmed vision, and occasionally hallucinations.[3,10] The acute effects are soon dissipated, but if the dose is sufficiently large or if several doses are administered, in some species, a Parkinsonian movement disorder develops (see below).

## Biochemical Effects

The acute biochemical changes attending MPTP-induced behavioral responses are consistent with release of peripheral catecholamines and initial central activation followed by inhibition of amine formation and metabolism in the brain. Plasma levels of norepinephrine and epinephrine are increased in rats;[8] cardiac and mesenteric artery norepinephrine levels are decreased in rats and mice.[11]

During the acute phase, alterations in biogenic amines and their metabolites in the rat and mouse brain appear to reflect diminished serotonin and dopamine metabolism. Levels of serotonin in the raphe nucleus and hypothalamus are increased and the deaminated metabolites of both dopamine and serotonin are decreased 15 min after MPTP administration. This could be due to diminished amine release by a direct action of MPTP[12] or it might reflect inhibition of monoamine oxidase.[13-15] Norepinephrine release, however, appears to be enhanced in both brain and at peripheral sympathetic nerve endings. Brain 3-methoxy-4-hydroxyphenylethylene glycol (MHPG) levels increase while norepinephrine levels decline.[16]

In rhesus monkeys, the ventricular cerebrospinal fluid (CSF) levels of homovanillic acid (HVA), 5-hydroxyindoleacetic acid (5-HIAA), and MHPG decline during the first day after MPTP administration and remain low for several weeks.[5] The acute, transient syndromes due to MPTP are clearly different from the chronic toxic effects that appear to occur in only some species and seem to be far more specific in targeting specific neurones for destruction (see below).

## Manifestations of Chronic MPTP Toxicity

While the acute effects of MPTP are similar among a wide variety of species, there are striking differences in manifestations and vulnerability to chronic toxic effects. In primates, including rhesus,[5] squirrel monkeys,[6] and marmosets,[7] there develops over a period ranging from 3 days to 3 weeks, increasingly severe bradykinesia, stooped posture, rigidity, episodes of "freezing," and some tremor. The degree of motor impairment that finally develops may vary from minimal symptoms to severe Parkinsonism. This variability in severity of the persistent motor effects may be related to the observation that over 80% of the dopaminergic neurons must be destroyed to elicit significant behavioral deficits. Vulnerability also appears to increase with age and females are more susceptible than males.

## Chronic Biochemical Effects of MPTP Toxicity

The biochemical effects observed are consistent with destruction of the nigro-striatal dopamine neurones. Whereas CSF levels of 5-HIAA and MHPG return almost to normal, levels of HVA remain low.[5] Attempts to produce a permanent Parkinsonian model in rats[9] and guinea pigs,[9] have not met with success. High doses of MPTP may produce transient motor effects, but biochemical and histological evidence for damage sufficiently extensive to result in a persistent Parkinsonian syndrome have not been obtained.

Mice, however, do appear to be affected,[17-20] and in some strains relatively low doses of MPTP (20 mg/kg) have produced marked decreases in brain dopamine that persists for long periods, but there appear to be relatively wide differences among strains in sensitivity to MPTP. In this species, however, the lesions are not confined to the nigro-striatal system. Dopamine levels in the nucleus accumbens (N. Acc.)[21] and norepinephrine levels in the striatum and frontal cortex are depressed.[18] There is, however, a gradual return, over months, of brain catecholamine levels in brain areas of mice.[19]

## Pathological Changes in MPTP-Treated Animals

The ages, treatment schedules, times after MPTP administration, and species of primate used all appear to influence the pathological findings obtained in brain catecholaminergic neurons. The dopaminergic neurons projecting to the striatum are consistently affected, but the extent of involvement and the degree of symptomatic improvement vary widely. In some primate species the locus coeruleus is almost always affected, whereas in others it appears to be spared.

In the only human known to have died after developing MPTP-induced Parkinsonism[3] there was extensive destruction of neurons in the substantia nigra, neuromelanin pigment was found in the extracellular spaces, and a single intracytoplasmic eosinophilic inclusion, similar to a Lewy body, was noted. The cells of the locus coeruleus appeared intact. In rhesus monkeys made Parkinsonism by repeated intravenous injections of MPTP, there was almost complete depletion of dopamine neurons in the substantia nigra pars compacta[21] with a marked decrease in the number of surviving neurons two months after MPTP treatment. There was a marked increase in the number of swollen catecholamine-fluorescent axons in the area above the substantia nigra compacta that projected toward the putamen via the globus pallidus. The dopaminergic terminal fibers in the striatum were almost completely absent up to 4 months after MPTP, but some preterminal axons appear to have persisted. The cells of the A10 area and their projections (including the fine terminals and varicosities) in the accumbens and olfactory tubercle appeared to be spared from any damage. In these rhesus monkeys the locus coeruleus appeared to have also been spared.

Forno et al.[22] reported that in squirrel monkeys treated with MPTP, the most severely damaged area is the medial portion of the substantia nigra with apparent sparing of the ventral tegmental area (A10). They found that five of six of these animals also had severe focal lesions in the locus coeruleus. Eosinophilic inclusions were also found, particularly in older animals. Mitchell et al.[23] found that in cynamologus monkeys MPTP also produces damage to the locus coeruleus; they found some damage to dopaminergic neurones in the ventral tegmental area, as well as severe damage to the substantia nigra. In this species, dopamine was depleted in the N. Acc. to the same extent as in the caudate and putamen. The pattern of neuronal damage in vervet monkeys also appears to be somewhat different than in other species. MPTP appeared to damage selectively the dopaminergic neurones of the A8 area[24] and the medial but not lateral region of the substantia nigra.[25] The central area of the substantia nigra was involved only in one severely Parkinsonian animal. In all treated animals, dopamine levels were markedly lowered in all areas of the striatum.

In the marmoset, as in other primates, MPTP causes a Parkinsonian syndrome[7] with depletion of dopamine in the caudate putamen and degeneration of neurones in the substantia nigra.[26] In addition there is, however, gliosis in the hypothalamus, suggesting that dopaminergic neurones of the A11–A14 areas may be affected.

Differences in regional specificity of MPTP toxicity have also been noted in strains of mice. Sundstrom et al.[27] compared four strains of mice: C57 BL/6, NMRI, CBA/Ca, and Swiss-Webster. After two doses (50 mg/kg, sc) of MPTP given 16 hr apart, and 7 days later, there was usually marked depletion of striatal dopamine: $-96\%$ in the C57 BL/6, $-92\%$ in the NMRI, and $-86\%$ in the CBA/Ca, but even after 10 doses of MPTP given daily for 10 days in Swiss-Webster mice, striatal dopamine was only $-74\%$. In all strains examined, the effects on mesencephalic dopamine were similar ($-36\%$ in CBA, $-45\%$ in NMRI, and $-52\%$ in C57 BL/6), but the effects on frontal cortex norepinephrine levels differed greatly, ranging from no significant depletion in C57 BL/6 to $-8\%$ in NMRI and $-61\%$ in CBA/Ca. Differences in vulnerability among Swiss-Webster mice obtained from different sources have also been reported.[29]

## MECHANISMS OF MPTP NEUROTOXICITY

Understanding the basis for differences in species vulnerability and tissue specificity of MPTP requires knowledge of the mechanisms that contribute to the neurotoxicity of MPTP. FIGURE 2 is a schematic representation of the factors that have been implicated in determining the effects of MPTP on neuronal survival. MPTP is a lipid soluble compound that easily penetrates membranes, including the blood–brain barrier. Markey et al.[32] showed that MPTP is rapidly metabolized to its quaternary amine derivative, 1-methyl-4-phenylpyridine (MPP+). This was a previously known plant toxin called cyperquat. The conversion of MPTP to MPP+ was first demonstrated in vitro in homogenates of rat[30] or monkey[29] brain, but has been subsequently shown to occur in many tissues. Because the oxidation of MPTP to MPP+ is mediated by a mitochondrial enzyme and is inhibited by drugs that block monoamine oxidase type B (MAO-B), but not those that block only MAO type A (MAO-A), it was concluded that MAO-B was the responsible enzyme.[30] The oxidation appears to occur in two steps, as shown in FIGURE 3, with 1-methyl-4-phenyl-3,4-dihydropyridine (MPDP+) as an intermediate. MPDP+ spontaneously dismutates to form MPTP and MPP+ or may be oxidized by

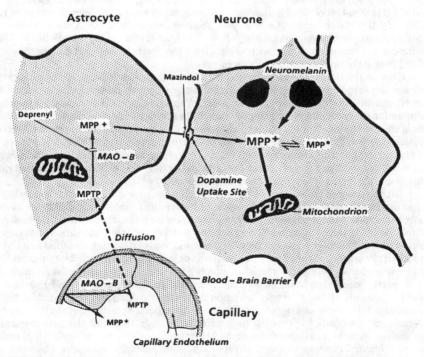

**FIGURE 2.** Schematic representation of the processes involved in targetting MPTP toxicity to dopaminergic neurones (see text).

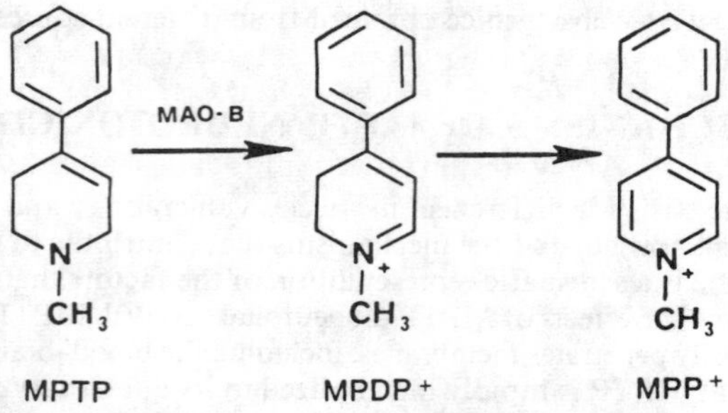

**FIGURE 3.** MPP⁺ (cyperquat) is formed by the MAO-B-mediated oxidation of MPTP to MPDP⁺. MPDP⁺ can auto-oxidize to MPP⁺, but MAO-B may accelerate this reaction.

MAO-B. Since blockade of MAO-B both prevents formation of MPP⁺ and blocks MPTP toxicity,[31,32] MPP⁺ is regarded as the active toxin. MPP⁺ was readily demonstrated to be toxic *in vitro*, after intravenous injection, or after local injection directly into the brain. In some species, however, MPP⁺ formation has been suggested to be protective. MPP⁺ does not easily penetrate the blood–brain barrier, so that its formation from MPTP in brain microvessels might prevent the precursor from entering the brain. Thus, MAO-B in small blood vessels and capillaries may act as an enzymatic barrier to penetration of MPTP into brain. Harik *et al.*[33] showed that in rats, which are resistant to MPTP, brain microvessels contain high levels of MAO-B and rapidly metabolize MPTP, whereas in humans the brain microvessels have low levels of MAO-B and metabolize MPTP at only one thirtieth the rate in rats.

Once in the brain, MPTP is available to MAO-B, which is localized in astrocytes or serotoninergic neurones.[34] MPP⁺ formed in astrocytes (or other MAO-B-containing cells) can slowly diffuse into the surrounding fluids. Since MPP⁺ is a substrate for dopamine and norepinephrine uptake sites,[35] these neurones and their axon terminals concentrate the toxin. Inhibition of dopamine uptake mechanisms prevents MPTP toxicity in mice,[36–38] and when given over a prolonged interval after MPTP, in monkeys.[39] This may explain the pattern of MPTP toxicity in mice in which noradrenergic as well as monkey dopaminergic neurones are targets, but does not explain the specificity of the toxin for nigro-striatal neurones in primates.

The occurrence of neuromelanin in the neurones of species (primates and dogs) that are most vulnerable to MPTP has led to attempts to relate neuromelanin to the mechanism of MPTP toxicity. Neuromelanin is a complex redox polymer resulting from the oxidation of dopamine (or other catechols) to quinones and subsequent deposition on lipofuscin. It accumulates with increasing age and is often regarded as a waste product. Possibly neuromelanin accumulates only in neurones with marginal ability to survive a toxic insult and is therefore merely a marker of vulnerability. Neuromelanin may participate in the toxic mechanism if its free radicals react with MPP⁺ to yield MPP˙ free radical, but attempts to demonstrate redox cycling and free radical formation from MPP⁺ have not suggested that this is an important mechanism in its toxicity. Neuromelanin binds MPP⁺ with high affinity,[40] suggesting that the neuromelanin granules may serve as a depot from which MPP⁺ can be maintained at toxic cytoplasmic levels. This view has been supported by the demonstration that chloroquin, which blocks MPP⁺ binding to neuromelanin, diminishes MPTP toxicity in monkeys.[41]

The accumulation of MPP⁺ by mitochondria and the consequent blockade of respiratory enzymes at complex I have been strongly implicated as the basis of the toxicity of MPTP (see reviews by Trevor *et al.*[42] and Nicklas *et al.*[43]).

The variability of the factors that influence the concentrations of $MPP^+$ in target cells and the considerable differences among potential target cells in their resistance to irreversible damage by $MPP^+$ to vital processes probably accounts for the variation in species and regional vulnerability to MPTP.

Since intravenously administered MPTP has a relatively short half-life and is converted to $MPP^+$, which does not readily penetrate the blood–brain barrier, it is possible by internal carotid artery infusion to expose one half of the brain to much higher concentrations of MPTP than becomes available to the contralateral side. Using this technique, monkeys have been made hemi-Parkinsonian.[44] Bradykinesia, flexed posture, dystonic movements, tremor, and cogwheel rigidity appear in the contralateral limbs. Spontaneous activity is attended by circling toward the chemically lesioned side. The motor abnormalities are reversed by treatment with L-DOPA/carbidopa and the direction of spontaneous rotation is reversed. Treatment with apomorphine, a dopamine agonist, produces prompt (within 5 min) reversal of the motor defect and dose-related circling away from the MPTP-treated side. This provides a useful method to assess efficacy of anti-Parkinsonian drugs. The biochemical changes on the MPTP-treated side are consistent with almost complete destruction of the neurones found on histological examination of the substantia nigra. Dopamine and tyrosine hydroxylase are markedly depleted from the caudate and putamen of the injected side, but are normal on the contralateral side. Dopamine uptake sites labeled with $^3H$-mazindole are virtually absent on the treated side, but there are increases in $D_2$ receptors as revealed by $^3H$-spiroperidol binding,[45] consistent with the motor effects of apomorphine previously described.

The pattern of alterations in brain glucose utilization as quantified by 2-14C-deoxyglucose autoradiography is a useful means of assessing metabolic alterations that occur at different stages after administration of MPTP and reflect the initial responses to MPTP-induced amine release as well as effects secondary to MPTP-induced destruction of dopaminergic neurones in the nigrostriatal pathway.

During the acute actions of MPTP (10–30 min after its intravenous injection, Palombo *et al.*[46] found that glucose utilization is decreased throughout the cerebral cortex and thalamus (by about 30–40%), with somewhat smaller decreases in the caudate–putamen (about 20%). The most striking changes are the *increases* in glucose utilization in the substantia nigra compacta (80% above control), the adjacent pigmented nuclei in the ventral tegmental area, and the ventral lamina of the inferior olive (+50%). Schwartzman and Alexander[47] examined glucose utilization in monkeys after several days of repeated treatment with MPTP when Parkinsonian features had developed. Decreases in glucose utilization appeared in the cerebral cortex and caudate–putamen, but increases were found in the globus palladus and both the pars compacta and pars reticulata of the substantia nigra. Mitchell *et al.*,[48] found increased glucose utilization in the globus pallidus, but not in the substantia nigra reticulata, at about 3 weeks. These observations appear to have reflected both acute and chronic effects of MPTP, since 3–5 months after MPTP-induced Parkinsonism, Porrino *et al.*[49] found reductions in glucose utilizations in the substantia nigra compacta, subthalamic nucleus, ventral tegmental area, and caudate–putamen. Decreases in metabolism in the frontal eye fields and medial dorsal nucleus of the thalamus were also evident. Only in the external segment of the globus pallidus was there an increase in glucose utilization. In these animals, the effects of L-DOPA were striking. Whereas L-DOPA has little effect on glucose utilization in normal animals, in doses that restore to normal the motor activity of MPTP–Parkinsonian animals, L-DOPA produces increases in cerebral metabolism in both areas rich in dopaminergic receptors (e. g., caudate–putamen) and nondopaminergic areas involved in motor function.[51] The rates of glucose utilization seen after L-DOPA far exceeded the normal rates in the affected regions. This is consistent with the increase in dopamine receptors previously described.

In addition to involvement of the dopaminergic neurones of the substantia nigra in monkeys, MPTP appears to produce changes in retinal function. Ghilardi *et al.*[51] showed that MPTP-treated Parkinsonian monkeys developed DOPA-reversible abnormalities in pattern electroretinogram and visually evoked potentials recorded as long as one year after treatment. Animals made hemi-Parkinsonian by infusion of MPTP into a carotid artery to treat the brain hemisphere with the drug, also have had the ipsilateral eye exposed to high levels of MPTP. In such monkeys alternating areas with high and low glucose utilization are found in brain of the occipital cortex in areas representing binocularly consistent with ocular dominance columns, but not in monocularly innervated cortical regions. The monocularly innervated areas contralateral to the infused side have low metabolic rates; L-DOPA induces marked increases in glucose uptake in hypometabolic columns, and thereby enhances the columnar differences in metabolic rate.[52] Thus the MPTP–Parkinsonian monkey is useful for demonstrating the alterations in cerebral metabolism (and presumably neuronal activity) that occur when dopaminergic neuronal activity of the nigrostriatal pathway is abolished. The availability of animal models in which dopaminergic neurones are selectively damaged has not only provided new information about the role of these neurones in visual and motor function, but has furnished a means for evaluating drug therapies and exploring neuronal tissue implants as means of reversing Parkinsonian deficits. Understanding mechanisms responsible for vulnerability of these specific neurones is hoped to provide insights regarding approaches to prevent or alleviate the progressive degenerative process that destroys these and other neurons. Thus, the tragic exposure of young drug addicts to a toxic contaminant of an illicit narcotic has resulted in a revitalization of research in Parkinson's disease.

## REFERENCES

1. CARLSSON, A. 1959. The occurrence, distribution, and physiological role of catecholamines in the nervous system. Pharm. Rev. 11: 490–493.
2. COOPER, J. R., F. E. BLOOM & R. H. ROTH. 1986. The Biochemical Basis of Neuropharmacology, 5th ed. Oxford Univ. Press. New York/ London.
3. DAVIS, G. C., A. C. WILLIAMS, S. P. MARKEY, M. H. EBERT, E. D. CAINE, C. M. REICHERT & I. J. KOPIN. 1979. Chronic Parkinsonism secondary to intravenous injection of meperidine analogues. Psychiatry Res. 1: 249–254.
4. LANGSTON, J. W., P. BALLARD, J. W. TETRUD & I. IRWIN. 1983. Chronic Parkinsonism in humans due to a product of meperidine-analog synthesis. Science 219: 979–980.
5. BURNS, R. S., C. C. CHIUEH, S. P. MARKEY, M. H. EBERT, D. M. JACOBOWITZ & I. J. KOPIN. 1983. A primate model of Parkinsonism: Selective destruction of dopaminergic neurons in the pars compacta of the substantia nigra by N-methyl-4-phenyl-1,2,3,6-tetrahydropyridine. Proc. Natl. Acad. Sci. U.S.A. 80: 4546–4550.
6. LANGSTON, J. W., L. S. FORNO, C. S. ROBERT & I. IRWIN. 1984. Selective nigral toxicity after systemic administration of 1-methyl-4phenyl-1,2,3,6-tetrahydropyridine (MPTP) in the squirrel monkey. Brain Res. 292: 390–394.
7. JENNER, P., N. M. RUPNIAK, S. ROSE, E. KELLY, G. KILPATRICK, A. LEES & C. D. MARSDEN. 1984. 1-methyl-4-phenyl-1,2,3,6-tetrahydropyridine-induced Parkinsonism in the common marmoset. Neurosci. Lett. 50: 85–90.
8. CHIUEH, C. C., S. P. MARKEY, R. S. BURNS, J. N. JOHANNESSEN, A. PERT & I. J. KOPIN. 1984. Neurochemical and behavioral effects of systemic and intranigral administration of N-methyl-4phenyl-1,2,3,6-tetrahydropyridine in the rat. Eur. J. Pharmacol. 100: 189–194.

9. CHIUEH, C. C., S. P. MARKEY, R. S. BURNS, J. N. JOHANNESSEN, D. M. JACOBOWITZ & I. J. KOPIN. 1984. Neurochemical and behavioral effects of in rat, guinea pig, and monkey. Psychopharmacol. Bull. **20**: 548–553.

10. BALLARD, P. A., J. W. TETRUD & J. W. LANGSTON. 1985. Permanent human parkinsonism due to 1-methyl-4 phenyl-1,2,3,6-tetrahydropyridine (MPTP): Seven cases. Neurology **35**: 949–956.

11. FULLER, R. W., R. A. HAHN, H. D. SNODDY & J. H. WIKEL. 1984. Depletion of cardiac norepinephrine in rats and mice by 1-methyl-4-phenyl-1,2,3,6-tetrahydropyridine (MPTP). Biochem. Pharmacol. **33**: 2957–2960.

12. SCHMIDT, C. J., L. A. MATSUDA & J. W. GIBB. 1984. *In vitro* release of tritiated monoamines from rat CNS tissue by the neurotoxic compound 1-methyl-1-phenyl-tetrahydropyridine. Eur. J. Pharmacol. **103**: 255–260.

13. SALACH, J. I., T. P. SINGER, N. CASTAGNOLI, JR. & A. TREVOR. 1984. Oxidation of the neurotoxic amine by monoamine oxidases A and B and suicide inactivation of the enzymes by MPTP. Biochem. Biophys. Res. Commun. **125**: 831–835.

14. FULLER, R.W. & S. K. HEMRICK-LEUCKE. 1985. Inhibition of types A and B monoamine oxidase by 1-methyl-4-phenyl-1,2,3,6-tetrahydropyridine. J. Pharmacol. Exp. Ther. **232**: 696–701.

15. MELAMED, E., M. B. YOUDIM, J. ROSENTHAL, I. SPANIER, A. UZZAN & M. GLOBUS. 1985. *In vivo* effect of MPTP on monoamine oxidase activity in mouse striatum. Brain. Res. **359**: 360–363.

16. ENZ, A., F. HEFTI & W. FRICK. 1984. Acute administration of 1-methyl-4 phenyl-1,2,3,6-tetrahydropyridine (MPTP) reduces dopamine and serotonin but accelerates norepinephrine metabolism in the rat brain. Effect of chronic pretreatment with MPTP. Eur. J. Pharmacol. **101**: 37–44.

17. HALLMAN, H., J. LANGE, L. OLSON, I. STRÖMBERG & G. JONSSON. 1985. Neurochemical and histochemical characterization of neurotoxic effects of 1-methyl-4-phenyl-1,2,3,6-tetrahydropyridine on brain catecholamine neurones in the mouse. J. Neurochem. **44**: 310–313.

18. HEIKKILA, R. E., A. HESS & R. C. DUVOISIN. 1984. Dopaminergic neurotoxicity of 1-methyl-4-phenyl-1,2,3,6-tetrahydropyridine in mice. Science **224**: 1451–1453.

19. HALLMAN, H., L. OLSON & G. JONSSON. 1984. Neurotoxicity of the meperidine analogue N-methyl-4-phenyl-1,2,3,6-tetrahydropyridine on brain catecholamine neurones in the mouse. Eur. J. Pharmacol. **97**: 133–136.

20. MELAMED, E., J. ROSENTHAL, M. GLOBUS, O. COHEN, Y. FRUCHT & A. UZZAN. 1985. Mesolimbic dopaminergic neurons are not spared by MPTP neurotoxicity in mice. Eur. J. Pharmacol. **114**: 97–100.

21. JACOBOWITZ, D. M., R. S. BURNS, C. C. CHIUEH & I. J. KOPIN. 1984. N-methyl-4-phenyl-1,2,3,6-tetrahydropyridine causes destruction of the nigrostriatal but not the mesolimbic dopamine system in the monkey. Psychopharmacol. Bull. **20**: 416–422.

22. FORNO, L. S., J. W. LANGSTON, L. E. DELANNEY, B. S. IRWIN & G. A. RICUARTE. 1986. Locus coeruleus lesions and eosinophilic inclusion in MPTP-treated monkeys. Ann. Neurol. **20**: 449–455.

23. MITCHELL, I. J., A. J. CROSS, M. A. SAMBROOK & A. R. CROSSMAN. 1985. Sites of the neurotoxic action of 1-methyl-4-phenyl-1,2,3,6-tetrahydropyridine in the macaque monkey include the ventral tegmental area and the locus coeruleus. Neurosci. Lett. **61**: 121–126.

24. DEUTCH, A. Y., J. D. ELSWORTH, M. GOLDSTEIN, K. FUXE, D. E. REDMOND, JR., J. R. SLADEK, JR. & R. H. ROTH. 1986. Preferential vulnerability of A8 dopamine neurons in the primate to the neurotoxin 1-methyl-4phenyl-1,2,3,6-tetrahydropyridine. Neurosci. Lett. **68**: 51–56.

25. ELSWORTH, J. D., A. Y. DEUTCH, D. E. REDMOND, JR., J. R. SLADEK, JR. & R. N. ROTH. 1987. Differential responsiveness to 1-methyl-4 phenyl-1,2,3,6-tetrahydropyridine toxicity in subregions of the primate substantia nigra and striatum. Life Sci. **40**: 193–202.

26. GIBB, W. R., A. J. LEES, P. JENNER & C. D. MARSDEN. 1986. The dopamine neurotoxin 1-methyl-4-phenyl-1,2,3,6-tetrahydropyridine (MPTP) produces histological lesions in the hypothalamus of the common marmoset. Neurosci. Lett. **65**: 79–83.

27. SUNDSTROM, E., I. STRÖMBERG, T. TSUTSUMI, L. OLSON & G. JONSSON. 1987. Studies of

the effect of 1-methyl-4 phenyl-1,2,3,6-tetrahydropyridine (MPTP) on central catechol-amine neurons in C57 BL/6 mice. Comparison with three other strains of mice.

28. HEIKKILA, R. E. 1985. Differential neurotoxicity of 1-methyl-4 phenyl-1,2,3,6-tetrahydro-pyridine (MPTP) in Swiss-Webster mice from different sources. Eur. J. Pharmacol. **117**: 131–133.

29. MARKEY, S. P., J. N. JOHANNESSEN, C. C. CHIUEH, R. S. BURNS & M. A. HERKENHAM. 1984. Intraneuronal generation of a pyridinium metabolite may cause drug-induced Par-kinsonism. Nature **311**: 464–467.

30. CHIBA, K., A. TREVOR & N. CASTAGNOLI, JR. 1984. Metabolism of the neurotoxic tertiary amine, MPTP, by brain monoamine oxidase. Biochem. Biophys. Res. Commun. **120**: 574–578.

31. LANGSTON, J. W., I. IRWIN, E. B. LANGSTON & L. S. FORNO. 1984. Pargyline prevents MPTP-induced parkinsonism in primates. Science. **225**: 1480–1482.

32. HEIKKILA, R. E., L. MANZINO, F. S. CABBAT & R. C. DUVOISIN. 1984. Protection against the dopaminergic neurotoxicity of 1-methyl-4-phenyl-1,2,3,6-tetrahydropyridine by mono-amine oxidase inhibitors. Nature **311**: 467–469.

33. HARIK, S. I., M. I. MITCHELL & R. N. KALARIA. Human susceptibility and rat resistance to systemic 1-methyl-4-phenyl-1,2,3,6-tetrahydropyridine (MPTP) neurotoxicity correlate with blood brain barrier monoamine oxidase B activity. Neurology **37**: 338–339.

34. WESTLUND, K. N., R. M. DENNEY, L. M. KOCHERSPERGER, R. M. ROSE & C. W. ABELL. 1985. Distinct monoamine oxidase A and B populations in primate brain. Science **230**: 181–183.

35. JAVITCH, J.A. & S. H. SNYDER. 1984. Uptake of MPP(+) by dopamine neurons explains selectivity of Parkinsonism-inducing neurotoxin, MPTP. Eur. J. Pharmacol. **106**: 455–456.

36. SUNDSTROM, E. & G. JONSSON. 1985. Pharmacological interference with the neurotoxic ac-tion of 1-methyl-4 phenyl-1,2,3,6-tetrahydropyridine (MPTP) on central catecholamine neurons in the mouse. Eur. J. Pharmacol. **110**: 293–299.

37. PILEBLAD, E. & A. CARLSSON. 1985. Catecholamine-uptake inhibitors prevent the neurotoxicity of 1-methyl-4 phenyl-1,2,3,6-tetrahydropyridine (MPTP) in mouse brain. Neuropharma-cology **24**: 689–692.

38. RICAURTE, G. A., J. W. LANGSTON, L. E. DELANNEY, I. IRWIN & J. D. BROOKS. 1985. Dopamine uptake blockers protect against the dopamine depleting effect of 1-methyl-4-phenyl-1,2,3,6-tetrahydropyridine (MPTP) in the mouse striatum. **59**: 259–264.

39. SCHULTZ, W., E. SCARNATI, E. SUNDSTROM, T. TSUTSUMI & G. JONSSON. 1986. The cate-cholamine uptake blocker nomifensine protects against MPTP-induced parkinsonism in monkeys. Exp. Brain Res. **53**: 216–220.

40. D'AMATO, R. J., Z. P. LIPMAN & S. H. SNYDER. 1986. Selectivity of the Parkinsonian neu-rotoxin MPTP: Toxic metabolite MPP$^+$ binds to neuromelanin. Science **231**: 987–989.

41. D'AMATO, R. J., G. M. ALEXANDER, R. J. SCHWARTZMAN, C. A. KITT, D. L. PRICE & S. H. SNYDER. 1987. Neuromelanin: A role in MPTP-induced neurotoxicity. Life Sci. **40**: 705–712.

42. TREVOR, A. J., N. CASTAGNOLI, JR., P. CALDERA, R. R. RAMSAY & T. P. SINGER. 1987. Bioactivation of MPTP: Reactive metabolites and possible biochemical sequelae. Life Sci. **40**: 713–719.

43. NICKLAS, W. J., S. K. YOUNGSTER, M. V. KINDT & R. E. HEIKKILA. 1987. MPTP, MPP$^+$ and mitochondrial function. Life Sci. **40**: 721–729.

44. BANKIEWICZ, K. S., E. H. OLDFIELD, C. C. CHIUEH, J. L. DOPPMAN, D. M. JACOBOWITZ & I. J. KOPIN. 1986. Hemiparkinsonism in monkeys after unilateral internal carotid ar-tery infusion of 1-methyl-4-phenyl-1,2,3,6-tetrahydropyridine (MPTP). Life Sci. **39**: 7–16.

45. JOYCE, J. N., J. F. MARSHALL, K. S. BANKIEWICZ, I. J. KOPIN & D. M. JACOBOWITZ. 1986. Hemiparkinsonism in a monkey after unilateral internal carotid artery infusion of 1-methyl-4-phenyl-1,2,3,6-tetrahydropyridine (MPTP) is associated with regional ipsilateral changes in striatal dopamine D-2 receptor density. Brain Res. **382**: 360–364.

46. PALOMBO, E., L. J. PORRINO, V. W. HO, A. M. CRANE, I. J. KOPIN & L. SOKOLOFF. 1987. Acute administration of MPTP increases local cerebral glucose utilization in the sub-stantia nigra of primates. Brain Res. In press.

47. SCHWARTZMAN, R. J. & G. M. ALEXANDER. 1985. Changes in the local cerebral metabolic

rate for glucose in the 1-methyl-4-phenyl-1,2,3,6-tetrahydropyridine (MPTP) primate model of Parkinson's disease. Brain Res. **358:** 137–143.

48. MITCHELL, I. J., A. J. CROSS, M. A. SAMBROOK & A. R. CROSSMAN. 1986. Neural mechanisms mediating 1-methyl-4-phenyl-1,2,3,6-tetrahydropyridine-induced Parkinsonism in the monkey: Relative contributions of the striatopalladal and striatonigral pathways as suggested by 2-doexyglucose uptake. Neurosci. Lett. **63:** 61–65.

49. PORRINO, L. J., R. S. BURNS, A. M. CRANE, E. PALOMBO, I. J. KOPIN & L. SOKOLOFF. 1987. Changes in local cerebral glucose utilization associated with Parkinson's syndrome induced by 1-methyl-4-phenyl-1,2,3,6-tetrahydropyridine (MPTP) in the primate. Life Sci. **40:** 1657–1664.

50. PORRINO, L. J., R. S. BURNS, A. M. CRANE, E. PALOMBO, I. J. KOPIN & L. SOKOLOFF. 1987. Local cerebral metabolic effects of L-Dopa to MPTP-induced Parkinsonism in monkeys. Proc. Natl. Acad. Sci. U.S.A. In press.

51. GHILARDI, M. F., I. BODIS-WOLLNER, E. CHUNG, M. ONOFRI & A. GLOVER. 1987. Visual electrophysiologic abnormalities correlate with the evolution of Parkinsonian signs (PS) in MPTP-treated monkeys. Neurology **37.**

52. PORRINO, L. J., V. W. HO, E. PALOMBO, C. KENNEDY, N. T. KUWABARA, D. G. COGAN, K. S. BANKIEWICZ & I. J. KOPIN. 1987. Columnar organization of metabolic activity in the striate cortex of hemiparkinsonian monkeys. Neurology **37.**

# The Roles of Glucocorticoid and Dopaminergic Systems in Delusional (Psychotic) Depression[a]

ALAN F. SCHATZBERG AND
ANTHONY J. ROTHSCHILD

*Affective Disease Program*
*Depression Research Facility*
*McLean Hospital*
*Belmont, Massachusetts 02178*

*Department of Psychiatry*
*Harvard Medical School*
*Boston, Massachusetts 02115*

## INTRODUCTION

Over the past five years, considerable attention has been paid to the study of hypothalamic–pituitary–adrenal (HPA) axis physiology in various psychiatric disorders, particularly depression. For many years, one major strategy has been the application of the Dexamethasone Suppression Test (DST) to diagnose depressed patients. In more recent years, several groups have explored the direct roles that corticotropin-releasing factor (CRF), adrenocorticotropin hormone (ACTH), and cortisol may play in the possible expression of mood disorders. For example, CRF infusions have been reported to induce stresslike reactions in rats[1] and anorexia and withdrawal in monkeys.[2] CRF levels in cerebrospinal fluid (CSF) have been reported to be elevated in some studies of severe depression,[3] and ACTH responses to CRF infusions are blunted in some depressed patients,[4] suggesting that increased CRF activity may play a key role in the development of depressive symptoms. Our group has explored whether cortisol's effects on dopaminergic systems could play a key role in the development of delusions in depressed patients. This approach is described in detail in this paper.

## DELUSIONAL (PSYCHOTIC) DEPRESSION

In recent years, numerous studies continue to point to delusional (psychotic) depression as being a distinct biological subtype with unique characteristics on a number of important dimensions in addition to symptom morphology: Morbidity and mortality, familial risk, treatment response, and biological characteristics.

One–two-year morbidity is higher in delusional depressives than in their nondelu-

[a] This work was supported in part by National Institutes of Mental Health Grant MH 38671 and a grant from the Poitras Charitable Foundation.

sional counterparts,[4,5] and the risk for death by suicide is some five times higher.[6] Follow-up studies on younger delusional depressives point to a linkage with bipolar disorder with relatively frequent bipolar outcomes in younger delusional patients.[7,8]

Recent family history data also suggest that delusional depression is linked to bipolar disorders. Patients with psychotic depression have an increased risk for bipolar disorder in their first-degree relatives,[9] and a recent study reported an increased risk of bipolar features in their children. In at least one of these studies, delusional depressives were mainly of the early onset subtype.[10] Delusional depressives also demonstrate significantly higher familial risk for depression than do nondelusional depressives,[11,12] and a higher risk for delusional depression in first-degree relatives.[11]

Treatment response studies further point to delusional depression being a distinct subtype of affective disorder. Psychotically depressed patients respond more favorably to electroconvulsive therapy (ECT) or combined tricyclic antidepressant–neuroleptic treatment than they do to tricyclic antidepressants (TCAs) alone.[13,14] The positive response to combined neuroleptic/TCA treatment suggests dopamine (DA) may play a role in delusional depression.

Delusionally depressed patients may be demarcated by a number of biological characteristics. Three recent studies[15-17] have reported psychotic depressives demonstrate elevated cerebrospinal fluid (CSF) levels of homovanillic acid (HVA) — a major metabolite of DA [and in some cases high levels of the serotonin metabolite, 5-hydroxyindoleacetic acid (5-HIAA) as well]. However, one recent small-scale study reported lower CSF HVA and 5-HIAA levels in delusionally depressed patients than in their nondelusional counterparts,[18] suggesting there may be two delusional subtypes. As elaborated on below, we have reported higher plasma-free DA levels in psychotic depressives than in their nondelusional counterparts or normal control subjects.[19]

Marked increases and disruptions in HPA axis activity have been reported in most, but not all, studies of this disorder.[20-25] For example, delusionally depressed patients demonstrate elevated urinary-free cortisol levels[20] and very high rates of DST nonsuppression.[21,22] Moreover, our group and others have reported that delusionally depressed patients also demonstrate markedly elevated postdexamethasone cortisol levels — for example, 4 p.m. postdexamethasone cortisol levels $\geq$10–15 µg/dl.[24,25] We have argued that high circulating cortisol levels increase dopamine activity both peripherally and centrally, leading to the development of delusions[26] (see below for further discussion). Other affective psychotic patients (i.e., psychotic manic patients) also demonstrate extremely elevated postdexamethasone cortisol levels.[25,27,28]

Studies by our group and others point to enlarged ventricle-to-brain ratios (VBRs) in psychotic depressives, and these could be related to elevated cortisol levels. Patients with Cushing's disease or those treated with glucocorticoids demonstrate enlarged ventricles that decrease in some patients over time with successful treatment or cessation of glucocorticoid administration.[29] UFC has been reported to correlate with VBRs in depressed patients,[30] and before us others had reported that psychotic depressives demonstrate higher VBRs than do nonpsychotic depressives.[31-33] Recently, we reported in a series of 22 unipolar depressed patients that VBRs were significantly higher in those patients with psychosis than in those without.[34] Moreover, the mean 4 p.m. postdexamethasone cortisol level in unipolar psychotic depressives was significantly higher than in unipolar nonpsychotic depressives; higher 4 p.m. predexamethasone cortisol levels were also observed in psychotic depressed patients (trend significance). We are currently pursuing follow-up studies to determine if enlarged ventricles in psychotic depressives are reversible with successful treatment.

In one recent sleep study, delusional depressives demonstrated shortened REM latency, decreased REM time, and poorer sleep efficiency when compared with nonpsychotic depressives or normal control subjects.[35] These differences were not due to age or agitation. Of interest, REM latency and REM time have been reported to be decreased by exposure to dexamethasone or to L-DOPA infusions,[35] suggesting increased cortisol and DA activity could underlie these sleep findings in delusionally depressed patients.

A number of studies have explored dopamine-β-hydroxylase (DBH) and platelet monoamine oxidase (MAO) activity. Unipolar psychotic depressives demonstrate lower DBH than do their unipolar nonpsychotic counterparts.[36,37] Meltzer and colleagues reported platelet MAO activity was higher in female psychotic than in female nonpsychotic depressed patients.[38] Recently, we reported significantly higher platelet MAO activity in a small group of delusional depressives than in a nondelusional, depressed comparison group.[39]

## CORTISOL AND DA

A number of observations point to glucocorticoids' increasing DA activity in man. Banki and colleagues reported that cerebrospinal fluid levels of homovanillic acid (HVA) were increased after dexamethasone administration.[40] Our group has reported that plasma-free dopamine levels in healthy controls were significantly increased after 1 mg of dexamethasone,[41] and Wolkowitz and colleagues have reported similar increases in plasma HVA levels.[42]

A number of studies in lower species point to glucocorticoids' increasing DA in various regions of the brain. For example, Markey and colleagues reported corticosterone increased DA concentrations in specific regions of the mouse brain.[43] Our group reported that in rats, acute intraperitoneal administration of dexamethasone results in significant increases in dopamine levels in the hypothalamus and nucleus accumbens; in contrast, 3,4-dihydroxyphenylacetic acid (DOPAC) was reduced in frontal, cortical regions.[44] Wolkowitz and colleagues reported that corticosterone administration significantly increased HVA concentrations in the rat caudate.[45]

Indirect evidence on glucocorticoids' effects on prolactin further suggest glucocorticoids may increase DA activity. Rats treated with dexamethasone demonstrate attenuated stress-induced increases in prolactin.[46,47] Patients treated with glucocorticoids or those with Cushing's disease show blunting of expected early a.m. rises in serum prolactin.[46,47] Although glucocorticoids' effects on prolactin have been inferred as occurring at the level of the pituitary, in these individuals TRH-induced increases in prolactin remain intact, suggesting glucocorticoids exert suprapituitary effects on prolactin as well.[49]

Although the exact mechanism by which glucocorticoids increase DA levels remains to be illuminated, there is mounting evidence that such increases may be mediated via effects on tyrosine hydroxylase. ACTH and glucocorticoids have been reported to increase tyrosine hydroxylase in various brain regions (including the locus ceruleus) in lower species.[50] Recently, monoclonal antibody studies have also pointed to important interactions between glucocorticoids and biogenic amine systems in brain and other organs. Harfstramd et al.[51] reported the colocalization of glucocorticoid receptors with receptors for tyrosine hydroxylase in dopaminegic neurons in the rat brain. Moreover, Towle and Evinger[52] reported that dexamethasone increased transcription of mRNA for tyrosine hydroxylase in the human adrenal. All these data point to an intimate role for glucocorticoids in the control of tyrosine hydroxylase activity.

## CORTISOL/DA IN PSYCHOTIC DEPRESSION

A few years ago, we hypothesized that the development of delusions in depressed patients was actually due to the patients' own enhanced cortisol activity and its effects on dopamine systems.[26] This hypothesis was based on a number of observations previously outlined, particularly that (a) psychotically depressed patients demonstrate marked disruption of the HPA axis with extremely elevated postdexamethasone cortisol levels; (b) glucocorticoids themselves increase dopamine and HVA levels in man and in the rat brain; and (c) Cushing's disease patients demonstrate relatively high prevalences of psychosis and other psychiatric symptoms.[53-55]

Recently, we have reported[19] on plasma cortisol and catecholamine levels in a small series of psychotic depressives ($N = 4$), nonpsychotic depressed counterparts ($N = 18$), and healthy controls ($N = 6$). Patients and controls were studied under drug-free conditions. Plasma was obtained for catecholamine and cortisol determinations at 4 p.m. on Day 1 and Day 2; a 1-mg dose of dexamethasone was administered at 11 p.m. on Day 1. In 19 of the patients, platelet monoamine oxidase was determined at 8 a.m. prior to dexamethasone administration.[39]

When psychotic and nonpsychotic depressives were combined into a single depressed group, they did not differ significantly from controls in predexamethasone cortisol, DA, epinephrine (EPI), or norepinephrine (NE) levels. Postdexamethasone, depressed patients demonstrated significantly lower ($F = 4.50$, $p = 0.04$) DA concentrations and higher cortisol levels (trend significance $F = 3.37$, $p = 0.078$).

In control subjects, DA levels were significantly higher ($t = 4.30$, $p < 0.01$) and cortisol levels were significantly lower ($t = 4.63$, $p < 0.01$) after dexamethasone than before. In depressed patients a much smaller, but significant, ($t = 2.37$, $p = 0.03$) increase in Da was observed after dexamethasone; cortisol was significantly lower after dexamethasone ($t = 3.85$, $p = 0.001$), although here too the magnitude of difference was significantly lower then in controls. These data suggest a relative blunting of dexamethasone-induced increases in DA and decreases in cortisol in depressed patients as compared with controls. Dexamethasone did not appear to affect NE or EPI in either patients or controls.

Seven of the 22 patients failed to suppress (4 of 4 delusional versus 3 of 18 nonpsychotic patients; Fisher exact test, $p = 0.005$). ANOVA with post-hoc Neuman–Keuls tests were performed comparing nonpsychotic patients, psychotic depressives, and healthy controls. As indicated in TABLE 1, psychotic depressed patients demonstrated significantly higher predexamethasone cortisol and dopamine than did the two remaining groups. Postdexamethasone, psychotic patients demonstrated significantly higher cortisol levels than did nonpsychotic patients or normal controls. DA levels were significantly lower in nonpsychotics than in the other two groups.

Platelet monoamine oxidase activity was significantly higher ($F = 7.64$, $p = 0.014$) in psychotic depressed patients (9.98 ± 1.95 nanomoles tryptamine deaminated/hr/mg protein) than in their nonpsychotic counterparts (6.54 ± 2.0 units).

We explored the effects of a number of variables on our DA/cortisol findings. Covarying for age differences, we still noted significant main effects for psychosis on DA and cortisol, with the exception of predexamethasone cortisol where diagnosis did not exert a significant effect but age did.

Covarying for severity [total score on the Hamilton Depression Rating Scale (HDRS)], significant main effects for psychosis were still observed on DA and cortisol both pre- and postdexamethasone. (Total HDRS scores did exert significant effects on pre- and postdexamethasone DA and postdexamethasone cortisol.) We also assessed

TABLE 1. Mean ± SD Pre- and Postdexamethasone Dopamine (DA) and Cortisol (COR) Levels in Psychotic and Nonpsychotic Depressed Patients and Normal Controls[a]

| | Psychotic (n = 4) | Nonpsychotic (n = 18) | Controls (n = 6) | ANOVA F | ANOVA p | Newman-Keuls |
|---|---|---|---|---|---|---|
| Predex COR[b] | 18.5 ± 3.1 | 11.2 ± 3.9 | 10.0 ± 5.9 | 4.6 | =0.02 | P vs. NP; P vs. C |
| Postdex COR | 17.5 ± 6.8 | 3.8 ± 6.0 | 1.5 ± 1.7 | 10.3 | <0.001 | P vs. NP; P vs. C |
| Predex DA[c] | 282.0 ± 24.8 | 50.7 ± 17.5 | 43.0 ± 9.8 | 79.8 | <0.001 | P vs. NP; P vs. C |
| Postdex DA | 278.5 ± 58.8 | 69.2 ± 30.1 | 175.3 ± 76.0 | 24.5 | <0.001 | P vs. NP; NP vs. C |

[a] From Rothschild et al.[19] Reproduced with permission.
[b] COR = µg/dl.
[c] DA = pg/ml.

severity by dividing our nonpsychotic patients by HDRS scores < or ≥ 18. More severely depressed nonpsychotic patients with HDRS scores ≥18 demonstrated lower ($F$ = 5.00, $p$ ± 0.04), predexamethasone DA levels (44.6 ± 9.5 pg/ml) than did patients with HDRS scores <18 (63.0 ± 23.8 pg/ml). No differences in postdexamethasone DA or pre- and postdexamethasone cortisol levels were noted. Thus, our findings were not merely due to psychotic depressives being more severely ill (see also below for correlational data).

A series of Pearson product–moment and Spearman rank–order correlations were determined between specific items on the HDRS and biological measures. Because of limitations of space, we emphasize symptom correlations that achieved significance ($p < 0.05$). Predexamethasone DA correlated significantly with depression ($r = 0.49$, $p = 0.01$), psychomotor retardation ($r = 0.50$, $p < 0.01$), and early insomnia ($r = 0.44$, $p < 0.03$), but not with agitation, psychic anxiety, or severity (total HDRS score). Predexamethasone norepinephrine correlated negatively and significantly with paranoia ($r = -0.40$, $p < 0.04$) and insight ($r = -0.45$, $p < 0.02$). Epinephrine correlated with obsessionality ($r = -0.40$, $p < 0.04$) and early insomnia ($r = 0.38$, $p < 0.05$). Cortisol also correlated significantly with depressed mood ($r = 0.43$, $p <0.03$), but (unlike DA) it also correlated positively with agitation and psychic anxiety ($r = 0.40$, $p <0.04$). Cortisol did not correlate with severity or psychomotor retardation. Platelet monoamine oxidase correlated significantly with psychomotor retardation ($r = 0.48$, $p = 0.02$), obsessionality ($r = -0.50$, $p = 0.016$), early insomnia ($r = 0.41$, $p < 0.05$), and lack of insight ($r = 0.40$, $p < 0.05$), but not with severity, depressed mood, agitation, or psychic anxiety. A number of trend correlations were observed, and these have been elaborated on elsewhere.[39]

The following correlations among biological measures achieved at least trend significance ($p < 0.09$) predexamethasone: cortisol/DA ($r = 0.48$, $p < 0.02$), cortisol/EPI ($r = 0.37$, $p < 0.05$), cortisol/MAO ($r = 0.36$, $p = 0.064$), and DA/EPI ($r = 0.31$, $p = 0.088$). When the four psychotic patients were excluded, only the cortisol/EPl correlation attained significance. These data point to intimate relationships among cortisol, DA, EPI, and MAO activity, with the cortisol/DA relationships largely occurring in or with the inclusion of psychotic depressives.

## DISCUSSION

Our preliminary findings indicate that cortisol and dopamine are elevated pre- and postdexamethasone in psychotic depressives compared with their nonpsychotic counterparts. They are consistent with our hypothesis that cortisol-induced increases in DA may play an important role in the pathogenesis of delusional symptoms in depressed and other affectively ill patients, although further studies are required to determine whether high cortisol/high DA are epiphemomena to or causes of psychosis (see below).

Findings of our group and others that glucocorticoids enhance catecholamine function is intriguing pathophysiologically, but one must ponder the physiological significance of such effects. In short, what purpose could steroidal increases of dopamine serve in the normal state? Such approaches could help our understanding of the development of affective psychotic states.

Recent studies from two groups suggest that DA may have important modulating functions of stress responses in lower species; by extension, steroidal increases of DA activity may actually represent key steps in limiting stress responses in various species including man. Gilam and colleagues[56] have reported that mesocorticolimbic dopamine neurons are activated in stressed animals. Moreover, they noted that increased

DA activity results in decreases in cholinergic neuronal activity in the hippocampus. They reported that apomorphine—a dopamine agonist—decreases both acetylcholine (ACh) release and choline uptake in the hippocampus of handled rats. In contrast, sulpiride—a $D_2$ antagonist—increased choline uptake and ACh release. Thus, in this paradigm, DA serves to limit ACh-mediated physiological responses to stress. ACh is well known to stimulate the HPA axis, resulting in increased glucocorticoid levels in blood.

In a different approach, Downs and colleagues[57] reported that in rats, DA depletion after 6-hydroxydopamine (6-HDA) administration results in supersensitive responses to physostigmine administration. These data point further to DA having a down-regulating effect on hippocampal ACh systems. Taken together, these two studies point to an important ACH/DA balance in stress responses in the rat and suggest that corticosteroids' increase of DA could reflect the organism's attempt to limit, or down-regulate, the stress-induced increases in cholinergic activity.

Glucocorticoids and ACTH increase of tyrosine hydroxylase (TH) activity in various tissues, including specific brain regions, could be a major clue in our understanding of why some patients decompensate under stress. TH and other catecholamine synthesizing enzymes [e.g., phenylethylmethyltransferase (PNMT)] have been shown to be under strong genetic control, and in the early experiments of Ciaranello and Barchas[58] not only were TH and PNMT activity under strong genetic control but glucocorticoid-induced increases in PNMT were also genetically controlled. In these studies, glucocorticoids' effects on TH activity were not explored. The recent observations of co-localization of TH and corticosteroid receptors in dopaminergic neurons further points to effects of steroids on TH at the level of the genome. Genomic effects of glucocorticoids were reported several years ago in studies of McEwen and colleagues,[59] and have been thought to be key ways in which environment and soma may interact, that is, glucocorticoids may mediate the translation of environmental impulses into somatic neurochemical responses. We have hypothesized[26] that disorders in regulating tyrosine hydroxylase could play a key role in placing individuals at risk for developing psychosis in the context of a depressive episode. Patients who are at particular risk for psychosis could be those who fail to modulate their corisol-induced increases in tyrosine hydroxylase. This could also help explain the possible linkage between psychotic depression (particularly early-onset type) and bipolar disorder.

Cortisol effects on DA and VBRs may prove of importance in understanding recent findings in other psychotic disorders, including schizophrenia. As previously indicated, we have observed both increased VBRs and elevated postdexamethasone cortisol levels in psychotic depressives. A number of groups have reported positive relationships between high plasma HVA levels and severity of schizophrenic symptoms on the one hand,[60] and between low CSF HVA and elevated VBRs on the other hand.[61] As discussed in David Pickar and colleagues' presentation at this meeting, CSF HVA and plasma HVA levels may relate in opposite directions to current severity.[62] HVA levels in the CSF of primates have recently been reported to reflect prefrontal DA activity,[63] and Weinberger et al. in this meeting and elsewhere have postulated that decreased prefrontal DA might underline schizophrenic processes.[64] In our acute experiments in rats we reported that dexamethasone reduced DOPAC in the frontal cortex but increased DA in the nucleus accumbens and hypothalamus.[44] Similar differential regional effects on DA concentrations have been reported for cocaine. Conceivably then cortisol effects on mesocorticolimbic DA systems could play important roles in various psychotic syndromes, including even some patients with schizophreniclike or schizoaffective disorders. Further studies in this area seem warranted.

Our data suggest that reducing plasma cortisol levels (or cortisol's effects on DA systems) in psychotic depressives (and perhaps in other psychotic patients) could help to reduce psychotic symptoms. Two possible approaches include: (1) blocking cortisol synthesis or (2) using specific glucocorticoid receptor blockers. Regarding the former, a number of agents (ketoconazole, metyrapone, and mitotane) have been reported to reduce depressive and other psychiatric symptoms in patients with Cushing's disease.[65-67] Glucocorticoid receptor blockers are not yet available for treatment of psychiatric patients. Dexamethasone administration might be inferred to be a treatment for those delusional patients who suppress on the DST but who show high predexamethasone cortisol levels; however, such an appproach might not lead to decreased DA activity. We are currently pursuing the use of ketoconazole and metryapone as possible treatment for psychotically depressed patients.

## ACKNOWLEDGMENT

Gale Dalrymple and Patricia Mancuso prepared the manuscript.

## REFERENCES

1. BRITTON, K. T., G. LEE, R. DANA, S. C. RISCH & G. F. KOOB. 1986. Life Sci. **39:** 1201–1286.
2. KALIN, N. K. & L. K. TAKAHASHI. 1988. Altered hypothalamic-pituitary adrenal regulation in animal models of depression. *In* Physiology and Pathaphysiology of the HPA axis: Psychiatric Implications. A. F. Schatzberg and C. B. Nemeroff, Eds. Raven Press. New York.
3. BANKI, C. M., G. BISETTE, M. ARATO, L. O'CONNOR & C. B. NEMEROFF. 1987. Am. J. Psychiatry **144:** 873–877.
4. GOLD P. W., G. CHRONSOS, C. KELLNER *et al.* 1984. Am. J. Psychiatry **141:** 615–627.
5. CORYELL, W., P. LAVORI, J. ENDICOTT, M. KELLER & M. VAN EERDEWEGH. 1984. Arch. Gen. Psychiatry **41:** 787–791.
6. ROOSE, S. P., A. H. GLASSMAN, T. WALSH, S. WOODRING & J. VITAL-HERNE. 1983. Am. J. Psychiatry **140:** 1150–1162.
7. AKISKAL, H. A., P. WALKER, V. R. PUZANTIAN, D. KING, T. L. ROSENTHAL & M. DRANON. 1983. J. Aff. Dis. **5:** 115–128.
8. STROBER, M. & G. CARLSON. 1982. Arch. Gen. Psychiatry **39:** 549–555.
9. WEISSMAN, M. M., B. A. PRUSOFF & K. R. MERIKANGAS. 1984. Am. J. Psychiatry **141:** 892–893.
10. WEISSMAN, M. M., V. WARNER, K. JOHN, B. A. PRUSOFF, K. R. MERIKANGAS, P. WICK-RAMARATINE & G. D. GAMMON. Neuropsychobiology. In Press.
11. LECKMAN, J. F., M. M. WEISSMAN, B. A. PRUSOFF, K. A. CARUSO, K. R. D. L. PAULS & K. K. KIDD. 1984. Arch. Gen. Psychiatry **41:** 833–838.
12. BOND, T. C., A. J. ROTHSCHILD, J. LERBINGER & A. F. SCHATZBERG. 1986. Biol. Psychiatry **21:** 1239–1246.
13. AVERY, D. & A. LUBRANO. 1979. Am. J. Psychiatry **136:** 559–562.
14. SPIKER, D. F., J. COFSKY WEISS, R. S. DEAHY, S. J. GRIFFIN, I. HANIN, J. F. NEIL, J. M. PEREL, A. J. RUSSI & P. H. SOLOFF. 1985. Am. J. Psychiatry **142:** 430–436.
15. AGREN, H. & L. TERENIUS. 1985. J. Aff. Dis. **9:** 25–34.
16. ABERG-WISTEDT, A., B. WISTEDT & L. BERTILSSON. 1985. Arch. Gen. Psychiatry **42:** 925.
17. BROWN, R. P., M. STIPETIC, J. KEILIP, M. STANLEY, B. STANLEY & J. J. MANN. 1987. Annual Meeting of The American Psychiatric Association. New Research Abstracts. NR. 11, p. 38.
18. SPIKER, D. F., P. A. BERGER, R. S. BEALY, K. F. FAULL, S. J. GRIFFIN, D. B. JARRETT & D. J. KUPFER. 1985. Biological Psychiatry. *In* O. Shagass *et al.*, Eds. Elsevier. Amsterdam/New York,

19. ROTHSCHILD, A. J., A. F. SCHATZBERG, P. J. LANGLAIS, J. E. LERBINGER, M. M. MILLER & J. O. COLE. 1987. Psychiatry Res. **20:** 143–153.
20. ANTON, R. F. 1987. Biol. Psychiatry **22:** 24–34.
21. RIHMER, Z., M. ARATO, E. SZADOCZKY, K. REVAI, E. DEMETER, S. GYORGY & P. UDVAR-HELYI. 1984. Br. J. Psychiatry **145:** 508–571.
22. LEVY, A. B. & S. L. STERN. 1987. Am. J. Psychiatry **144:** 472–475.
23. NELSON, J. C. & M. B. BOWERS. 1978. Arch. Gen. Psychiatry **35:** 1321–1328.
24. SCHATZBERG, A. F., A. J. ROTHSCHILD, J. B. STAHL, T. C. BOND, A. H. ROSENBAUM, S. B. LOFGREN, R. A. MACLAUGHLIN, M. SULLIVAN & J. O. COLE. 1983. Am. J. Psychiatry **140:** 88–91.
25. EVANS, D. L. & C. B. NEMEROFF. 1987. J. Psychiatr. Res. **21:** 185–194.
26. SCHATZBERG, A. F., A. J. ROTHSCHILD, P. J. LANGLAIS, E. T. BIRD & J. O. COLE. 1985. J. Psychiatr. Res. **19:** 57–64.
27. ARANA, G. W., P. J. BARREIRA, B. M. COHEN, J. F. LIPINSKI & D. FOGELSON. 1983. Am. J. Psychiatry **140:** 1521–1523.
28. KRISHNAN, K. R. R.,, J. R. T. DAVIDSON, K. RAYASAM, K. S. TANAS, F. S. SHOPE & S. PELTON. 1987. Biol. Psychiatry **22:** 618–628.
29. HEINZ, E. R., R. M. POST, R. SAWARD & P. W. GOLD. 1984. Arch. Gen. Psychiatry **41:** 279–286.
30. KELLNER, C. H., D. R. RUBINOW, P. W. GOLD & R. M. POST. 1983. Psychiatry Res. **8:** 191–197.
31. SCHLEGEL, S. & K. KRETZSCHMAR. 1987. Biol. Psychiatry. **22:** 4–14.
32. LUCHINS, D. J. & H. Y. MELTZER. 1983. Biol. Psychiatry **18:** 1197–1198.
33. TARGUM, S. D., L. N. ROSEN, L. E. DELISI, D. R. WEINBERGER & C. M. CITRIN. 1983. Biol. Psychiatry **18:** 1329–1336.
34. ROTHSCHILD, A. J., F. BENES, B. WOODS & A. F. SCHATZBERG. 1987. Neuroendocrinol. Lett. **9:** 147.
35. THASE, M. E., D. J. KUPFER & R. F. ULRICH. 1986. Arch. Gen. Psychiatry **43:** 886–893.
36. MATUZAS, W., H. Y. MELTZER, E. H. UHLENHUTH, R. M. GLASS & C. TONG. 1982. Biol. Psychiatry **17:** 1415–1425.
37. MOD, L., Z. RIHMER, I. MAGYAR, M. ARATO, A. ALFOLDI & G. BAGDY. 1986. Psychiatry Res. **19:** 331–333.
38. MELTZER, H. Y., R. C. ARORA, H. JACKMAN, G. PSCHEIDT & M. D. SMITH. 1980. Schizophrenia Bull. **6:** 213–219.
39. SCHATZBERG, A. F., A. J. ROTHSCHILD, P. J. LANGLAIS, J. E. LERBINGER, J. J. SCHILDKRAUT & J. O. COLE. 1987. Psychiatry Res. **20:** 155–164.
40. BANKI, C. M., M. ARATO, Z. PAPP & M. KURCZ. 1983. Pharmacopsychiatry **16:** 77–81.
41. ROTHSCHILD, A. J., P. J. LANGLAIS, A. F. SCHATZBERG, F. X. WALSH, J. O. COLE & E. D. BIRD. 1984. J. Psychiatry Res. **18:** 217–223.
42. WOLKOWITZ, O. M., M. E. SUTTON, A. R. DORAN, R. LABARCA, A. ROY, J. W. THOMAS, D. PICKAR & S. M. PAUL. 1985. Psychiatry Res. **16:** 101–109.
43. MARKEY, K. A., A. C. TOWLE & P. Y. SZE. 1982. Endocrinology **111:** 1159–1163.
44. ROTHSCHILD, A. J., P. J. LANGLAIS, A. F. SCHATZBERG, M. M. MILLER, M. S. SALOMAN, J. E. LERBINGER, J. O. COLE & E. D. BIRD. 1985. Life Sci. **36:** 2491–2501.
45. WOLKOWITZ, O. M., M. SUTTON, M. KOULU, R. LABARCA, L. WILKINSON, A. DURAN, R. HANGER, D. PICKAR & J. CRAWLEY. 1986. Eur. J. Pharmacol. **122:** 329–338.
46. COPINSCHI, G., M. L'HERMITE, R. LE CLERCQ, J. GOLDSTEIN, L. VANHAELST, E. VIRASORO & C. ROBYN. 1975. J. Clin. Endocrinol. Metab. **40:** 442–449.
47. EUKER, J. S., J. MEITES & G. D. RIEGLE. 1975. Endocrinology **96:** 85–92.
48. OSTERMAN, P. O., J. FAGINS & L. WIDE. 1977. Acta Endocrinol. **84:** 237–247.
49. KRIEGER, D. T., P. J. HOWANITZ & A. G. FRANTZ. 1976. J. Clin. Endocrinol. Metab. **42:** 260–272.
50. MARKEY, K. A. & P. Y. SZE. 1984. Neuroendocrinol. **38:** 269–275.
51. HARFSTRAMD, A., L. FAYE, L. F. CINTRA, M. AGNATI, M. ARONSON, M. ZOLI, I. KITAYAMA & J. A. GUSTAVSSON. 1987. Abstracts, 6th Int. Catecholamine Symp. p. 22.
52. TOWLE, A. C. & T. H. EVINGER. 1987. Neuroendocrinol. Lett. **9:** 223–224.
53. REGESTEIN, Q. R., L. I. ROSE & G. H. WILLIAMS. 1972. Arch. Int. Med. **130:** 114–117.
54. GIFFORD, S. & J. G. GUNDERSON. 1970. Medicine **49:** 397–411.

55. STARKMAN, M. N., D. E. SCHTEINGART & M. A. SCHORK. 1981. Psychosom. Med. **43**: 3–18.
56. GILAD, G. M., V. H. GILAD & J. M. RABEY. 1986. Life Sci. **39**: 2387–2393.
57. DOWNS, N. S., K. T. BRITTON, D. M. GIBBS, G. F. KOOB & N. R. SWERDLOW. 1986. Biol. Psychiatry **21**: 775–786.
58. BARCHAS, J. D., R. D. CIARANELLO, S. KESSLER & D. A. HAMBURG. 1975. *In* Genetic Research In Psychiatry. R. R. Fieve, D. Rosenthal, and H. Brill, Eds.: 27–62. Johns Hopkins Press. Baltimore.
59. MCEWEN, B. S., P. G. DAVIS, B. PARSONS & D. PFOFF. 1979. Ann. Rev. Neurosci. **2**: 65–112.
60. PICKAR, D., R. LABARCA, A. R. DORAN, O. M. WOLKOWITZ, A. ROY, A. BREIER, M. LINNOILA & S. M. PAUL. 1986. Arch. Gen. Psychiatry **43**: 669–676.
61. VAN KAMMEN, D. P., L. S. MANN, D. E. STEINBERG, M. SCHEININ, P. T. NINAN, S. R. MARDER, W. B. VAN KAMMEN, R. O. REIDER & M. LINNOILA. 1983. Science **220**: 974–977.
62. PICKAR, D., A. BREIER & J. KELSOE. 1988. Plasma homovanillic acid as an index of central dopaminergic activity: Studies in schizophrenic patients. This volume.
63. ELSWORTH, J. D., D. J. LEAHY, R. H. ROTH & D. E. REDMOND. 1987. J. Neural. Trans. **68**: 51–62.
64. WEINBERGER, D., K. F. BERMAN & T. N. CHASE. 1988. Mesocortical dopaminergic function and human condition. This volume.
65. JEFFCOATE, W. J., J. J. SILVERSTONE, C. R. W. EDWARDS & G. M. BESSER. 1979. Q. J. Med. **48**: 465–472.
66. STARKMAN, M. N., D. E. SCHTEINGART & A. SCHORK. 1986. Psychiatry Res. **19**: 177–188.
67. ANGELI, A. & R. FRAIRIA. 1985. Lancet **1**: 821.

# Localization of Mu Opioid and Neurotensin Receptors within the A10 Region of the Rat

R. P. DILTS AND P. W. KALIVAS

*Department of Veterinary Comparative Anatomy, Pharmacology, and Physiology*
*Washington State University*
*Pullman, Washington 99154–6520*

## INTRODUCTION

Recently it has been demonstrated that mu opioid receptor agonists produce a potent stimulation of the A10 dopaminergic cell group, including the ventral tegmental area (VTA).[1] In contrast, delta receptor agonists are relatively ineffective. To study the anatomical basis for this effect we employed quantitative receptor autoradiography. Additionally, to study whether the enhanced dopaminergic activity caused by mu agonists involves direct stimulation of dopaminergic perikarya or whether the increased output was caused by other neuronal elements within the mesencephalic tegmentum, we utilized unilateral injections of the neurotoxins 6-hydroxydopamine (6-OHDA) and quinolinic acid (QUIN), respectively.

## METHODS

The highly selective ligand, $^{125}$I-Tyr-D-Ala-Gly-N-MePhe-Gly(ol) (DAGO), was prepared by lactoperoxidase iodination and purified by reverse-phase HPLC using a 14% acetonitrile 40-mM $H_3PO_4$, 50-mM triethylamine, and 10-mM acetate mobile phase. $^{125}$I-Tyr$^3$-neurotensin (NT-3) was prepared in a similar fashion employing 21% acetonitrile in the mobile phase with subsequent trypsin digest[2] used to identify eluent-containing pure NT-3. As described elsewhere,[3] adjacent 16–18-μm cryostat sections of fresh-frozen rat brains were subjected to modified autoradiographic procedures using 0.2 nanomoles of ligand. Unilateral injections of 7.5–10-μg 6-OHDA (free base) in 1.2–1.5 μl of 0.2% ascorbate were infused over a 20–30-min period in male Sprague-Dawley rats (250–350 g) pretreated with desmethylimipramine (DMI, 30 mg/kg, ip) at A/P 2.9 M/L 0.7 D/V 2.7 from the interaural line in accordance with the atlas of Pellegrino *et al*.[4] Likewise, injections of 300 nanomoles of quinolinic acid in 1.5-μl phosphate buffered saline were performed, except rats were not pretreated with DMI.

## RESULTS

Analysis of DAGO binding within the A10 region showed a moderate density of receptors, 5–20 fmol/mg protein, within the nucleus parabrachialis pigmentosa, the

472

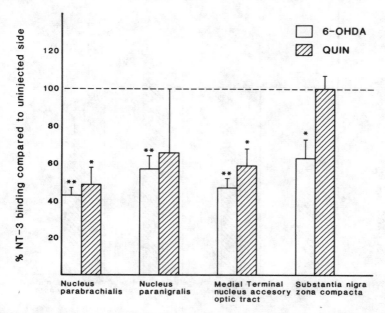

**FIGURE 1.** Comparison of 6-OHDA and QUIN treatments on neurotensin binding within the mesencephalic tegmentum. Values were obtained by a comparison of densities for treated/untreated sides and are expressed as the mean ± S.E.M. *$p < 0.05$ by paired t-test following normalization of data ($n = 4$).**$p < 0.01$.

nucleus paranigralis, and the interfascicular nucleus. Increased binding density was observed within the substantia nigra, zona compacta, and the area immediately circumscribing the fasciculus retroflexus. Highest levels of DAGO binding exist within the medial terminal accessory nucleus of the optic tract. In an adjacent section, NT-3 binding achieved the highest levels, 40 fmol/mg protein, in the lateral aspect of the nucleus paranigralis adjacent to the medial terminal accessory nucleus of the optic tract.

Unilateral treatment with 6-OHDA failed to alter DAGO binding within the A10 region while invoking a 60% unilateral loss of neurotensin receptors within the VTA (FIG. 1).[5] Unilateral administration of QUIN produced a maximal 70% loss of DAGO binding within the lesioned area with a concomitant reduction in NT-3 binding (FIG. 2).

## DISCUSSION

These results provide an anatomical basis whereby mu opioid receptor-mediated events may enhance the output of the A10 dopaminergic cell group in response to intra-VTA injections of opioid agonists. Furthermore, they provide evidence that the enhanced output of the dopaminergic neurons caused by mu receptor activation is medi-

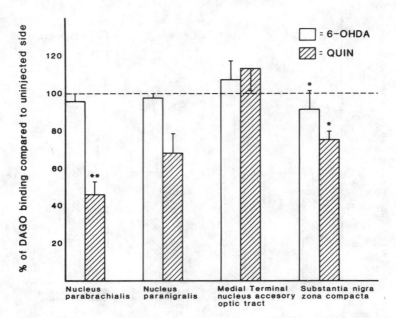

**FIGURE 2.** Comparison of 6-OHDA and QUIN treatments on DAGO binding within the mesencephalic tegmentum. Values were obtained by a comparison of densities for treated/untreated sides and are expressed as the mean ± S.E.M. *$p < 0.05$ by paired two-tailed t-test following normalization of data ($n = 4$). **$p < 0.01$.

ated, at least in part, by a group of nondopaminergic neurons intrinsic within the A10 region of the rat.

## REFERENCES

1. LATIMER, L. G., P. DUFFY & P. W. KALIVAS. 1987. Mu opioid receptor involvement in enkephalin activation of dopamine neurons in the ventral tegmental area. J. Pharmacol. Exp. Ther. In press.
2. SADOUL, J. L., J. MAZELLA, S. AMAR, P. KITABGI & J. P. VINCENT. 1984. Preparation of neurotensin selectively iodinated on the Tyrosine 3 residue. Biological activity and binding properties on mammalian neurotensin receptors. Biochem. Biophys. Res. Comm. **120:** 812–819.
3. MASKOWITZ, A. S. & R. R. GOODMAN. 1984. Light microscopic autoradiographic localization of mu and delta opioid binding sites in the mouse central nervous system. J. Neurosci. **4:** 1331–1342.
4. PELLEGRINO, L. K., A. S. PELLEGRINO & A. J. CUSHMAN. 1979. A Stereotaxic Atlas of the Rat Brain. Plenum. New York.
5. PALACIOUS, J. M. & M. M. KUHAR. 1981. Neurotensin receptors are located on dopamine-containing neurones in rat midbrain. Nature **294:** 587–589.

# Inhibition of Endogenous Dopamine Release from the Ventromedial Mesencephalon after Daily Cocaine or Morphine

PATRICIA DUFFY[a] AND PETER W. KALIVAS

*Deparment of Veterinary Comparative Anatomy,*
*Pharmacology and Physiology*
*Washington State University*
*Pullman, Washington 99164-6520*

Drugs of abuse as diverse in pharmacological action as cocaine and morphine have been shown to produce behavioral sensitization such that subsequent administration of these drugs results in a greater psychomotor stimulant effect than the initial injection.[1,2] While the pharmacological mechanism of action of cocaine and morphine is different, both drugs increase mesocorticolimbic dopamine (DA) neurotransmission. Cocaine prevents reuptake of DA into the presynaptic terminal, thereby increasing the concentration of DA in the synaptic cleft,[3] and local injection of opioids into the A10 DA region increases terminal fields' mesocorticolimbic DA metabolism.[4] Based upon the similarity between these drugs at increasing mesocorticolimbic DA neurotransmission and the production of behavioral sensitization we designed a study to evaluate the effect of daily peripheral morphine or cocaine administration on the *in vitro* release of endogenous DA from tissue slices of the ventromedial mesencephalon (containing the A10 and A9 DA perikarya), the nucleus accumbens, and striatum.

Male Sprague-Dawley rats were injected for three days with cocaine (15 mg/kg, ip) or five days with morphine (10 mg/kg, ip), and two to three weeks later the rats were decapitated and tissue slices (210 µm) prepared from the ventromedial mesencephalon, nucleus accumbens, and striatum using a McIlwain tissue chopper. It was necessary to pool the tissue from two rats to obtain measureable unstimulated release of endogenous DA from the ventromedial mesencephalon. The tissue slices were pipetted into a superfusion chamber adapted from Fallon *et al.*[5] The superfusion medium consisted of 5 mM KCl, 120 mM NaCl, 1.3 mM $Na_2HPO_4$, 10 mM $NaHCO_3$, 5 mM D-glucose, 25 mM Hepes, 1.2 mM $MgCl_2$, 2.4 mM $CaCl_2$. To provoke the release of endogenous DA, the potassium concentration was increased to between 10 and 60 mM by equimolar substitution of KCl for NaCl. The experiments were performed at 37°C and the effluent accumulated in 5% trichloroacetic acid (0.5 ml) over ten-min periods. The tissue was washed for 25 to 30 min at a flow rate of 0.5 ml/min, and collection of samples begun at a flow rate of 0.2 ml/min for the remainder of the experiment. After collection of a sample to measure basal release, the high potassium perfusate was presented for 6 min in the next 10-min sample, followed by at least two 10 min collections with the 5-mM perfusate. The tissue was then removed from the superfu-

---

[a] To whom correspondence should be addressed.

**TABLE 1.** Effect of Increasing Potassium Concentration on *in Vitro* DA Release

| Pretreatment | Concentration of Potassium | | | | | |
|---|---|---|---|---|---|---|
| | 10 | 20 | 30 | 40 | 50 | 60 |
| Ventromedial mesencephalon | | | | | | |
| Saline | — | 110 ± 5 | — | 163 ± 17.5 | 195 ± 11.3 | 294 ± 22.3 |
| Cocaine | — | — | — | 101 ± 10.4[a] | 113 ± 6.8[b] | 240 ± 23.7 |
| Morphine | — | — | — | 98 ± 8.5 | 106 ± 5.7[b] | 136 ± 15.1[b] |
| Nucleus accumbens | | | | | | |
| Saline | 150 ± 10.4 | — | 535 ± 42.7 | — | — | 978 ± 122.8 |
| Cocaine | 238 ± 36.7[a] | — | 656 ± 40.8 | — | — | 1131 ± 173.5 |
| Morphine | 163 ± 18.8 | — | 656 ± 76.5 | — | — | 1156 ± 301 |

[a] $p < 0.05$, comparing cocaine and morphine pretreatment with saline pretreatment using a one-way analysis of variance followed by a Newman-Keuls test for multiple comparisons.
[b] $p < 0.01$.

sion chamber and the protein content determined using Folin reagent. The DA content of the release samples was measured using high-pressure liquid chromatography with electrochemical detection. Five hundred microliters of the sample were added to the high-performance liquid chromatography (HPLC) system, and the mobile phase, octadecylsilane (ODS) column, and data analysis used are described elsewhere.[6]

TABLE 1 shows the percent of change in DA release observed in the second tube (containing the high potassium superfusate) compared with the first collection tube. Note that DA release was more difficult to elicit from the ventromedial mesencephalon than from the nucleus accumbens. In the ventromedial mesencephalon, potassium was significantly less effective in releasing DA from the ventromedial mesencephalon of rats pretreated with daily cocaine or morphine. In contrast, in the nucleus accumbens there was only a slight enhancement of potassium-evoked DA release in cocaine-pretreated rats at 10 mM, but not 30 or 60 mM KCl. No effect of either pretreatment on potassium-induced DA release was measured in the striatum, and no effect was observed on basal release (data not shown).

These data demonstrate that following daily pretreatment with cocaine or morphine at doses capable of producing behavioral sensitization[1,2] the DA perikarya are refractory to potassium-induced release of DA. In contrast the effect of drug pretreatment was minimal in the terminal fields examined. Since daily morphine or cocaine produce postmortem changes indicative of increased DA neurotransmission in the mesocorticolimbic terminal fields,[6,7] it was surprising that the primary effect observed was in the DA cell bodies. However, a decrease in the capacity of the DA perikarya to release DA in response to depolarization could explain the increase in terminal field DA neurotransmission. Less somatodendritic DA release would result in less autoreceptor stimulation, and since stimulation of the somatodendritic autoreceptors has been shown to decrease the firing frequency of DA neurons,[8] less autoreceptor activation produced by diminished DA release in drug-sensitized rats would increase neuronal activity and concomitant DA release in the terminal fields. Finally, the increase in DA neurotransmission in the terminal fields would result in greater behavioral hyperactivity in response to acute morphine or cocaine challenge.

## REFERENCES

1.  POST, R. M. & H. ROSE. 1976. Increasing effects of repetitive cocaine administration in the rat. Nature 260: 731–732.
2.  BABBINI, M. & W. M. DAVIS. 1972. Time-dose relationships for locomotor activity effects of morphine after acute or repeated treatment. Br. J. Pharmacol. 46: 213–224.
3.  REITH, M. E. A., B. E. MEISLER, H. SERSHEN & A. LASTHA. 1986. Structural requirements for cocaine congeners to interact with dopamine and serotonin uptake sites in the mouse brain and to induce stereotyped behavior. Biochem. Pharmacol. 35: 1123–1129.
4.  KALIVAS, P. W. 1985. Interactions between neuropeptides and dopamine neurons in the ventromedial mesencephalon. Neurosci. Biobehav. Rev. 9: 573–587.
5.  O'FALLON, J. V., R. W. BROSEMER & J. W. HARDING. 1981. The Na, K-ATPase: A plausible trigger for voltage-dependent release of cytoplasmic neurotransmitters. J. Neurochem. 36: 369–378.
6.  KALIVAS, P. W. & P. DUFFY. 1987. Sensitization to repeated morphine injection in the rat: Possible involvement of A10 dopamine neurons. J. Pharmacol. Exp. Ther. 241: 201–212.
7.  KALIVAS, P. W., P. DUFFY, L. A. DUMARS & C. SKINNER. 1987. Behavioral and neurochemical effects of acute and daily cocaine administration in rats. J. Pharmacol. Exp. Ther. 245: 485–492.
8.  ROTH, R. H. 1984. CNS dopamine autoreceptors: Distribution, pharmacology and function. Ann. N.Y. Acad. Sci. 430: 27–53.

# Effects of Neurotensin on Dopamine Release in the Nucleus Accumbens: Comparisons with Atypical Antipsychotic Drug Action[a]

CHARLES D. BLAHA,[b,c,d] ANTHONY G. PHILLIPS,[c]
HANS C. FIBIGER,[d] AND ROSS F. LANE[d,e]

*Departments of [c]Psychology, [d]Psychiatry, and [e]Chemistry*
*University of British Columbia*
*Vancouver, British Columbia, Canada V6T 1Y7*

The tridecapeptide neurotensin (NT) and dopamine (DA) have been shown to be co-localized in mesolimbic neurons. The observation that intracerebroventricular (icv) administration of NT produces behavioral effects similar to those of atypical antipsychotic drugs (e.g., blockade of locomotor activity but not stereotypy induced by amphetamine) has prompted hypotheses about the role of NT in the etiology of schizophrenia.[1] Using *in vivo* electrochemical techniques,[2] we have previously shown that classical antipsychotic drugs [e.g., haloperidol (HAL) and chlorpromazine] increase the release of DA in both the accumbens and striatum of the rat, sites of mesolimbic and nigro-striatal DA nerve terminals, respectively. In contrast, atypical antipsychotic drugs [e.g., clozapine (CLOZ) and thioridazine] selectively increase the release of DA within the accumbens.[2,3] The present study compares the effects of NT with those of HAL and CLOZ on DA release in the posteromedial accumbens and anterodorsal striatum of chloral hydrate anesthetized rats (stereotaxic coordinates as previously described[2,3]). In an effort to understand the mechanisms of the action of NT on DA release, the effects of NT and these antipsychotics in combination with a direct (apomorphine) and an indirect (*d*-amphetamine) DA agonist were also examined.

Our initial studies have shown that icv administration of NT (0.1 to 10 µg/10 µl) induces an immediate dose-dependent increase in basal DA release in the accumbens, whereas release of DA in the striatum was unaffected by NT at these doses (Phillips *et al.*, this volume). Similar to the effects observed with a dose of 0.5 µg of NT, CLOZ (20 mg/kg, sc) administration produced comparable increases in DA release in the accumbens while having no effect on DA release in the striatum (FIG. 1A and 1B). In contrast, HAL (0.5 mg/kg, sc) administration produced increases in DA release in both brain regions (FIG. 1A and 1B).

[a] This work was supported in part by MRC Program Grant 23 and in part by U.S. Public Health Service Grant NS 13556.
[b] To whom correspondence should be addressed.

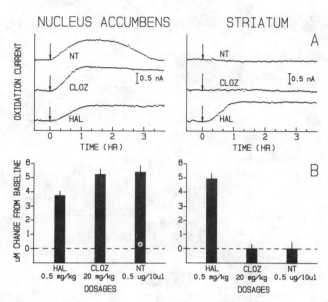

**FIGURE 1.** (**A**) Representative chronoamperometric recordings depicting the time courses of the differential effects of neurotensin (NT), clozapine (CLOZ), and haloperidol (HAL) administration on DA release in the nucleus accumbens and striatum of anesthetized rats. (**B**) Corresponding maximum change from basal values in DA concentration following administration of each compound. Larger doses of NT (5.0–10.0 μg) also proved ineffective in the striatum (Phillips *et al.*, this volume). Chronoamperometric responses were obtained by applying a potential pulse for 1 sec from $-0.10$ V to $+0.25$ V vs. Ag/AgCl to the recording electrode at 1-min intervals. For clarity, every second measurement is shown. Bars show mean values ± S.E.M. from 9 to 10 animals per drug group. CLOZ and HAL were injected subcutaneously and NT intracerebroventricularly at the dosages indicated below each bar.

Gammabutyrolactone (GBL) is known to block DA neuronal impulse flow[4] and induce concomitant reductions in basal DA release.[3] GBL (200 mg/kg, ip) injected 80 min after NT (0.5 or 1 μg, icv) immediately reversed the stimulatory effects of the peptide on DA release in the accumbens (FIG. 2B). In addition, 40 min pretreatment with GBL completely prevented these effects of NT (FIG. 2C). Both the CLOZ- and HAL-induced increases in DA release in this brain region were similarly affected by GBL. Systemic apomorphine (50 μg/kg, iv) was also effective in antagonizing both NT- and antipsychotic-induced changes in DA release (FIG. 2D). In addition, d-amphetamine (AMP, 1 mg/kg, iv), administered at the peak of the stimulatory effects of either NT or the antipsychotic drugs, produced a further increase in DA release that was comparable in magnitude to that produced after AMP administration alone (FIG. 2E).

These results provide direct *in vivo* evidence that (1) at the doses tested, NT selectively stimulates mesolimbic DA release, (2) these effects of NT on DA release and its interactions with GBL and DA agonists parallel the effects of atypical antipsychotic drugs, suggesting the possibility of a common mechanism of action, (3) the inability of NT to alter the magnitude of AMP-induced increases in DA release in the accumbens

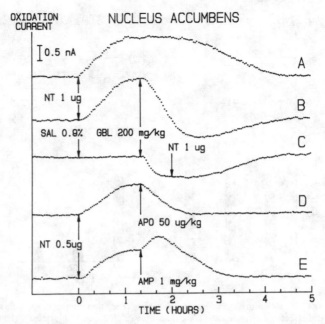

**FIGURE 2.** Chronoamperometric recordings showing the time courses of **(A)** the stimulatory effects of neurotensin (NT, 1.0 µg/10 µl, icv) alone on DA release in the nucleus accumbens and **(B)** the reversal and **(C)** blockade of these effects by gamma-butyrolactone (GBL, 200 mg/kg, ip). Note that administration of apomorphine (APO, 50 µg/kg, iv) also completely reversed NT-induced (0.5 µg/10 µl, icv) increases in DA release **(D)**, whereas a challenge injection of *d*-amphetamine (AMP, 1 mg/kg, iv) produced a further increase in DA release **(E)** that did not differ significantly in magnitude to that produced by AMP administration alone. The stimulatory effects of both haloperidol and clozapine on DA release in the nucleus accumbens were similarly affected by GBL, APO, or AMP (data not shown). Chronoamperometric conditions as in FIGURE 1. Responses are representative from 5 animals per treatment. SAL: 0.9% saline.

strongly suggests that the previously reported icv NT blockade of AMP-elicited behaviors is mediated at sites postsynaptic to the DA nerve terminal, and (4) the ability of NT to both selectively enhance the release of DA and antagonize mesolimbic DA neurotransmission suggests a mechanism consistent with antipsychotic drug action.[1]

## REFERENCES

1. NEMEROFF, C. B. 1986. Psychoneuroendocrinology **11:** 15–37.
2. LANE, R. F. & C. D. BLAHA. 1986. Ann. N.Y. Acad. Sci. **473:** 50–69.
3. LANE, R. F. & C. D. BLAHA. 1987. Brain Res. **408:** 317–320.
4. WALTERS, J. R., R. H. ROTH & G. AGHAJANIAN. 1973. J. Pharmacol. Exp. Ther. **186:** 630–639.

# Effects of Chronic Neuroleptic Administration on Nigrostriatal and Mesocorticolimbic Dopamine Release: Analysis Using *in Vivo* Voltammetry[a]

ROSS F. LANE[b] AND CHARLES D. BLAHA[c]

*Institute of Neuroscience*
*and*
*Department of Chemistry*
*University of Oregon*
*Eugene, Oregon 97403*

Electrophysiological studies reported by Bunney and co-workers[1,2] and confirmed by White and Wang[3,4] have shown that repeated administration of typical neuroleptics [i.e., those antipsychotic drugs associated with a high incidence of extrapyramidal side effects (EPSE) such as haloperidol (HAL)] results in a marked decrease in the number of spontaneously firing dopamine (DA) neurons in the substantia nigra zona compacta (A9) and ventral tegmental (A10) areas, whereas atypical antipsychotics [those associated with a low incidence of EPSE such as clozapine (CLOZ) and thioridazine (THIO)] inactivate only A10 DA neurons. Direct intracellular recordings from identified DA cells inactivated after repeated neuroleptic treatment have established that the reduction in DA cell activity is due to the development of depolarization block and that apomorphine (APO) administration restores spontaneous activity in these neurons.[5] We have used *in vivo* voltammetry[6-8] to investigate the effects of chronic treatment of both typical and atypical neuroleptics on basal DA release in striatum and nucleus accumbens of the rat, sites of nigrostriatal and mesolimbic DA nerve terminals, respectively. Experimental design and drug protocols are described in detail elsewhere.[6-8] FIGURE 1 shows that repeated treatment with HAL, chlorpromazine, and ( − )-sulpiride significantly reduced the basal release of DA in both striatum and accumbens. In contrast, CLOZ and THIO decreased basal DA release only in the accumbens. Metoclopramide treatment at a dose sufficient to induce EPSE but not antipsychotic action[4,6,8] produced effects that were opposite from those of CLOZ and THIO in that DA release was decreased only in the striatum. These effects appeared to be due to selective DA receptor blockade, since repeated treatment with promethazine, ( + )-sulpiride, and desipramine, drugs with no antipsychotic efficacy or EPSE,[1,2] failed to alter basal DA release in either brain region (FIG. 1). In all cases where decreases in DA release were observed, APO injection reversed these decreases to values that

[a] This work was supported by U.S. Public Health Service Grants NS 13556 and MH 17148.
[b] Present address: Departments of Chemistry and Psychiatry, University of British Columbia, Vancouver, British Columbia, Canada V6T 1Y6.
[c] Present address: Departments of Psychology and Psychiatry, University of British Columbia, Vancouver, British Columbia, Canada V6T 1Y7.

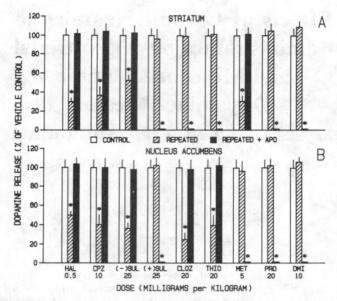

**FIGURE 1.** The effects of repeated (21-day) treatment with antipsychotic and nonantipsychotic drugs on basal dopamine (DA) release in rat striatum (**A**) and nucleus accumbens (**B**). Note that in every case where repeated drug treatment had no effect on DA release, injection of apomorphine (APO, 100 µg/kg, iv) completely inhibited DA release, whereas in every case showing a decrease in DA release, APO administration reversed these decreases to values that did not differ significantly from vehicle-treated controls. *Bars* show mean values ± S.E.M. from six rats per drug group and are expressed as a percentage of the mean basal DA release value measured in vehicle-treated controls. This value is designated as 100% (*open bars*). *Numbers beneath abscissa* represent drug doses and were chosen on the basis of clinical doses equivalent to HAL at 0.5 mg/kg. *Asterisks* indicate a significant difference ($p < 0.001$) from vehicle (VEH) controls. Abbreviations: HAL, haloperidol; CPZ, chlorpromazine; (−)-SUL, (−)-sulpiride; (+)-SUL, (+)-sulpiride; CLOZ, clozapine; THIO, thioridazine; MET, metoclopramide; PRO, promethazine; and DMI, desipramine.

did not differ significantly from vehicle-treated controls (FIG. 1). When not observed, APO reduced DA release to undetectable values, as seen in control animals. As discussed previously,[6–8] we propose that the effects of APO on the reductions in DA release result from its ability to reactivate (repolarize) DA neurons displaying depolarization block.[1,5]

Previous work has provided evidence that the anticholinergic and/or the α-noradrenergic (NE) blocking properties of CLOZ and THIO may underlie their relative inabilities to induce EPSE.[6,9] Thus, the anticholinergic drug trihexyphenidyl (THP) or the $\alpha_1$-NE antagonist prazosin (PRAZ) was combined with HAL in an attempt to elucidate the differential regional effects of CLOZ and THIO on DA release. Chronic coadministration with HAL of either THP or PRAZ resulted in a differential effect on striatal and accumbens DA release identical to that observed with chronic CLOZ or THIO alone. Thus, chronic treatment with these combinations of drugs decreased basal DA release in the accumbens but had no effect (vs. controls) in the striatum

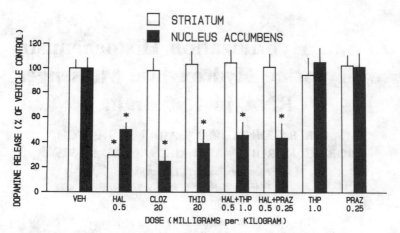

**FIGURE 2.** Effects of repeated (21 day) administration of haloperidol (HAL), trihexyphenidyl (THP), prazosin (PRAZ), and their combinations (HAL + THP and HAL + PRAZ) on basal dopamine (DA) release in rat striatum and nucleus accumbens. Note that chronic coadministration with HAL of either THP or PRAZ decreases DA release in accumbens but has no effect in the striatum, a profile identical to that observed with chronic CLOZ or THIO alone. *Bars* show mean values ± S.E.M. from six rats per drug group and are expressed as a percentage of the mean basal DA release value measured in vehicle-treated controls. This value is designated as 100% (*open bars*). *Asterisks* indicate a significant difference ($p < 0.001$) from vehicle (VEH) controls. Other conditions as in legend of FIGURE 1.

(FIG. 2). These decreases were again inferred to be due to induction of depolarization block of A10 DA cell firing,[5,9] since APO again restored DA release to control levels. Repeated treatment with THP or PRAZ did not alter DA release in either brain region. These data suggest that anticholinergic and/or $\alpha_1$-NE receptor blocking properties of CLOZ and THIO may, in part, mediate their differential effects on nigrostriatal and mesolimbic DA neurotransmission. The results further suggest that *in vivo* voltammetry may prove useful in comparing the sites and mechanisms of action of typical and atypical neuroleptics in an effort to find differences between the neuronal elements involved in clinical efficacy and those involved in side-effect induction.

## REFERENCES

1. BUNNEY, B. S. & A. A. GRACE. 1978. Life Sci. **23:** 1715–1728.
2. CHIODO, L. A. & B. S. BUNNEY. 1983. J. Neurosci. **3:** 1607–1619.
3. WHITE, F. J. & R. Y. WANG. 1983. Life Sci. **32:** 983–993.
4. WHITE, F. J. & R. Y. WANG. 1983. Science **221:** 1054–1057.
5. GRACE, A. A. & B. S. BUNNEY. 1986. J. Pharmacol. Exp. Ther. **238:** 1092–1100.
6. LANE, R. F. & C. D. BLAHA. 1986. Ann. N.Y. Acad. Sci. **473:** 50–69.
7. LANE, R. F. & C. D. BLAHA. 1987. Brain Res. Bull. **18:** 135–139.
8. BLAHA, C. D. & R. F. LANE. 1987. Neurosci. Lett. **78:** 199–204.
9. CHIODO, L. A. & B. S. BUNNEY. 1985. J. Neurosci. **5:** 2539–2544.

# In Situ Hybridization Histochemistry of Tyrosine Hydroxylase Messenger RNA in Rat Brain

FRANK BALDINO, JR.,[a,b,d] ARIEL Y. DEUTCH,[c]
ROBERT H. ROTH,[c] AND MICHAEL E. LEWIS[b,d]

[b]Medical Products Department
E. I. Dupont de Nemours and Co.
Wilmington, Delaware 19898

[c]Department of Pharmacology and Psychiatry
Yale University School of Medicine
New Haven, Connecticut 06520

Catecholamines are synthesized in neurons located in several nuclei throughout the central nervous system (CNS). Many of these neurons, particularly the mesencephalic and rhombencephalic cell groups, project to distant regions of the CNS and play a critical role in a number of functions of the nervous system. Tyrosine hydroxylase (TH) is the rate-limiting enzyme in catecholamine biosynthesis, and factors that influence the expression of this enzyme are likely to influence catecholamine function.

The recent cloning of a cDNA coding for rat TH[1] has made it possible to investigate the regulation of the mRNA coding for this enzyme. Recent anatomical studies have utilized in situ hybridization techniques to address these issues.[2,3] The purpose of this study was to use a synthetic oligodeoxynucleotide probe to localize mRNA for TH to single neurons in situ.

Adult male Sprague-Dawley rats (250–300 g) were perfused transcardially and processed for immunohistochemistry and in situ hybridization according to previously published methods.[4,5] For northern blot experiments, total and poly (A)$^+$ RNAs from rat brain stem were isolated, transferred to nitrocellulose, and hybridized with a 30 base [$^{32}$P]-labeled probe complementary to the 3' coding region of TH mRNA. The probe was labeled on its 5' end with [gamma-$^{32}$P] ATP and T4 polynucleotide kinase. Under these conditions a single species of RNA approximately 2.2 kb in length was detected, which is consistent with the published size of TH mRNA.[1] In addition, the hybridization signal obtained in the poly (A)$^+$ lane was considerably more intense than that for total RNA (data not shown).

In tissue sections, catecholamine cell groups were defined by both the presence of TH immunoreactive material and hybridization signal with an oligonucleotide probe labeled with either [$^{125}$I]dCTP or [$^{35}$S]dATP. Individual neurons containing TH mRNA were characterized by a dense collection of silver grains over the cytoplasm, with little or no labeling over the nucleus. Specific labeling for both protein and mRNA was

---

[a] To whom correspondence should be addressed.
[d] Present address: Cephalon, Inc., 145 Brandywine Parkway, West Chester, Pennsylvania 19380.

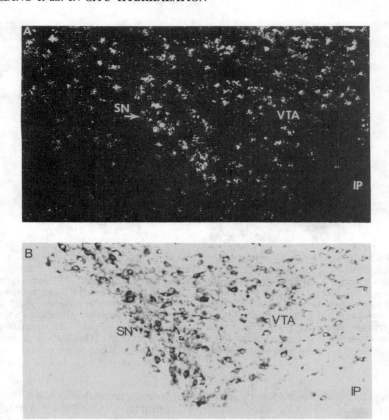

**FIGURE 1.** (**A**) Dark-field photomicrograph depicting the distribution of tyrosine hydroxylase mRNA in the substantianigra (SN). (**B**) Bright-field photomicrograph illustrating the distribution of TH-immunoreactive material in the same region of the SN. VTA: ventral tegmental area; IP: interpeduncular nucleus. Bar = 100 μm. Methods: A 30 base oligodeoxynucleotide complementary to a portion of the 3' coding region of TH mRNA was prepared according to previously published methods.[4,5] The oligomer was synthesized on an Applied Biosystems (Model 380A) DNA synthesizer and purified by reverse-phase HPLC on a μBondapak C18 column (Waters Associates). The 30-mer was labeled on its 3' end with [125I]dCTP or [35S]dATP and terminal deoxynucleotidyl transferase and separated on a Nensorb column (Dupont NEN) according to previously published methods.[5] The final activity of the probe was approximately $10^9$ counts per minute (cpm)/μg. Brain sections were fixed and cut according to the methods detailed in FIGURE 2. For *in situ* hybridization, sections were rinsed in diethylpyrocarbonate (1 μl/5 ml), incubated with Proteinase K (1 μg/ml in 20 mM tris-HCl, 2 mM $CaCl_2$, pH 7.4) for 15 min at 37°C) and incubated in hybridization buffer [2X SSC, 10X Denhardts solution, 50% formamide, yeast tRNA (85 ng/ml) and 0.1% denatured salmon sperm DNA] at 37°C for one hour. Sections were hybridized overnight with labeled probe (1.5 × $10^6$ cpm per slide, diluted in hybridization buffer) at 37°C. Slides were then washed to a final stringency of 0.5X SSC at 37°C, air dried, and either exposed to X-ray film or dipped in NTB2 nuclear track emulsion (Kodak) diluted 1:1 with $dH_2O$. Slides were exposed for 4 weeks in light-proof boxes at 4°C. Development was performed with Kodak D19 for 2 min at 16°C, washed in $dH_2O$ for 30 sec, and followed by 5 min fixation with Kodak fixer at 16°C. The slides were then washed in $dH_2O$ for 30 minutes, counterstained, dehydrated, and coverslipped.

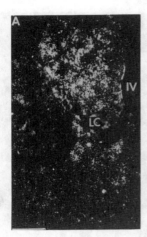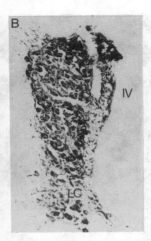

**FIGURE 2.** (A) Dark-field photomicrograph illustrating the distribution of neurons containing TH mRNA in the locus coeruleus (LC). IV indicates the fourth ventricle. Bar = 200 μm. On the right is a bright-field photomicrograph (**B**) illustrating the distribution of TH-immunoreactive neurons at this level of the locus coeruleus. Methods: Colchicine-treated (75 μg) rats were perfused with phosphate-buffered saline (pH 7.0) followed by 4% paraformaldehyde in 0.1 M sodium phosphate buffer containing 0.1 M lysine-HCl and 0.01 M sodium periodate. The brains were cryoprotected overnight in 30% sucrose. Transverse 30-μm sections containing the regions of interest were cut on a freezing microtome and processed for *in situ* hybridization, or immunohistochemistry using the avidin-biotin method and diaminobenzidine as the chromogen.

found in neurons in several regions, including the ventral tegmental area (A10 cell group), the retrorubral field (A8), subcoeruleus (A6), ventral lateral medulla (C1/A1), the incertohypothalamic cell group (A14–A15), as well as in the arcuate nucleus. The strongest hybridization signal was found in the substantianigra (SN) (A9) and the locus coeruleus (A6). Tyrosine hydroxylase immunoreactive neurons in the SN are present in the pars compacta; only a few scattered TH-positive neurons are observed in the zona reticulata (FIG. 1B). The distribution of hybridization signal observed with either X-ray film or emulsion autoradiography was essentially identical to that observed with immunohistochemistry and was generally limited to the zona compacta of the SN (FIG. 1A). In the locus coeruleus, the autoradiographic signal appeared as a dense cellular collection of grains over both small- and large-diameter neurons (FIG. 2). Specific labeling was not observed in the cerebellum or cerebral cortex.

The results of this study demonstrate the utility of synthetic radiolabeled oligodeoxynucleotide probes in the detection of specific TH mRNA within individual neurons *in situ*. The distribution of hybridization signal (mRNA) paralleled the distribution of TH-immunoreactive material in all regions of the rat brain. Future efforts will focus on factors that influence the expression of TH mRNA.

## REFERENCES

1.  GRIMA, B., A. LAMAROUX, F. BLANOT, N. FAUCON BIGUET & J. MALLET. 1985. Complete coding sequence of rat tyrosine hydroxylase mRNA. Proc. Natl. Acad. Sci. U.S.A. **82:** 617–621.

2. SCHALLING, M., T. HÖKFELT, B. WALLACE, M. GOLDSTEIN, D. FILER, C. YAMIN & D. H. SCHLESINGER. 1986. Tyrosine 3-hydroxylase in rat brain and adenal medulla: Hybridization histochemistry and immunohistochemistry combined with retrograde tracing. Proc. Natl. Acad. Sci. U.S.A. **83:** 6208–6212.
3. BEROD, A., N. FAUCON BIGUET, S. DUMAS, B. BLOCH & J. MALLET. 1987. Modulation of tyrosine hydroxylase gene expression in the central nervous system visualized by in situ hybridization. Proc. Natl. Acad. Sci. U.S.A. **84:** 1699–1703.
4. WOLFSON, B., R. W. MANNING, L. G. DAVIS, R. ARENTZEN & F. BALDINO, JR. 1985. Co-localization of corticotropin releasing factor and vasopressin mRNA in neurons after adrenalectomy. Nature **315:** 59–61.
5. LEWIS, M. E., R. ARENTZEN & F. BALDINO, JR. 1986. Rapid high resolution in situ hybridization histochemistry with radioiodinated synthetic oligonucleotides. J. Neurosci. Res. **16:** 117–124.

# Neurotensin Stimulates the Phosphorylation of Caudate Nucleus Synaptosomal Proteins[a]

SCOTT T. CAIN, MURRAY ABRAMSON, AND
CHARLES B. NEMEROFF

*Departments of Psychiatry and Pharmacology*
*Duke University Medical Center*
*Durham, North Carolina 27710*

A considerable literature has developed that documents the ability of the brain–gut tridecapeptide neurotensin (NT) to modulate brain dopaminergic (DA) neurotransmission in the central nervous system (CNS).[1] Defining the molecular signal transduction events coupled to the binding of NT to its receptor is an integral step in delineating the mechanisms of NT/DA interactions in the CNS. Our laboratory is now in the process of characterizing the role of protein phosphorylation in mediating the NT signal.

Adult male rats were decapitated and the caudate nucleus rapidly dissected and homogenized in 0.32 M sucrose. A crude synaptosomal fraction was prepared by centrifugation and resuspended in 150 mM Hepes buffer pH 7.1, containing 24 mM $MgCl_2$ and 0.5 mM EGTA. The lysed synaptosomes were preincubated at 30°C for 1 minute and then with $NT_{1-13}$ or vehicle for 5 minutes. ATP (containing $[\gamma^{32}P]ATP$, specific activity approximately 4000–5000 Ci/mM) was added for 1 minute before the reaction was quenched in SDS-denaturing solution. The final reaction concentrations were 50 mM Hepes, 8 mM $MgCl_2$, 1 mM $CaCl_2$, 0.17 mM EGTA, and 10 µM ATP. The phosphorylated proteins were separated on 10% SDS-polyacrylamide gels. The gels were fixed in acetic acid/methanol, stained with Coomassie Blue, and vacuum dried. Autoradiographs were prepared from the dried gels and phosphate incorporation into individual proteins quantitated by microdensitometry.

NT (0.75 µM) preincubation for 5 minutes increased the phosphate incorporation into proteins with approximate molecular weights of 76,000, 72,000, and 49,000 (FIG. 1). Phosphorylation of the 76 and 72 kd proteins was nearly 40% greater after NT preincubation ($p < 0.05$ and $p < 0.01$, respectively), while phosphorylation of the 49 kd protein increased approximately 20% ($p < 0.05$). We subsequently determined that the *in vitro* phosphorylation of each of these proteins was enhanced in the presence of calcium and phosphatidylserine (PS, 100 µg/ml, FIG. 2). It is interesting to note that the phosphorylation of a prominent protein of 59 kd, which is not altered by NT, is also not influenced by Ca/PS (FIGS. 1 and 2).

We have now demonstrated that NT alters the phosphorylation of multiple protein substrates in caudate nucleus synaptosomes. Our evidence that calcium/PS stimulates phosphate incorporation into 76, 72, and 49 kd substrates indicates that the calcium/phospholipid-dependent protein kinase (protein kinase C) regulates the phos-

[a] This work was supported by National Institute of Mental Health Grants MH-39415 and MH-15177.

**FIGURE 1.** NT preincubation increases the *in vitro* phosphorylation of 76,000, 72,000, and 49,000 protein substrates. Lysed caudate nucleus synaptosomes were prepared and phosphorylated in the presence or absence of 0.75 μM NT, as described in the text. Phosphorylated proteins were separated on 10% polyacrylamide gels and autoradiographs prepared from the dried gels. Phosphate incorporation into individual proteins was quantitated densitometrically. ($n = 3$.)

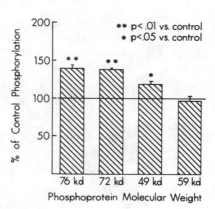

phorylation of these proteins. Our results are thus consistent with those demonstrating the coupling of NT receptors to phosphatidylinositol hydrolysis.[2] Future experiments will examine the hypothesis that NT receptors located on nigro-striatal dopaminergic terminals are coupled to PI hydrolysis, and thus alter DA synthesis and release by activating protein kinase C and the phosphorylation of specific protein substrates. We are also currently in the process of further characterizing the NT-sensitive substrates and correlating NT structure activity of the phosphorylation effect with the biological and receptor binding potency of NT and its fragments.

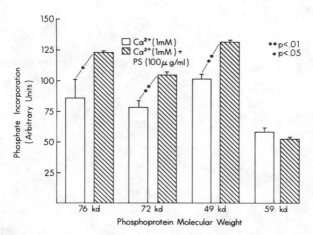

**FIGURE 2.** Phosphorylation conditions were identical to those described above except that samples were phosphorylated in the presence of either 1 mM $CaCl_2$ or combined 1 mM $CaCl_2$/100 μg/ml phosphatidylserine (PS). Phosphatidylserine potentiates the phosphorylation of the NT-sensitive 76, 72, and 49 kd protein substrates, but not a non-NT-stimulated 59 kd protein. ($n = 3$.)

## ACKNOWLEDGMENTS

Gratitude is expressed to Shelia Walker for assistance in the preparation of this manuscript.

## REFERENCES

1. NEMEROFF, C. B. & S. T. CAIN. 1985. Trends Pharmacol. Sci. **6:** 201–205.
2. GOEDERT, M., R. D. PINNOCK, C. P. DOWNES, P. W. MANTYH & P. C. EMSON. 1984. Brain Res. **323:** 193–197.

# Facilitory and Inhibitory Effects of Nucleus Accumbens Amphetamine on Feeding

LOIS M. COLLE AND ROY A. WISE

*Center for Studies in Behavioral Neurobiology*
*Concordia University*
*Montreal, Quebec, Canada H3G 1M8*

Amphetamine, once used for the treatment of obesity, has both facilitory and inhibitory effects on feeding. While high doses inhibit feeding, low doses can facilitate it. Facilitory and inhibitory effects are each associated with dopaminergic synaptic actions; facilitory effects occur in response to amphetamine microinjections into the caudate[1] and the nucleus accumbens,[2] while inhibitory effects result from higher doses in the accumbens.[2,3] The present study was designed to provide dose-response information and to compare *d*- and *l*-amphetamine isomers administered in each of the two sites.

The effects of intraperitoneal dosages of 0.0625 to 2.0 mg/kg on intake of sweetened mash in 16-hr food-deprived rats are shown in FIGURE 1. A significant increase was seen with 0.125 mg/kg, and significant decreases were seen with 0.5, 1.0, and 2.0 mg/kg; the other doses did not produce statistically significant differences from control levels of feeding.

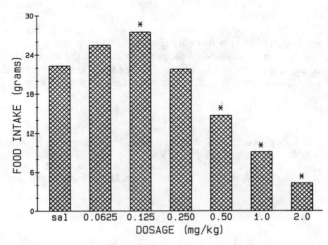

**FIGURE 1.** The effects of systemic amphetamine on food intake. *Asterisks* denote statistical significance.

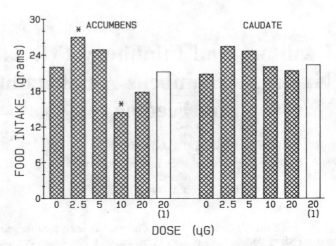

**FIGURE 2.** The effects of centrally administered amphetamine on food intake. *Asterisks* denote statistical significance. *Hatched histograms*: *d*-amphetamine; *open histograms*: *l*-amphetamine.

The effects of caudate and nucleus accumbens injections of 2.5, 5.0, 10.0, and 20.0 μg of *d*-amphetamine and 20 μg of *l*-amphetamine are shown in FIGURE 2. Only the nucleus accumbens injections of 2.5 and 10 μg of *d*-amphetamine produced statistically reliable effects; the 2.5 μg dose increased feeding while the 10.0 μg dose decreased it. There were no significant effects of *l*-amphetamine injected into either site. These doses of *d*- but not *l*-amphetamine similarly influence eating induced by lateral hypothalamic electrical stimulation.

The differential effects of the two isomers confirm that both the facilitation and the inhibition of feeding by these amphetamine injections involve dopaminergic actions; the two isomers are equipotent in their noradrenergic actions.[4] The greater effectiveness of nucleus accumbens injections suggests that both facilitory and inhibitory effects are triggered in this nucleus; spread of drug up the cannula shaft — the most frequent path of drug efflux — would carry the drug to the less sensitive injection site in the caudate. It is not clear whether the caudate injections act within the caudate or diffuse to the accumbens to cause their weak facilitory effects on feeding.

## REFERENCES

1. WINN, P., S. F. WILLIAMS & L. J. HERBERG. 1982. Psychopharmocology **78**: 336–341.
2. EVANS, K. R. & F. J. VACCARINO. 1986. Pharm. Biochem. Behav. **25**: 1149–1151.
3. CARR, G. D. & N. WHITE. 1986. Pharm. Biochem. Behav. **25**: 17–22.
4. WISE, R. A. & B. J. HOFFER. 1977. Physiol. Behav. **18**: 1005–1009.

# Influence of Neurotensin on Endogenous Dopamine Release from Explanted Mesoaccumbens Neurons *in Vitro*: Selective Activation of Somatodendritic Receptor Sites[a]

M. DUFF DAVIS[b,c] AND CLINTON D. KILTS[d]

*Departments of Psychiatry[c] and Pharmacology[d]*
*Duke University Medical Center*
*Durham, North Carolina 27710*

## INTRODUCTION

Ventromedial mesencephalic dopamine neurons are implicated in the etiology of certain psychiatric and motor disorders.[1] They receive synaptic input from a variety of impinging afferent elements. Cholinergic, GABAergic, serotonergic, catecholaminergic, and peptidergic (e.g., substance P, neurotensin, enkephalin) terminals, among others, may each provide a neurotransmitter or neuromodulatory role in the overall regulation of dopaminergic function and/or the manifestation of physiologic dysfunction. In addition, humoral agents may factor into this equation, as well. With present *in vivo* and *in vitro* methodologies, it is difficult at best to delineate the relative contribution of each of these components in this elaborate circuitry and which are critical in establishing predominant control over this dopamine system. In order to unravel some of these complexities, we have sought in this study to develop a simplified explant of the mesolimbic dopamine neuronal population that preserves the cell body-to-terminal continuum and that facilitates the examination of some of the basic neuropharmacology of dopamine neurons. Initially, we have focused on the effects of neurotensin (NT) on neurotransmitter release from the mesoaccumbens projection, as its receptor topography and physiological and behavioral responses on this neuronal population have been at least partially characterized.[2]

## METHODS AND MATERIALS

Immediately following decapitation, the brains of young (20–30 day old), male Sprague-Dawley rats were removed and chilled in ice-cold buffer. After 1 to 2 minutes, each

[a] This work was supported in part by National Institute of Mental Health Grant MH-39967, in part by Public Health Service National Research Service Award MH-15115, and in part by a grant from the United Way and the Gorrell Family Endowment.
[b] To whom correspondence should be addressed.

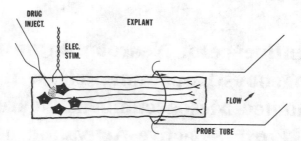

**FIGURE 1.** Schematic diagram of the explant perifusion method employed in this study. Neuronal cell bodies of the ventral tegmental and substantia nigra pars compacta (VTA–SNC) nuclei are depicted on the left with their terminal projections in the nucleus accumbens on the right. Dopamine is released from these endings into the surrounding media, which is then taken up by the "probe" tube and fed directly into the HPLC apparatus for catecholamine determinations. Alterations in the rate of basal dopamine release are monitored in response to administration of test agents or electrical stimulation to the VTA–SNC region.

brain was removed and two coronal cuts made, the first at a plane just rostral to the head of the caudate nucleus, the second at a plane just rostral to the brain stem. With the resulting brain block oriented caudal-face up, a sharpened, stainless-steel cannula (0.8 mm, id) was driven into the tissue with the aid of a vibrating pencil. The cannula was first guided through the lateral border of the ventral tegmental area (VTA) where it met the substantia nigra pars compacta (SNC), and then successively along the medial forebrain bundle and the nucleus accumbens, where it finally exited out the rostral face of the brain block. The explant, collected as an elongated cylindrical piece of tissue within the cannula (encompassing, in one contiguous unit, the A10 dopamine cell bodies, their axons, and terminal projections), was gently blown out into a small chamber where it was anchored and perifused with warm, oxygenated Earle's balanced salt media. The accumbens end of the explant was inserted partway into the end of a probe tube that, in turn, was connected to a peristaltic pump. The pump withdrew media surrounding the tissue and fed it directly into an automated high-pressure liquid chromatograph (HPLC) for the electrochemical detection of released dopamine (FIG. 1).

## RESULTS

Electrical field stimulation (1–30 Hz) of the explant VTA–SNC region evoked a frequency-dependent increase in baseline dopamine release from the nucleus accumbens. Administration of neurotensin (0.01–1.0 μM) to the perifusion media elicited a concentration-dependent elevation in dopamine (50–250% above control), but not serotonin efflux. During continuous infusion of neurotensin, the elevated dopamine level was sustained for up to 30 minutes, followed by a recovery to pretest levels, and there appeared to be no tachyphylaxis upon subsequent peptide administration. This effect was blocked by coadministration with TTX (1.0 μM), a neurotoxin that inhibits the formation of sodium-dependent action potentials. Following explant hemisection, which severs the axons in the medial forebrain bundle (MFB), neurotensin was ineffective in initiating dopamine release (FIG. 2).

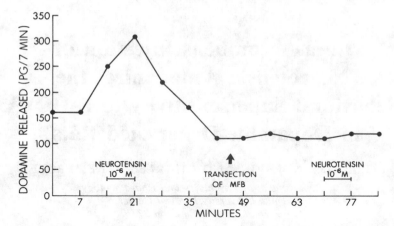

**FIGURE 2.** Profile of dopamine release from a single mesoaccumbens explant. Neurotensin (1.0 µM) administered to the perifusion media induced an elevation in neurotransmitter release from the intact, but not the medial forebrain bundle-lesioned (MFB), explant. This is suggestive of a somatodendritic, as opposed to a terminal, site of neurotensin receptor activation.

## DISCUSSION

Neurotensin binding sites have been identified in the VTA–SNC dopamine cell body area, with little or no receptors localized to mesolimbic terminal membranes in the nucleus accumbens.[3,4] Microinjection of neurotensin into the VTA *in vivo* initiates a pronounced elevation of dopamine metabolites in the nucleus accumbens.[5] Our results corroborate these observations by demonstrating a preferential pharmacological activation of mesoaccumbens dopamine neurons via somatodendritic, as opposed to terminal, neurotensin receptors. Furthermore, these studies address the utility of the explant procedure in the isolation of discrete neuronal pathways, and we are continuing to explore this model in the potential application to the extirpation of other neurotransmitter systems.

### REFERENCES

1. FLUCKIGER, E., E. E. MULLER & M. O. THORNER, EDS. 1985. The Dopaminergic System. Springer-Verlag. Berlin/New York.
2. DAVIS, M. D. & C. B. NEMEROFF. 1987. *In* Receptors and Ligands in Psychiatry. A. K. Sen and T. Lee, Eds. Cambridge Univ. Press. London/New York. In press.
3. QUIRION, R., C. C. CHUIEH, H. D. EVERIST & A. PERT. 1985. Brain Res. **327:** 385–389.
4. HERVE, D., J. P. TASSIN, J. M. STUDLER, C. DANA, P. KITABGI, J. P. VINCENT, J. GLOWINSKI & W. ROSTENE. 1986. Proc. Natl. Acad. Sci. U.S.A. **83:** 6203–6207.
5. KALIVAS, P. W. 1985. Neurosci. Biobehav. Rev. **9:** 573–587.

# Intra-Accumbens Injection of Neurotensin Antagonizes the Behavioral Supersensitivity to L-DOPA in Dopamine-Denervated Rats[a]

GREGORY N. ERVIN AND CHARLES B. NEMEROFF

*Departments of Psychiatry and Pharmacology*
*Duke University Medical Center*
*Durham, North Carolina 27710*

There is much evidence that neurotensin (NT), an endogenous tridecapeptide, modulates activity of the mesolimbic dopamine (DA) system.[1] Intra-accumbens injections of NT antagonize the behavioral arousal associated with activation of mesolimbic dopamine (DA) neurons, produced either by relatively low doses of amphetamine,[2] by intra-accumbens injections of DA,[3] or by bilateral injections of NT into the ventral tegmental area.[4] Endogenous NT is present throughout the cortex and limbic forebrain, along with NT receptors that are present both on DA terminals and elsewhere.[5] Are the behavioral effects of intra-accumbens NT due to an effect on NT receptors that are on DA terminals in or around the nucleus accumbens, or on NT receptors postsynaptic to DA terminals? To investigate this we observed the behavioral effects of intra-accumbens NT on rats treated with L-DOPA (ip). In our group of rats, limbic forebrain DA receptors were supersensitive because of the selective destruction of ascending DA neurons. In these rats with preferential DA receptor supersensitivity, but not in intact controls, L-DOPA induces behavioral arousal.[6]

Male CD rats (Charles River, Raleigh, N.C.), weighing 275–300 g, were pretreated with desipramine (25 mg/kg, ip), anaesthetized with sodium pentobarbital (25 mg/kg, ip), and mounted in a stereotaxic instrument with the upper incisor bar 5 mm above the interaural line. Bilateral injections were made in the anterolateral hypothalamus (A7.0, RL2.0, and 8.0 mm down from dura) of: (1) 9 μg (free base) 6-hydroxydopamine HCl (6-OHDA) and 0.6 μg ascorbic acid; or (2) ascorbic acid alone. Ascorbic acid, with or without 6-OHDA, was injected over 90 sec in 3 μl of 0.9% NaCl; the cannula was left in place 30 sec after the injection. Then all rats were implanted with guide cannulae aimed bilaterally at the nucleus accumbens (N. Acc.) (A9.4, RL1.5, and 4.0 mm down from dura). Injection cannulae of 28 gauge were cut to extend 2.0 mm beneath the guide cannulae into the nucleus accumbens. At 0700 hr on days 21 and 28 after surgery, all rats were placed in photocell cages (43 × 43 × 21 cm; Optomex 3/831, Columbus Instruments). At 1000 hr, half of the rats received an intra-accumbens injection of 5 μg NT (Bachem) in 1 μl, and half were held but no cannula was inserted. The rats then received intraperitoneal injections of L-DOPA (50 mg/kg) and were returned to their cages. For the following 2 hr, rats were observed for 30 sec every 10

---

[a]This work was supported by National Institute of Mental Health Grant MH-39415.

**TABLE 1.** Effects of Intra-Accumbens Neurotensin on L-DOPA-Induced Behaviors in 6-Hydroxydopamine- and Control-Treated Rats

| Behavior | Ascorbic Acid | | 6-OHDA | |
|---|---|---|---|---|
| | − NT | + NT | − NT | + NT |
| Locomotion and rearing | 1.4 | 0.4 | 10.4 | 1.8* |
| | (± 0.66) | (± 0.25) | (± 1.52) | (± 0.63) |
| General activity | 263 | 181 | 1285 | 362* |
| (photocell counts) | (± 35) | (± 45) | (± 198) | (± 70) |
| Sniffing | 3.9 | 2.0 | 16.9 | 6.0* |
| | (± 0.89) | (± 0.56) | (± 1.30) | (± 1.37) |
| Resting and sleep | 19.0 | 22.4 | 10.2 | 20.8* |
| | (± 1.58) | (± 2.09) | (± 1.97) | (± 1.17) |

NOTE: Behavioral score ($\bar{x}$ ± S.E.M.).
* $p < 0.05$.

min. Each 30-sec observation period was divided into three 10-sec time samples, and the incidence of the following behaviors was scored as described elsewhere:[2] (1) locomotion; (2) rearing; (3) sniffing; (4) grooming of head and forepaws; (5) grooming of hindlimbs and body; (6) resting throughout a 10-sec time sample; (7) sleeping throughout a 10-sec time sample. In addition, the number of photocell interruptions was used as a measure of general activity. On test day 28, each rat received the accumbens treatment opposite to that which it had received on test day 21. Behavioral scores following L-DOPA with or without NT were compared with the two-way, matched-pair t-test.

Following L-DOPA, ascorbic-acid-treated rats rested or slept, but showed few other behaviors (TABLE 1). All 6-OHDA-treated rats rested or slept significantly less, and showed significant sniffing and locomotion and/or rearing. The L-DOPA-induced arousal in 6-OHDA rats was antagonized by intra-accumbens NT. (Grooming behaviors were infrequent; NT had no consistent effect, and data are not presented.) The behavioral supersensitivity to L-DOPA in 6-OHDA rats is behavioral evidence for severe DA denervation and DA receptor supersensitivity. Because intra-accumbens injections of NT antagonize this behavioral supersensivity, NT must antagonize dopaminergic function postsynaptic to DA terminals.

**REFERENCES**

1. NEMEROFF, C. B. & S. T. CAIN. 1985. Trends Pharmacol. Sci. **6:** 201–205.
2. ERVIN, G. N., L. S. BIRKEMO, C. B. NEMEROFF & A. J. PRANGE, JR. 1981. Nature **291:** 73–76.
3. KALIVAS, P. W., C. B. NEMEROFF & A. J. PRANGE, JR. 1984. Neuroscience **11:** 919–930.
4. KALIVAS, P. W., C. B. NEMEROFF & A. J. PRANGE, JR. 1981. Brain Res. **229:** 525–529.
5. QUIRION, R., C. C. CHIUHEH, H. D. EVERIST & A. PERT. 1985. Brain Res. **327:** 385–389.
6. ERVIN, G. N., J. S. FINK, R. C. YOUNG & G. P. SMITH. 1977. Brain Res. **132:** 507–520.

# Regulation of Mesolimbic Dopamine Tracts by Cyclo(Leu-Gly)[a]

J. Z. FIELDS,[b] R. SAMI,[b] J. M. LEE,[b]
F. DELEON-JONES,[c] AND R. F. RITZMANN[c]

[b]Research Service
Hines VA Hospital
Hines, Illinois 60141

[c]Department of Psychiatry
Olive View Medical Center
Sylmar, California 91342

According to the dopamine (DA) hypothesis of schizophrenia, suppression of meso-limbic DA neurotransmission should be therapeutic. Therefore, we have been studying oligopeptides such as prolyl-leucyl-glycinamide (MIF, PLG) and cyclo (leucyl-glycyl) (CLG), a diketopiperazine, that appear to be dopaminergic neuromodulators and may be capable of just such a suppression.

Our previous report[1] showed that a single CLG injection (8 mg/kg, sc) to naive, male, Sprague-Dawley rats up-regulated striatal $D_2$ DA receptors. This was seen four days later (a) as an increase in apomorphine (0.5 mg/kg, ip) induced stereotypy (continuous sniffing), and (b) as a peptide-induced leftward shift in the curve for DA inhibition of [3H]spiroperidol (0.075-nM) binding to striatal membranes. The Ki for DA binding to the $D_2$-high site decreased from 81 to 1 nM. In the hypothalamus, on the other hand, after a single injection of CLG, $D_2$ DA receptors were down-regulated. This was seen as (a) a weaker hypothermic response to apomorphine (4 mg/kg), and (b) a shift of the DA inhibition curve several orders of magnitude to the right.

The main point of the current report is that the effect of CLG on the mesocor-ticolimbic DA tract turned out to be similar to CLG effects on the hypothalamus and opposite to CLG effects turned on the striatum. Rats were treated as previously stated with CLG. Four days later, we monitored amphetamine (1.5 mg/kg, ip) -induced locomotion. Following an acclimation period of 20 min, locomotor activity was automatically recorded (as counts per five minute time bin) for 30 minutes using the radiofrequency field capability of Stoelting Electronic Activity Monitors. Although there was no change in spontaneous locomotion (observed during the acclimation period), we did observe a 30 to 60% decrease ($p < 0.05$) in amphetamine-stimulated locomotor activity in the CLG-treated animals. Under these conditions the simultaneous incidence of intense continuous sniffing or other oral stereotypies (licking, gnawing) was less than 1%, thus ensuring that the decrease in locomotion was not due to suppression by other stereotypic behaviors that can emerge at higher doses of DA mimetics.

Increasing or decreasing the CLG dose (range 2 to 24 mg/kg) diminished the down-regulatory effect of 8-mg/kg CLG on amphetamine-induced locomotion. This bell-

[a] This work was supported in part by grants from the Veterans Administration.

498

shaped or invert-U-shaped dose response curve is typical for a number of the pharmacological actions of CLG and related peptides.

We also observed the effects of 8-mg/kg CLG on striatum and nucleus accumbens after only 1 day following a single injection of CLG. We found a quantitatively similar up-regulation in the nigro-striatal DA tract and down-regulation in the mesolimbic DA tract. Surprisingly, increasing the dose to 24 mg/kg produced the opposite effect in the striatum from that seen at 8 mg/kg. That is, apomorphine-induced stereotypic sniffing after the 24-mg/kg dose was significantly ($p < 0.05$) decreased.

CLG also down-regulated mesolimbic DA receptors in a model of mesolimbic supersensitivity. Haloperidol (1 mg/kg, sc) or vehicle was injected daily for 21 days to male Swiss-Webster mice. Compared to controls, there was a hyperlocomotor response to a challenge dose of apomorphine (1 mg/kg, ip) 48 hours following the last dose of haloperidol (87% increase in activity compared to vehicle-treated control animals, $p < 0.05$). Daily coadministration of CLG (2 mg/kg, sc) along with the haloperidol completely inhibited the development of this supersensitivity.

Although prevention of the development of mesolimbic supersensitivity is an exciting finding, most schizophrenics are first diagnosed with what is presumed to be an already established dopaminergic supersensitivity.[2] Thus it will be important to determine whether CLG can reverse an already established behavioral supersensitivity to dopamine.

## REFERENCES

1. LEE, J. M., R. F. RITZMANN & J. Z. FIELDS. 1984. Cyclo(Leu-Gly) has opposite effects on D-2 dopamine receptors in different brain areas. Peptides **5:** 7–10.
2. WONG, D. F., H. N. WAGNER *et al.* 1987. Positron emission tomography reveals elevated D2 dopamine receptors in drug/naive schizophrenics. Science **234:** 1558–1563.

# Effects of Phencyclidine on Ventral Tegmental A10 Dopamine Neurons in Rats with Lesions of the Prefrontal Cortex, Accumbens, and Dorsal Raphe Nuclei

ANGELO CECI AND EDWARD D. FRENCH[a]

*Maryland Psychiatric Research Center*
*University of Maryland*
*Baltimore, Maryland 21228*

Phencyclidine (PCP) is a well-known drug of abuse that can produce in man symptoms that mimic those seen in schizophrenia. While the exact mechanism by which PCP elicits its psychotomimetic effects is unknown, there is substantial evidence from animal studies linking the behavioral effects of PCP to dopamine-containing pathways, with the A10–mesolimbic–mesocortical components playing a major role in this regard.[1,2] Also, these same dopaminergic components are considered of pivotal importance in the self-administration of drugs of abuse.[3,4] Thus, a knowledge of the site and mechanism of action by which PCP influences the activity of the midbrain A10 cells may provide some insights into the pathophysiology of schizophrenia and possibly identify those processes subserving PCP's reinforcing properties. In the present study we examined the effects of PCP on the activity of A10 neurons in animals with lesions of the nucleus accumbens, prefrontal cortex, and dorsal raphe nucleus; structures containing high concentrations of PCP binding sites and/or providing putative afferents to the ventral tegmental area (VTA).

Standard extracellular recording techniques were used in chloral hydrate anesthetized rats to measure single-unit activity of presumptive A10 dopamine neurons within the VTA and their response to incremental iv doses of PCP.[5] In naive or sham-lesioned control animals, PCP produced a characteristic dose-dependent biphasic (increase/decrease) change in A10 firing rates with a peak effect in activity occurring at 1 mg/kg (FIG. 1). In rats with a kainic acid lesion of the nucleus accumbens, the overall response of A10 neurons to PCP was markedly augmented with a noticeable resistance to slowing of activity at higher doses (FIG. 1). Excitotoxic lesions of the prefrontal cortex, however, only slightly attenuated the overall response to PCP and did not alter the dose-dependent biphasic pattern (data not shown). In marked contrast, radio-frequency lesions of the dorsal raphe nucleus (FIG. 1) prevented almost completely PCP-induced changes in A10 firing rates. None of the effects could be related to baseline firing rates, which were not significantly different between the various groups.

These results provide the first evidence that some structures may differentially regu-

[a] Present address: Department of Pharmacology, Department of Medicine, Health Sciences Center, The University of Arizona, Tucson, Arizona 85724.

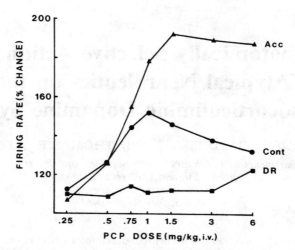

**FIGURE 1.** Effects of PCP on the activity of A10 dopamine neurons in animals with lesions of the accumbens (Acc) and dorsal raphe nuclei (DR). Neuronal responses in sham-lesioned and naive animals were not significantly different and were combined to serve as the control group (Cont). PCP dose is expressed as a cumulative amount and changes in firing as a percent of the basal rate. Activity changes were averaged across 8–12 animals per treatment group.

late and modify particular components of PCP's characteristic effect on the activity of A10 dopamine neurons. In particular, nucleus accumbens lesions augmented PCP's actions apparently by interfering with the rate-decreasing effects of the higher doses presumably mediated through postsynaptic elements within the accumbens. However, the prefrontal cortex seems to have little or no direct influence on the response of A10 cells to PCP, even though it may also be a primary site of action for PCP as inferred from its high concentration of PCP binding sites. Although dorsal raphe lesions were particularly efficacious against PCP-induced changes in A10 firing, further studies employing more selective lesioning methods will be needed to specifically implicate a serotoninergic involvement. Nevertheless, our findings, like those of others, would suggest that serotonin-containing systems may play a prominent role in PCP's central actions.[6] In a broader sense, these studies may yield some insights into specific neurobiological processes underlying PCP's psychotomimetic as well as reinforcing properties in man.

## REFERENCES

1. FRENCH, E. D. & G. VANTINI. 1984. Psychopharmacology **82:** 83–88.
2. FRENCH, E. D., C. PILAPIL & R. QUIRION. 1985. Eur. J. Pharmacol. **116:** 1–9.
3. SPYRAKI, C., H. C. FIBIGER & A. G. PHILLIPS. 1982. Brain Res. **253:** 185–193.
4. ROBERTS, D. C. S. & G. F. KOOB. 1982. Pharmacol. Biochem. Behav. **17:** 901–904.
5. FRENCH, E. D. 1986. Neuropharmacology **25:** 241–248.
6. NABESHIMA, T., K. YAMADA, K. YAMAGUCHI, M. HIRAMATSU & T. KAMEYAMA. 1983. Eur. J. Pharmacol. **91:** 455–462.

# Anatomically Selective Action of Atypical Neuroleptics on the Mesocorticolimbic Dopamine System

ELIOT L. GARDNER[a,b,d] AND THOMAS F. SEEGER[c]

*Departments of Psychiatry,[a] Neuroscience,[b] and Pharmacology[c]*
*Albert Einstein College of Medicine*
*1300 Morris Park Avenue*
*Bronx, New York 10461*

Both the antipsychotic action and the neurological (motoric) side effects of neuroleptic drugs are believed to result from blockade of brain dopamine (DA) receptors, the antipsychotic action resulting from mesocorticolimbic (A10) DA blockade, and the motoric side effects from nigro-striatal (A9) DA blockade. The atypical neuroleptic clozapine is a superior antipsychotic, but devoid of motoric side effects.[1] To examine whether this clinically atypical profile results from anatomic DA site-specificity, we studied functional DA up-regulation following chronic neuroleptic administration, using ana-

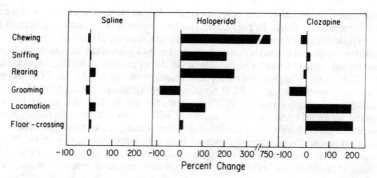

**FIGURE 1.** Percent change in apomorphine-induced mesocorticolimbic-mediated and nigro-striatal-mediated behaviors following 3 weeks of daily chronic administration of haloperidol (1 mg/kg/day), clozapine (20 mg/kg/day), or saline. The chewing, sniffing, and rearing behaviors, as measured in the present experiments, are dopaminergic (DA) stereotypies mediated by selective DA activation of the nigro-striatal (A9) DA system.[2,4,5] The locomotion and lateral floor-crossing behaviors, as measured in the present experiments, are DA stereotypies mediated by selective DA activation of the mesocorticolimbic (A10) DA system.[2,4,5] The grooming behavior is a non-stereotypic, non-DA-mediated behavior that decreases in duration as total DA-mediated stereotypies increase; it was included as a behavioral control. As can be seen, chronic saline had no effect on any A9- or A10-mediated behavior, chronic haloperidol (a classical or typical neuroleptic) significantly affected both the A9 and A10 DA systems, and chronic clozapine (an atypical neuroleptic) affected only the A10 (mesocorticolimbic) DA system.

---

[d] To whom correspondence should be addressed.

**FIGURE 2.** Differential effects of the typical neuroleptic haloperidol and the atypical neuroleptic clozapine on electrical intracranial self-stimulation (ICSS) from mesocorticolimbic (A10) and nigro-striatal (A9) dopaminergic (DA) brain loci. For these experiments, rats were implanted with brain stimulation electrodes in the ventral tegmental area (A10 nucleus) or substantia nigra pars compacta (A9 nucleus) and trained to self-administer ICSS. Three weeks of daily injections of haloperidol (1 mg/kg/day), clozapine (20 mg/kg/day), or saline were then given. Postneuroleptic ICSS testing was resumed on day 3 after the last drug injection, and continued at 2- to 6-day intervals for the next 32 days. As can be seen, chronic saline had no effect on either A9- or A10-mediated ICSS, chronic haloperidol (a classical or typical neuroleptic) significantly affected both A9 and A10 DA-modulated ICSS, and chronic clozapine (an atypical neuroleptic) affected only A10 (mesocorticolimbic) DA-modulated ICSS.

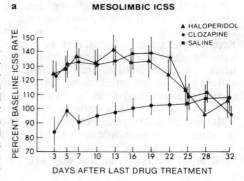

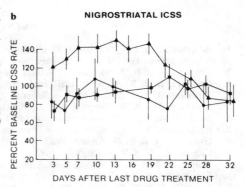

tomically specific probes of the A9 and A10 systems. To these ends, we adapted the paradigms of DA agonist-induced stereotypy[2] and electrical intracranial self-stimulation (ICSS) of brain DA loci.[3] For the stereotypy experiments, apomorphine-induced chewing, sniffing, and rearing (mediated by A9 DA activation[2,4,5]) and total locomotion and lateral floor-crossing (mediated by A10 DA activation[2,4,5]) were measured before and after 3 weeks of daily haloperidol, clozapine, or saline. For the ICSS experiments, rats were trained to perform stable baseline ICSS of either the ventral tegmental area (A10 DA nucleus) or substantia nigra pars compacta (A9 DA nucleus), and then given 3 weeks of daily haloperidol, clozapine, or saline.

In the stereotypy experiments, after 3 weeks of chronic haloperidol, apomorphine produced intense stereotypy, with large augmentation of both A9- and A10-mediated behaviors (FIG. 1). Three weeks of chronic clozapine produced no change in A9-mediated behaviors, but produced large augmentation of A10-mediated behaviors (FIG. 1). In the ICSS experiments in rats with A10 electrodes, 3 weeks of chronic haloperidol produced a robust increase in ICSS, as did 3 weeks of chronic clozapine (FIG. 2a). In contrast, rats with A9 ICSS electrodes showed postneuroleptic enhancement only after chronic treatment with haloperidol (FIG. 2b). In these A9 animals, 3 weeks of chronic clozapine produced no significant effect (FIG. 2b). Clozapine's lack of effect on A9 ICSS is also in marked contrast to the strong effects of other classical neuroleptics on A9 ICSS.[6,7]

These findings appear strongly suggestive of a functional selectivity of clozapine for the A10 DA system, a conclusion supported by a broad range of other behavioral, biochemical, and electrophysiological data.[8-10] We therefore suggest that clozapine's atypical clinical profile derives from mesocorticolimbic DA site-specificity of action. Recently, two groups reported that the addition of trihexyphenidyl to haloperidol imparts clozapine-like A10 site-specificity to haloperidol in electrochemical and single-neuron electrophysiological recording studies.[11,12] Preliminarily, we do not observe any shift in haloperidol's profile in our paradigms following the addition of atropine. Further, we question whether clozapine's atypicality derives from its anticholinergic potency, in view of anticholinergic-induced therapeutic reversal in psychotic patients treated with standard neuroleptics,[13,14] in marked contrast to the superior therapeutic efficacy of clozapine. We therefore conclude that clozapine's mesocorticolimbic site-specificity derives from other, as yet unknown, pharmacological properties. The elucidation of these properties is crucial, and may well yield superior antipsychotic drugs.

## REFERENCES

1. ACKENHEIL, M. & H. HIPPIUS. 1977. Clozapine. *In* Psychotherapeutic Drugs. E. Usdin and L. S. Forest, Eds.: 923–956. Dekker. New York.
2. COSTALL, B. & R. J. NAYLOR. 1977. Adv. Behav. Biol. **21:** 47–76.
3. CORBETT, D. & R. A. WISE. 1980. Brain Res. **185:** 1–15.
4. PIJNENBERG, A. J. J. & J. M. VAN ROSSUM. 1973. J. Pharm. Pharmacol. **25:** 1003–1005.
5. KELLY, P. H., P. W. SEVIOUR & S. D. IVERSEN. 1975. Brain Res. **94:** 507–522.
6. EICHLER, A. J., S. M. ANTELMAN & A. E. FISHER. 1976. Neurosci. Abstr. **2:** 848.
7. ETTENBERG, A. & R. A. WISE. 1976. Psychopharmacol. Commun. **7:** 117–124.
8. HUFF, R. M. & R. N. ADAMS. 1980. Neuropharmacology **19:** 587–590.
9. CHIODO, L. A. & B. S. BUNNEY. 1983. J. Neurosci. **3:** 1607–1619.
10. WHITE, F. J. & R. Y. WANG. 1983. Science **221:** 1054–1057.
11. CHIODO, L. A. & B. S. BUNNEY. 1985. J. Neurosci. **5:** 2539–2544.
12. LANE, R. F. & C. D. BLAHA. 1986. Ann. N.Y. Acad. Sci. **473:** 50–69.
13. SINGH, M. M. & S. R. KAY. 1975. Psychopharmacologia **43:** 103–113.
14. SINGH, M. M., S. R. KAY & L. A. OPLER. 1987. Psychol. Med. **17:** 39–48.

# Electrical Stimulation of Medial Prefrontal and Cingulate Cortex Elicits Bursting in a Small Population of Mesencephalic Dopamine Neurons

R. F. GARIANO[a] AND P. M. GROVES[b,c]

*Departments of Neuroscience[a] and Psychiatry[b]*
*School of Medicine*
*University of California, San Diego*
*La Jolla, California 92093*

Midbrain dopamine (DA) neurons fire spontaneously in a slow irregular or in a burst pattern. Bursts consist of two or more action potentials with an average interspike

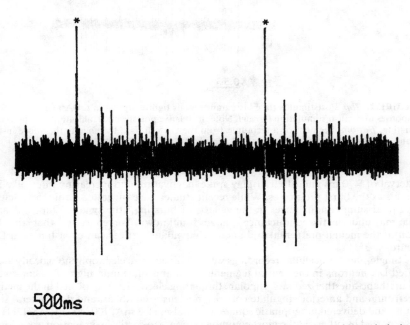

**FIGURE 1.** Recording from a mesencephalic DA neuron showing two consecutive cortical stimuli (*), each followed by bursts. Note the interspike interval of approximately 75 ms and spike inactivation.

[c] To whom correspondence should be addressed.

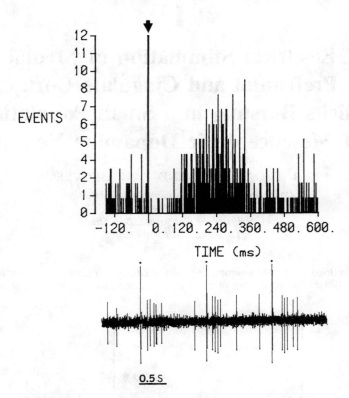

**FIGURE 2.** *Top.* Poststimulus time histogram reveals tight coupling in a DA neuron of burst responses to cortical stimulation (*arrow*). Note the relative poststimulus inhibition that precedes bursting. *Bottom.* Segment of a recording from the DA cell used to generate the above histogram, showing three consecutive cortical stimuli (*).

interval of $\cong$70 ms and often display spike inactivation and increasing interspike intervals as the burst progresses. While recent studies have suggested a role for calcium and potassium conductances in the genesis of bursting,[1] the synaptic input, if any, that may underlie the conductance changes is unknown. We report here that stimulation of the medial prefrontal and anterior cingulate cortices can elicit bursts in DA neurons.

Single-unit extracellular recordings were obtained from electrophysiologically identified DA neurons in the ventral tegmental area and substantia-nigra pars compacta of urethane-anesthetized rats. Bipolar stimulating electrodes were placed in the medial prefrontal and anterior cingulate cortices, nucleus accumbens, and dorsolateral striatum, and delivered monophasic square wave pulses (1–3 mA, 100–400 μs, 0.5–1.0 Hz). As reported by others,[2,3] the most common response to cortical stimulation was a long-lasting inhibition, occasionally interrupted by an excitatory response. A small percentage of DA neurons ($n = 13$) responded with bursts consisting of 3–7 spikes with an interspike interval of $\cong$70 ms (FIG. 1). The evoked bursts often displayed spike inactivation and progressively longer interspike intervals. Poststimulus time histograms were constructed to determine the coupling of the burst to the stimulus, as shown in FIGURE 2. We have seen cortically induced bursts in midbrain DA neurons with a wide range of firing rates and that were antidromically identified as projecting to striatum, accumbens, or prefrontal cortex. Relatively high stimulus current intensities were employed, suggesting that the relevant cortical elements are of high threshold or that current spread to more lateral cortical tissue might be required. Bursting was never seen in response to striatal or accumbens stimulation.

These data appear to be the first example of a brain region that can evoke bursting in DA neurons. Corticomesencephalic fibers as well as indirect routes via striatum, globus pallidus and subthalamic nucleus might mediate this effect. It seems likely that synaptic input is required for spontaneous bursts as well, since bursts are not seen in DA cells recorded in the de-afferented slice preparation.[4,5] It may be relevant that the evoked bursts were preceded by an inhibition (mean duration = 181 ± 27 ms; FIG. 2), possibly mediated by activation of striato-nigral and pallidonigral fibers. Whether the inhibition is necessary for genesis of the evoked bursts or is a coincidental concomitant of cortical stimulation is unclear; however, DA cells are reported to possess a low-threshold calcium spike that is activated at hyperpolarized membrane potentials and that in other brain regions gives rise to bursting activity.[6]

It has been speculated that bursts deliver large amounts of DA to circumscribed postsynaptic loci and affect the release of co-stored neuropeptides from DAergic terminals.[1] Our results suggest a specific means by which the frontal cortex can influence these effects in a small proportion of DA neurons.

## REFERENCES

1. GRACE, A. A. & B. S. BUNNEY. 1984. J. Neurosci. **4:** 2877–2890.
2. NAKAMURA, S. et al. 1979. Japan J. Physiol. **29:** 353–357.
3. THIERRY, A. M., J. M. DENIAU & J. FEGER. 1979. Neurosci. Lett. **15:** 103–107.
4. SANGHERA, M. K., M. E. TRULSON & D. C. GERMAN. 1984. Neuroscience **12:** 793–801.
5. SILVA, N. L. & B. S. BUNNEY. 1986. Soc. Neurosci. Abstr. **12:** 1517.
6. LLINAS, R., S. A. GREENFIELD & H. JAHNSEN. 1984. Brain Res. **294:** 127–132.

# Microdialysis in the Nucleus Accumbens during Feeding or Drugs of Abuse: Amphetamine, Cocaine, and Phencyclidine[a]

LUIZ HERNANDEZ, FRANCIS LEE,
AND BARTLEY G. HOEBEL

*Department of Psychology*
*Princeton University*
*Princeton, New Jersey 08544*

## INTRODUCTION

Microdialysis provides a valuable new tool for studying the function of dopamine (DA) systems. We have devised a small, removable probe that facilitates microdialysis during behavior in freely moving rats.[1] Earlier techniques showed that the DA metabolite, 3,4-dihydroxyphenylacetic acid (DOPAC), increased in the nucleus accumbens (N. Acc.) during free feeding, but not tube feeding.[2] DA changes could not be detected, perhaps because both extracellular and intracellular DA were measured together postmortem. In a similar study the DOPAC/DA ratio in N. Acc. tissue increased after eating a nutritive meal, but not saccharin.[3] Recently, microdialysis in the striatum (STR) showed increased DA during feeding at spaced intervals, but not free feeding.[4] We used microdialysis in the N. Acc. to measure DA and metabolites during free feeding, bar-pressing for food, and stimulation-induced feeding, then compared the effects with drugs of abuse.

## MONOAMINE RELEASE DURING FEEDING

Microdialysis was performed with a $0.2 \times 3.0$-mm probe perfused at 1 μl/min to obtain 20-min samples from the N. Acc. (A 10, L 1.2, V 7 perpendicular below cortex) assayed by high-performance liquid chromatography (HPLC) with electrochemical detection.[1] Five rats with implanted guideshafts were partially food deprived to 80% of normal body weight. When these rats were given food pellets to eat, extracellular DA, DOPAC, and homovanillic acid (HVA), but not 5-hydroxyindoleacetic acid (5-HIAA), increased significantly. DA increased from 7 pg/sample before eating to 10 pg/sample afterward. Thus DA turnover in the N. Acc. might be related, in part, to feeding in underweight rats.

[a] This work was supported in part by U.S. Public Health Service Grant DA-03597 and in part by the Campbell Soup Company.

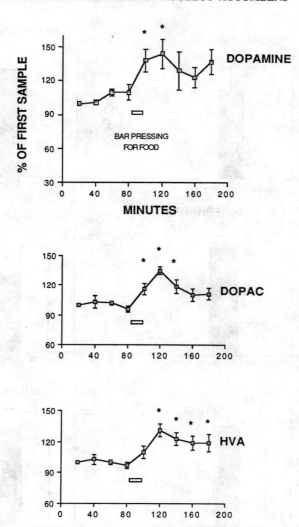

**FIGURE 1.** When hungry rats were given the opportunity to bar press for food pellets, extracellular dopamine, DOPAC, and HVA increased in the nucleus accumbens. (*$p < 0.05$ relative to baseline.)

## DEPRIVATION-INDUCED FEEDING

Seven, normal-weight, pretrained rats were food deprived for 20 hours, then allowed 20 min to press a lever for food pellets. DA, DOPAC, and HVA increased significantly during responding and eating. DA and its metabolites remained increased in the 20 min afterward when the rat was not eating (see Fig. 1).

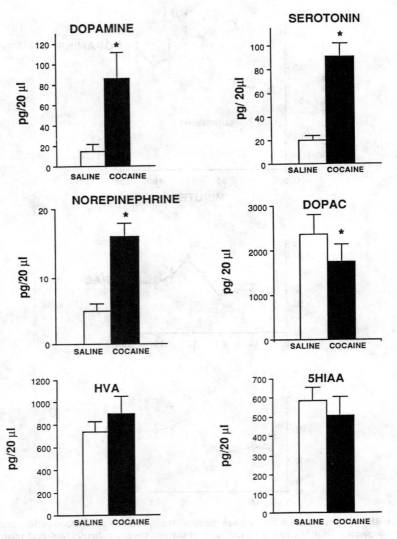

**FIGURE 2.** Effect of cocaine (20 µg in 0.5 µl) on a 20-min microdialysis sample taken 10 min after unilateral injection in the N. Acc. compared to the effect of saline injected at the same site in counterbalanced order. Cocaine increased DA, 5-HT, and norepinephrine while decreasing DOPAC. (*$p < 0.05$ relative to saline control.)

## STIMULATION-INDUCED FEEDING

Four rats, neither underweight nor deprived, were stimulated with unilateral, monopolar, perifornical lateral hypothalamic (A 6.5, L 1.5, V 7.5) current (0.1 ms, 100 Hz, 0.1–0.2

mA) to induce feeding. Again, extracellular DA, DOPAC, and HVA increased significantly, and the changes persisted afterwards. The same effect was obtained using stimulation or self-stimulation without food available. This is consistent with our earlier studies that suggested that lateral hypothalamic (LH) stimulation, which induces both feeding and self-stimulation, mimics the appetite whetting properties of food.[5-7]

## MONOAMINE RELEASE DURING LOCAL INJECTION OF THREE DRUGS OF ABUSE

Microdialysis was performed before and after injecting amphetamine (4 µg in 0.5 µl) or saline directly into the N. Acc. and the ventral STR of six freely moving rats by temporarily removing the microdialysis probe. The DA baseline increased (N. Acc.: from 9 pg/sample before injection to 147 pg/sample after; STR: 16 pg before to 409 pg after). Serotonin (5-HT) also increased (N. Acc.: from 8 pg before to 120 pg after; vSTR: 4 pg before to 200 pg after). DOPAC decreased significantly reflecting decreased DA metabolism likely due to the reuptake blocking properties of the drug. Cocaine (20 µg) increased extracellular DA and 5-HT fivefold in the N. Acc. and also doubled norepinephrine; DOPAC decreased; HVA and 5-HIAA were unchanged (FIG. 2). Phencyclidine (20 µg) increased DA 10-fold, doubled 5-HT at both sites, and decreased DOPAC.

These microdialysis experiments corroborate that the mesolimbic DA pathway functions as part of a self-administration system for both food and drugs of abuse.[8] The direct measurements of extracellular DA demonstrate for the first time that feeding behavior in normal rats increases extracellular DA concentration in the N. Acc.

### REFERENCES

1. HERNANDEZ, L., B. G. STANLEY & B. G. HOEBEL. 1986. Life Sci. **39:** 2629–2637.
2. HEFFNER, T. G., J. A. HARTMAN & L. S. SEIDEN. 1980. Science **208:** 1168–1170.
3. BLACKBURN, J. R., A. G. PHILLIPS & H. C. FIBIGER. 1986. Pharmacol. Biochem. Behav. **25:** 1095–1100.
4. CHURCH, W. H., J. B. JUSTICE, JR. & D. B. NEILL. 1986. Brain Res. **412:** 397–399.
5. MURZI, E., L. HERNANDEZ & T. BAPTISTA. 1986. Physiol. Behav. **36:** 829–834.
6. HOEBEL, B. G. 1985. Am. J. Clin. Nutr. **42:** 1133–1150.
7. HOEBEL, B. G. 1988. *In* Stevens' Handbook of Experimental Psychology. Atkinson *et al.*, Eds.
8. WISE, R. A. & M. A. BOZARTH. 1987. Psychol. Rev. **94:** 169–472.

# The Effect of Isolation Rearing and Stress on Monoamines in Forebrain Nigrostriatal, Mesolimbic, and Mesocortical Dopamine Systems

R. R. HOLSON, S. F. ALI, AND A. C. SCALLET

*Division of Reproductive and Development Toxicology*
*National Center for Toxicological Research*
*Jefferson, Arizona 72079*

Isolation rearing in primates produces bizarre stereotypies, self-mutilation, and asocial behavior. Humans in acute isolation sometimes experience thought disorders and hallucinations. Both syndromes bear superficial resemblance to schiziform disorders in humans. This resemblance may be more than coincidental. It has been hypothesized that schizphrenics suffer from an abnormality in the dopamine (DA) system of the brain, one perhaps localized in the prefrontal cortex.[1] Similarly, abnormalities in the prefrontal cortical DA system have been reported in isolate rodents.[2] Thus, animals reared in isolation may resemble human schizophrenics neurochemically as well as behaviorally.

We report here two experiments designed to further investigate the relationship between isolation rearing, stress, and the mesolimbic and mesocortical DA systems. In the first experiment, the subjects were reared in transparent plastic cages in isolation or in pairs from weaning (21 days) to 90 days of age. At that time, subjects were exposed to a 0-, 5-, or 20-minute forced swim in 25°C water, then sacrificed. The brains were quickly removed, and frontal pole, caudate nucleus, and nucleus accumbens were dissected out for analysis by high-pressure liquid chromatography, as previously described.[3] In experiment 2, grouped subjects were reared as previously stated (but 3 per cage), while isolates were housed in more restrictive hanging metal cages. At 90 days of age, all subjects were sacrificed within less then 2 minutes of removal from the home cage. The brains were dissected into the mesial frontal cortex, nucleus accumbens plus olfactory tubercle, hypothalamus, amygdala, and entorhinal cortex, then assayed as previously.

Isolation did not affect regional content of serotonin or its major metabolite in either experiment (data not shown). Neither experiment produced evidence for isolation-induced abnormalities in the forebrain DA system outside of prefrontal cortex (TABLES 1 and 2). In experiment 1, stress had no effect on concentrations of DA, diphenylacetic acid (DOPA), or homovanillic acid (HVA; TABLE 1). However, in both experiments isolation lowered frontal concentrations of DOPAC and HVA (TABLES 1 and 2).

It is concluded that, as previously reported,[2] isolation rearing reduces levels of DA metabolites in mesial frontal cortex. This effect is not seen in other DA-rich regions of the forebrain, nor is it seen in serotonin systems. Thus the reduction in DA metabolites in isolate prefrontal cortex is both robust and highly specific. This reduction does not seem to be a reflection of altered responsivity to stress. Isolation rearing may be

**TABLE 1.** Experiment 1: The Effects of Rearing Condition and Stress on Regional Concentrations of Dopamine and Major Metabolites

| Stress Duration | Rearing Condition | Frontal Pole | | | Nucleus Accumbens | | | Caudate Nucleus | | |
|---|---|---|---|---|---|---|---|---|---|---|
| | | DA | DOPAC | HVA | DA | DOPAC | HVA | DA | DOPAC | HVA |
| 0 minute | Isolation | 33.1 ±6.5 (8) | 6.5 ±0.9 (7) | 6.3 ±0.6 (7) | 716.5 ±92.5 (8) | 262.9 ±14.0 (8) | 56.1 ±8.4 (8) | 1280.5 ±159.3 (8) | 199.8 ±39.3 (8) | 73.4 ±6.4 (8) |
| | Social | 37.6 ±6.8 (8) | 8.0 ±1.3 (8) | 7.4 ±0.4 (8) | 503.8 ±39.5 (7) | 246.6 ±34.0 (7) | 32.5 ±7.8 (6) | 1428.3 ±109.2 (8) | 167.1 ±10.5 (8) | 70.9 ±3.8 (8) |
| 5 minutes | Isolation | 34.4 ±3.9 (8) | 7.0* ±0.8 (8) | 6.2* ±0.4 (7) | 622.1 ±52.9 (8) | 210.1 ±24.0 (8) | 32.0 ±2.7 (8) | 1269.3 ±130.2 (8) | 225.1 ±39.3 (8) | 71.1 ±4.8 (8) |
| | Social | 46.5 ±7.0 (7) | 11.1 ±1.1 (8) | 7.6 ±0.3 (8) | 674.1 ±122.8 (8) | 277.0 ±24.3 (8) | 49.1 ±3.9 (7) | 1428.4 ±47.6 (8) | 178.7 ±9.9 (8) | 70.9 ±2.9 (8) |
| 20 minutes | Isolation | 25.4 ±3.5 (8) | 9.3 ±1.8 (8) | 6.8* ±0.2 (8) | 753.9 ±90.5 (8) | 275.7 ±24.0 (8) | 68.8* ±17.8 (8) | 1542.2 ±65.5 (8) | 202.4 ±10.4 (8) | 79.2 ±3.5 (8) |
| | Social | 42.5 ±8.6 (8) | 10.1 ±1.2 (7) | 8.6 ±0.4 (8) | 642.2 ±69.3 (8) | 270.3 ±21.4 (8) | 47.0 ±3.9 (7) | 1245.0 ±105.0 (8) | 250.2 ±51.2 (8) | 80.5 ±8.1 (8) |
| Average over stress conditions | Isolation | 32.0 ±2.6 (24) | 7.6* ±0.7 (22) | 6.4* ±0.2 (22) | 697.5 ±46.0 (24) | 249.6 ±13.1 (24) | 52.3 ±7.1 (24) | 1364.0 ±73.6 (24) | 204.1 ±18.1 (24) | 74.6 ±2.9 (24) |
| | Social | 41.7 ±4.1 (23) | 9.7 ±0.7 (23) | 7.8 ±0.2 (24) | 611.0 ±50.7 (23) | 265.4 ±14.8 (23) | 43.4 ±3.3 (20) | 1367.2 ±53.7 (8) | 198.7 ±18.6 (8) | 74.1 ±3.1 (8) |

NOTE: All figures are in nanograms per 100-mg brain wet weight, plus or minus the standard error of the mean. Number of subjects in parentheses. (*Significant difference between rearing conditions, $p < 0.05$, 2-tailed t-test.)

**TABLE 2.** Experiment 2: The Effect of Isolation Rearing on Dopamine and Metabolite Concentration

| Brain Region | Rearing Condition | DA | DOPAC | HVA |
|---|---|---|---|---|
| Mesial frontal cortex | Social | 22.6 ± 4.4 (24) | 7.3 ± 0.8 (24) | 5.1 ± 0.6 (24) |
| | Isolation | 15.0 ± 1.5 (24) | 5.6 ± 0.4† (24) | 3.6 ± 0.2* (24) |
| Entorhinal Cortex | Social | 4.1 ± 0.5 (24) | 1.4 ± 0.1 (23) | Not detectable |
| | Isolation | 3.6 ± 0.4 (24) | 1.4 ± 0.3 (23) | Not detectable |
| Amygdala | Social | 53.8 ± 4.4 (24) | 14.2 ± 0.9 (24) | 4.9 ± 0.4 (24) |
| | Isolation | 52.1 ± 3.5 (24) | 12.5 ± 0.8 (24) | 4.2 ± 0.4 (24) |
| Hypothalamus | Social | 41.6 ± 2.4 (24) | 15.4 ± 1.1 (24) | 3.0 ± 0.3 (19) |
| | Isolation | 40.6 ± 3.4 (24) | 14.5 ± 1.3 (24) | 2.9 ± 0.3 (19) |
| Nucleus accumbens + olfactory tubercle | Social | 170.6 ± 12.6 (24) | 45.9 ± 4.2 (24) | 9.1 ± 0.7 (22) |
| | Isolation | 160.7 ± 15.0 (24) | 42.9 ± 3.9 (24) | 8.2 ± 0.7 (20) |

NOTE: Values in nanograms per 100-mg brain wet weight, ± S.E.M. Number of subjects in parentheses. (*$p < 0.05$; †$p < 0.06$, 2-tailed t-test.)

a convenient method for producing the abnormalities in prefrontal cortex suspected to accompany schizophrenia in humans.

## REFERENCES

1. LEVIN, S. 1984. Frontal lobe dysfunctions in schizophrenia. 1. Eye movement impairments. 2. Impairments of psychological and brain functions. J. Psychiat. Res. **18**: 27–72.
2. BLANC, G., D. HERVE, H. SIMON, A. LISOPORAWSKI, J. GLOWINSKI & J. P. TASSIN. 1980. Response to stress of mesocortical-frontal dopaminergic neurones in rats after long-term isolation. Nature **284**: 265–267.
3. ALI, S. F., J. M. CRANMER, P. T. GOAD, W. SLIKKER, JR., R. D. HANDISUR & M. F. CRANMER. 1983. Trimethyltin-induced changes of neurotransmitter levels and brain receptor binding in the mouse. Neurotoxicology **4**: 29–36.

# Alterations in Neurotensin- and Bombesin-like Immunoreactivity in MPTP-Treated Mice[a]

BETH LEVANT,[b,c] GARTH BISSETTE,[d]
YUKA-MARIE PARKER,[d] AND CHARLES B. NEMEROFF[c,d]

*Departments of Pharmacology[c] and Psychiatry[d]*
*Duke University Medical Center*
*Durham, North Carolina 27710*

1-methyl-4-phenyl-1,2,3,6-tetrahydropyridine (MPTP) is a neurotoxin that causes destruction of nigrostriatal dopamine (DA) neurons and subsequent symptoms resembling Parkinson's disease (PD) in humans and subhuman primates. The MPTP-treated mouse has recently been proposed as an animal model of PD.[1] In a previous study, we demonstrated decreases in the regional brain concentrations of the neuromodulatory peptides neurotensin (NT) and bombesin (BOM) in human patients with idiopathic PD.[2] One goal of these studies was to determine whether this murine model is an appropriate model of PD with respect to neuropeptide alterations. Adult, male, Swiss-Webster mice were injected daily with MPTP (30 mg/kg, ip) for 5 consecutive days. The mice were killed on day 10, the brains rapidly removed, dissected into 12 regions, and frozen. Brain regions were extracted and assayed for NT and BOM by sensitive and specific radioimmunoassays previously described in detail.[3,4] When compared to controls, the concentration of NT was decreased in the frontal cortex ($p < 0.01$), caudate ($p < 0.01$), and preoptic area ($p < 0.02$) of the MPTP-treated animals. An increase in BOM concentration was found in the amygdala ($P < 0.04$), whereas a decrease in the concentration of this peptide was observed in the preoptic area ($P < 0.05$) of the MPTP-treated animals (TABLE 1). Specificity of the DA neuronal degeneration was verified by reversal-phase HPLC assay[5] of caudate samples for DA, 3,4-dihydroxyphenylacetic acid (DOPAC), homovanillic acid (HVA), 5-hydroxytryptamine (5-HT), and 5-hydroxyindoleacetic acid (5-HIAA) (FIG. 1). Caudate DA, DOPAC, and HVA concentrations were decreased to 12% ($p \ll 0.01$), 28% ($p \ll 0.01$), and 42% ($p < 0.01$) of control, respectively. A decrease in 5-HT concentration to 69% of control ($p < 0.02$) was found, while 5-HIAA exhibited a nonsignificant increase to 118% of control, indicating a slight increase in 5-HT turnover. Although substantial depletion of striatal DA was observed in the MPTP-treated mice, the brain regions exhibiting changes in NT and BOM concentration differed substantially from those demonstrated in human idiopathic PD (IPD), where a decrease in NT was observed in the hippocampus and decreases in BOM concentration were found in the caudate and globus pallidus. The young mature MPTP-treated mouse would therefore appear not to be a satisfactory model of human PD with respect to neuropeptide

[a] This work was supported in part by National Institute of Mental Health Grant MH39415 and in part by the Scottish Rite Schizophrenia Research Foundation.
[b] To whom correspondence should be addressed.

**TABLE 1. Regional Neurotensin and Bombesin Concentrations in MPTP-Treated Mice**

| Brain Region | Neurotensin | | | | Bombesin | | | |
|---|---|---|---|---|---|---|---|---|
| | Control | | MPTP | | Control | | MPTP | |
| | x̄ ± S.E.M. | (n) | x̄ ± S.E.M. | (n) | x̄ ± S.E.M. | (n) | x̄ ± S.E.M. | (n) |
| Hypothalamus | 848.87 ± 48.62 | (11) | 799.76 ± 32.46 | (11) | 31.47 ± 2.43 | (10) | 37.23 ± 3.95 | (10) |
| Frontal cortex | 32.02 ± 2.48 | (11) | 20.13 ± 1.24 | (11)[a] | ND | | ND | |
| Cerebellum | 31.75 ± 2.77 | (11) | 28.16 ± 2.76 | (12) | ND | | ND | |
| Olfactory tubercles | 173.92 ± 18.64 | (10) | 183.67 ± 9.30 | (13) | ND | | ND | |
| Nucleus accumbens | 155.50 ± 21.34 | (11) | 139.59 ± 8.40 | (11) | ND | | ND | |
| Hippocampus | 37.34 ± 5.60 | (12) | 31.27 ± 2.02 | (11) | 8.53 ± 1.32 | (11) | 8.12 ± 1.17 | (10) |
| Substantia nigra/ ventral tegmental area | 229.41 ± 7.49 | (12) | 215.94 ± 11.68 | (13) | 6.58 ± 2.45 | (12) | 5.73 ± 3.56 | (12) |
| Septal area | 312.25 ± 16.17 | (11) | 292.16 ± 23.21 | (13) | 11.95 ± 2.33 | (10) | 17.61 ± 3.47 | (12) |
| Amygdala | 209.21 ± 18.03 | (12) | 168.45 ± 17.60 | (12)[b] | 3.66 ± 0.57 | (13) | 5.60 ± 1.72 | (12)[d] |
| Caudate | 142.13 ± 22.64 | (12) | 74.67 ± 10.06 | (11)[c] | ND | | ND | |
| Preoptic area | 1180.72 ± 111.10 | (12) | 862.48 ± 48.87 | (12) | 12.33 ± 2.44 | (13) | 6.21 ± 0.81 | (10)[e] |
| Globus pallidus | 186.15 ± 20.17 | (12) | 178.16 ± 25.22 | (12) | ND | | ND | |

NOTE: In the brain regions in which BOM was detectable, values below the detectable concentration were interpreted as the lowest detectable value for statistical calculations. NT and BOM concentrations are expressed as pg/mg protein. ND–Not Detectable.

[a] $p < 0.01$.
[b] $p < 0.01$.
[c] $p < 0.02$.
[d] $p < 0.03$.
[e] $p < 0.04$.

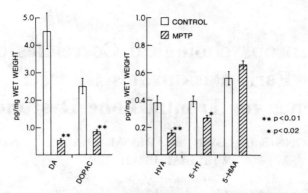

**FIGURE 1.** Effect of MPTP on DA, 5-HT, and their metabolites in the mouse caudate nucleus.

changes. Recent data, however, indicate that aged mice are more vulnerable to the effects of MPTP.[6] MPTP-induced alterations in peptidergic neurons should therefore be studied in aged mice.

## REFERENCES

1. HEIKKILA, R. E., A. HESS & R. C. DUVOISIN. 1984. Science **224:** 1451–1453.
2. BISSETTE, G., C. B. NEMEROFF, M. W. DECKER, J. S. KIZER, Y. AGID & F. JAVOY-AGID. 1985. Ann. Neurol. **17:** 324–328.
3. BISSETTE, G., C. RICHARDSON, J. S. KIZER & C. B. NEMEROFF. 1984. J. Neurochem. **43:** 283–287.
4. DECKER, D. W., A. C. TOWLE, G. BISSETTE, R. A. MUELLER, J. M. LAUDER & C. B. NEMEROFF. 1985. Brain Res. **342:** 1–8.
5. KILTS, C. D., G. R. BREESE & R. B. MAILMAN. 1981. J. Chromatog. **225:** 347–357.
6. LANGSTON, J. W., L. E. DELANNEY & I. IRWIN. 1986. Soc. Neurosci. Abst. **12:** 91.

# Neuropsychological Correlates of Early Parkinson's Disease: Evidence for Frontal Lobe Dysfunction

BONNIE E. LEVIN,[a] MARIA M. LLABRE,[b] AND
WILLIAM J. WEINER[a]

[a]Department of Neurology
University of Miami School of Medicine
Miami, Florida 33101

[b]Department of Educational and Psychological Studies
University of Miami
Coral Gables, Florida 33124

Patients with Parkinson's disease have been shown to exhibit a wide spectrum of neuropsychological deficits. However, it is unclear whether these cognitive impairments result from the dysfunction of specific neuroanatomical pathways. Furthermore, the order of appearance of the deficits and their relationship to the pathophysiology of PD are unknown. A major methodologic problem is that most investigators have collapsed their data across disease duration, combining subjects with Parkinson's disease ranging anywhere from 6 months to 33 years. The purpose of the present study was to identify the neuropsychological changes in patients with Parkinson's disease of less than two years duration.

The neuropsychological test performance of 32 patients with early Parkinson's disease (mean symptom duration 1.8 years) was compared with 32 normal controls matched on age, sex, and education. Parkinson subjects were evaluated in terms of stage of Parkinson's disease,[1] degree of disability (Comprehensive Motor Disability Scale), and independence in tasks of daily living (Northwestern Activities of Daily Living). All subjects received a comprehensive battery of neuropsychological tasks sampling five domains: language, visuospatial/constructive skills, attention and memory, judgment and reasoning and ability to shift set.

On language-related subtests, the PD group's performance was significantly more impaired than controls on a measure of verbal fluency [$t(62) = -2.46, p < 0.01$], months backwards [$t(62) = -1.76, p < 0.05$], and proverb interpretation [$t(62) = -3.06, p < 0.01$]. All other language skills (word retrieval, conceptual reasoning, and the ability to recite rote learned automatized information in sequence) did not differ between PD and control groups. For visuospatial functions, the PD group's performance did not differ from controls on tasks assessing visuospatial and perceptual judgments. However, Parkinsonian's ability to complete more complex spatial/constructive tasks involving integration of stimuli, such as recognizing faces [$t(62) = -2.56, p < 0.01$], discriminating between embedded line drawings of objects [$t(62) = -2.16, p < 0.05$] and geometric designs [$t(62) = -2.71, p < 0.01$], and constructing three-dimensional block designs [$t(62) = -2.40, p < 0.05$] was significantly more impaired than matched control subjects.

On tasks assessing attention, the PD group was significantly more impaired than controls on digit [$t(62) = -1.84$, $p < 0.05$] and block (visual) span [$t(62) = -1.75$, $p < 0.05$] and the ability to shift set on a card-sorting task [$t(62) = -1.75$, $p < 0.05$]. Performance was significantly impaired on all memory tasks. Compared to controls, the PD group's performance was significantly impaired on immediate and delayed recall of verbal discourse material and word lists ($p < 0.0001$ for all tasks) and geometric designs [$t(62) = -1.86$, $p < 0.05$].

Our findings suggest that Parkinson's disease of less than 2 years duration is already associated with significant neuropsychological deterioration. PD patients experience impaired performance on tasks of frontal lobe function. These include deficiencies in initiating, sustaining, and shifting between cognitive sets, formulating abstractions, and generating well-organized problem-solving strategies.

Luria[2] has suggested that frontal lobe patients may also do poorly on spatial tasks, not because of a primary visuospatial or perceptual disturbance but because of a higher level problem with planning, impulsivity, and a failure to self-monitor. The finding that the PD group did not significantly differ from controls on the more basic visuospatial and perceptual assembly tasks supports this hypothesis. By contrast, Parkinson patients were impaired on those tasks that rely on the ability to organize and integrate visuospatial material (encoding embedded figures and geometric designs, solving a complex facial-recognition task, and generating organized visuoconstructive strategies).

Although memory functions are traditionally assigned to the temporal lobes, Luria has suggested that frontal lobe damage may interfere with the organization of strategies for the retrieval of encoded memories. The improved memory performance after cueing suggests that the information was encoded correctly but the deficit involved accurate retrieval.

It is well recognized that the PD is caused by degeneration of mesolimbic and mesocortical dopaminergic systems. Dopamine transmission is required for normal frontal lobe function, and dopaminergic dysfunction produces deficits that resemble focal frontal lobe damage. We propose that the early cognitive deficits in PD may result from dysfunction of subcortical dopaminergic pathways projecting to the frontal lobes.

## REFERENCES

1.  HOEHN, M. M. & M. D. YAHR. 1967. Parkinsonism: Onset, progression and mortality. *Neurology* 17: 427–442.
2.  LURIA, A. R. 1980. Higher Cortical Functions in Man, 2nd ed. Basic Books. New York.

# Distinct Dopamine Terminal Areas Controlling Behavioral Activation and Reward Value of Hypothalamic Stimulation

DARRYL NEILL

*Department of Psychology*
*Emory University*
*Atlanta, Georgia 30322*

In the research reported here, I have taken the approach that, by combining a discriminant behavioral analysis with local manipulation of brain DA systems, the motoric/arousal functions of DA can be separated from the reward function for intracranial self-stimulation (ICSS).

We use the autotitration ICSS procedure. In my version, the intensity of hypothalamic stimulation is stepped down 3 μA upon every fifth depression of a stimulation lever. The rat is free to travel to another lever that, when depressed, resets the intensity to the maximum value for that rat. The rat then returns to the stimulation lever and the stepping-down process starts anew.

Because injections of the DA receptor blocker haloperidol into nucleus accumbens septi (NAS) reduce ICSS in the more typical single-lever procedure, we expected that such injections would produce earlier resetting; that is, the rats would no longer tolerate low currents. We found, however, that intra-NAS haloperidol injections produced *later* resetting.[1] Recently, we have found the same later resetting to follow injections of the catecholamine neurotoxin 6-hydroxydopamine (6-OHDA) into NAS. My interpretation of these data is that DA in NAS has little to do with the reward of hypothalamic stimulation. Instead, NAS DA is involved in setting a general activational level. Injection of haloperidol into NAS produces a sluggish rat that will bar-press but is less likely to reset.

Systemic injections of haloperidol produce earlier resetting and reduce single-lever responding; that is, they reduce reward value. Because of our results with NAS, we have searched for a DA terminal region that regulates reward value. I report here that this region seems to be in a zone encompassing portions of the amygdala and overlying "central" neostriatum. Injections of 6-OHDA that deplete this region of DA have little effect on the general activational level of the rat as measured in activity devices. However, these injections produce much earlier resetting in autotitration and reduce single-lever ICSS. The rats look rather unexcited by the stimulation and in autotitration repeatedly respond on the reset lever, a phenomenon usually seen when the current is drastically reduced.

In conclusion, we find that DA in NAS has an activational function; DA in central striatum/amygdala seems to regulate the reward value of hypothalamic stimulation.

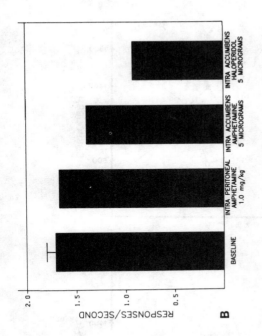

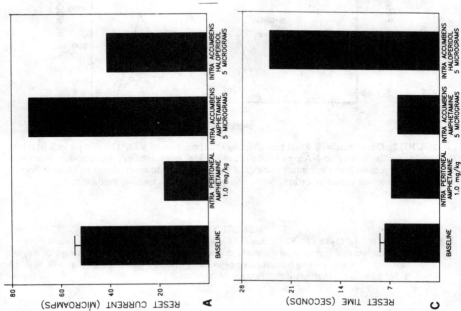

**FIGURE 1.** Data from a single rat (84–185) illustrating the effect of injections of the DA agonist amphetamine and the DA antagonist haloperidol into the NAS on three parameters of autotitration ICSS. **(A)** Mean reset intensity; **(B)** mean response rate; **(C)** mean reset time. Note that while intraperitoneally injected amphetamine produces *later* resetting, intra-NAS injection produces *earlier* resetting. Dose-response studies have shown that this unexpected effect of intra-NAS injections occurs at all doses (0.125–5 μg) tested.

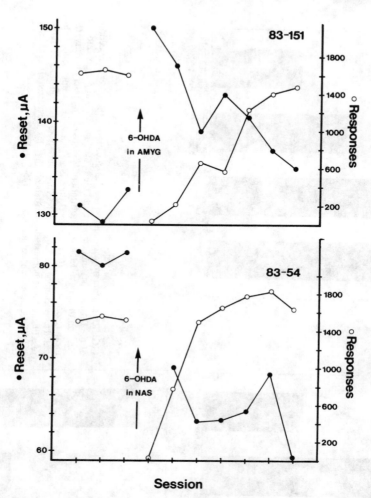

**FIGURE 2.** Data from individual rats showing that injection of 6-OHDA (5.6 µg in 2 µl 0.1% ascorbic acid vehicle) into NAS, as with the haloperidol in FIGURE 1, produces later resetting. The same injection into the central nucleus of the amygdala, however, seems to blunt ICSS reward and produce earlier resetting. Note that both injections reduce response rate.

**REFERENCE**

1. NEILL, D. B., L. GAAR, A. S. CLARK & M. D. BRITT. 1982. "Rate-free" measures of self-stimulation and intracranial microinjections: Evidence toward a new concept of dopamine and reward. *In* The Neural Basis of Feeding and Reward. B. Hoebel and D. Novin, Eds.: 289–297. Haer Institute. Brunswick, Maine.

# Increased Motivation to Self-Administer Apomorphine following 6-Hydroxydopamine Lesions of the Nucleus Accumbens

DAVID C. S. ROBERTS AND G. VICKERS

*Department of Psychology*
*Carleton University*
*Ottawa, Ontario, Canada, K1S 5B6*

## INTRODUCTION

We have previously shown that 6-hydroxydopamine (6-OHDA) -induced lesions of mesolimbic DA cell bodies[1] or DA terminals in the nucleus accumbens[2] cause extinction of intravenous cocaine self-administration. These data are consistent with the idea that cocaine is an indirect acting agonist at dopamine (DA) receptors, and that the presynaptic element is necessary for cocaine to have a reinforcing effect. By contrast, the self-administration rate of apomorphine (APO), a direct DA agonist, is not affected by 6-hydroxydopamine lesions of the accumbens. Indeed, the same lesioned animals that fail to respond for cocaine injections have been shown to self-administer apomorphine at prelesion rates.[2]

The failure of DA denervation to affect the rate of apomorphine self-administration has been puzzling. If the reinforcing action of apomorphine is mediated via stimulation of DA receptors in the accumbens, and if 6-OHDA lesions induce DA receptor supersensitivity, then the rewarding effects of apomorphine should be enhanced, and some change in apomorphine intake would be expected. The implication is that either DA receptors do not mediate the reinforcing effects of apomorphine or, more likely, the rate of self-administration does not reflect reward strength. We have therefore reinvestigated the effect of 6-OHDA lesions on apomorphine self-administration using a progressive ratio schedule of reinforcement.

## MATERIALS AND METHODS

Rats were prepared with chronically indwelling jugular cannulae and trained to self-administer apomorphine on a progressive ratio schedule. At the beginning of each session, rats earned an injection of apomorphine with only a few lever responses, but with each infusion the requirements of the schedule increased. The "breakpoint" was established each day, and was defined as the last reinforcement ratio completed in the 5-hour session. (The ratios were such that it was unusual for an animal to earn an infusion in the last hour.) When tested following surgery, most animals in the 6-OHDA group showed dramatic increases in their breakpoints, whereas no consistent changes

523

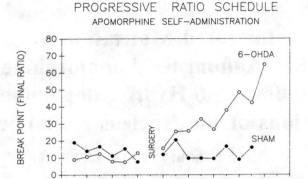

**FIGURE 1.** The effect of 6-OHDA lesions of the nucleus accumbens on breakpoints determined during apomorphine self-administration. Each point represents the daily mean of 6-OHDA or control groups.

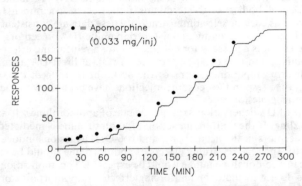

**FIGURE 2.** Record of a 6-OHDA-treated animal self-administering apomorphine. The *line* represents the cumulative responses and the *dots* represent infusions. The final ratio achieved in this case was 47.

were observed in the control group. FIGURE 1 shows the mean final ratios achieved by groups of 6-OHDA lesioned and control rats before and after surgery. These data demonstrate that 6-OHDA-treated animals show an increased motivation to self-administer apomorphine that progresses daily after the lesion and may parallel the development of supersensitive DA receptors.

### REFERENCES

1. ROBERTS, D. C. S. & G. F. KOOB. 1982. Pharmacol. Biochem. Behav. **17:** 901–904.
2. ROBERTS, D. C. S., M. E. CORCORAN & H. C. FIBIGER. 1977. Pharmacol. Biochem. Behav. **6:** 615–620.

# A Study of the Interactions of Pimozide, Morphine, and Muscimol on Brain Stimulation Reward: Behavioral Evidence for Depolarization Inactivation of A10 Dopaminergic Neurons

PIERRE-PAUL ROMPRÉ AND ROY A. WISE

*Center for Studies in Behavioral Neurobiology*
*Concordia University*
*Montreal, Quebec, Canada H3G 1M8*

Electrophysiological experiments have revealed that systemic administration of dopaminergic antagonists or local administration of morphine increases the firing rate of A10 dopaminergic neurons.[1,2] Sustained excitation of these neurons can result in depolarization inactivation, and, in this case, dopaminergic cell firing can be paradoxically reinitiated by local application of gamma-aminobutyric acid (GABA), an inhibitory neurotransmitter.[1] The present experiments represent a behavioral parallel for these electrophysiological studies.

In the first experiment, we tested the ability of central injection of morphine to reverse attenuation of brain stimulation reward by a systemic injection of pimozide. Rats were implanted with a stimulating electrode in the medial brain stem and a guide cannula in the area of the A10 dopaminergic neurons. Brain-stem self-stimulation (SS) was first stabilized and tests were made in the following order: (1) determination of baseline SS threshold; (2) systemic injection of pimozide (0.35 mg/kg, ip) or its vehicle and determination of SS threshold 4.5 hours later for 30 minutes; (3) central injection of morphine (1.25, 2.5, and 5.0 μg/0.25 μl) or its vehicle and repeated determination of SS threshold for 90 minutes; (4) systemic injection of naloxone (2.0 mg/kg, ip) or its vehicle and repeated determination of SS threshold for 60 minutes. SS threshold was significantly increased by pimozide. Morphine was found effective in reversing the effect of pimozide and naloxone blocked the reversal effect of morphine (FIG. 1, top panel). However, in some cases morphine, instead of reversing the effect of pimozide, completely abolished self-stimulation (FIG. 1, bottom panel). This unexpected result might reflect a depolarization inactivation of the A10 dopaminergic cells due to a combined action of pimozide and morphine on A10 firing rate. To test this hypothesis, we studied the ability of muscimol (a GABA agonist) to reinitiate SS behavior after administration of pimozide and morphine.

The following tests were made after stabilization of SS behavior: (1) determination of baseline SS threshold; (2) systemic injection of pimozide (0.175 or 0.35 mg/kg, ip) and determination of SS threshold 4.5 hours later for 30 minutes; (3) central injection

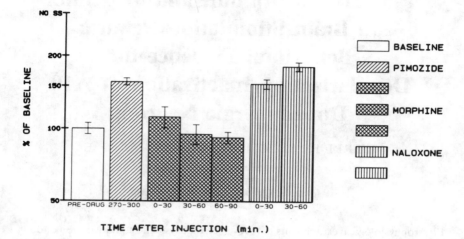

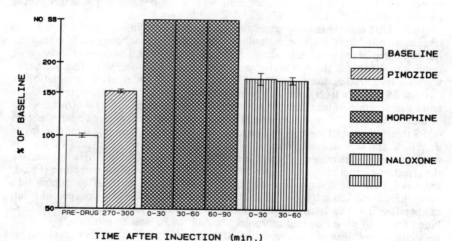

**FIGURE 1.** Interactions between pimozide, morphine, and naloxone on brain-stem self-stimulation threshold of rat P6 (*top panel*) and rat P7 (*bottom panel*). Results are expressed as percentage of predrug (*baseline*).

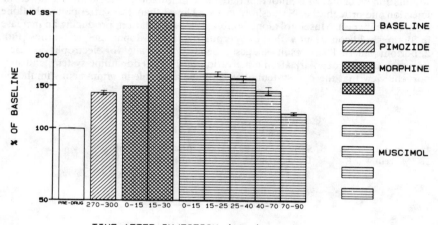

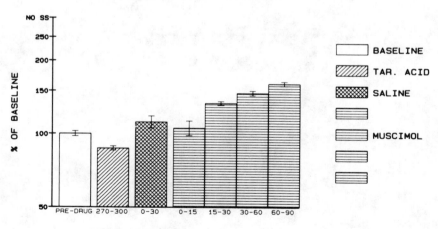

**FIGURE 2.** *Top panel*: Interactions between pimozide, morphine, and muscimol on brain-stem self-stimulation threshold. *Bottom panel*: The effect of muscimol injection into the ventral tegmental area on brain-stem self-stimulation threshold. Results are expressed as percentage of predrug (*baseline*).

of morphine (2.5–5.0 µg/0.25 µl) and repeated determination of SS threshold for 30 minutes; (4) central injection of muscimol (12.5–25 ng/0.25 µl) or its vehicle and repeated determination of SS threshold for 90 minutes. As expected, pimozide increased SS threshold, and morphine at these dose combinations completely abolished self-stimulation behavior. Muscimol reinitiated self-stimulation 15 to 30 minutes after the injection and brought the SS threshold to a level lower than it was after pimozide alone (FIG. 2, top panel). Muscimol alone inhibited self-stimulation, producing an increase in SS threshold consistent with the hyperpolarization of dopaminergic neurons (FIG. 2, bottom panel). These results suggest a behavioral parallel for electrophysiological demonstration of depolarization inactivation of the A10 dopamine system, and support the view that the A10 system plays an important role in brain-stem stimulation reward.

## REFERENCES

1.  CHIODO, L. A. & B. S. BUNNEY. 1983. J. Neurosci. **8:** 1607–1619.
2.  MATTHEWS, R. T. & D. C. GERMAN. 1984. Neuroscience **11:** 617–625.

# Pharmacology of Dopamine-Induced Electrophysiological Responses in the Rat Prefrontal Cortex: $D_1$- or $D_2$-Mediated?

## SUSAN R. SESACK[a] AND BENJAMIN S. BUNNEY[b,c]

*Departments of Pharmacology[a] and Psychiatry[b]*
*Yale University School of Medicine*
*New Haven, Connecticut 06510–8066*

Cells in the deep layers of the medial prefrontal cortex (PFC) have been shown to be inhibited by iontophoretically applied dopamine (DA)[1] and by stimulation of cortically projecting DA neurons in the ventral tegmental area (VTA).[2,3] Pharmacological studies have demonstrated that the receptor mediating the inhibitory effects of DA is distinct from adrenergic receptors and is uniquely dopaminergic.[4] However, the subtype of DA receptor involved ($D_1$ or $D_2$) has not yet been determined. Therefore, single-unit extracellular recording and microiontophoretic techniques were used to complete the pharmacological characterization of the receptor mediating DA-induced inhibition in the PFC.

**TABLE 1.** Effect of Selective Dopamine Receptor Antagonists on Dopamine-Sensitive Neurons in the Medial PFC

| | Reversible Antagonism of DA Inhibition | No Effect |
|---|---|---|
| $D_2$ antagonist ( − )sulpiride ($n = 30$) | 25 (83%) | 5 (17%) |
| $D_1$ antagonist SCH 23390 ($n = 12$) | 3 (25%) | 9 (75%) |

Studies using selective antagonists revealed that the $D_2$ selective blocker, ( − )sulpiride, but not the $D_1$ selective blocker, SCH 23390, antagonized DA's inhibitory effects on the majority of cells tested (TABLE 1). Surprisingly, the results of experiments examining the effects of iontophoretically applied selective agonists revealed that neither the $D_2$ selective agonist, LY 171555, nor the $D_1$ selective agonist, SKF 38393, inhibited the majority of DA-sensitive PFC neurons (TABLE 2). The nonselective agonist, pergolide, did, however, produce inhibitory effects on most DA-sensitive cells tested (TABLE 2).

Though unexpected, the lack of effect of selective DA agonists suggested that combined stimulation of $D_1$ and $D_2$ receptors might be necessary to inhibit DA-sensitive cells in the PFC. Coadministration of $D_1$ and $D_2$ agonists has been reported to induce

---

[c] To whom correspondence should be addressed.

**TABLE 2.** Effect of Selective Dopamine Receptor Agonists on Dopamine-Sensitive Neurons in the Medial PFC

|  | Inhibition | Inhibition Followed by Excitation | Excitation | No Effect |
|---|---|---|---|---|
| $D_2$ selective |  |  |  |  |
| LY 171555 |  |  |  |  |
| ($n = 62$) | 3 (5%) | 3 (5%) | 2 (3%) | 54 (87%) |
| $D_1$ selective |  |  |  |  |
| SKF 38393 |  |  |  |  |
| ($n = 46$) | 4 (9%) | 2 (4%) | 1 (2%) | 39 (85%) |
| $D_2$ selective + $D_1$ selective |  |  |  |  |
| LY 171555 + SKF 38393 |  |  |  |  |
| ($n = 17$) | 0 | 0 | 0 | 17 (100%) |
| $D_1/D_2$ nonselective |  |  |  |  |
| pergolide |  |  |  |  |
| ($n = 28$) | 18 (64%) | 0 | 0 | 10 (36%) |

potentiated responses in the globus pallidus and nucleus accumbens.[5,6] However, co-iontophoresis of LY 171555 and SKF 38393 did not inhibit DA-sensitive PFC cells (TABLE 2).

In contrast to the results of iontophoretic experiments, it was found that intravenous injection of LY 171555 (in doses as low as 5 µg/kg) did inhibit DA-sensitive neurons in the PFC. Systemic administration of SKF 38393 produced only weak inhibition, even in doses up to 20 mg/kg. Furthermore, these doses of SKF 38393 did not potentiate the response of PFC neurons to subthreshold doses of LY 171555.

Thus, experiments with locally or systemically administered agonists failed to provide evidence for a potentiating interaction between $D_1$ and $D_2$ receptors in the PFC. While the observed effects of iontophoretically applied antagonists and intravenously administered agonists suggest that DA is acting on a receptor with $D_2$ characteristics, the lack of effect of locally applied agonists suggests that the DA receptor in the PFC may not conform to the pharmacological definition of either $D_1$ or $D_2$ subtypes.

## REFERENCES

1. BUNNEY, B. S. & G. K. AGHAJANIAN. 1976. Life Sci. **19:** 1783–1792.
2. FERRON, A., A. M. THIERRY, C. LE DOUARIN & J. GLOWINSKI. 1984. Brain. Res. **302:** 257–265.
3. THIERRY, A. M., C. LE DOUARIN, J. PENIT, A. FERRON & J. GLOWINSKI. 1986. Brain. Res. Bull. **16:** 155–160.
4. BUNNEY, B. S. & L. A. CHIODO. 1984. *In* Monoamine Innervation of Cerebral Cortex. L. Descarries, T. R. Reader, and H. H. Jasper, Eds.: 263–277. Alan Liss. New York.
5. CARLSON, J. H., D. A. BERGSTROM & J. R. WALTERS. 1986. Brain. Res. **400:** 205–218.
6. WHITE, F. J. 1987. Eur. J. Pharmacol. **135:** 101–105.

# Rat Mesocortical Dopaminergic Neurons Are Mixed Neurotensin/Dopamine Neurons: Immunohistochemical and Biochemical Evidence

J. P. TASSIN,[a] P. KITABGI,[b] G. TRAMU,[c]
J. M. STUDLER,[a] D. HERVÉ,[a] F. TROVERO,[a]
AND J. GLOWINSKI[a]

[a]INSERM U. 114
Collège de France
Paris, France

[b]Laboratoire de Biochimie
Centre National de la Recherche Scientifique
Nice, France

[c]INSERM U. 156
Lille, France

In 1984, Hökfelt et al.[1] demonstrated the presence of neurotensin (NT), a tridecapeptide isolated by Leeman and co-workers,[2] in some dopaminergic (DA) cell bodies of the rat ventral tegmental area (VTA). However, projection sites of these mixed neurons remain to be identified. Although an NT projection from the VTA to the nucleus accumbens has been described,[3] the endogenous peptide content in limbic areas as well as in the striatum is not affected by destruction of the DA neurons following an intracerebroventricular injection of 6-hydroxydopamine (6-OHDA).[4] Nevertheless, the striking similarity of distribution between NT binding sites and $D_1$ receptors in the prefrontal cortex (FIG. 1) indicates that a mixed NT/DA innervation could occur in this region, and led us to examine the effects of a 6-OHDA lesion of the VTA on the endogenous NT concentrations in the forebrain DA areas. We present here biochemical and immunohistochemical evidence that most of the DA mesocortical neurons contain NT.

Bilateral injections of 6-OHDA into the VTA (4 µg in 1 µl), which induced important decreases of DA in the prefrontal cortex (− 84%), in the nucleus accumbens (− 95%), and in the anterior striatum (− 78%), had no effect on the NT-immunological material[5] contained in the nucleus accumbens and the anterior striatum, but produced a 70% decrease in NT content in the prefrontal cortex. Because 6-OHDA lesions of the VTA affect also noradrenergic (NA) ascending fibers (64% decrease in NA content in the prefrontal cortex), we have verified that lesions of NA fibers alone did not change NT levels in the prefrontal cortex.[6]

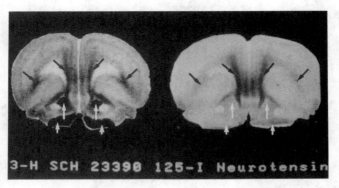

**FIGURE 1.** Autoradiographic analysis of the distribution of dopaminergic ($D_1$) receptors and neurotensin binding sites in the anterior cerebral cortex. Note the similarity between the distributions in the medial and rhinal prefrontal cortices (*black arrows*) and the differences in the nucleus accumbens and the olfactory tubercles (*white arrows*). ($^3$H-SCH 23390: 2.5 nM; Specific activity: 85 Ci/mmole). ($^{125}$I-NT: 0.1 nM; Specific activity: 2000 Ci/mmole.) (Obtained in collaboration with W. Rostène, INSERM U. 55, Paris.)

Immunohistochemistry[7] performed on these NA-depleted animals showed that, in the prefrontal cortex, almost all the fibers reacting with the antibody against tyrosine hydroxylase were also anti-NT positive (FIG. 2).

If the presence of a mixed NT/DA mesocortical pathway can be demonstrated in man, this could provide an anatomical substratum for the biological theory of schizophrenia. Indeed, an increase of NT concentrations in the Brodman's area 32[8] as well as a decrease of NT in the cerebrospinal fluid of schizophrenic patients have been described.[9] Moreover, the development of drugs that bind on NT receptors may help to act differentially on DA transmission in limbic and cortical structures and therefore have important clinical applications.

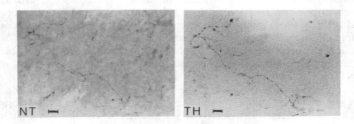

**FIGURE 2.** Successive stainings of the same prefronto–cortical section according to the elution-restaining procedure.[7] Cortical beaded fibers were first stained for neurotensin (NT) and, following decolorizing and antibody elution, for tyrosine-hydroxylase (TH). *Black bars* correspond to 10 μm.

## REFERENCES

1. HÖKELFT, T., B. J. EVERITT, E. THEODORSSON-NORHEIM & M. GOLDSTEIN. 1984. J. Comp. Neurol. **222:** 543–559.
2. CARRAWAY, R. & S. E. LEEMAN. 1973. J. Biol. Chem. **248:** 6854–6861.
3. KALIVAS, P. W. & J. S. MILLER. 1984. Brain Res. **300:** 157–160.
4. BISSETTE, L., L. JENNES, A. J. PRANGE, G. R. BREESE & C. B. NEMEROFF. 1984. Soc. Neurosci. Abstr. **9:** 290.
5. CARRAWAY, R. & S. E. LEEMAN. 1976. J. Biol. Chem. **251:** 7035–7044.
6. STUDLER, J. M. *et al.* 1988. Neuropeptides **11:** 95–100.
7. TRAMU, G., A. PILLEZ & J. LEONARDELLI. 1978. J. Histochem. Cytochem. **26:** 322–324.
8. NEMEROFF, C. B., W. W. YOUNGBLOOD, P. J. MANBERG, A. J. PRANGE, JR. & J. S. KIZER. 1983. Science **221:** 972–975.
9. WIDERLÖV, E. *et al.* 1982. Am. J. Psychiatry **139:** 1122–1126.

# Comparison of the Effects of Selective $D_1$ and $D_2$ Receptor Antagonists on Sucrose Sham Feeding and Water Sham Drinking[a]

L. H. SCHNEIDER,[b] D. GREENBERG,
AND G. P. SMITH

*New York Hospital-Cornell Medical Center*
*White Plains, New York 10605*

In recent experiments, we demonstrated that $D_1$ and $D_2$ dopaminergic (DA) receptor antagonists decreased the sham feeding of sucrose solutions in a dose-related manner.[1-3] We interpreted these results as evidence that central DA synaptic activity at $D_1$ and $D_2$ receptors was necessary for the normal ingestive response to the orosensory stimulation provided by sucrose during sham feeding. Futhermore, we hypothesized that the DA activity was necessary for the normal sensory and/or hedonic processing of the sucrose stimulation rather than for the motor responses of mouth opening, licking, and swallowing.

To test our hypothesis, we investigated the effect of $D_1$ and $D_2$ antagonists on the sham drinking response to water in the water-deprived rat. Since rats use the same motor responses to sham drink water as they do to sham feed sucrose, we reasoned that if the decrease of sucrose sham feeding by $D_1$ and $D_2$ antagonists was due to a motor deficit, then the $D_1$ and $D_2$ antagonists should produce the same dose-related decrease in water sham drinking as in sucrose sham feeding. We report here that the $D_1$ and $D_2$ antagonists had differential effects on the sham feeding of sucrose and the sham drinking of water. This result is consistent with a necessary role for central DA in the normal processing of sensory and/or hedonic effects of orosensory stimulation by sucrose during sham feeding.

Twelve male Sprague-Dawley rats (315–375 g) were chronically implanted with a stainless-steel gastric cannula.[2] About two weeks after surgery, testing began. During a test, the cannula was open; this allowed ingested fluid to drain out of the stomach, thus removing the postingestive effects of the liquids while retaining their orosensory effects. Rats were tested for sham feeding a 10% sucrose solution after a 4-hr 45-min food deprivation (SF; water *ad libitum*) and, on separate days, for sham drinking water after an 18-hr water deprivation (SD; pellets *ad libitum*). (Although the rat emits the same ingestive movements during sham feeding and sham drinking and thus, both could be considered sham drinking, we prefer to differentiate the ingestive response on the basis of its functional relationship to deprivation state.) Under these condi-

[a] The work of one of the authors (L. H. C.) was supported by Grant MH90400, and the work of another of the authors (G. P. S.) was supported by Grant MH15455.
[b] To whom correspondence should be addressed.

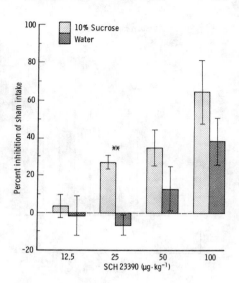

**FIGURE 1.** The effects of SCH 23390 on sucrose sham feeding (*light pattern*, n = 5) and water sham drinking (*dark pattern*, n = 6). Data are mean ± S.E.M. percent inhibition from intake after vehicle injection on preceding day. After vehicle injections, sucrose intake was 41.8 ± 5.0 ml and water intake was 43.1 ± 2.2 ml. SCH 23390 significantly ($p < 0.05$) decreased sucrose intake after doses ≥ 25 µg · kg⁻¹ and decreased water intake at 100 µg · kg⁻¹. **$p < 0.001$, 25 µg · kg⁻¹ decreased sucrose intake significantly more than water intake.

tions, 30-min sham intakes (mean ml ± S.E.M., n = 12) were 41.0 ± 2.6 for sucrose and 36.7 ± 3.2 for water. (Note that shorter periods of water deprivation produced smaller water intakes). Since these mean intakes were not significantly different, rats were distributed between the experimental SF and SD groups (n = 6 each) on the basis of their rank-ordered intakes. After rats were adapted to vehicle injection ip at −15 min, the experiment proper consisted of testing first the effects of the $D_2$ antagonist, (-)-raclopride (0.3, 0.2, 0.1, and 0.4 mg/kg) and then the $D_1$ antagonist, SCH 23390 (50, 25, 12.5, and 100 µg/kg) on the SF and SD groups. Data analyses were conducted on the percent inhibition of 30-min sham intakes by drug treatments from control (vehicle) test on the day preceding the drug test. We used one-way ANOVAs to determine the effect of each antagonist on percent inhibition of sucrose and water and two-way ANOVAs to compare the effect of one antagonist on sucrose and water intake. The threshold dose of antagonist for inhibiting sucrose and water intakes was determined by comparing the intakes on the preceding control day with the intakes on the test day by a matched-pairs t-test. The relative effects of a single dose of antagonist on sucrose and water intake were determined by t-test. All tests were two-tailed and $p < 0.05$ was considered significant.

Although SCH 23390 and (-)-raclopride decreased the sham intake of water and sucrose, the threshold dose of both drugs for the decrease of sucrose intake was less than the threshold dose for the decrease of water intake (FIGS. 1 and 2). The differential results with (-)-raclopride extends previous results[2,4] with pimozide and haloperidol.

Since the intakes of sucrose and water after vehicle injections were not significantly different (see legends for FIGS. 1 and 2), it is reasonable to assume that the ingestive movements were equivalent in the two-test situations. Thus, the differential effects of (-)-raclopride and SCH 23390 on sucrose and water intake were probably not due to a motor deficit produced by the drugs. We conclude that the differential effects are further evidence for our hypothesis that central DA synaptic activity at $D_1$ and $D_2$ receptors is necessary for the normal processing of the sensory and/or hedonic effects of the orosensory simulation by sucrose during sham feeding.

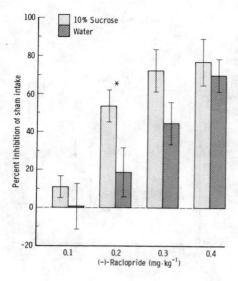

**FIGURE 2.** The effect of (-)-raclopride on sucrose sham feeding (*light pattern, n = 6*) and water sham drinking (*dark pattern, n = 6*). Data are mean ± S.E.M. percent inhibition from intake after vehicle injection on preceding day. After vehicle injections, sucrose intake was 40.1 ± 4.7 and water intake was 36.0 ± 2.8. (-)-raclopride significantly ($p < 0.05$) decreased sucrose intake after doses $\geq 0.2$ mg · kg$^{-1}$ and decreased water intake after doses $\geq 0.3$ mg · kg$^{-1}$ *$p$ < 0.05, 0.2 mg · kg$^{-1}$ decreased sucrose intake more than water intake.

The ability of larger doses of both SCH 23390 and (-)-raclopride to decrease the sham drinking of water implicates central $D_1$ and $D_2$ receptors in the normal ingestive response to water in the water-deprived rat. This is consistent with much previous work using less specific $D_2$ antagonists,[5] and with the effect of SCH 23390 on real drinking of water.[6] The failure of Gilbert and Cooper[6] to decrease real drinking of water with the specific $D_2$ antagonist sulpiride was probably the result of the low doses they used.

It is not possible to conclude from our results whether the decrease in sham drinking was the result of a motor, sensory, and/or hedonic deficit. The fact that it took a larger dose of both antagonists to reduced water intake than sucrose intake suggests that the sham drinking of water released more dopamine at some $D_1$ and $D_2$ receptor sites than the sham drinking of sucrose did, but available neurochemical evidence for real water intake[7] is not consistent with this suggestion. A search for increased dopaminergic activity during sham drinking may be worthwhile.

The present study supports the involvement of both $D_1$ and $D_2$ receptor mechanisms in the normal sham feeding of sucrose and sham drinking of water. Thus, it extends to these ingestive behaviors the idea derived from the pharmacological analysis of the stereotyped behavioral and basal ganglia neuronal electrophysiological responses to DA agonists[8] that both $D_1$ and $D_2$ receptor mechanisms must be activated concurrently for endogenous DA to produce normal effects.

## ACKNOWLEDGMENTS

The authors wish to thank Drs. L. Iorio and A. Barnett of Schering Corporation, Bloomfield, N.J., for their gift of SCH 23390, and Drs. C. Kohler and S. Ogren of Astra Lakemeda, Sodertalje, Sweden, for their gift of (-)-raclopride. We are also grateful to Mrs. Marion Jacobson and Mrs. Jane Magnetti for processing the manuscript.

## REFERENCES

1. GEARY, N. & G. P. SMITH. 1985. Pimozide decreases the positive reinforcing effect of sham-fed sucrose in the rat. Pharmacol. Biochem. Behav. **22:** 787–790.
2. SCHNEIDER, L. H., J. GIBBS & G. P. SMITH. 1986. D-2 selective receptor antagonists suppress sucrose sham feeding in the rat. Brain Res. Bull. **17:** 605–611.
3. SCHNEIDER, L. H., J. GIBBS & G. P. SMITH. 1986. Selective D-1 or D-2 receptor antagonists inhibit sucrose sham feeding in rats. Appetite **7:** 294–295.
4. XENAKIS, A. & A. SCLAFANI. 1981. The effects of pimozide on the consumption of a palatable saccharin-glucose solution in the rat. Pharmacol. Biochem. Behav. **15:** 435–442.
5. ROWLAND, N. & D. J. ENGLE. 1977. Feeding and drinking interactions after acute butyrophenone administration. Pharmacol. Biochem. Behav. **7:** 295–301.
6. GILBERT, D. B. & S. J. COOPER. 1987. Effects of the dopamine D-1 antagonist SCH 23390 and the D-2 antagonist sulpiride on saline acceptance-rejection in water-deprived rats. Pharmacol. Biochem. Behav. **26:** 687–691.
7. LUTTINGER, D. & L. S. SEIDEN. 1981. Increased hypothalamic norepinephrine metabolism after water deprivation in the rat. Brain Res. **208:** 147–165.
8. WALTERS, J. R., D. A. BERGSTROM, J. H. CARLSON, T. N. CHASE & A. R. BRAUN. 1987. D-1 dopamine receptor activation required for postsynaptic expression of D-2 agonist effects. Science **236:** 719–722.

# Index of Contributors